CECIL REVIEW OF GENERAL INTERNAL MEDICINE

4TH EDITION

Edited by

LLOYD H. SMITH, Jr., M.D.

Professor of Medicine and Associate Dean,
University of California, San Francisco, School of Medicine,
San Francisco, California

JAMES B. WYNGAARDEN, M.D.

Director, National Institutes of Health,
Bethesda, Maryland

1989

W. B. SAUNDERS COMPANY

Harcourt Brace Jovanovich, Inc.

Philadelphia, London, Toronto, Montreal, Sydney, Tokyo

W. B. SAUNDERS COMPANY
Harcourt Brace Jovanovich, Inc.

The Curtis Center
Independence Square West
Philadelphia, PA 19106

Library of Congress Cataloging-in-Publication Data

Cecil review of general internal medicine / edited by Lloyd H. Smith, Jr., James B. Wyngaarden.—4th ed.
p. cm.
Includes bibliographies.
ISBN 0-7216-2464-2
1. Internal medicine—Examinations, questions, etc.
I. Smith, Lloyd H., 1924– II. Wyngaarden, James B., 1924–

RC46.T35 1985b Suppl.

616'.0076—dc19 88-6582

Acquisition Editor: John Dyson

Production Manager: Frank Polizzano

Manuscript Editor: Donna Walker

Listed here is the latest translated edition of this book together with the language of the translation and the publisher:

Portuguese—*Third Edition*—DISCOS CBS Industria e Comercio Ltda. Rio de Janeiro, Brazil

CECIL REVIEW OF GENERAL INTERNAL MEDICINE ISBN 0-7216-2464-2

Last digit is the print number: 9 8 7 6 5 4 3 2 1

CONTRIBUTORS

NATHAN M. BASS, M.D., Ph.D
Assistant Professor of Medicine, University of California, San Francisco, School of Medicine; Attending Physician, University of California, San Francisco Hospitals and Clinics, San Francisco, California

CHRISTOPHER C. BENZ, M.D.
Assistant Professor of Medicine, Cancer Research Institute, University of California, San Francisco, School of Medicine; Attending Physician, University of California, San Francisco Hospitals and Clinics, San Francisco, California

EDWARD E. BONDI, M.D.
Associate Professor of Dermatology, Hospital of the University of Pennsylvania, Philadelphia, Pennsylvania

MICHAEL H. BOWMAN, Ph.D., M.D.
Assistant Professor of Medicine (Neurology), Department of Medicine, Duke University Medical Center, Durham, North Carolina

JAMES K. BROWN, M.D.
Associate Professor of Medicine and Associate Staff, Cardiovascular Research Institute, University of California, San Francisco, School of Medicine; Assistant Chief, Respiratory Care Section, Department of Medicine, Veterans Administration Medical Center, San Francisco, California

JURRIEN DEAN, M.D.
Senior Investigator, Laboratory of Cellular and Developmental Biology, National Institute of Diabetes and Digestive and Kidney Diseases, National Institutes of Health, Bethesda, Maryland

KENNETH R. FEINGOLD, M.D.
Associate Professor of Medicine, University of California, San Francisco, School of Medicine; Chief, Endocrine-Metabolism Clinic, Veterans Administration Medical Center, San Francisco, California

BARRIE J. HURWITZ, M.D.
Associate Professor, Department of Medicine (Neurology) and Assistant Professor, Department of Community and Family Medicine, Duke University Medical Center; Attending Neurologist, Duke University Medical Center, Durham, North Carolina

JOHN B. IMBODEN, JR., M.D.
Assistant Professor, Department of Medicine, University of California, San Francisco, School of Medicine; Staff Physician, Veterans Administration Medical Center, San Francisco, California

RICHARD D. KLAUSNER, M.D.
Chief, Cell Biology and Metabolism Branch, National Institute of Child Health and Human Development, National Institutes of Health, Bethesda, Maryland

ROBERT F. KLEIN, M.D.
Associate, Department of Endocrinology, Geisinger Medical Center, Danville, Pennsylvania

RODGER A. LIDDLE, M.D.
Assistant Professor of Medicine, Duke University School of Medicine, Durham, North Carolina

CHARLES A. LINKER, M.D.
Associate Clinical Professor of Medicine, University of California, San Francisco, School of Medicine; Attending Physician, University of California, San Diego Hospitals and Clinics, San Francisco, California

HENRY MASUR, M.D.
Associate Professor of Clinical Medicine, George Washington University School of Medicine, Washington, D.C.; Deputy Director, Critical Care Medicine Department, Clinical Center, National Institutes of Health, Bethesda, Maryland

DOUGLAS L. PACKER, M.D.
Assistant Professor of Medicine, Division of Cardiology, Duke University School of Medicine, Durham, North Carolina

ALLAN S. POLLOCK, M.D.
Assistant Professor of Medicine, University of California, San Francisco, School of Medicine; Chief of Outpatient Dialysis and Renal Clinics, Veterans Administration Medical Center, San Francisco, California

CHARLES E. REESE, M.D.
Clinical Instructor in Medicine, University of California, San Francisco, School of Medicine; Attending Physician, University of California, San Francisco Hospitals and Clinics, San Francisco General Hospital, San Francisco, California

DAVID G. WARNOCK, M.D.
Professor of Medicine, University of Alabama School of Medicine, Birmingham, Alabama

ROBERT A. WAUGH, M.D.
Associate Professor of Medicine, Duke University School of Medicine; Attending Physician, Duke University Hospital, Durham, North Carolina

PREFACE

The scope of medicine, much like Einsteinian space, has no discrete boundaries. In the student this open-ended nature of the discipline evokes anxiety, for there are no limits—no margins that define when clinical medicine has been successfully mastered. During the years devoted to basic science, such an open-ended commitment does not appear to pertain, for there are lecture notes, syllabi, and standard textbooks that collectively encompass that portion of biochemistry or of histology that the student is expected to know. The clinical years, however, dispel any sense of certainty. How much should we know about hypertension, for example? As much as can be learned within the limits of the time, energy, and resourcefulness that one can devote to the demanding profession of medicine. To understand this single pathologic condition we must be cognizant of selective elements of epidemiology, physiology, biochemistry, pathology, pharmacology, and many of the specialties of internal medicine (cardiology, nephrology, endocrinology, neurology, etc.). The subject carries us further into preventive medicine, public health, and public policy. Similar ramifications spread out endlessly from all clinical problems. The physician must be primarily concerned with the unique individuality of the patient, whose welfare cannot be defined as the simple integral of these formidable disciplines into which biomedical science has been conveniently but arbitarily segregated. It has been said that M.D. stands for "moderately done," in contrast to Ph.D., which stands for "phenomenally done." It is this continuing sense of incompletion that is the main defense against complacency, the dry rot of our profession.

There are many ways in which to learn medicine. Each student or physician will differ in the methods by which he or she learns most easily and effectively. Education has been defined as what you have left when you have forgotten the facts. "The facts" are nowhere more transient than in medicine, so that a premium must be placed on education as defined above. This includes the ability to reason effectively from data that are often incomplete. This manual has been developed as a series of questions that test both knowledge and the ability to utilize it effectively in clinical medicine. As such it is designed to reinforce the use of knowledge already obtained from other sources or of skills already obtained through experience. The form of a question is a challenge that requires that we assess what we know or, more important, what we do not know about the topic at hand. It crystallizes a problem set and demands that we take a position. Answers are supplied not only to indicate what is correct or incorrect but also to offer a rational explanation for these choices. This book has been constructed primarily to assist in the education or continuing education of medical students in advanced clerkships, house staff, internists, family physicians, or anyone who wishes to maintain competency in internal medicine. Both its content and form make it useful also to physicians preparing for certification or recertification by the American Board of Internal Medicine.

The *Cecil Textbook of Medicine* has been the standard definitive textbook of medicine in the United States since its introduction more than sixty years ago (1927). For convenience most of the references in the answer section have been directed to the eighteenth edition of *Cecil,* of which this is a companion book. Other useful general references are included as well. Through these references each topic can be pursued in much more depth than allowed within the confines of this book.

This is the fourth edition of *Review of General Internal Medicine.* It has been extensively revised since the third edition, with seven new contributors and approximately 900 new questions. The supporting references have been updated as well, both those relating to the eighteenth edition of *Cecil* and those relating to other standard sources. We would like to express special gratitude to our colleagues at the Duke University Medical Center, at the University of California, San Francisco, and at the National Institutes of Health for their excellent contributions in preparing these self-assessment exercises in the respective disciplines of internal medicine.

In all phases of revising this book Ms. Judith Serrell and Ms. Margaret Quinlan have been invaluable colleagues. Ms. Ann Petracek has brought special editorial skills to this project as well. At the W. B. Saunders Company we have benefitted from the general guidance of John Dyson and the production skills of Lorraine Kilmer. We are indebted to all of these individuals for the skill and resourcefulness that they have brought to this enterprise.

LLOYD H. SMITH, JR., M.D.
JAMES B. WYNGAARDEN, M.D.

CONTENTS

INSTRUCTIONS

This book is designed to provide a comprehensive review of internal medicine in the form of a self-assessment examination. The format enables you to answer the questions, to quickly determine which ones you got right and wrong, and then to review those questions you answered incorrectly. The examination is divided into 11 Parts. These Parts may be taken individually, in any order. To take advantage of this book's special features, we suggest the following steps:

1. Tear out the answer sheet (located on perforated pages at the end of the book) for the Part you want to use.

2. Take the test, recording your answers on the answer sheet. Note that there are three different question types used; be sure to read and follow the directions for each of them.

3. To quickly determine how many questions you answered correctly, compare your answers with the answer key (pp. 269–275). On your answer sheet, circle any questions you may have missed.

4. For a detailed discussion of questions answered incorrectly, refer to the Answers following the questions in each Part. References to Wyngaarden and Smith: *Cecil Textbook of Medicine* (18th ed.) and to other sources are provided for more extensive review. As time permits, reading the discussions of questions you answered correctly should also prove beneficial.

No criteria for deciding "how well" you did are provided because we believe that in a self-assessment examination you are the best judge. Read the discussions of the questions you missed and decide for yourself why you answered incorrectly, whether you should have known the answer, and whether the material deserves further study.

No time limits have been set, and no harm will be done by taking a Part over several days. We recommend that you do not look up any answers until you have completed the entire Part. In order to get maximal benefit from this style of review, it is essential that you treat the questions as you would questions in a "real" examination. Don't just "take a stab" at a question because you know the answer is easy to look up. Reading the answers is not an adequate substitute for taking as much time as you need and doing your best on each question.

PART 1

CARDIOVASCULAR DISEASES

DOUGLAS L. PACKER and ROBERT A. WAUGH

DIRECTIONS: For questions 1 to 69, choose the ONE BEST answer to each question.

1. Each of the following results in a decrease in contractility EXCEPT

   A. ischemia
   B. acidosis
   C. beta endorphins
   D. elevated P_{CO_2}
   E. arterial hypoxia

2. Hypoxia produces vasoconstriction in which of the following vascular beds?

   A. Coronary circulation
   B. Cerebral circulation
   C. Splanchnic bed
   D. Renal arteries
   E. None of the above

3. Each of the following is a potential mediator of vasoconstriction during systemic shock EXCEPT

   A. hypoxia
   B. prostacyclin
   C. thromboxane A_2
   D. angiotensin
   E. vasopressin

4. Each of the following increases the tendency for fluid extravasation EXCEPT

   A. increased postcapillary sphincter tone
   B. histamines
   C. decreased plasma oncotic pressure
   D. endothelial cell damage
   E. bradykinin

5. Each of the following cellular pathophysiologic processes occurs in the shock state EXCEPT

   A. increase in sodium/potassium ATPase activity
   B. increase in insulin-mediated glucose uptake in muscle
   C. precipitation of calcium in the mitochondria
   D. cellular swelling
   E. depletion of ATP and cyclic AMP

6. Each of the following maternal conditions is associated with an increased incidence of congenital heart disease EXCEPT

   A. rubella during the first trimester
   B. smoking
   C. alcoholism
   D. diabetes
   E. congenital heart disease

7. Circulatory changes typically occurring following birth include each of the following EXCEPT

   A. fall in pulmonary vascular resistance
   B. rise in systemic vascular resistance
   C. abrupt rise in pulmonary blood flow
   D. fall in left atrial volume and pressure
   E. functional constriction of the ductus arteriosus

8. Congenital heart defects, typically accompanied by an increased risk of bacterial endocarditis, include each of the following EXCEPT

   A. ventricular septal defect
   B. patent ductus arteriosus
   C. stenotic bicuspid aortic valve
   D. hypertrophic obstructive cardiomyopathy (IHSS)
   E. atrial septal defect

9. The most useful finding for distinguishing an ostium primum from a secundum atrial septal defect is

   A. systolic ejection murmur at the upper left sternal border
   B. fixed split second heart sound
   C. right atrial enlargement on chest roentgenogram
   D. left axis deviation on ECG
   E. none of the above

10. Persistent patent ductus arteriosus occurs with higher likelihood in each of the following EXCEPT

    A. female infants
    B. premature infants
    C. infants born at high altitudes
    D. infants born to mothers with first-trimester rubella
    E. infants born to mothers with first-trimester toxoplasmosis

11. The most common aortic malformation accompanying tetralogy of Fallot is

    A. right-sided aortic arch
    B. coarctation of the aorta
    C. congenital aortic stenosis
    D. bicuspid aortic valve
    E. aortic ectasia

12. Which of the following is NOT a typical feature of coarctation of the aorta?

    A. Associated with Turner's syndrome
    B. Commonly associated with a bicuspid aortic valve
    C. Affects males more frequently than females

D. The lesion typically occurs proximal to the left subclavian artery
E. May predispose to aortic rupture during the third trimester of pregnancy

13. Each of the following congenital anomalies is accompanied by a strong possibility of multiple other cardiac defects EXCEPT

A. asplenia syndrome
B. isolated levocardia
C. dextrocardia with situs inversus
D. dextroversion with situs solitus
E. polysplenia syndrome

14. Each of the following findings is seen in the setting of Eisenmenger's syndrome EXCEPT

A. elevated pulmonary vascular resistance
B. predominant left to right shunting
C. clubbing
D. polycythemia
E. increased risk of sudden death

15. Each of the following typically worsens the symptoms of mitral stenosis EXCEPT

A. vigorous exercise
B. significant fever
C. atrial fibrillation
D. first-trimester pregnancy
E. second-trimester pregnancy

16. A brisk peripheral pulse is expected with each of the following EXCEPT

A. thyrotoxicosis
B. mitral stenosis
C. mitral regurgitation
D. cardiac beriberi
E. aortic insufficiency

17. Each of the following pathophysiologic processes causes an increased loudness of the first heart sound EXCEPT

A. thyrotoxicosis
B. mitral stenosis
C. sinus tachycardia
D. acute aortic insufficiency
E. atrial septal defect

18. Which of the following auscultatory findings of mitral stenosis is the most suggestive of severe disease?

A. The presence of an S_3
B. A loud opening snap
C. A diminished P_2
D. A short A_2–opening snap interval
E. None of the above

19. Classic echocardiographic findings in patients with mitral stenosis include each of the following EXCEPT

A. left atrial enlargement
B. increased echogenicity of the mitral valve
C. decrease in the E to F slope of the mitral valve
D. prominent A wave of the mitral valve
E. mitral valve leaflet tethering

20. Prudent medical therapy for a completely asymptomatic 37-year-old housewife with no children at home who has mitral stenosis and atrial fibrillation would include each of the following EXCEPT

A. careful follow-up during any pregnancy
B. endocarditis prophylaxis for dental procedures
C. control of the ventricular response rate during atrial fibrillation
D. prophylactic anticoagulation
E. prophylaxis for rheumatic fever

21. The leading cause of mitral regurgitation is

A. mitral valve prolapse
B. rheumatic heart disease
C. coronary artery disease with papillary muscle dysfunction
D. cardiomyopathy with marked left ventricular dilatation
E. connective tissue disease

22. Elevated left atrial pressures typically occur in each of the following conditions EXCEPT

A. moderate mitral stenosis
B. chronic mitral regurgitation
C. marked left ventricular dysfunction following an acute myocardial infarction
D. hypertrophic obstructive cardiomyopathy
E. atrial myxoma

23. The clinical finding most suggestive of a poor prognosis in a patient with aortic stenosis is

A. syncope
B. angina
C. congestive heart failure
D. complex ventricular ectopy
E. left bundle branch block

24. Each of the following physical examination findings is consistent with severe calcific aortic stenosis EXCEPT

A. pulsus parvus et tardus
B. systolic thrill at the upper right sternal border
C. a loud ejection sound
D. decreased second heart sound
E. late-peaking systolic ejection murmur

25. Elective valve replacement is usually recommended for which one of the following asymptomatic patients?

A. A 12-year-old boy with congenital aortic stenosis and a valve area of 0.4 cm^2/m^2
B. A 19-year-old man with 3+ mitral regurgitation
C. A 36-year-old woman with mitral stenosis and a valve area of 1.1 cm^2
D. A 39-year-old woman with Ebstein's malformation of the tricuspid valve
E. A 46-year-old man with 3–4+ aortic regurgitation

26. Treatment with high-dose long-acting nitrates is potentially dangerous in

A. aortic sclerosis
B. aortic regurgitation
C. mitral regurgitation
D. idiopathic congestive cardiomyopathy
E. hypertrophic obstructive cardiomyopathy

27. Patients with which one of the following are most likely to show significant improvement in left ventricular function following valve replacement?

A. Mitral stenosis
B. Mitral regurgitation
C. Aortic regurgitation
D. Aortic stenosis
E. None of the above

28. Volume overload of the left ventricle is typically produced by each of the following EXCEPT

A. aortic regurgitation
B. mitral regurgitation
C. patent ductus arteriosus
D. ventricular septal defect
E. atrial septal defect

29. Which of the following valvular abnormalities is most likely to be congenital in origin?

A. Mitral stenosis
B. Tricuspid stenosis
C. Aortic stenosis
D. Pulmonic stenosis
E. None of the above

30. Each of the following is a direct determinant of increased oxygen consumption EXCEPT

A. increased heart rate
B. increased contractility
C. increased wall tension
D. increased wall thickness
E. increased systolic blood pressure

31. The most common reason for recurrent angina following coronary bypass grafting is

A. graft occlusion
B. incomplete revascularization at surgery
C. progression of intrinsic coronary artery disease
D. postoperative ventricular hypertrophy
E. none of the above

32. Which of the following testing modalities is LEAST likely to provide early documentation of an acute myocardial infarction?

A. Electrocardiogram
B. LDH isoenzymes
C. Thallium-201 scanning
D. Technetium pyrophosphate scanning
E. CPK isoenzymes

33. Which one of the following is included among appropriate indications for temporary pacemaker insertion in the setting of an acute myocardial infarction?

A. New right bundle branch block
B. High-grade type I second-degree AV block
C. New left bundle branch block with P-R prolongation
D. Accelerated idioventricular rhythm
E. None of the above

34. The blood supply to the anterior hemifascicle of the AV conduction system is most like that of the

A. left posterior hemifascicle
B. His bundle
C. right bundle branch
D. AV node
E. left anterior papillary muscle

35. Each of the following arrhythmias is commonly observed with digitalis toxicity EXCEPT

A. sinus tachycardia
B. atrial tachycardia with block
C. frequent PVC's
D. type I second-degree AV block
E. junctional tachycardias

36. Antiarrhythmic agents that might be useful in slowing the ventricular response rate during atrial fibrillation include each of the following EXCEPT

A. digoxin
B. propranolol
C. verapamil
D. diltiazem
E. quinidine

37. The incidence of peripheral emboli following conversion from atrial fibrillation to normal sinus rhythm in the absence of mitral valve disease approaches

A. 2%
B. 8%
C. 10%
D. 15%
E. 30%

38. Which of the following antiarrhythmic agents is LEAST likely to prolong the Q-T interval?

A. Pronestyl
B. Quinidine
C. Disopyramide
D. Flecainide
E. Amiodarone

39. Factors favoring the diagnosis of ventricular tachycardia include each of the following EXCEPT

A. QRS duration greater than 0.14 sec
B. 12-lead ECG showing left axis deviation
C. triphasic QRS pattern in V_1 (rSr')
D. fusion or capture beats
E. VA dissociation

40. Each of the following decreases antegrade conduction across the accessory pathway in the Wolff-Parkinson-White syndrome EXCEPT

A. quinidine
B. procainamide
C. flecainide
D. disopyramide
E. verapamil

41. In patients with hypertrophic obstructive cardiomyopathy, which antiarrhythmic agent carries the highest risk of a deleterious effect in treating atrial fibrillation?

A. Beta blockers
B. Verapamil
C. Amiodarone
D. Disopyramide
E. Digoxin

42. In hypotension, which of the following vascular beds has the greatest autoregulatory capacity for maintaining blood flow?

A. Hepatic
B. Skeletal muscle
C. Mesenteric
D. Splenic
E. Cerebral

43. In acute hemorrhagic shock, which of the following is most important in producing an IMMEDIATE beneficial rightward shift in the oxygen-hemoglobin dissociation curve?

A. Increased red cell 2,3-diphosphoglyceric acid
B. Hypoxia
C. Anemia
D. Acidosis
E. Hypophosphatemia

44. Each of the following statements concerning ventricular septal defects is true EXCEPT

A. If small, they are compatible with normal longevity
B. They are associated with an increased incidence of aortic regurgitation
C. Their rarity in older adults is most likely due to the mortality of affected subjects at an earlier age
D. Formation of an aneurysm in the membranous septum is a well-documented mechanism of spontaneous closure
E. A moderate-sized ventricular septal defect with normal pulmonary vascular resistance imposes a volume load primarily on the left ventricle

45. Each of the following statements concerning left ventricular outflow tract obstruction is true EXCEPT

A. Poor ventricular function does not contraindicate repair of a stenotic aortic valve
B. The presence of an aortic ejection sound suggests that the problem is valvular
C. If blood pressure is significantly higher in the right arm than in the left, supravalvular aortic stenosis is suggested
D. A palpable fourth heart sound favors the diagnosis of hypertrophic obstructive cardiomyopathy (idiopathic hypertrophic subaortic stenosis, IHSS)
E. Subvalvular membranous aortic stenosis is strongly associated with aortic regurgitation

46. Which of the following is NOT likely to be responsible for converting stable angina pectoris to an unstable syndrome?

A. Platelet aggregation at the site of a plaque
B. Coronary artery spasm superimposed on a coronary arterial plaque
C. Hemorrhage into an atherosclerotic plaque
D. Increased concentration of thromboxane at the plaque site
E. Increased concentration of prostacyclin at the plaque site

47. Each of the following statements concerning sudden death and myocardial infarction is true EXCEPT

A. Most patients resuscitated from sudden death do not evolve acute myocardial infarction
B. Most patients dying acutely of transmural myocardial infarction show evidence of acute coronary occlusion
C. Recent studies suggest that thrombosis is *not* a primary factor in patients dying of myocardial infarction
D. Approximately 20% of patients with acute myocardial infarction suffer infarct extension within the first five days
E. If more than 40% of the left ventricle has been damaged irreversibly by myocardial infarction, patients are at very high risk for left ventricular failure and cardiogenic shock

48. Each of the following statements concerning the treatment of tachyarrhythmias in association with Wolff-Parkinson-White accessory conduction is true EXCEPT

A. Digoxin should be used with great caution, if at all, in treating atrial fibrillation
B. A 1:1 relationship between atrial and ventricular complexes is usual
C. Propranolol is useful primarily because it slows conduction over the accessory pathway
D. In a nonhypotensive patient, the treatment of choice for a reciprocating AV junctional tachycardia is intravenous verapamil
E. Surgical division of the accessory pathway can "cure" a reciprocating tachycardia

49. The most important effect of angiotensin II on blood pressure is via

A. arteriolar vasoconstriction
B. release of catecholamines from the adrenal medulla
C. stimulation of the CNS vasomotor center
D. stimulation of aldosterone secretion
E. renal diuretic effects

50. Electrocardiography is LEAST helpful in which of the following clinical situations?

A. Assessing a patient with runs of rapid heart action
B. Estimating the serum digoxin level
C. Diagnosing an intraventricular conduction defect
D. Assessing the status of AV conduction
E. Assessing the function of an artificial pacemaker

51. Which of the following complications of cardiac catheterization is the most serious?

A. Ventricular tachycardia
B. Aortic dissection
C. Complete heart block
D. Bleeding at the groin puncture site
E. Loss of pulse below the arterial access site

52. In which of the following should cardiac catheterization NOT be considered?

A. A 14-year-old boy with increasing cyanosis. The echo-Doppler findings are typical of tetralogy of Fallot with moderate to severe infundibular pulmonary stenosis and mild aortic regurgitation.
B. An asymptomatic 40-year-old male airline pilot with a Bruce protocol stage IV positive ETT at a heart rate of 152 bpm and a reversible anterior wall perfusion defect on rest/exercise thallium imaging.
C. An asymptomatic 42-year-old, sedentary man with classic bedside and echo-Doppler findings of

aortic stenosis. The Doppler predicts a 70 mm Hg peak gradient and a 46 mm Hg mean gradient with a normal cardiac output.
D. A 56-year-old man with an ETT that is positive early in stage II of the Bruce protocol at a heart rate of 106 bpm. He has typical stable angina and several risk factors for coronary artery disease.
E. A 56-year-old man with aortic regurgitation, a blood pressure of 156/50 mm Hg, and increasing dyspnea on exertion with the recent onset of paroxysmal nocturnal dyspnea

53. Which one of the following patients is at LEAST risk for the development of post–cardiac catheterization renal dysfunction?

A. A patient whose dye load is 6 cc/kg body weight
B. A patient on chronic diuretic therapy for hypertension
C. A 38-year-old diabetic male on glipizide therapy
D. A 48-year-old man with severe mitral regurgitation
E. A 49-year-old woman with multiple myeloma

54. Which of the following arrhythmias most likely reflects digoxin toxicity?

A. Atrial fibrillation with an irregularly irregular ventricular rhythm at 130–140 per minute
B. Atrial flutter with a regular ventricular rhythm at 150 per minute
C. AV node re-entry tachycardia (PAT) with a regular atrial and ventricular rate of 190 per minute
D. Multifocal atrial tachycardia (MAT) with an irregularly irregular atrial rhythm at 130–150 per minute and a 1:1 ventricular response
E. Atrial fibrillation with a regular ventricular rhythm at 76 per minute

55. The LEAST effective of the myocardial compensatory mechanisms to maintain cardiac output in congestive heart failure is

A. increased heart rate
B. ventricular dilatation
C. ventricular hypertrophy
D. increased contractility
E. release of atrial natriuretic hormone

56. In a patient with pulmonary hypertension, which of the following interventions is likely to result in the greatest drop in the pulmonary artery pressure?

A. Closed mitral valve commissurotomy in a patient with severe mitral stenosis (mitral valve area = 0.6 cm^2)
B. Weight loss of 150 pounds in a 350-pound patient with pickwickian syndrome
C. Anticoagulant therapy with Coumadin in a patient with multiple pulmonary emboli
D. Closure of a ventricular septal defect in a patient with Eisenmenger's syndrome
E. Antibiotic therapy in a patient with cystic fibrosis and acute bronchitis

57. In a patient with primary pulmonary hypertension, exertional syncope is most likely due to

A. right ventricular ischemia and dysfunction
B. paroxysmal atrial fibrillation with a rapid ventricular response
C. inability to sufficiently augment cardiac output during exercise
D. ventricular tachycardia with a heart rate of 200 per minute or greater
E. dilatation of the central venous reservoir

58. In a 68-year-old man, which of the following is the most important predictor of the future risk for ischemic heart disease?

A. HDL cholesterol of 46 mg/dl
B. Total cholesterol of 206 mg/dl
C. Fasting blood sugar of 110 mg/dl
D. Systolic blood pressure of 178 mm Hg
E. History of myocardial infarction in his mother at age 57

59. Which of the following statements concerning radiation-induced heart disease is NOT correct?

A. Pericardial disease is the most common manifestation of radiation injury
B. Bundle branch block and/or atrioventricular block is common
C. Accelerated atherosclerosis occurs in the experimental animal model
D. Clinically detectable cardiac injury occurs in about 5% of patients receiving 4000 rads or more to the mediastinum
E. Myocardial fibrosis and ventricular dysfunction sufficient to cause congestive heart failure occur

QUESTIONS 60–61

A 46-year-old woman presents for evaluation of fatigue of 18 months' duration and of malaise, episodic dyspnea, and fever that began about eight months ago. She had an episode of slurred speech and difficulty swallowing two months ago; it resolved spontaneously and she did not seek medical attention. Although she has no history of PND or orthopnea, increasing nocturia has occurred over the past 4–6 weeks. During medical examination a year ago, a doctor heard a murmur and told her that she "must have had rheumatic fever" although she cannot remember any such history. She has no palpitations or syncope, and the remainder of the medical history is negative. On physical examination, temperature is 37.9°C and pulse is 80 per minute and regular. Blood pressure is 118/78 mm Hg with no postural change. There are no petechiae or splinter hemorrhages and the optic fundi are normal. The neck veins are remarkable for an elevated mean venous pressure (12 cm H_2O) with a normal morphology. Carotid pulses are normal with no bruits. Chest examination shows bibasilar inspiratory rales more prominent at the right base. Cardiovascular examination is remarkable for a palpable pulmonary artery impulse and a sustained impulse at the lower left sternal edge. No separate apical impulse is felt. The first heart sound is soft, and the second heart sound is single and accentuated at the upper left sternal edge. No extrasystolic sounds are noted. There is a variable diastolic sound approximately 100 msec after S_2 that is best heard at the apex in the left lateral decubitus position. There is an apical holosystolic high-frequency plateau-shaped murmur and a brief early diastolic rumble at the apex. No gallops are noted. The abdomen is free of masses and bruits and there is 1–2+ pitting edema of both lower extremities. Chest roentgenogram shows left atrial enlargement and interstitial pulmonary edema. Electrocardiogram shows left atrial enlargement and nonspecific ST-T wave changes. Echocardiogram (long axis, diastolic and systolic frames) is shown in the accompanying figures on page 6. The scale indicators are 1.0 cm.

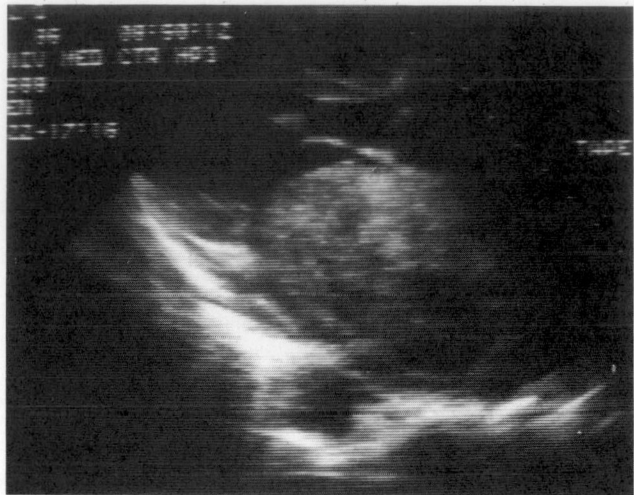

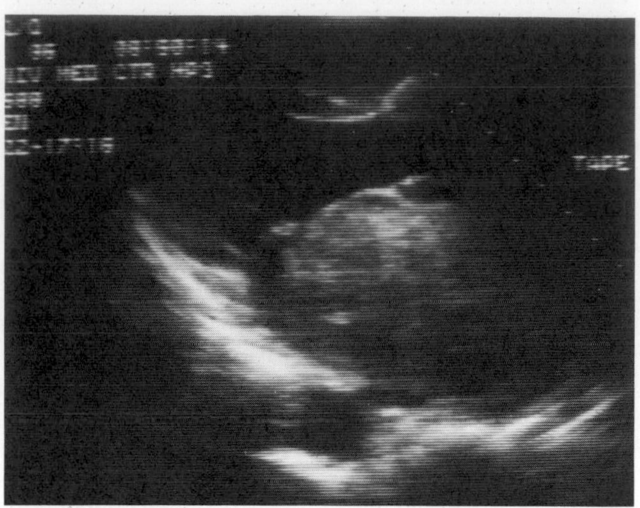

60. Based on the history, physical examination, and laboratory data, what is the most likely diagnosis?

A. Left atrial myxoma
B. Mitral valve endocarditis with vegetation
C. Marked mitral annular calcification with mitral regurgitation
D. Left atrial calcification due to longstanding severe mitral regurgitation
E. Rheumatic mitral valve disease with severe stenosis and a ball valve thrombosis

61. Which of the following should be your next step in the evaluation/management of this patient?

A. Surgery as soon as possible
B. Balloon valvuloplasty of the mitral valve
C. A six-week course of antibiotics with periodic repeat echocardiography
D. Cardiac catheterization, including transseptal puncture, to measure left atrial pressure
E. Cardiac catheterization with pulmonary angiography and use of the levophase to analyze the left side of the heart

QUESTIONS 62–63

A 46-year-old man is evaluated for "spells." For three years he has had periodic "gray-outs" occurring during and following exercise. These have never progressed to overt loss of consciousness, but the patient has been quite careful to limit his activity and, with the advent of symptoms, to cease whatever he is doing immediately and sit down until the symptoms pass. He has not had any associated palpitations and has never had any chest pain. He has noted a mild increase in dyspnea over the past 6–8 months but attributes this to his two-pack per day cigarette smoking habit and increasing weight gain. He has no PND/orthopnea or edema, and there is no prior history of rheumatic fever. A murmur was first noted in his 20's, and he has received variable and conflicting advice concerning limiting his physical activity and bacterial endocarditis prophylaxis. On some occasions, physicians have evidently not heard anything abnormal. The remainder of his history is negative. On physical examination he is well developed, overweight, and in no distress. His pulse is 68 per minute with occasional premature beats. His blood pressure is 150/102 mm Hg in both arms with no postural change. Optic fundi show arteriolar narrowing and an increased arteriolar light reflex. The venous pulse in the neck is grossly unremarkable. There are no neck bruits. A couple of examiners found the carotid upstroke slightly brisk. The chest is clear to percussion and auscultation. The apical impulse is palpable only in the left lateral decubitus position with a presystolic as well as a sustained systolic impulse. No other precordial impulses are noted. On auscultation, the first heart sound is normal. The second heart sound shows prominent expiratory splitting that narrows during inspiration. There is a prominent apical fourth heart sound and a harsh Grade 2–3/6 medium frequency, diamond-shaped murmur that begins after S_1 and peaks in late systole. The murmur is maximal at the lower left sternal edge and well heard at the base and the apex. The murmur softens with squatting and accentuates with standing back up. It is louder after a premature beat. There are no diastolic murmurs and no S_3 is noted. The abdomen is free of masses and bruits. The femoral, dorsalis pedis, and posterior tibial pulses are symmetric and easily palpable, and there is no radial-femoral pulse delay. A chest roentgenogram shows probable left ventricular hypertrophy with clear lung fields. No intracardiac calcifications are noted. An electrocardiogram shows an axis of minus 40 degrees, left atrial enlargement, and left ventricular hypertrophy with strain. The echocardiogram (long axis, diastolic and systolic frames) is shown in the accompanying figures on page 7. The scale indicators are 1.0 cm.

62. Based on the history, physical examination, and laboratory data, what is the most likely diagnosis?

A. Congestive cardiomyopathy with mitral regurgitation
B. Calcific aortic stenosis
C. Subvalvular membranous aortic stenosis
D. Hypertrophic obstructive cardiomyopathy
E. A bicuspid aortic valve with congenital commissural fusion

63. Which therapy would you elect at this point?

A. Aortic valve replacement
B. Mitral valve replacement
C. Septal myectomy
D. Beta blocker
E. Digitalis and verapamil

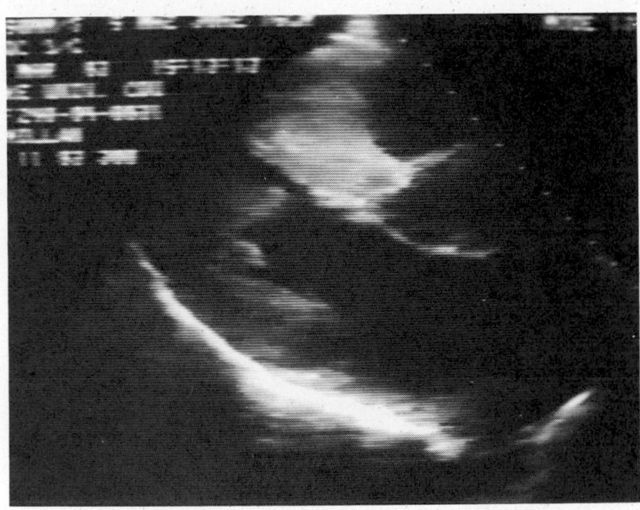

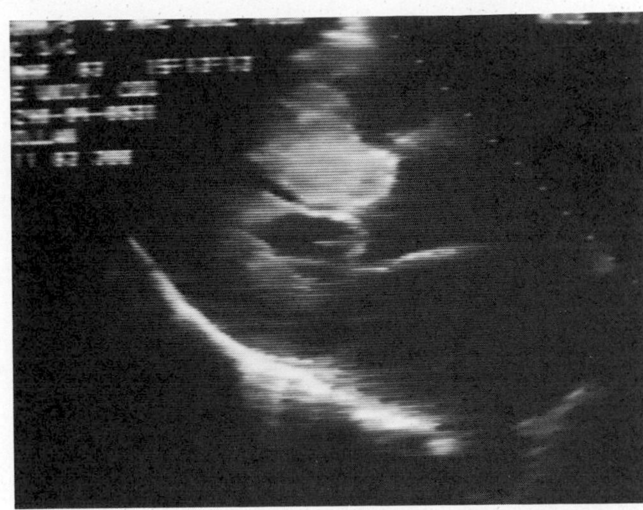

64. Which of the following statements concerning ventricular function is NOT true?

A. Atrial contraction normally contributes a boost of approximately 20% to the stroke volume
B. The geometry of the right ventricle explains its ability to handle a large volume of blood at a low pressure
C. Atrial dilatation and hypertrophy occur in response to decreased ventricular compliance
D. The apex of the left ventricle is thinner because its radius of curvature is greater, thus normalizing wall stress
E. In the left ventricle, major shortening occurs circumferentially

65. The most important factor modulating arterial blood pressure is

A. cardiac output
B. peripheral vascular resistance
C. ventricular contractility
D. cardiac preload
E. heart rate

66. The most important extrinsic factor controlling systemic arteriolar peripheral vascular resistance is

A. level of circulating catecholamines
B. level of circulating prostaglandins
C. degree of stretch of vascular smooth muscle
D. tissue metabolites
E. neurogenic tone

67. Which one of the following is most predictive of left ventricular failure?

A. Cardiomegaly to palpation
B. A murmur of mitral regurgitation
C. A left ventricular S_3
D. Arterial pulsus alternans
E. Electrocardiographic evidence of left ventricular hypertrophy

68. In a 45-year-old woman with a 15-year history of untreated hypertension (diastolic blood pressure 100 mm Hg), which of the following would be most unusual?

A. Electrocardiographic evidence of left ventricular hypertrophy
B. Arteriolar narrowing on funduscopic examination
C. History of a prior myocardial infarction
D. Serum creatinine of 2.6 mg/dl
E. Carotid bruit

69. Each of the following statements concerning cold-induced arterial vasospasm is true EXCEPT

A. Most patients have no associated recognizable cause
B. Beta blockers are likely to improve symptoms in patients with Raynaud's disease
C. In patients with coronary artery spasm, there is an increased incidence of Raynaud's disease and migraine headache
D. An attack of Raynaud's phenomenon is initially indicated by pallor
E. In double-blind, controlled trials, nifedipine has shown to be an effective treatment for Raynaud's disease

DIRECTIONS: For questions 70 to 120, you are to decide whether EACH choice is true or false. Any combination of answers, from all true to all false, may occur. Mark the answer sheet "T" or "F" in the space provided.

70. In patients with cardiogenic shock complicating a myocardial infarction, which of the following statements regarding intra-aortic balloon counterpulsation is/are true?

A. It contributes to decreased systolic arterial pressure
B. It has been shown to increase coronary artery blood flow
C. It produces a significant improvement in survival
D. It is effective in reducing afterload in patients with ventricular septal defect or papillary muscle dysfunction
E. It is a temporizing measure prior to surgical revascularization

71. Which of the following statements concerning congenital complete heart block is/are true?

A. The majority of patients have other cardiac abnormalities contributing to the heart block
B. It occurs more frequently in infants born to mothers with systemic lupus erythematosus
C. It rarely ocurs in a familial form
D. It is accompanied by marked symptoms during the first two decades of life
E. When an isolated finding, it is accompanied by a poor prognosis

72. Afterload reduction is usually beneficial in which of the following settings?

A. Mitral regurgitation
B. Aortic regurgitation
C. Ischemic cardiomyopathy
D. Congestive cardiomyopathy
E. Aortic stenosis

73. Which of the following statements pertaining to HDL levels is/are true?

A. They are significantly higher in men than in women
B. They are typically decreased by jogging
C. They are reduced in the presence of diabetes mellitus
D. They are inversely related to LDL levels
E. They are decreased by small amounts of alcohol consumption

74. Which of the following statements regarding the hemodynamic effects of nitroglycerin (NTG) is/are true?

A. It dilates medium-sized penetrating coronary vessels
B. It improves coronary blood flow and distribution
C. It dilates systemic veins, resulting in a decreased venous return
D. It causes a reflex decrease in heart rate
E. It decreases end-diastolic volume, thereby reducing wall tension

75. Which of the following statements pertaining to exercise stress testing is/are true?

A. 1–2 mm of upsloping ST-segment depression is considered indicative of ischemia
B. The incidence of false-positive tests is lower in women than in men
C. Exercise stress testing is accompanied by a 40–50% false-negative rate
D. A stage I positive exercise stress test suggests the likelihood of severe coronary artery disease
E. A focal region of ischemia is strongly indicated by an accumulation of thallium-201 in that distribution

76. Which of the following statements pertaining to cigarette smoking is/are true?

A. It has been shown to reduce HDL levels in adult men
B. It may result in direct constriction of coronary vessels
C. Nicotine has no demonstrable effect on blood pressure
D. Nicotine contained in cigarette smoke produces little increase in heart rate
E. Carbon monoxide contained in cigarette smoke makes oxygen more available at the tissue level

77. Which of the following statements regarding coronary artery bypass grafting (CABG) is/are true?

A. It has a mortality rate of 3–5%
B. It is accompanied by a 20–30% perioperative infarction rate
C. It is effective in improving symptoms in up to 90% of patients
D. It is accompanied by a first-year vein graft occlusion rate of 10–20%
E. It improves longevity in patients with three-vessel coronary disease who have abnormal left ventricular function

78. Which of the following statements regarding sudden death in the over-30 age group is/are true?

A. It is usually precipitated by an acute myocardial infarction
B. A minority of patients have coronary artery disease
C. The recurrence rate for resuscitated patients is greater than 75% in the first year
D. A pulmonary process is responsible for one third of the episodes
E. Patients at risk may be identified by the presence of single or multiple cardiac risk factors

79. Which of the following statements regarding atrioventricular block below the His bundle region is/are true?

A. Escape rhythms typically show wide QRS complexes
B. It typically has a worse prognosis than AV block occurring within the AV node
C. It is typically aggravated by vagal stimulation
D. It presents as type I second-degree AV block on the surface electrocardiogram
E. It is accompanied by escape rhythms with rates of 50–60 bpm

80. Which of the following statements regarding the mechanism of action of digoxin is/are true?

A. It has a centrally mediated vagal action on the heart
B. It results in slowing of AV nodal conduction

C. It decreases refractoriness of the AV node
D. It increases refractoriness of atrial tissue
E. It results in slowing of the intrinsic sinus rate

81. Which of the following statements about procainamide is/are true?

A. It undergoes acetylation in the liver
B. It has a quinidine-like alpha-blocking effect
C. It is relatively contraindicated in patients with renal insufficiency
D. Typical procainamide-induced lupus adversely affects the lung, brain, and kidney
E. Fewer than one third of patients treated with procainamide develop a positive FANA in the first year of therapy

82. Which of the following statements regarding pericarditis is/are true?

A. It occurs in up to 40% of patients with systemic lupus erythematosus
B. In rheumatoid arthritis, pericarditis usually occurs only when other systemic manifestations of this illness are present
C. Dressler's syndrome typically occurs 2–5 days following myocardial infarction
D. Dressler's syndrome is usually refractory to treatment with nonsteroidal anti-inflammatory agents
E. Prevalence of pericarditis is greater in patients with progressive systemic sclerosis (scleroderma) than in those with systemic lupus erythematosus

83. Which of the following statements regarding thrombolytic therapy with streptokinase for an acute myocardial infarction is/are true?

A. Streptokinase is less likely than urokinase to induce an allergic response
B. Timely streptokinase therapy results in an improved long-term survival rate
C. Streptokinase administered intravenously is as effective as when administered directly into the coronary artery
D. Intravenous thrombolytic therapy with streptokinase is less effective than with tissue plasminogen activator
E. Patients treated with intravenous streptokinase within 8 hours of the onset of a myocardial infarction show a 70% reperfusion rate

84. Which of the following statements regarding flecainide is/are true?

A. It is metabolized in the liver to multiple active metabolites
B. It produces Q-T prolongation similar to quinidine and procainamide
C. It can be used safely in patients with marked ventricular dysfunction
D. It produces fewer side effects than amiodarone but is less effective in controlling sustained ventricular tachycardia
E. The incidence of proarrhythmic effects of flecainide is dependent on the integrity of ventricular function and the arrhythmia being treated

85. Which of the following statements concerning rheumatic heart disease is/are true?

A. The decline in the incidence of rheumatic fever predated the introduction of antibiotic therapy
B. The severity of residual rheumatic heart disease following attacks of acute rheumatic fever has remained constant over the past two decades
C. The most important risk factors for developing rheumatic fever are the climate and socioeconomic status
D. Recurrent rheumatic fever is prevented by daily oral penicillin or monthly bicillin injections
E. The prevalence of rheumatic heart disease in the United States population is less than 0.5%

86. Which of the following statements concerning the epidemiology of coronary artery disease is/are true?

A. In men, its incidence begins to exceed that of women only after the age of 45 years
B. Weight loss is an independent factor in decreasing the risk for coronary artery disease
C. The increased incidence of coronary artery disease in smokers is secondary to the inhalation of nicotine and carbon monoxide
D. It takes approximately two years following the cessation of cigarette smoking for the associated increased risk of coronary artery disease to disappear almost completely
E. Measurement of HDL and LDL cholesterol levels gives more prognostic information concerning the risk of coronary artery disease than the total cholesterol determination alone

87. Which of the following has/have been shown to reduce the risk of death from coronary artery disease?

A. Lowering the total cholesterol level
B. Addition of water softeners to the water supply
C. Tight control of the blood sugar in juvenile-onset diabetes
D. Control of mild hypertension in women under the age of 50
E. Control of moderate to severe hypertension in both sexes

88. In addition to correction of digitalis dosage, which of the following is/are included in the treatment of digitalis toxicity?

A. Correction of hypokalemia
B. Prophylactic suppression therapy with lidocaine or procainamide (Pronestyl), even if no ventricular arrhythmias are present
C. Treatment of digitalis-induced atrial tachycardia with synchronized cardioversion
D. Treatment of heart block, a slow heart rate, and hyperkalemia with placement of a temporary pacemaker
E. Treatment of ventricular bigeminy with digoxin-specific antibodies

89. Which of the following is/are included among complications of intracardiac congenital shunts?

A. Syncope
B. Brain abscess
C. Cyanosis and polycythemia
D. Pulmonary vascular disease
E. Ventricular volume overload and failure

90. Which of the following statements concerning aortic regurgitation is/are correct?

A. Both the mid-diastolic rumble of aortic regurgitation (Austin Flint murmur) and the diastolic rumble of mitral stenosis increase in response to amyl nitrite inhalation

B. Etiologic factors include rheumatic fever, Reiter's syndrome, and rheumatoid arthritis
C. In a patient with acute aortic regurgitation, progressive softening of the first heart sound (in the absence of an increase in P-R interval) is an ominous prognostic sign
D. A systolic thrill in the carotid artery identifies concomitant aortic stenosis
E. Even with severe shock regurgitation, exercise capacity is typically well maintained

91. Which of the following statements concerning patients with acute myocardial infarction is/are true?

A. Prophylactic beta-blocker therapy is likely to improve the prognosis
B. Prophylactic lidocaine decreases the risk of ventricular fibrillation
C. Prophylactic anticoagulation decreases the risk of systemic embolization
D. Intracoronary streptokinase six hours after the onset of pain is likely to reduce the risk of death
E. Pericardial friction rub is a *contraindication* to anticoagulation

92. Which of the following is/are determinant(s) of ventricular wall stress (force/cross-sectional area)?

A. Intraventricular pressure
B. Ventricular wall thickness
C. The viscosity of pericardial fluid
D. Rheologic characteristics of ejected blood
E. The radius of curvature of the left ventricular wall

93. Which of the following indicate(s) abnormal cardiac performance (pressure/function)?

A. A mean left atrial pressure (or pulmonary capillary wedge pressure) of 21 mm Hg
B. An aortic root systolic pressure of 180 mm Hg
C. A mean central venous pressure of 4 mm Hg
D. A pulmonary artery peak systolic pressure of 48 mm Hg
E. An ejection fraction of 58%

94. Which of the following is/are associated with vagally mediated decreases in heart rate?

A. Painful stimuli
B. Nausea and vomiting
C. Intubation of the trachea
D. Decreased arterial pulse pressure
E. Facial immersion in water

95. Which of the following is/are characteristic of a normal venous pulse in the neck?

A. An estimated mean venous pressure of 6 cm H_2O
B. A pulsation that is both visible and palpable
C. An X descent that is deeper than the Y descent
D. A fall in the venous pressure with inspiration
E. A higher pressure in the external as compared to the internal jugular veins

96. Which of the following exert(s) a predominant hemodynamic effect by changing ventricular preload?

A. The administration of intravenous fluids
B. The administration of nitroglycerin
C. The administration of digoxin
D. The Mueller maneuver
E. Upright isotonic exercise

97. Which of the following is/are accurate concerning the risks of cardiac catheterization?

A. The risk of death from right heart catheterization is about 0.01%
B. The risk of death from coronary angiography is about 0.1%
C. The risk of systemic embolization is diminished by concomitant administration of heparin
D. The risk of major morbidity with left heart catheterization is about 0.2%
E. Coronary angiography is contraindicated with a history of allergy to contrast media

98. Which of the following statements concerning rest/exercise radionuclide angiography (MUGA—first pass) is/are true?

A. Their sensitivity for detecting coronary artery disease is higher than that of treadmill exercise testing
B. They are the only noncatheterization techniques for measuring exercise changes in left ventricular function
C. The specificity of a negative test for excluding coronary artery disease is higher than a negative, adequate treadmill exercise test
D. A drop in the exercise ejection fraction of 5% or more reliably identifies coronary artery disease
E. The sensitivity and predictive accuracy for the diagnosis of coronary artery disease are comparable to rest/exercise thallium perfusion imaging

99. Which of the following statements concerning digitalis is/are true?

A. The historic status of this drug is disproportionate to its current importance as a pharmacologicagent
B. The serum level of digoxin typically increases with concomitant quinidine administration
C. An improvement in renal function typically lowers the serum digoxin concentration
D. Digoxin toxicity is defined by a serum level greater than 2.0 ng/ml
E. Treatment with digoxin antibody fragments is indicated for life-threatening arrhythmias due to digoxin toxicity

100. Which of the following is/are included in the ECG criteria for left ventricular hypertrophy?

A. A QRS duration of 0.17 second
B. An R wave of 3.6 mV in leads V_5 and/or V_6
C. A mean QRS axis more negative than minus 30 degrees
D. ST-segment depression and T-wave inversion in leads I, aVL, V_5, and V_6
E. A P-R interval of 0.30 second

101. Which of the following peripheral adaptations for sustaining cardiac output in congestive heart failure exert(s) an effect primarily via the Frank-Starling mechanism?

A. Peripheral arteriolar vasoconstriction
B. Peripheral venoconstriction
C. Redistribution in organ blood flow
D. Increased levels of atrial natriuretic hormone
E. Expansion of circulating blood flow

102. Which of the following measurements is/are necessary at the time of cardiac catheterization to calculate the area of a stenotic valve?

A. The peak pressure difference across the valve
B. The cardiac output
C. The heart rate
D. The time per minute that blood flows across the obstruction
E. dP/dT in the downstream chamber

103. Which of the following is/are typical of malignant hypertension?

A. Hematuria
B. Proteinuria
C. Left ventricular enlargement
D. Retinal hemorrhages and papilledema
E. Schistocytes on peripheral blood smear

104. In mild hypertension, which of the following complications has/have been shown to be reduced by antihypertensive therapy?

A. Retinopathy
B. Myocardial infarction
C. Cerebral vascular accident
D. Left ventricular hypertrophy
E. Sudden death

105. Which of the following has/have been shown to prevent high blood pressure?

A. Isometric exercise
B. Reduced sodium intake
C. Reduction of stress
D. Reduction of body weight
E. Increased potassium intake

106. Which of the following is/are considered normal blood pressure(s)?

A. A systolic blood pressure of 138 mm Hg
B. A systolic blood pressure of 155 mm Hg
C. A diastolic blood pressure of 84 mm Hg
D. A diastolic blood pressure of 88 mm Hg
E. A diastolic blood pressure of 98 mm Hg

107. Which of the following is/are initial therapies of choice for mild to moderate hypertension according to the 1984 Joint National Committee on the Detection, Evaluation and Treatment of High Blood Pressure?

A. Vasodilators
B. Beta blockers
C. Calcium blockers
D. Thiazide diuretics
E. Angiotensin-converting enzyme inhibitors

QUESTIONS 108–111

A 56-year-old white man presents for evaluation of increasing dyspnea on exertion. He smokes two packs of cigarettes daily, has gained 40 pounds since the age of 18, and was advised on a pre-employment physical examination two years ago that blood pressure, blood glucose, and cholesterol were all elevated. He has no history of chest pain, paroxysmal nocturnal dyspnea, orthopnea, or edema. He drinks 6–8 ounces of alcohol daily and receives allopurinol for "gout." He is also taking ibuprofen for low back pain and tolbutamide, 250 mg before breakfast and dinner, for his glucose level.

The patient is 70.5 in tall and weighs 246 pounds. Pulse rate is 90 per minute and regular. Blood pressure is 172/98 mm Hg in both arms seated with no postural change. No buffalo hump, moon facies, or skin striae are noted. The eye grounds show arteriolar narrowing, focal spasm, an increased arteriolar light reflex, and one small flame-shaped hemorrhage in the temporal quadrant of the left eye. The thyroid is not enlarged. Chest examination shows decreased breath sounds and scattered wheezing. The venous pulse in the neck is normal. The carotid pulses are large but have a normal upstroke and one systolic peak. The remainder of the pulses are intact, and there is no radial-femoral pulse delay. The apex impulse and the first heart sound are normal. The aortic component of the second heart sound is loud. No gallops or murmurs are noted. The abdomen is obese with no obvious mass. No bruit is noted. There is no peripheral edema and the neurologic examination, except for a mild resting tremor, is intact.

108. Which of the following factors is/are the most likely causes of the dyspnea in this patient?

A. Obesity
B. Deconditioning
C. Alcoholic cardiomyopathy
D. An unrecognized myocardial infarction
E. Chronic obstructive pulmonary disease

109. Which of the following is/are among the major remediable risk factors for the development of ischemic heart disease that need consideration in this patient?

A. Diabetes
B. Cigarette smoking
C. Hypertension
D. Hypercholesterolemia
E. Hyperuricemia

110. An ECG, blood urea nitrogen urinalysis, and serum electrolytes were all normal. Roentgenogram showed low diaphragms, normal pulmonary vascularity, and a normal heart size. A fasting blood glucose was 130 mg/dl, and the total cholesterol was 252 mg/dl. Which of the following is/are NOT among likely causes of the hypertension in this patient?

A. Cushing's syndrome
B. Primary aldosteronism
C. Coarctation of the aorta
D. Polycystic kidney disease
E. Congenital adrenal hyperplasia

111. You decide to initiate pharmacologic treatment with propranolol 20 mg orally four times daily. You also advise the patient to stop smoking and lose weight. Which additional measure(s) would you also advise in the care of this patient?

A. Reduce alcohol intake to 1–2 ounces per day
B. Avoid processed meats/cheeses and anything that tastes salty, and do not add salt at the table
C. Restrict fat intake to no more than 30% of daily calories, and substitute polyunsaturated vegetable fats for saturated animal fats whenever possible
D. Discontinue ibuprofen
E. Add regular isotonic exercise to the daily routine

112. Which of the following is/are likely to effect more than a transient increase in cardiac output?

A. Infusion of isoproterenol (Isuprel)
B. Valsalva maneuver
C. Constriction of the systemic veins
D. Atrial pacing to a heart rate of 120 per minute
E. Changing position from upright to supine

113. Which of the following is/are among the beneficial effects of digoxin in congestive heart failure?

A. Enhanced contractility
B. Systemic venous vasodilatation
C. Systemic arteriolar vasodilatation
D. Reflex increase in the heart rate
E. Direct natriuretic effects on the kidney

114. In a 56-year-old patient with mildly symptomatic congestive heart failure due to a congestive cardiomyopathy, which of the following is/are included in the initial treatment?

A. Restriction of dietary sodium and, if necessary, caloric intake
B. Rest (and/or moderation of activity), along with correction of any precipitating factors
C. Diuretic therapy
D. Vasodilator therapy
E. Administration of digitalis

115. Which of the following statements concerning arterial hypertension is/are true?

A. Hypertensive patients die mainly from myocardial infarction, stroke, peripheral vascular disease, or renal failure
B. Among hypertensive patients, most deaths occur in those individuals with the highest blood pressure levels
C. Symptoms from high blood pressure are usually not of themselves an important part of the hypertensive disease spectrum
D. Given two groups of persons 40–49 years of age, the relative risk for stroke in a group with diastolic blood pressures higher than 104 mm Hg is 10 times greater than that of a group with diastolic blood pressures lower than 85 mm Hg
E. Given two 40-year-old men with normal ECG's, the risk of coronary artery disease in a nonsmoker who has systolic blood pressure of 195 mm Hg, cholesterol of 185 mg/dl, and a normal fasting blood sugar is greater over an eight-year period than that in a smoker who has systolic blood pressure of 105 mm Hg, cholesterol of 335 mg/dl, and an elevated fasting blood sugar

116. Which of the following statements concerning hypertensive individuals is/are correct?

A. A single estimate of urinary VMA level is 98% accurate in detecting a pheochromocytoma
B. The overall incidence of renal artery stenosis causing mild hypertension is less than 1%
C. Treatment of isolated systolic hypertension in the elderly lowers the incidence of hypertensive complications
D. The ingestion of certain cheeses by patients taking monoamine oxidase inhibitors is a well-documented cause of hypertension
E. When hypertension is due to fibromuscular hyperplasia of the renal arteries, balloon dilatation is particularly successful

117. Which of the following is/are true of pericarditis?

A. Patients in whom the pericardium is absent have a high likelihood of right heart failure
B. Blood in the pericardium is a necessary prerequisite for the subsequent development of the postpericardiectomy syndrome
C. An inspiratory drop in arterial blood pressure that is greater than 10 mm Hg is pathognomonic of pericardial tamponade
D. Large pericardial effusions are *not* associated with pericardial friction rub
E. Kussmaul's sign is typical of constrictive pericarditis

118. Which of the following statements concerning diseases of the aorta is/are correct?

A. The one-year survival rate for patients with dissecting aortic aneurysm is less than 10%
B. Repair of a ruptured abdominal aortic aneurysm is associated with a mortality rate of less than 20%
C. Symptomatic patients with abdominal aortic aneurysms 5 cm in diameter or less can be followed medically
D. The VDRL test is accurate in identifying syphilitic aortitis in all age groups
E. The majority of patients with dissection of the thoracic aorta have peripheral pulse inequalities

119. Which of the following statements concerning arteriosclerosis obliterans is/are correct?

A. Pallor of the sole of the foot upon mild elevation indicates a severe reduction in arterial blood flow
B. Arterial vasodilator therapy is an effective therapeutic modality
C. An exercise-induced drop in systolic dorsalis pedis arterial pressure is characteristic of significant arterial obstruction
D. A patient who has sudden paralysis of one or both lower extremities should be evaluated for acute arterial obstruction
E. In a patient with arteriosclerosis obliterans and rest pain, a regular exercise program is indicated

120. Which of the following statements concerning venous thrombosis is/are correct?

A. Patients with thrombophlebitis are frequently asymptomatic
B. Prophylactic therapy with small doses of aspirin decreases the incidence of postoperative thrombophlebitis
C. Major risk factors for the development of thrombophlebitis include venostasis, venous vessel wall injury, and a hypercoagulable state
D. Among the surgical operations with the highest risk for postoperative thrombophlebitis are prosthetic hip replacement and prostatectomy
E. The most accurate test for the diagnosis of thrombophlebitis is scanning with radioisotope-labeled fibrinogen

DIRECTIONS: Questions 121 to 195 are matching questions. For each numbered item, choose the most likely associated lettered item from those provided. Each numbered item has ONLY ONE answer. Within each set of questions, each lettered item may be the answer to one, more than one, or none of the numbered items.

QUESTIONS 121–125

For each of the following patient histories, select the hemodynamic data (A–E) with which it is most consistent.

	PCWP	RAP	CO	A-Vo_2 diff	MVo_2	SVR
A.	11	1	1	1	1	11
B.	1	1	1	1	1	11
C.	1–	–	11	11	11	1–
D.	11	1	1	1–	1–	1
E.	1–	11	11	11	11	11

121. A 20-year-old man with increasing dyspnea, a Grade 3/6 holosystolic murmur at the lower left sternal border with radiation to the right chest, large pulmonary arteries, and left ventricular enlargement on chest roentgenogram.

122. A 40-year-old woman with a known history of diabetic ketoacidosis who presents with profound weakness, lethargy, a temperature of 39.0°C, sinus tachycardia, and evidence of a urinary tract infection.

123. A 65-year-old man with a history of exertional chest pain who developed severe substernal chest pressure 24 hours ago. He now has marked resting dyspnea and pallor, and diminished pulses, rales, and an S_3 on physical examinations.

124. A 68-year-old woman with chest pain and marked nausea and vomiting, whose skin is cold and clammy. Examination shows elevated neck veins, intermittent cannon A waves, and a pulse rate of 50 per minute. ECG shows ST elevation in rV_1 and rV_4.

125. A 75-year-old woman with a history of peptic ulcer disease and a four-day history of "black stools." She presented after a single syncopal episode and currently has a blood pressure of 90/70 mm Hg supine with a sitting pressure of 78/50 mm Hg.

QUESTIONS 126–130

In the following questions, select the hemodynamic response most likely to occur with the given pharmacologic agent.

	HR	SVR	PCWP	CO	BP
A.	1	1–	1–	1	1–
B.	1–	11	1	1–	11
C.	1	11	1–	1–	11
D.	11	11	11	1	1–
E.	1	1	1	11	1

126. Norepinephrine

127. Dobutamine

128. Nitroprusside

129. Dopamine

130. Isoproterenol

QUESTIONS 131–135

Match the following antiarrhythmic agents with their characteristic accompanying side effect:

A. Quinidine
B. Digoxin
C. Procainamide
D. Amiodarone
E. Flecainide

131. Ectopic atrial tachycardia with block

132. Thrombocytopenia

133. Drug-induced lupus erythematosus

134. Aggravation of congestive heart failure

135. Interstitial lung disease and/or alveolitis

QUESTIONS 136–140

Match the following neck vein morphologies with the appropriate accompanying pathophysiologic process:

A. Atrial-septal defect
B. Tricuspid stenosis
C. Tricuspid regurgitation
D. Constrictive pericarditis

136. Typical "M" or "W" shape with a rapid "Y" descent

137. Prominent A and V waves with an intervening "X" descent

138. Prominent "C-V" wave

139. Increased jugular venous distention with inspiration

140. Giant A waves with a slow "Y" descent

QUESTIONS 141–146

For each of the following patients, select the most appropriate laboratory test to be obtained after a thorough history and physical examination.

A. Doppler echocardiography
B. Time motion/two-dimensional echocardiography
C. Phonocardiography
D. Chest roentgenography
E. Chest fluoroscopy

141. A febrile patient with a new high-frequency diastolic decrescendo murmur at the lower left sternal border

142. A patient with an enlarged area of precordial dullness to percussion

143. A 46-year-old patient with an undetermined degree of aortic stenosis

144. A patient with suspected intracardiac calcification

145. A patient with a strong family history of hypertrophic cardiomyopathy and sudden death

146. An asymptomatic patient with severe aortic regurgitation who is seen for annual follow-up examination

QUESTIONS 147–150

For each of the following patients receiving chronic digitalis therapy, select the most appropriate decision concerning further pharmacologic therapy.

A. Continue digoxin therapy unchanged
B. Increase the dose of digoxin
C. Decrease or hold further doses of digoxin
D. Change to another digitalis preparation
E. Add propranolol or verapamil to the regimen

147. A 45-year-old woman who has known rheumatic heart disease, paroxysmal atrial fibrillation, and chronic furosemide therapy; she returns with a new onset of nausea. Potassium level is 3.0 mEq/L. Electrocardiogram shows a regular atrial rate of 140 per minute with a 2:1 ventricular response.

148. A 49-year-old man who has chronic atrial fibrillation and normal ventricular function; ventricular rate is 140 per minute and irregularly irregular. Digoxin level is 0.3 ng/ml.

149. A 65-year-old man who has mitral regurgitation, an ejection fraction of 70%, and chronic atrial fibrillation; ventricular response is 130 per minute and irregularly irregular. Electrolytes are normal; digoxin level is 2.1 ng/ml.

150. A 65-year-old woman who has chronic atrial fibrillation due to coronary artery disease with compensated congestive heart failure. She has mild exertional dyspnea but is comfortable at rest. Heart rate is 82 per minute at rest, increasing to 98 per minute when climbing one flight of stairs. Ventricular response is irregularly irregular. Digoxin level is 1.5 ng/ml.

QUESTIONS 151–155

For each of the following clinical findings, select the most likely appearance on chest roentgenogram.

A. Normal pulmonary vascularity
B. Increased pulmonary vascularity
C. Decreased pulmonary vascularity

151. Ostium primum atrial septal defect

152. Ebstein's anomaly of the tricuspid valve

153. Tetralogy of Fallot

154. Tricuspid atresia

155. Partial anomalous pulmonary venous return

QUESTIONS 156–160

For each of the following patients, select the most appropriate course of management.

A. Commissurotomy of the valve
B. Prosthetic tissue valve replacement
C. Prosthetic mechanical valve replacement
D. Institution of indicated medical management; deferment of surgery

156. A 14-year-old boy with aortic stenosis who is asymptomatic. Cardiac catheterization shows no aortic valve calcification; valve area is 0.4 cm^2/m^2.

157. A 24-year-old man who has calcific aortic stenosis and a calculated valve area of 0.5 cm^2/m^2. He has mild dyspnea, no chest pain, and exertional syncope.

158. A 28-year-old woman in normal sinus rhythm who has moderate pulmonary hypertension and mitral stenosis. Cardiac catheterization shows that the mitral valve area is 0.7 cm^2; no valvular calcification is noted. The patient receives diuretics and continues to have orthopnea and dyspnea during mild exertion.

159. A 52-year-old woman with chronic atrial fibrillation who receives digoxin therapy and has well-controlled ventricular response. She is dyspneic during ordinary activities. Cardiac catheterization shows mild mitral stenosis and 3+ mitral regurgitation; the ejection fraction is 46% and the A-Vo_2 difference is 7.2 ml/dl. There is moderate pulmonary hypertension.

160. A 64-year-old man with longstanding aortic regurgitation who suffers primarily from fatigue. Cardiac catheterization shows 4+ aortic regurgitation, mild elevation in left atrial and pulmonary artery pressures, and an A-Vo_2 difference of 6.2 ml/dl. The ejection fraction is 42%. The patient has a history of diverticulosis with gastrointestinal bleeding; the precise site of bleeding has never been documented, despite extensive evaluation.

QUESTIONS 161–164

For each of the following heart disease conditions, select the most typical descriptions of the precordial pulse.

A. Inferolaterally displaced, enlarged, and hyperdynamic apical impulse with no other palpable precordial impulses
B. A tapping, nondisplaced apical impulse with a sustained impulse at the lower left sternal edge
C. A nondisplaced, enlarged, sustained apical impulse with a palpable presystolic component
D. A laterally displaced, sustained, systolic impulse with a palpable early diastolic impulse and a late systolic impulse at the lower left sternal edge
E. A sustained systolic impulse at the third left intercostal space, 8 cm to the left of the midsternal line, with a palpable presystolic component

161. Severe mitral regurgitation with well-maintained left ventricular function

162. Severe aortic regurgitation with well-maintained left ventricular function

163. Moderate mitral stenosis

164. Moderate aortic stenosis with well-maintained left ventricular function

QUESTIONS 165–169

For each of the following clinical situations, select the most likely description of the carotid pulse.

A. A normal carotid pulse
B. A dicrotic carotid pulse
C. A bisferious carotid pulse
D. A spike and dome carotid pulse
E. A slow rising carotid pulse
F. Pulsus paradoxus

165. A 16-year-old boy with hypertrophic obstructive cardiomyopathy

166. A 38-year-old woman with breast cancer, peripheral edema, and a large pericardial effusion

167. A 38-year-old male alcoholic with an ejection fraction of 15%

168. A 49-year-old woman with severe aortic regurgitation

169. A 49-year-old man with severe calcific aortic stenosis

QUESTIONS 170–174

For each of the following clinical situations, select the most likely electrocardiographic change.

A. P-R prolongation
B. ST-segment elevation
C. ST-segment shortening
D. Prominent u waves
E. Peaked, tall T waves
F. Q-T prolongation

170. Pericarditis

171. Hyperkalemia

172. Digoxin therapy

173. Quinidine therapy

174. Hypercalcemia

QUESTIONS 175–180

For each of the following clinical situations choose the most appropriate ECG method of evaluation. Assume that the clinical circumstances warrant further evaluation.

A. 24-hour ambulatory ECG monitoring
B. Transtelephonic ECG telemetry
C. Electrophysiologic stimulation/monitoring with intracardiac catheter techniques
D. Esophageal electrocardiography
E. His bundle electrocardiography
F. ECG signal averaging

175. A patient with daily bouts of palpitations lasting 1–3 minutes

176. An older patient who is being treated with digoxin for shortness of breath develops episodic dizziness and presyncope. A 12-lead ECG shows RBBB and an axis of minus 70 degrees. On subsequent bedside monitoring in the hospital, there is 2:1 AV block with an atrial rate of 100 per minute.

177. A patient with a narrow QRS tachycardia that is regular at a rate of 150 per minute. There is no response to vagal interventions, and a 12-lead ECG fails to define atrial activity.

178. A patient with rare (1–2 times per month) bouts of rapid heart action lasting 1–3 minutes

179. A patient with a wide (0.14 second) QRS tachycardia at 136 per minute. There is a 1:1 relationship between the P's and QRS's.

180. A patient with WPW syndrome and three bouts of rapid heart action over the past year, each associated with syncope

QUESTIONS 181–185

For each of the following potential side effects, select the most likely causative antihypertensive drug.

A. Propranolol
B. Nifedipine
C. Guanethidine
D. Hydrochlorothiazide
E. Captopril
F. Hydralazine

181. Impotence

182. Lupus-like reaction

183. Peripheral edema

184. Loss of sense of taste

185. Bronchospasm

QUESTIONS 186–190

For each of the following physical findings, select the most likely corresponding echocardiogram (A–E). Each echo is

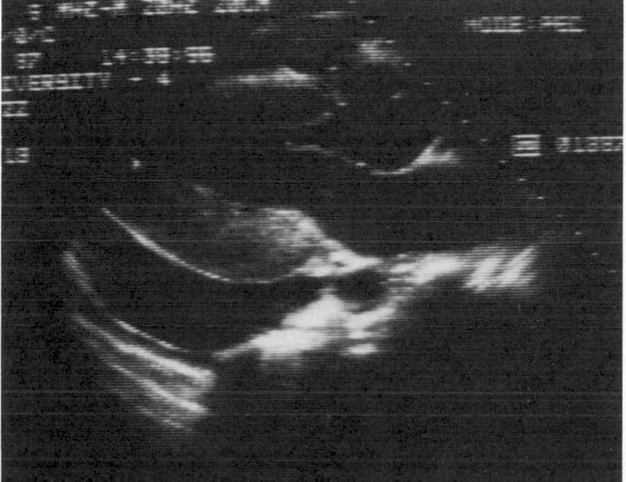

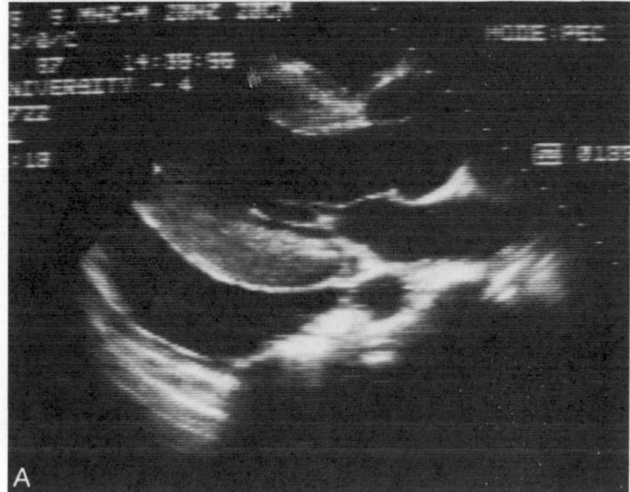

A

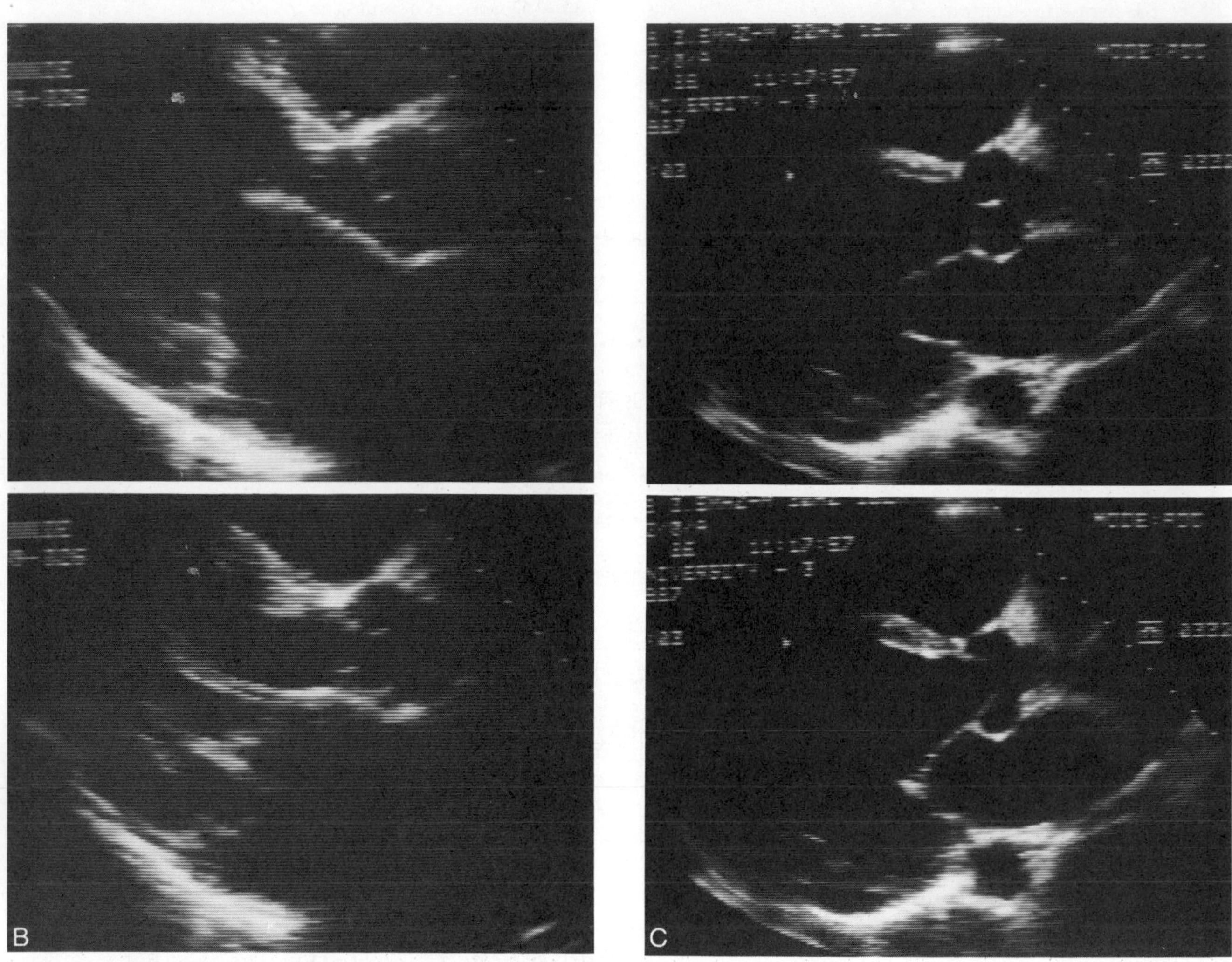
B
C

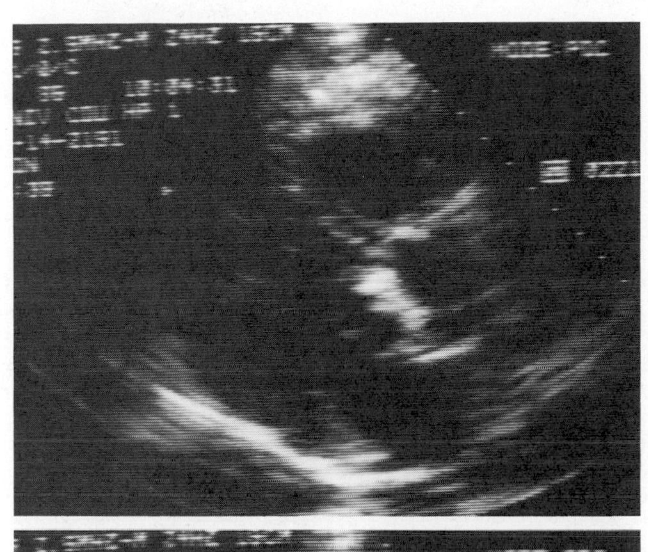

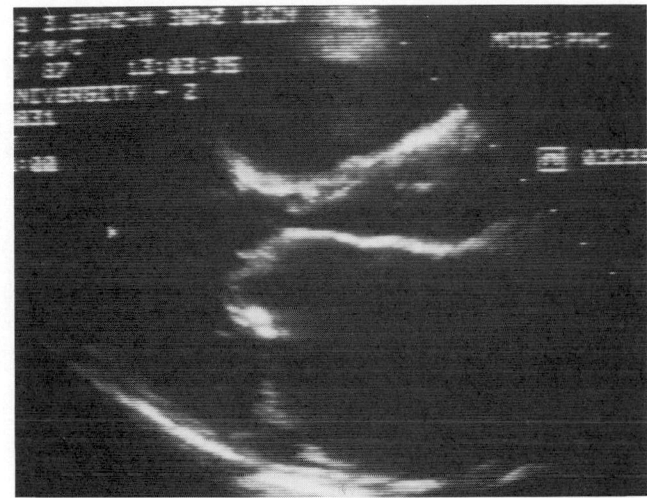

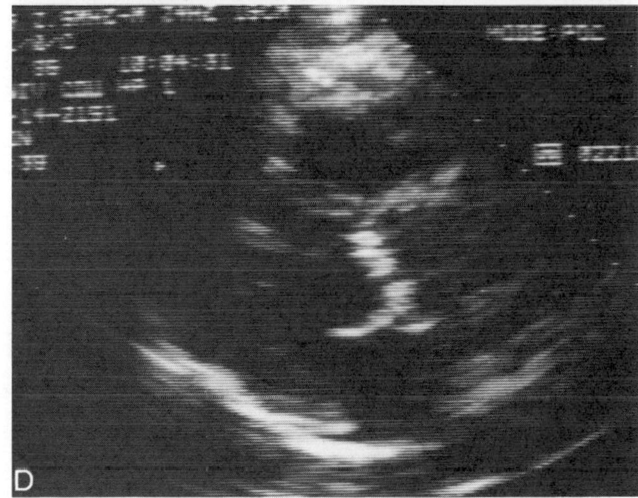
D

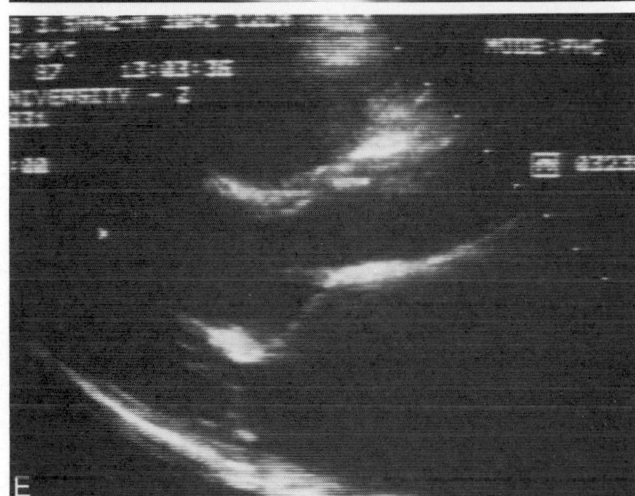
E

a parasternal long-axis view of the same patient in diastole (upper row) and systole (lower row). The scale indicators are 1.0 cm.

186. Apical late systolic, high-frequency crescendo murmur

187. Apical long diastolic rumble

188. Apical harsh, midsystolic, diamond-shaped murmur

189. Distant heart sounds at the apex

190. Apical S_3, S_4, and high-frequency holosystolic murmur

QUESTIONS 191–195

For each of the following rhythm strips (A–E), select the most accurate electrocardiographic description.

191. Second-degree AV block, type undetermined

192. Second-degree AV block, type I

193. Second-degree AV block, type II

194. Third-degree AV block

195. No evidence of pathologic AV block

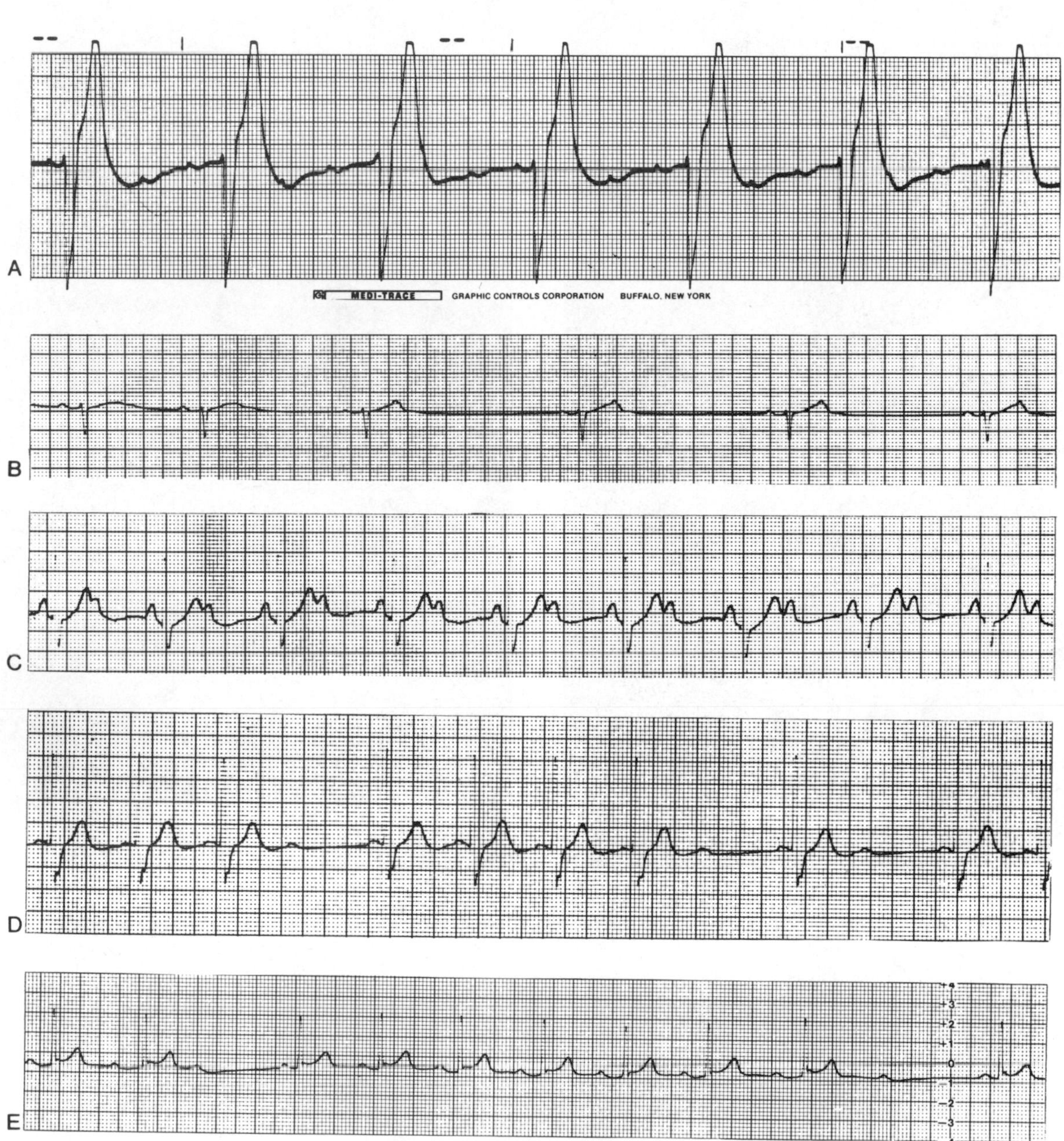

PART 1

CARDIOVASCULAR DISEASES

ANSWERS

1.(D) Acidosis results from anaerobic metabolism with generation of lactate, from decreased renal perfusion with accumulation of organic acids, and possibly from hypoventilation of certain pulmonary segments leading to respiratory acidosis. The development of acidosis results in a reduced myocardial contractility. Myocardial ischemia along with hypoxia also produces a decrease in contractility. Beta endorphins may also be released and contribute either directly or indirectly to myocardial depression and shock. Hypercapnia per se has not been demonstrated to result in any further decrease in myocardial contractility. *(Cecil, Ch. 44)*

2.(C) In the presence of hypoxia the coronary, cerebral, and renal vascular beds undergo vasodilatation, in part due to a direct, vascular effect. In contrast, hypoxia activates chemoreceptors causing a sympathetic vasoconstrictor response in the skeletal muscle, skin, and splanchnic beds, thus permitting the redistribution of blood to the vital organs with higher oxygen demand. *(Cecil, Ch. 44)*

3.(B) In the setting of systemic shock, hypoxia may result in vasoconstriction of the skeletal, skin, and splanchnic vascular beds. In addition, in platelets endoperoxides are converted to thromboxane A_2, which causes vasoconstriction and platelet aggregation. Vasopressin may be released from the posterior pituitary, primarily in response to changes in osmolality, and also plays an important vasoconstrictor role in the circulatory response to shock. The renin-angiotensin system may be activated in response to a fall in arterial blood pressure or an increase in sympathetic discharge to the kidney, which likewise may result in peripheral vasoconstriction. In contrast, prostacyclin, which is synthesized in vascular wall endothelial cells, is a powerful vasodilator and inhibitor of platelet aggregation. *(Cecil, Ch. 44)*

4.(E) The venules, or postcapillary resistance vessels, may be relatively more reactive to catecholamines that activate constrictor alpha receptors than the precapillary resistance vessels. This differential effect increases hydrostatic pressure further and may contribute to intravascular fluid loss. Histamines may also play an important role in regulating vascular tone and capillary permeability, favoring fluid extravasation. Endothelial cell damage and a decrease in plasma oncotic pressure also favor extravascular fluid loss. In contrast, bradykinin appears to participate in the local regulation of blood flow and produces vasodilation and hypotension without contributing directly to fluid extravasation. *(Cecil, Ch. 44)*

5.(B) In the setting of shock, an increase in membrane permeability to sodium and water, causing cellular swelling, is noted initially. This is followed by an increase in sodium/potassium-ATPase activity in an attempt to drive sodium out of the cell. Increased membrane ATPase activity eventually leads to the depletion of ATP and cyclic AMP. The latter may lead to alterations in the cellular response to insulin, glucagon, catecholamines, and other hormones. In animals that have been subjected to hemorrhagic shock, insulin-mediated glucose uptake by muscle is reduced. *(Cecil, Ch. 44)*

6.(B) Maternal smoking throughout pregnancy can damage the umbilical artery and vein and the vessels of the placental villi. As a result, the placenta may be relatively small and poorly vascularized, birth weights are low for gestational age, and the risk of first-trimester abortion, stillbirth, prematurity, or prenatal mortality may be increased. Nevertheless, an increased risk for congenital heart defects has not been described. In contrast, an increased incidence of congenital heart disease has been observed in the offspring of women who contract rubella during the first trimester of pregnancy. These offspring may show pulmonary valve stenosis, peripheral pulmonary artery stenosis, and persistent patent ductus arteriosus. The offspring of diabetic women are also at greater risk for a variety of congenital heart defects. Approximately one half of the offspring of alcoholic mothers have congenital heart disease: typically, left to right shunts. The prevalence of congenital heart disease in the children of women with congenital heart disease ranges between 2 and 5%. *(Cecil, Ch. 49)*

7.(D) Circulatory changes occurring shortly after birth include a marked fall in pulmonary vascular resistance as pulmonary vessels enlarge and dilate in response to the increased oxygen tension to which they are exposed. A rise in systemic vascular resistance with elimination of the lower-resistance placental circulation is noted. An abrupt rise in pulmonary blood flow, resulting in a rise in left atrial volume and pressure, also occurs, facilitating functional closure of the foramen ovale. Functional constriction of the ductus arteriosus in response to the effects of vasoactive substances and an elevated arterial Po_2 also occurs. *(Cecil, Ch. 45)*

8.(E) Many congenital heart lesions are accompanied by an increased risk of bacterial endocarditis, in part due to the presence of a high pressure gradient and turbulent blood flow. Because of these factors, patients with ventricular septal defect, patent ductus arteriosus, bicuspid aortic valve, and hypertrophic obstructive cardiomyopathy may show a higher risk for bacterial endocarditis. In contrast, the risk of endocarditis in patients with atrial septal defects is very low, and prophylaxis is not usually required. *(Braunwald, Ch. 34)*

9.(D) Patients with either an ostium primum or secundum atrial septal defect may present with a systolic ejection murmur at the upper left sternal border due to increased blood flow through the right ventricular outflow track. In addition, both may demonstrate fixed splitting of the second heart sound as well as right atrial enlargement on chest roentgenogram. In addition, with a primum defect, a cleft tricuspid valve may cause significant tricuspid regurgitation and further contribute to the right atrial enlargement. The electrocardiogram of the ostium primum defect, however, is distinctive in that a superior, counterclockwise frontal plane loop (left axis deviation), along with varying degrees of right ventricular hypertrophy, is observed. The presence of the left axis deviation on ECG, therefore, suggests the presence of an ostium primum defect. *(Cecil, Ch. 49)*

10.(E) During fetal life pulmonary arterial blood flows through the ductus arteriosus to the descending aorta for oxygenation in the placenta. Soon after birth, physiologic occlusion of the ductus occurs owing to the marked increase in arterial oxygen tension that accompanies the onset of ventilation and changes in the metabolism of vasoactive substances, especially prostaglandins. In the normal baby, anatomic closure is generally complete several weeks after birth. Persistent patency of the ductus arteriosus, however, is more frequent in females, in premature infants, in infants born at higher altitudes, and in infants whose first trimester of intrauterine life is complicated by maternal rubella. Infants born to mothers with first-trimester toxoplasmosis have not been shown to have a higher incidence of persistent patent ductus arteriosus. *(Cecil, Ch. 49)*

11.(A) In addition to the four characteristic components of tetralogy of Fallot, the ascending aorta may be displaced anteriorly (dextroposed) and the aortic arch may be right-sided in 20% of patients. Coarctation of the aorta, congenital aortic stenosis, a bicuspid aortic valve, and aortic ectasia do not occur with any increased frequency in these patients compared to those without tetralogy of Fallot. *(Cecil, Ch. 49)*

12.(D) Coarctation of the aorta may be manifest by the narrowing of the aortic lumen at one of several sites along the aorta. By far, the most common site of discrete obstruction is immediately distal to the origin of the left subclavian artery. The lesion is more common in males and accounts for 70% of all cardiac anomalies in patients with Turner's syndrome. A biscuspid aortic valve is also frequently observed in patients with coarctation. Although pregnancy may be well tolerated, coarctation predisposes a patient to aortic rupture during the third trimester of pregnancy. Because of the risk of aortic rupture and infective endocarditis, coarctectomy is advised in early childhood, preferably between the ages of three and five years. *(Cecil, Ch. 49; Braunwald, Ch. 49)*

13.(C) Isolated levocardia is accompanied by varying degrees of anomalous position of the abdominal viscera, so that situs inversus is partial or complete. Severe cardiac malformations are usual, including various combinations of anomalies of systemic and pulmonary venous return, atrioventricular canal defects, pulmonic stenosis or atresia, and defects of the atrial and ventricular septa. The asplenia syndrome, characterized by the absence of a spleen, is likewise accompanied by complex, severe cardiac malformations. The polysplenia syndrome may have complex severe cardiac malformations, but the cardiovascular abnormalities are typically less frequent and are not as complex as with the asplenia syndromes. Isolated dextroversion may likewise be accompanied by other cardiac abnormalities, while dextrocardia with situs inversus is usually associated with a normally functioning heart. *(Cecil, Ch. 49)*

14.(B) Eisenmenger's syndrome occurs most frequently with ventricular septal defect but may also occur with atrial septal defect and patent ductus arteriosus. It is associated with marked elevation of pulmonary vascular resistance, with reversed or bidirectional intracardiac or aortopulmonary shunting. Pulmonary vascular disease is the hallmark of this syndrome, and the site of the shunt is incidental. Medial hypertrophy of the pulmonary artery and arterioles is present and is associated with cellular, fibrotic, and fibroelastic intimal reactions. Because of the underlying physiology, hypoxia, cyanosis, polycythemia, and clubbing may be present. Patients with Eisenmenger's syndrome are at increased risk for syncope and sudden death between the ages of 20 and 40 years. *(Cecil, Ch. 49; Braunwald, Ch. 26)*

15.(D) Mitral stenosis, with fusion of the mitral valve leaflets and cordal tethering, presents an impedance to left atrial emptying. Patients with moderate to severe mitral stenosis may be further compromised by the development of atrial fibrillation, with a rapid ventricular response rate and further impairment of left atrial emptying. The tachycardia and increased cardiac output of vigorous exercise or a marked elevation of body temperature may also be poorly tolerated; they may precipitate or worsen pulmonary congestion. The first trimester of pregnancy, however, is prior to the increase in intravascular volume and is usually well tolerated. *(Cecil, Ch. 52)*

16.(B) Patients with significant aortic insufficiency, thyrotoxicosis, or cardiac (wet) beriberi may present in a high output state, during which peripheral pulses may be prominent. In chronic mitral regurgitation with well-maintained ventricular function, the peripheral pulses may be rapid in upstroke and of short duration. This pulse abnormality is due to the rapid contraction of the left ventricle as it ejects a large volume of blood into the low-pressure, dilated left atrium. In contrast, patients with mitral stenosis may demonstrate a diminished pulse pressure and narrowing of the pulse pressure due to the reduced stroke volume. *(Cecil, Ch. 52)*

17.(D) Several factors are important in determining the intensity of the first heart sound, including the ability of the atrioventricular valves to close, their mobility, and the velocity of their closing movement. A high velocity of closure has been found to correlate with a loud S_1, while slow velocity of closure correlates with a soft S_1. The position of the valve immediately prior to systole may also be important, with a louder S_1 generated when the valve is fully open at the onset of ventricular systole. The presence of a short P-R interval, as expected with thyrotoxicosis and sinus tachycardia, favors this valvular position. Such patients also have increased contractility, and both factors contribute to a louder S_1. Patients with mitral stenosis also display a loud first heart sound related to valvular thickening and the fact that the valve is held open by the diastolic transmitral valve pressure gradient until an abrupt high-velocity closing movement of the valve apparatus is produced by ventricular systole. Similarly, in patients with an atrial septal defect, S_1 may be increased, since the valve is held open by augmented flow from the right atrium to the right ventricle until closure finally occurs with ventricular systole. In contrast, with severe acute aortic insufficiency, preclosure of the atrioventricular valves may occur and S_1 may be diminished or absent. *(Braunwald, Ch. 3)*

18.(D) Patients with severe mitral stenosis have a marked impediment to left atrial emptying and ventricular filling. As a result, an S_3, which is typically generated by rapid ventricular filling of an overfilled ventricle in early diastole, does not occur. The presence of a left ventricular S_3 virtually excludes the presence of significant mitral stenosis. With increasingly severe mitral stenosis, pulmonary hypertension may develop, leading to accentuation of the pulmonic sound. While an opening snap may be heard with mild to moderate mitral stenosis, its intensity may actually diminish with progression of the disease. Inasmuch as the opening snap is generated by the opening of the mitral valve, higher atrial pressures accompanying more severe mitral stenosis would be expected to exceed ventricular pressures earlier in diastole, thus producing an earlier mitral valve opening snap. Of the auscultatory findings listed, the short A_2–opening snap interval is most consistent with severe disease. *(Cecil, Ch. 52)*

19. (D) The echocardiogram is extremely useful in demonstrating the presence of mitral stenosis with left atrial enlargement, increased echogenicity from mitral valve leaflet thickening, enlargement of the right ventricle, a diminutive mitral valve A wave, a reduced mitral valve E to F slope, a paradoxically moving posterior mitral leaflet, and central tethering of the mitral leaflets: all typical features of rheumatic mitral valve disease. *(Feigenbaum, pp. 249–262)*

20. (E) Patients with mitral stenosis are at increased risk for late sequelae including thromboemboli, particularly in the presence of coexisting atrial fibrillation and an enlarged left atrium. These patients should therefore be prophylactically anticoagulated. Because patients with mitral stenosis also have a higher risk of bacterial endocarditis, antibiotic prophylaxis at the time of dental procedures should be administered. Atrial fibrillation with a rapid ventricular response rate may also worsen already compromised left atrial emptying, and the rate should be controlled with restoration of sinus rhythm where possible or with medications directed at diminishing AV nodal conduction. Although the first trimester of pregnancy is usually well tolerated, additional symptoms may accompany the increased blood volume in the second and third trimesters of pregnancy. Women with mitral stenosis, therefore, should be followed extremely closely during pregnancy and intervention made where necessary. Patients with a history of rheumatic fever are at higher risk for recurrent rheumatic fever with or without the presence of mitral stenosis. Prophylactic antibiotics for prevention of recurrent rheumatic fever have therefore been recommended for patients with rheumatic fever who are under the age of 35. Older patients may continue to receive prophylactic therapy if they are consistently exposed to a higher risk of streptococcal infection (working with school-age children, in the military service, or in medical or allied health positions). *(Braunwald, Chs. 33 and 54)*

21. (A) Although rheumatic heart disease, coronary artery disease with papillary muscle dysfunction, and cardiomyopathy with marked left ventricular dilatation may lead to mitral regurgitation, mitral valve prolapse is the leading cause of mitral regurgitation. Connective tissue disease may also result in redundancy of the mitral valve, leading to mitral regurgitation. Nevertheless, the prevalence of mitral valve disease resulting from connective tissue disorders is low. *(Cecil, Ch. 52)*

22. (B) Patients with moderate mitral stenosis or an atrial myxoma may demonstrate elevated pulmonary capillary wedge pressures due to impaired left atrial emptying. In addition, patients with marked left ventricular dysfunction following an acute myocardial infarction may develop elevated left ventricular end-diastolic and pulmonary capillary wedge pressures due to marked systolic dysfunction. Patients with hypertrophic obstructive cardiomyopathy likewise show elevated pulmonary wedge pressures due to impaired diastolic function as well as concomitant mitral regurgitation. Although patients with acute mitral regurgitation may develop prominent V waves and accompanying left atrial pressure elevation, the mean left atrial pressure in chronic mitral regurgitation may remain within the normal range until late in the disease course, owing to the enlarged compliant left atrium and pulmonary veins as well as the increase in compliance properties of the volume-loaded left ventricle. *(Cecil, Ch. 52)*

23. (C) The cardinal symptoms of aortic stenosis commence most commonly in the sixth decade of life and include angina, syncope, and congestive heart failure. In the absence of treatment, the prognosis becomes poor once these symptoms become manifest. Survival curves show that the interval from the onset of symptoms to the time of death is approximately two years in patients with heart failure, three years in those with syncope, and five years in those with angina. The presence of left bundle branch block morphology on ECG and/or complex ventricular ectopy has not been identified as an indicator of a poor prognosis in aortic stenosis. *(Frank et al.; Braunwald, Ch. 33)*

24. (C) The severity of aortic stenosis may be discerned from the physical examination. Although an ejection sound may be present early in aortic stenosis, with progressive thickening and fusion of the aortic valve leaflets, the ejection sound may be lost. Similarly, the second heart sound may be significantly diminished. As the transvalvular gradient increases, the systolic ejection murmur peaks progressively later in systole. Significant stenosis may also be accompanied by pulsus parvus et tardus. An important physical finding is the detection of a palpable systolic thrill (vibration) over the primary aortic area which can be brought out with the patient in the sitting position during full expiration. Appreciation of this thrill correlates with a gradient across the valve of more than 40 mm Hg. *(Cecil, Ch. 49)*

25. (A) Elective valve replacement is usually not recommended for asymptomatic adults with mitral stenosis, aortic stenosis, mitral regurgitation, aortic regurgitation, or Ebstein's malformation. In contrast, asymptomatic young patients with congenital aortic stenosis have significant risk of sudden death. Surgical treatment is indicated when the obstruction is severe, as judged by a systolic gradient of 70 mm Hg or more or a calculated effective aortic valve area less than 0.5 cm^2/m^2 of body surface area. Because of the risk of sudden death in children and adolescents with critical stenosis, surgery is advised even if the patient is asymptomatic. It is also unwise to allow these patients to participate in competitive sports. *(Cecil, Ch. 49)*

26. (E) Long-acting nitrates produce peripheral venous dilatation, resulting in a decrease in venous return and therefore preload. This may be beneficial in disease entities accompanied by elevated left ventricular end-diastolic pressures. In addition, long-acting nitrates may reduce afterload, thus further improving forward ventricular output. Their use may be beneficial in dilated cardiomyopathies of idiopathic, ischemic, or valvular etiology. In hypertrophic obstructive cardiomyopathy, however, ventricular filling is compromised owing to poor diastolic relaxation, and excessive preload reduction by diuresis or nitrates may be detrimental. Furthermore, afterload reduction can increase the gradient across the outflow tract, creating further systolic impairment. As a result, long-acting nitrates in this disease may be hazardous. *(Braunwald, Ch. 42)*

27.(D) Because mitral stenosis primarily represents an impediment to left atrial emptying and, therefore, ventricular filling, left ventricular function is not usually impaired even in the presence of significant mitral stenosis. Improvement in ventricular function following valve replacement for mitral regurgitation or aortic regurgitation is a function of preoperative ventricular function. Preoperative left ventricular end-systolic dimensions exceeding 55 mm, shortening of the left ventricular diameter by less than 30%, elevated levels of end-diastolic radius/wall thickness ratios, and end-systolic stress correlate with poor postoperative left ventricular function. Ventricular performance returns to normal, however, more frequently in patients with aortic stenosis than in those with aortic regurgitation. The increased left ventricular mass may be reduced toward normal within 18 months. *(Braunwald, Ch. 33)*

28.(E) Because of the increased blood flow accompanying left to right shunting, both patent ductus arteriosus and ventricular septal defect result in left ventricular volume overload. In addition, the lesions of aortic and mitral regurgitation present an increased blood volume to the left ventricle. In contrast, an atrial septal defect results in increased blood flow and volume to the right atrium and ventricle as well as the pulmonary vascular system. The shunt at the left atrial level prevents excessive volume overload of the left ventricle. *(Cecil, Chs. 49 and 52)*

29.(D) Although aortic stenosis may be congenital, the majority of cases of aortic stenosis are acquired. Similarly, mitral and tricuspid stenosis are more typically caused by rheumatic fever and are rarely, if ever, of a congenital origin. Stenotic lesions of the pulmonic valve are almost always caused by congenital malformations and may be seen in the offspring of mothers contracting rubella during the first trimester of pregnancy. *(Cecil, Ch. 52; Braunwald, Ch. 33)*

30.(D) Direct determinants of oxygen consumption include an increase in heart rate, contractility, and myocardial wall tension. The determinants are also affected by a variety of factors, including afterload. In contrast, an increase in wall thickness results in a decrease in myocardial wall tension and a resulting decrease in oxygen consumption. *(Braunwald, Ch. 14)*

31.(C) Although graft occlusion and incomplete revascularization at surgery may contribute to recurrent angina following coronary artery bypass grafting, progression of intrinsic coronary artery disease remains the most common reason for redevelopment of postoperative angina. Postoperative ventricular hypertrophy has not been shown to be a relevant contributor to recurrent angina. *(Cecil, Ch. 51.1)*

32.(D) Hyperacute T wave changes or ST elevation is observed on the surface ECG within the first hour of a myocardial infarction. Similarly, CPK isoenzymes increase in the sera of patients within approximately 2 hours, peak in 10–12 hours, and often return to normal within 24 hours after the event. LDH isoenzymes may also be abnormal within the first 24–48 hours of a myocardial infarction. Thallium-201 scanning, a "cold spot" imaging technique, approaches a sensitivity of approximately 90% when used within 24 hours after an acute myocardial infarction. In contrast, technetium-99m stannous pyrosphosphate accumulates in irreversibly damaged myocardium 1–5 days after an infarction. *(Cecil, Ch. 51.2)*

33.(C) The development of a new right bundle branch block in the absence of a left anterior or posterior hemifascicular block is not considered to be an appropriate indication for temporary pacing in the setting of an acute myocardial infarction. In addition, accelerated idioventricular rhythms and type I second-degree AV block do not mandate temporary pacing. In contrast, the development of new left bundle branch block with P-R prolongation is an acceptable indication for temporary pacemaker insertion following an infarction. *(Braunwald, Ch. 23)*

34.(C) The His bundle derives its blood supply from two sources: the AV nodal artery and the first septal perforator of the left anterior descending branch of the left coronary artery. In 50% of cases, the right bundle branch has a twofold blood supply: the AV nodal artery and the first septal perforator of the left anterior descending coronary artery. In the other 50%, the right bundle branch derives its blood from a single source, the first septal perforator of the left anterior descending coronary artery. The anterior fascicle of the left bundle branch has the same blood supply as the right bundle branch, accounting for the frequent association of right bundle branch with left anterior fascicular block during acute myocardial infarction involving the septum. The left anterior papillary muscle is usually supplied by a branch of the left anterior descending coronary artery. *(Cecil, Ch. 45)*

35.(A) Common arrhythmic manifestations of digitalis intoxication include ectopic atrial tachycardia with block, frequent premature ventricular contractions, junctional tachycardias, bidirectional tachycardias, and type I second-degree AV block. Sinus tachycardia as a manifestation of digitalis toxicity is extremely uncommon. *(Cecil, Ch. 45; Braunwald, Ch. 17)*

36.(E) Many antiarrhythmic agents depress conduction in the atrioventricular node and may, therefore, be useful in slowing the ventricular response rate during atrial fibrillation. Cardiac glycosides such as digoxin, beta blockers such as propranolol, and calcium channel blockers such as verapamil and diltiazem may all be helpful in reducing the ventricular response rate. In contrast, quinidine, either through a direct effect or a vagolytic effect in combination with slowing of the atrial rate and less concealed conduction into the AV node, may cause actual acceleration of conduction through the atrioventricular node during atrial flutter or atrial fibrillation. *(Cecil, Ch. 45; Braunwald, Ch. 38)*

37.(A) The indications for anticoagulation prior to cardioversion of atrial fibrillation have remained controversial. Those patients with mitral stenosis, a history of recent or recurrent emboli, a prosthetic mitral valve, cardiac enlargement, and/or congestive heart failure are at higher risk for embolization and should probably be anticoagulated for 3–6 weeks prior to cardioversion. Most series, however, report a 2% incidence of peripheral emboli following conversion to sinus rhythm in patients without known mitral valve disease. *(Cecil, Ch. 45; Braunwald, Ch. 21)*

38.(D) Antiarrhythmic agents have traditionally been divided into classes based on a variety of electrophysiologic effects. For example, the type Ia agents (quinidine, disopyramide, and procainamide) produce prolongation of refractoriness manifest on the surface ECG by lengthening of the Q-T interval. Type Ib agents, such as lidocaine, tocainide, and mexiletine, shorten the Q-T interval. In contrast, the new type Ic agents, such as flecainide, encainide, propafenone, and lorcainide, have little effect on the Q-T interval. Amiodarone, like the type Ia agents, also prolongs the Q-T interval. *(Cecil, Ch. 45; Braunwald, Ch. 21)*

39.(C) The diagnosis of ventricular tachycardia is favored by the appearance of VA dissociation with a faster ventricular than atrial rate. The presence of fusion or capture beats is also indicative of ventricular tachycardia. In addition, a QRS duration greater than 0.14 second and significant left axis deviation have been shown to be predictive of a ventricular origin for a wide complex tachycardia. In contrast, the triphasic right bundle branch block QRS pattern in V_1 may be more characteristic of a supraventricular arrhythmia with aberrancy. *(Wellens et al)*

40.(E) The type Ia agents (quinidine, procainamide, and disopyramide), along with the newer type Ic agents (flecainide and encainide), produce prolongation of the refractoriness as well as a slowing of conduction in accessory pathways. In contrast, digoxin may cause enhancement of antegrade conduction across the accessory pathway in up to one third of patients. Verapamil similarly enhances conduction across the accessory AV connection in a significant percentage of patients. *(Gulamhusein et al)*

41.(E) In addition to producing a salutary effect on atrial fibrillation by conversion to sinus rhythm and/or slowing of the ventricular response, treatment with beta blockers, verapamil, amiodarone, or disopyramide may have a beneficial effect on the diastolic dysfunction observed in patients with hypertrophic cardiomyopathy. As a result, each of these agents can be used in treating accompanying atrial arrhythmias, with the one exception of avoiding the use of verapamil when there is concomitant pulmonary hypertension. In contrast, the positive inotropic effect of digoxin may further aggravate the already impaired ventricular filling or left ventricular outflow tract obstruction observed in hypertrophic cardiomyopathy. *(Braunwald, Ch. 42; Hurst, pp. 1206–1207)*

42.(E) In addition to the cerebral circulation, the coronary circulation has comparable autoregulatory capabilities. *(Cecil, Ch. 44)*

43.(D) In acute shock, acidosis is the most potent factor shifting the oxygen-hemoglobin dissociation curve to the right and facilitating continuing oxygenation at reduced P_{O_2} levels. Hypercapnia (not listed) may also shift the curve to the right acutely. On a more chronic basis, anemia, hypoxia, and acidosis also increase the 2,3-diphosphoglyceric acid concentrations in the red blood cells and shift the oxygen-hemoglobin dissociation curve to the right. Hypophosphatemia may actually decrease 2,3-diphosphoglyceric acid levels and, therefore, oxygen delivery. *(Cecil, Ch. 44)*

44.(C) Although large ventricular septal defects are a cause of premature mortality, this by no means explains the rarity of the lesion in the older adult population; spontaneous closure, occasionally via formation of an aneurysm of the membranous interventricular septum, is considered a likely factor. Uncomplicated septal defects (with normal pulmonary artery pressure) impose a volume load on the left heart: The right ventricle becomes significantly involved primarily when the pulmonary pressure begins to rise. The membranous interventricular septum is just beneath the right coronary cusp of the aortic valve, and a defect in this area may lead to loss of cusp support with resulting prolapse of the cusp and aortic regurgitation. *(Cecil, Ch. 49)*

45.(D) A palpable fourth heart sound may be found with all varieties of ventricular outflow tract obstruction, and its presence does not favor a particular diagnosis. The development of abnormal left ventricular function, while an ominous prognostic sign, does not contraindicate repair; postoperative left ventricular function may improve markedly following relief of the outflow tract obstruction. Because of a jet effect, patients with supravalvular aortic stenosis may have blood pressure of 10 mm Hg or more higher in the right arm than in the left. This does not occur in valvular or subvalvular aortic stenosis. Although aortic ejection sounds may be seen with aortic root dilatation, they are much more common in aortic valve disease; an aortic ejection sound particularly favors congenital aortic valve involvement. With membranous subaortic stenosis, the ejection jet may damage the aortic valve leaflets, the presumed mechanism for the associated aortic regurgitation. *(Cecil, Chs. 49, 52, and 53)*

46.(E) Prostacyclin, in addition to being a vasodilator, inhibits platelet aggregation; both factors promote coronary blood flow and relieve myocardial ischemia. *(Cecil, Ch. 51.1)*

47.(C) There are very convincing data, particularly from the more recent intracoronary streptokinase investigations, that thrombosis plays a very important primary role in the production of myocardial infarction. *(Cecil, Chs. 47 and 51.2)*

48.(C) Propranolol has little or no effect on most accessory pathways. Digoxin may increase conduction velocity over the accessory pathway, increase the ventricular response, and actually cause ventricular fibrillation. Because the accessory pathway is part of the loop in reciprocating tachycardia, any degree of AV or VA block is typically associated with termination of the tachyarrhythmia, and the usual ventricular-atrial relationship is 1:1. Intravenous verapamil is effective in terminating reciprocating tachycardias in probably 80 to 90% of patients; it is the treatment of choice as long as the blood pressure is well maintained. Surgical division of the accessory pathway is a well-documented mechanism of permanent cure, although careful patient selection is necessary. *(Cecil, Ch. 45)*

49.(D) Although angiotensin II is one of the most potent vasoconstrictors known, its dominant effect on blood pressure is probably via its stimulation of aldosterone secretion, in turn an important regulator of salt and water homeostasis. Similarly, although it is a potent stimulator of catecholamine release via both the CNS and the adrenal medulla, this is probably not important in the day-to-day regulation of blood pressure. It has no important direct renal diuretic action. *(Cecil, Ch. 41)*

50.(B) Although certain arrhythmias such as an ectopic atrial tachycardia and type I second-degree AV block may be seen with digitalis toxicity, the electrocardiogram is not a particularly accurate way to estimate the serum digoxin level. All the other cited uses of the electrocardiogram (including ambulatory electrocardiography) are valid. *(Cecil, Chs. 42.2 and 43, Fig. 42–2)*

51.(B) Aortic dissection is by far the most serious complication of cardiac catheterization, typically necessitating emergency operative repair that frequently has to be carried out in the setting of uncorrected underlying heart disease (coronary or otherwise). Ventricular tachycardia can usually be handled by lidocaine and/or cardioversion, while complete heart block is typically transient and effectively handled by temporary transvenous pacing. Some bleeding at the groin puncture site is inevitable, and small hematomas are frequent and usually of no significance. Large hematomas occasionally occur and require operative evacuation, but, again, this is not a major complication. Similarly, the pulses distal to the arterial access site are frequently diminished or lost but can be restored by either anticoagulation or operative extraction of the offending clot. *(Cecil, Ch. 42.5)*

52.(C) Patients A, B, D, and E are all candidates for cardiac catheterization. In a patient with an early positive treadmill test and classic angina, a majority of cardiologists would probably recommend coronary angiography in order to define the higher risk patients with severe coronary artery disease. The combination of aortic regurgitation and symptoms of heart failure probably identifies the need to consider aortic valve replacement and this patient, therefore, is also a candidate for catheterization. Patient A, with tetralogy of Fallot and increasing cyanosis, is a candidate for complete operative repair. The increasing cyanosis is likely due to worsening infundibular pulmonary stenosis with increasing right to left shunting across the ventricular septal defect. Although it may be argued that the echo-Doppler study can accurately diagnose the important physiologic abnormalities, some of these patients have an anomalous origin of the left anterior descending coronary artery from the right coronary such that it courses over the right ventricular outflow tract and can interfere with reconstruction of the infundibulum, constituting one reason to proceed to catheterization and angiography. Further evaluation of the mechanism and severity of the aortic regurgitation is another reason for catheterization. Although patient B is reportedly asymptomatic (note that the continued livelihood of pilots depends on being asymptomatic), the combination of a positive ETT and a reversible thallium perfusion defect strongly supports the possibility of coronary artery disease. Coronary angiography is recommended for definitive diagnosis and, if CAD were present or angiography were refused, this refusal would be grounds for revocation of a commercial pilot's license. In the patient with typical aortic stenosis, the severity is probably moderate but more importantly, he is asymptomatic and it will be difficult to make him feel better with an intervention. Catheterization should be delayed until the patient is believed to be an operative candidate (i.e., the advent of symptoms). Even then, the main reason to perform catheterization (given the accuracy of the echo-Doppler study in defining ventricular function and valvular involvement and severity) would be to visualize the coronary arteries. *(Cecil, Chs. 42.5 and 49, Table 42–6; Braunwald, Ch. 11)*

53.(D) Of these patients, the man with severe mitral regurgitation is at lowest risk. The risk of renal dysfunction increases with the absolute quantity of the dye load (and the type of dye), and it is recommended that a total contrast load be kept below 3 cc/kg body weight and, in high-risk patients, that non-ionic contrast media be used. The risk also increases with dehydration (e.g., chronic diuretic therapy), diabetes, and multiple myeloma. *(Cecil, Ch. 42.5)*

54.(E) Digitalis rarely, if ever, causes atrial flutter/fibrillation, multifocal atrial tachycardia, or AV node re-entry tachycardia; these are not likely digitalis toxic arrhythmias. Digitalis is commonly used in the milieu of patients with these arrhythmias, however, and recognition of concomitant toxicity is important. In MAT, patients usually have significant pulmonary dysfunction, hypoxia, and therapy with xanthine derivatives as the underlying cause. The arrhythmia can prove very resistant to primary antiarrhythmic therapy, although some patients may respond to verapamil. It is most important to differentiate MAT from atrial fibrillation, as the ventricular rate with the latter may slow with increase in digitalis; it rarely does with the former, and giving increased doses of digoxin frequently results in toxicity. With atrial fibrillation, increasing AV block could be one sign of possible digitalis toxicity. With a further elevation in the serum digoxin level, complete AV block with a regular junctional escape pacemaker may occur. Therefore, in addition to inordinate ventricular slowing, regularization of the ventricular rate is a hallmark of digitalis toxicity in the setting of atrial fibrillation. With further toxicity, the escape junctional pacer may speed (E). Increasing ventricular ectopy is another possible indicator of digitalis toxicity but also commonly reflects underlying ventricular dysfunction independent of the digoxin level. *(Cecil, Chs. 43 and 45)*

55.(D) All the compensatory mechanisms for maintaining cardiac output with the advent of congestive heart failure will eventually become inadequate. Atrial natriuretic hormone is a peptide secreted by atrial cells in response to atrial stretch. It has a variety of beneficial effects in congestive heart failure, including vasodilation, diuresis, and natriuresis. An increase in contractility due to the reflex increase in sympathetic nervous system activity is the least effective compensatory mechanism. *(Cecil, Ch. 43; Bates et al)*

56.(B) Why some of these patients develop alveolar hypoventilation with resulting hypoxia and reflex pulmonary hypertension and others, with equal obesity, do not is unknown. The underlying pulmonary parenchyma, however, is typically normal in such patients, and weight loss may entirely reverse any measurable elevation in pulmonary artery pressure. The other interventions enjoy variable success in the relief of pulmonary hypertension, with mitral valve commissurotomy probably the second most effective therapy. The reversibility is dependent upon the chronicity of the pulmonary hypertension and the resulting fixed changes in the pulmonary arterial vasculature. Closure of a ventricular septal defect in a patient with pulmonary vascular disease (Eisenmenger's syndrome) is contraindicated and will not lower the pulmonary artery pressure. Indeed, the surgery carries a very high mortality risk, and the pulmonary vascular resistance continues to increase postoperatively. Anticoagulant therapy in patients with multiple pulmonary emboli, particularly if the situation is chronic, may stabilize the situation but rarely allows the pulmonary artery pressure to return to normal. This is to be contrasted with the situation resulting from acute pulmonary embolus, wherein a remarkable decrease in the pulmonary pressure results from fibrinolysis of the clot. Treatment of bronchitis in patients with pulmonary parenchymal disease, such as cystic fibrosis, lowers the pulmonary artery pressure somewhat, but significant pulmonary hypertension typically persists. *(Cecil, Ch. 48)*

57.(C) The mechanism of syncope is analogous to that occurring in patients with aortic stenosis, wherein the stenosis prevents a significant increase in cardiac output during exercise. With exercise-induced reflex systemic arteriolar vasodilatation, there is resulting hypotension, a fall in blood pressure, and syncope. Although paroxysmal atrial fibrillation with a rapid ventricular response and ventricular tachycardia are possible, they are not the most likely explanation; and right ventricular ischemia/dysfunction and venodilatation have no proven role in syncope in this particular syndrome. *(Cecil, Ch. 48)*

58.(D) An elevated blood pressure (systolic, diastolic, or both) and significant cigarette smoking remain the most potent prognostic variables for the future development of ischemic heart disease. Also of note is the synergistic effect of additional risk factors (e.g., hypercholesterolemia, diabetes) for a given blood pressure level. *(Cecil, Ch. 47)*

59.(B) Although they have been reported, these are rare complications of myocardial irradiation. They presumably result from myocardial fibrosis and secondary involvement of the conduction system, although primary radiation injury is possible and has not been disproven. Accelerated atherosclerosis does appear to be a real entity, and angina, myocardial infarction, and sudden death in young patients have all been reported. At doses above 4000 rads, the likelihood of cardiac involvement increases, with as many as 50% of patients receiving 6000 rads or more developing carditis. In addition to myocardial fibrosis and ventricular dysfunction, valvular dysfunction has also been reported. In the case of mitral regurgitation, it is sometimes difficult to separate primary valvular injury from valvular dysfunction associated with concomitant ventricular dysfunction. *(Cecil, Ch. 53)*

60.(A) The echocardiogram below shows a large left atrial tumor (asterisk). This tumor was also shown to arise from the interatrial septum, typical of left atrial myxoma. Although heart involvement by malignancy does occur, intracavitary tumors are most commonly myxomas, with rhabdomyosarcoma a much less frequent etiology. This patient's history is typical, with a combination of systemic symptoms and symptoms arising from the disruption of mitral valve function with both regurgitation and stenosis. There is no underlying rheumatic mitral valve involvement (note the thin, nontethered anterior mitral valve leaflet—arrow), and rheumatic mitral valve disease with a ball valve thrombus is not present. Neither is there any evidence of atrial calcification or involvement of the mitral valve annulus. *(Cecil, Chs. 52 and 55)*

61.(A) This patient has a left atrial tumor that is most likely a benign myxoma. While "benign" is an appropriate description of the cell type, it may be "malignant" in its potential for death/disability. In addition to creating valvular dysfunction, it has probably been a source of at least one embolus to the brain. She has no history of angina and the echo-Doppler study showed no evidence of any other heart disease. She can be safely taken to the operating room without a heart catheterization. Indeed, catheterization in such patients can be fraught with problems, mainly related to catheter trauma of the left atrial mass with resulting embolization. *(Cecil, Ch. 55)*

62.(D) This patient's clinical presentation is typical of hypertrophic obstructive cardiomyopathy. The history of exertional and postexertional presyncope relates to one of the presumed mechanisms for syncope in this condition, wherein the cardiac output is unable to increase in response to exercise-induced peripheral arteriolar vasodilatation. In some patients, concomitant ventricular arrhythmias may be playing a role, but there are no hints of that in this patient. The physical examination is typical in that the carotid upstroke is normal to brisk and there is a prominent apical atrial or A wave due to augmented atrial systole. This is a hallmark of the disease, wherein diastolic dysfunction and stiffness play a very prominent role. The physical examination is also typical, with an outflow tract murmur that is relatively late peaking and that shows dynamic variability. The murmur softens during squatting because augmented venous return increases preload and ventricular size, while the increase in afterload distends the left ventricular outflow tract. Both hemodynamic effects contribute to softening of the murmur, and their reversal with standing augments obstruction and the murmur. The echocardiogram is classic for a hypertrophic obstructive cardiomyopathy. In this particular case, the hypertrophy is relatively symmetric (note the thickened septum [IVS] and posterior left ventricle [PLV]). The systolic frame shows unequivocal movement of the anterior mitral valve leaflet (arrow) into the left ventricular outflow tract (LVO), creating a mid to late systolic obstruction to blood flow. Note also the enlarged left atrium (LA) reflecting concomitant mitral regurgitation. *(Cecil, Chs. 52 and 53; Vanden Belt et al, pp. 197–207)*. See illustrations on page 26.

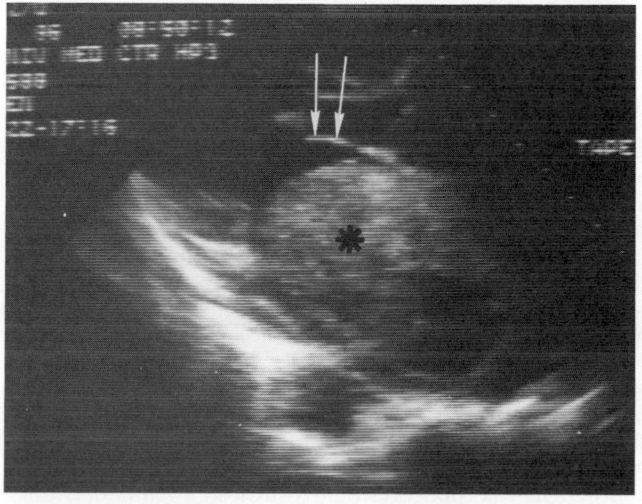

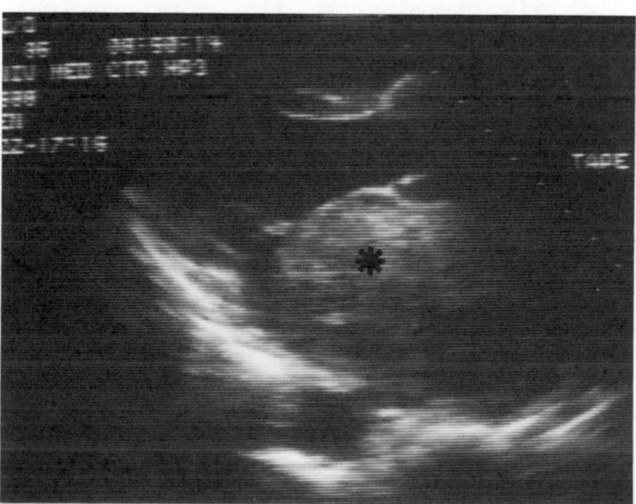

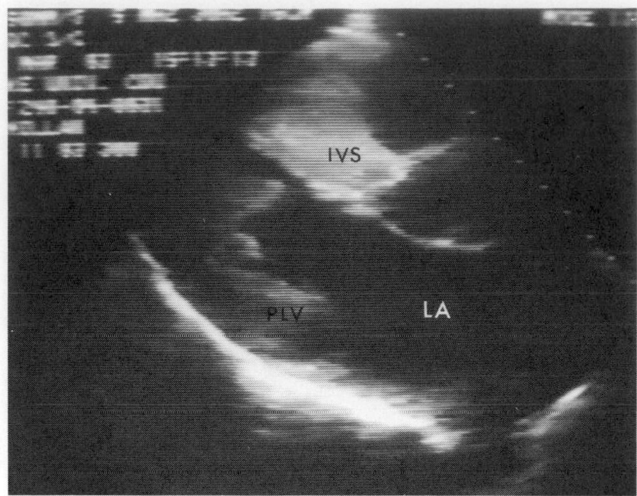

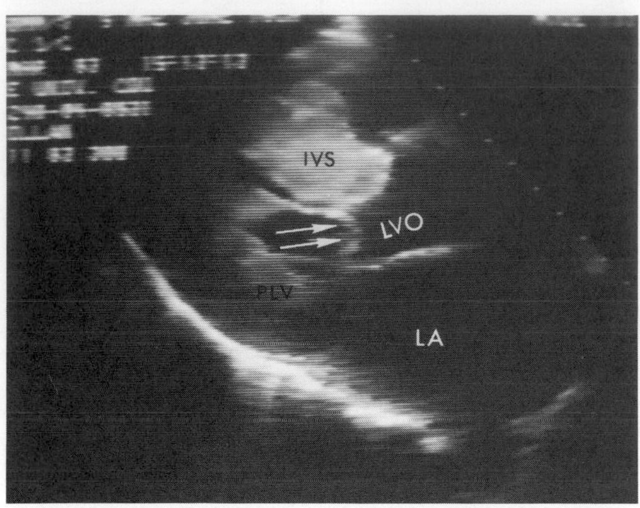

63. (D) A trial of beta-blocker therapy is a reasonable first step. This patient's aortic valve is functioning normally and does not need to be replaced. Replacement of the mitral valve has been advocated by some investigators, as, with resection of the anterior mitral valve leaflet, the obstruction is removed. In addition, whatever mitral regurgitation was present as a function of the abnormal traction on the anterior mitral leaflet is also corrected by mitral valve replacement. In most instances, however, it is not clear that surgery affects the natural history of the disease, and, indeed, there is some controversy concerning how important obstruction is in the overall syndrome. In this particular patient, an initial trial of beta-blocker therapy with careful follow-up of his functional status is indicated. *(Cecil, Ch. 53)*

64. (D) The apex of the left ventricle is thinner because its radius of curvature is less; this smaller radius–thinner wall relationship "normalizes" wall stress. With decreased left ventricular compliance (e.g., hypertrophic cardiomyopathy), there is atrial myofiber hypertrophy, and the resulting augmented atrial systole may contribute even more than the normal 20% boost to stroke volume. The right ventricle contracts in a bellows-like action, an extremely efficient method of ejecting a large volume of blood at low pressure. Most of the change in left ventricular volume during systole does occur by shortening of the minor (or circumferential) axis. Changes in the major (or long) axis are much less. *(Cecil, Ch. 41)*

65. (B) Although an increase in cardiac output can contribute to an increase in blood pressure, the arteriolar vascular resistance is by far the most important determinant of blood pressure. Contractility, preload, and heart rate are all determinants of cardiac output; they are not, therefore, primary factors in modulating blood pressure. *(Cecil, Chs. 41 and 47)*

66. (E) Circulating hormones are among the extrinsic factors regulating systemic arteriolar vascular resistance, but the most important factor is neurogenic tone mediated through various baro- and chemoreceptors. Tissue metabolites and the degree of stretch of vascular smooth muscle are *intrinsic* factors important in autoregulation of organ blood flow. *(Cecil, Ch. 41)*

67. (D) Cardiomegaly, a mitral regurgitation murmur, an S_3, and electrocardiographic left ventricular hypertrophy may all exist in the absence of heart failure. Pulsus alternans, however, accurately reflects left ventricular failure. *(Cecil, Chs. 42.2 and 43)*

68. (D) Mild to moderate hypertension, especially in this age group, characteristically leaves renal function relatively unimpaired, particularly as reflected by casual BUN/creatinine determination. *(Cecil, Ch. 47)*

69. (B) Beta-blocker therapy may actually cause vasospasm by blocking beta$_2$-mediated peripheral vasodilatation. The remainder of the statements are true. Calcium blockers appear to be a particularly valuable adjunct to treatment of this condition. *(Cecil, Ch. 57)*

70. (A—True; B—True; C—False; D—True; E—True) Intra-aortic balloon counterpulsation may be valuable in cardiogenic shock complicating myocardial infarction because of an afterload-reducing effect. The systemic arterial systolic pressure may be reduced and coronary artery blood flow may increase. This may be particularly helpful as an afterload-reducing measure in patients with ventricular septal defects or papillary muscle dysfunction and significant mitral regurgitation. It may also serve as a temporizing measure prior to surgical revascularization but has not been shown to produce any significant improvement in overall survival. *(Cecil, Ch. 44)*

71. (A—False; B—True; C—False; D—False; E—False) Congenital heart block may be caused by a variety of lesions affecting the atrioventricular node or bundle of His. Patients with congenital heart block without associated cardiac malformations may be asymptomatic for many years because of the presence of a stable junctional pacemaker under autonomic control. Hereditary or familial congenital heart block may be inherited as an autosomal dominant trait. Because of the stability of the junctional escape rhythm, the overall prognosis of patients with congenital complete heart block is good. Many do not require permanent pacing. Mothers with systemic lupus erythematosus and other connective tissue diseases give birth to children with a surprisingly high incidence of congenital heart block. In about 70% of children with complete AV block, the lesion is isolated, while the remainder may have other associated complex cardiac malformations such as ventricular inversion or single ventricle. *(Braunwald, Chs. 30 and 31; Cecil, Ch. 52)*

72. (A—True; B—True; C—True; D—True; E—False) An increased or inappropriate afterload may be a further impediment to ventricular emptying in a variety of pathophysiologic states, including mitral and aortic regurgitation, left ventricular dysfunction due to coronary artery disease, and congestive cardiomyopathy. These patients may respond well to pharmacologic afterload reduction. In contrast, afterload reduction in the presence of the fixed outflow tract obstruction of aortic stenosis may increase the gradient across the aortic valve, requiring increased left ventricular work for maintenance of cardiac output. In addition, coronary perfusion pressure can decrease, and these factors lead to further ventricular compromise. Afterload-reduction therapy is therefore relatively, if not absolutely, contraindicated in patients with aortic stenosis. *(Cecil, Ch. 52)*

73. (A—False; B—False; C—True; D—False; E—False) The risk of coronary heart disease is inversely related to the level of high density lipoprotein cholesterol. HDL levels are significantly higher in women than in men at all age levels, are reduced by the presence of diabetes mellitus, are increased by regular exercise such as jogging, and are not predictably related to levels of LDL in the same individual. HDL levels may be slightly increased with the consumption of small amounts of alcohol, although whether this involves the "protective fraction" of HDL or is beneficial in decreasing the risk of coronary disease remains unproven. *(Cecil, Ch. 50)*

74. (A—True; B—True; C—True; D—False; E—True) The beneficial effect of nitroglycerin appears to be related to its ability to dilate medium-sized penetrating, and occasionally epicardial, coronary vessels and thus improve coronary blood flow and its distribution. Nitroglycerin also dilates systemic veins, thus decreasing venous return to the heart, the ventricular end-diastolic volume, and wall tension. Oxygen demand is therefore reduced. The effect of nitroglycerin on heart rate in patients without heart failure is to increase the heart rate. This is potentially detrimental to the extent that it increases myocardial oxygen consumption. In the aggregate, the other beneficial effects usually dominate and relieve angina. *(Cecil, Ch. 51.1)*

75. (A—False; B—False; C—False; D—True; E—False) Exercise stress testing may be of value in the diagnosis of coronary artery disease. Furthermore, an exercise stress test that is positive in stage I suggests a higher prevalence of either left main or three-vessel coronary artery disease. The stress test result is considered positive if associated with a flat or downsloping ST-segment depression of 0.1 mV or greater 0.08 sec after the QRS-ST junction. In women, false-positive results occur in up to 20–30% of patients. False-positive results may also occur with electrolyte abnormalities, digoxin therapy, left ventricular hypertrophy, and conduction abnormalities. Rather than an accumulation of thallium-201, a focal region of ischemia is suggested by a cold spot or the absence of thallium uptake in a given distribution. The incidence of false-negative results with adequate exercise and multi-lead ECG analysis is around 10–15%. *(Cecil, Ch. 51.1; McNeer et al)*

76. (A—False; B—True; C—False; D—False; E—False) Avoidance of cigarette smoking by patients with angina is crucial. The nicotine in cigarettes increases heart rate and blood pressure, and the carbon monoxide that is inhaled may result in a shift in the oxyhemoglobin dissociation curve, making oxygen less available at the tissue level. Nicotine may also result in direct constriction of coronary vessels. Cigarette smoking, however, has not been clearly shown to reduce HDL levels in any patient population. *(Cecil, Chs. 50 and 51.1)*

77. (A—False; B—False; C—False; D—True; E—True) Coronary artery bypass grafting in most centers that publish their results carries an operative mortality rate of less than 2%. Nevertheless, the risk of perioperative myocardial infarction, as determined by changes in the electrocardiogram, is estimated to be from 1–10%. Complete relief of anginal pain is achieved in more than two thirds of patients following CABG. The vein graft occlusion rate during the first year varies from 10–20%. In addition to the improvement in quality of life, coronary artery bypass grafting improves longevity in patients with left main and, to a lesser extent, three-vessel coronary disease with abnormal left ventricular function. *(Cecil, Chs. 51.1 and 51.3)*

78. (All are False) Most cases of sudden cardiac death are not related to an identifiable acute myocardial infarction, which is detected electrocardiographically in less than 30% of patients hospitalized after resuscitation from ventricular fibrillation. Nevertheless, the majority of individuals have extensive coronary artery disease, including more than two thirds with multiple vessel involvement. However, the risk factors for atherosclerosis do not singly or in combination identify a subset of patients prone to sudden death. A pulmonary etiology for sudden death occurs in well under one third of any series. The recurrence rate in resuscitated patients is 20–60% during the first year. *(Cecil, Ch. 46)*

79. (A—True; B—True; C—False; D—False; E—False) Type II second-degree AV block is typically associated with bundle branch block morphology of the conducted beat and wide QRS escape beats. Conduction failure occurs in an "all or none" fashion, and type II second-degree AV block, while uncommon, is a more ominous finding because of a higher incidence of progression to complete heart block. In addition, the site of block is in the Purkinje system; the subsidiary escape pacemaker in this setting is likely to be a slow, unstable ventricular rhythm. This type of block is typically due to diffuse degenerative processes involving the His-Purkinje system but can also be observed in the course of a myocardial infarction. The vagus nerve has little or no effect on conduction in the His-Purkinje system. *(Cecil, Ch. 45)*

80. (A—True; B—True; C—False; D—False; E—False) Digoxin exerts a centrally mediated vagal action on the heart. Direct effects include slowing of conduction in the AV node, prolongation of refractoriness in the AV node, and a decrease in refractoriness of atrial tissue. All these effects in concert have important implications for the treatment of supraventricular tachycardia, especially atrial fibrillation/flutter. By decreasing the refractoriness of atrial tissue, atrial flutter can be "converted" to more rapid atrial fibrillation, which results in slowing of the ventricular response due to the phenomenon of concealed AV node conduction. In the normal heart, however, digoxin has little effect on the intrinsic sinus rate. *(Cecil, Ch. 45)*

81. (A—True; B—False; C—True; D—False; E—False) Procainamide has a short half-life of 2–4 hours and is 40–70% excreted unchanged by the kidneys. The remaining drug is acetylated in the liver to *N*-acetyl procainamide (NAPA). Patients may show fast or slow acetylation of the parent compound. Unlike quinidine, procainamide has no alpha-blocking effect and has a much weaker vagolytic effect. The *N*-acetyl metabolite is excreted exclusively by the kidneys and may accumulate in the presence of advanced renal insufficiency. As a result, treatment with procainamide may be relatively contraindicated in patients with advancing renal insufficiency. A systemic lupus erythematosus–like syndrome has been described in association with procainamide. Unlike typical lupus, the syndrome induced by procainamide spares the brain and kidney and shows no predilection for females. Nevertheless, fevers, arthritis, and hemorrhagic pericarditis have been observed. At least 75% of patients on procainamide therapy will develop antinuclear antibodies, but only one third of these will develop the lupus-like syndrome. The latter is more common in patients who are slow acetylators of the drug. *(Cecil, Ch. 45)*

82. (A—False; B—True; C—False; D—False; E—False) Pericarditis may result from a variety of pathophysiologic processes. One variety, due directly to epicardial necrosis and inflammation, may occur 2–5 days following an acute myocardial infarction. In contrast, a second form of pericardial involvement (post–myocardial infarction pericarditis, or Dressler's syndrome), typically occurs weeks to months following the acute infarction. The syndrome is usually self-limited and can be treated with analgesics or nonsteroidal anti-inflammatory agents. On occasion this process may become so repetitive that it is necessary to rely on a tapering course of steroids for treatment. Clinical signs of typical acute pericarditis may be seen in approximately 3% of patients with rheumatoid arthritis, even though autopsy series indicate that at least 10% of these patients may have an inflammatory response in the pericardium. In such patients pericarditis occurs most commonly when the basic disease process is active and particularly when rheumatoid nodules and markedly elevated titers of serum rheumatoid factor are present. Forty per cent of documented cases of lupus erythematosus may likewise show pericardial involvement. The diagnosis can be reasonably inferred when LE cells and anti-DNA antibodies are detectable in the blood. In addition, other connective tissue disorders such as periarteritis nodosa and progressive systemic sclerosis have been reported to show associated pericarditis, although significantly less often than in patients with rheumatoid arthritis or systemic lupus erythematosus. *(Cecil, Ch. 54)*

83. (A—False; B—True; C—False; D—True; E—False) Allergic reactions occur because streptokinase is a foreign, bacteria-derived protein. Streptokinase antibody titers clearly occur after treatment with streptokinase, are significant after day 7, and persist for 4–6 months. Such antibodies may interfere with efficacy and may cause allergic side effects if streptokinase is administered again. An allergic response to urokinase, a human-derived protein, is extremely unusual. Intracoronary administration of streptokinase results in thrombolysis in 60–80% of patients. Although reports detailing response to intravenous streptokinase have been variable, multiple studies have demonstrated thrombolytic reperfusion rates of 30–75%, suggesting a decreased response to intravenous streptokinase. Additionally, the administration of intracoronary streptokinase has been shown to reduce one-year mortality among patients with acute myocardial infarction in whom coronary artery reperfusion occurred. Recent studies have also demonstrated greater reperfusion efficacy with intravenous tissue plasminogen activator than with intravenous streptokinase. The response to any thrombolytic agent, however, is a function of time of administration following the onset of the acute myocardial infarction. The highest reperfusion rate with streptokinase occurs when it is administered within 4–6 hours of the onset of symptoms (the earlier, the better); the response following administration 6–8 hours after the onset of symptoms is dramatically diminished. *(Hurst, pp. 967–968, 1916–1922; Lee et al)*

84. (A—False; B—False; C—False; D—True; E—True) Flecainide, a type Ic agent (like encainide, lorcainide, and propafenone), produces little effect on the Q-T interval, unlike the type Ia drugs (quinidine, procainamide, and disopyramide), which classically prolong the Q-T interval. Flecainide produces minimal side effects and may be better tolerated than the type Ia agents in long-term use. Although it is highly effective in the treatment of ventricular ectopy or nonsustained ventricular tachycardia, it appears to be less effective than amiodarone in controlling sustained, more malignant, ventricular arrhythmias. Although flecainide is metabolized in the liver, its metabolites do not appear to have significant antiarrhythmic efficacy. Flecainide, like disopyramide, may have deleterious effects on myocardial contractility and aggravate heart failure in patients with underlying ventricular dysfunction. Furthermore, patients with poor ventricular function appear to be at higher risk for the development of the proarrhythmic effect from flecainide. Similarly, patients with underlying sustained ventricular tachycardia have fewer complications from flecainide therapy than when this agent is administered to patients with nonsustained ventricular tachycardia or simple ventricular ectopy. *(Morganroth et al; Roden and Woolsey)*

85. (A—True; B—False; C—False; D—True; E—True) The onset of the decline in rheumatic fever predated the introduction of antibiotics, but once effective therapy for streptococcal infections became available, the trend accelerated. The severity of the disease, at least in the United States, has also declined progressively. Although climate and socioeconomic status are risk factors, the most important risk factor is a previous beta-hemolytic streptococcal throat infection. Secondary prevention programs with penicillin are very effective in preventing recurrence of rheumatic fever. It is estimated that fewer than 1.1 million persons in the United States have rheumatic heart disease. *(Cecil, Ch. 40)*

86. (A—False; B—False; C—False; D—True; E—True) The incidence of coronary artery disease in men is consistently higher than in women from about age 35 on. Although obesity of more than 10% over ideal body weight is probably an independent risk factor for the development of coronary artery disease in patients under 50 years of age, there is no evidence that weight loss alone corrects the risk. The exact pathophysiology of cigarette smoking in the development of coronary artery disease is unclear, but it is encouraging that the increased risk almost disappears within two years following the cessation of cigarette smoking. Fractionation of cholesterol into its HDL and LDL components does appear to give additional prognostic information. Recent data have called into question whether modest daily consumption of alcohol can raise the HDL level. *(Cecil, Chs. 40 and 50)*

87. (A—True; B—False; C—False; D—False; E—True) A number of studies have documented that control of moderate to severe hypertension decreases the risk of mortality from coronary artery disease. In women under the age of 50 with mild hypertension, however, this point has not been proved, owing to the small number of subjects and the low morbidity rate. Although there is some evidence that tight blood sugar control in juvenile-onset diabetes can decrease some vascular (e.g., ophthalmologic) complications, there are no data for a similar protective effect in preventing death from coronary artery disease. Similarly, although water hardness may be a lesser risk factor for coronary artery disease, there are no data to support that modifying water hardness decreases the risk. A recent multicenter trial has demonstrated that lowering of serum cholesterol in men, with a combination of diet and cholestyramine, has a favorable impact on coronary artery disease mortality rate. *(Cecil, Ch. 40; Lipid Research Clinics Program)*

88.(A—True; B—False; C—False; D—True; E—True) In the absence of significant ventricular ectopy, prophylactic arrhythmia suppression therapy is not indicated. A digitalis-induced atrial tachycardia is typically due to an atrial ectopic pacemaker; it is unlikely to respond to cardioversion. The cardioversion itself may elicit malignant ventricular arrhythmias. In addition, a rapid ventricular response to the atrial tachycardia is usually not a problem, as there is invariably some associated AV block. Correction of hypokalemia alone may eliminate digitalis toxic arrhythmias. Heart block and hyperkalemia, particularly with hypotension, may necessitate temporary pacemaker therapy. Digoxin-specific antibodies are a new treatment modality that may be used for serious arrhythmias unresponsive to conventional antiarrhythmic drugs. *(Cecil, Chs. 43 and 45)*

89.(All are True) All are complications of congenital shunt lesions. *(Cecil, Ch. 49)*

90.(A—False; B—True; C—True; D—False; E—True) Amyl nitrite inhalation helps to differentiate the Austin Flint rumble (it softens) from the mitral stenosis rumble (it increases). A systolic thrill in the carotid artery may be found with isolated aortic regurgitation with no measurable gradient. Softening of S_1 reflects premature mitral valve closure and, if not due to first-degree heart block, identifies severe acute regurgitation with a very high left ventricular end-diastolic pressure. With exercise and a corresponding decrease in the diastolic interval, the degree of aortic regurgitation may actually diminish; this helps maintain excellent exercise capacities in patients with significant aortic regurgitation. *(Cecil, Ch. 52; Braunwald, Ch. 33)*

91.(A—True; B—True; C—True; D—False; E—True) Three randomized trials document the efficacy of beta-blocker therapy in favorably influencing the long-term prognosis of patients surviving acute myocardial infarction. It has been proved unequivocally that prophylactic lidocaine decreases the likelihood of ventricular fibrillation, but more recent data question the risk/benefit ratio of treating all suspected myocardial infarctions with prophylactic lidocaine; it remains a matter of individual preference. Although anticoagulants decrease the risk of systemic embolization, they increase the risk of hemorrhagic complications; routine anticoagulants are generally not indicated. In high-risk patients (those with large anterior myocardial infarctions and/or congestive heart failure), cautious, carefully controlled anticoagulant therapy may be beneficial. There is no evidence that streptokinase administered intravenously this late in myocardial infarction favorably influences the chance of survival. Indeed, a number of studies in which the drug was given even earlier failed to show a favorable influence. Anticoagulating a patient with pericardial friction rub risks the development of hemorrhagic pericardial effusion with tamponade. *(Cecil, Ch. 46)*

92.(A—True; B—True; C—False; D—False; E—True) Wall stress is defined by the Laplace relation, wherein it is directly related to intraventricular pressure and the radius of wall curvature and is inversely related to wall thickness. *(Cecil, Ch. 41)*

93.(A—True; B—True; C—False; D—True; E—False) The normal mean left atrial pressure (or pulmonary capillary wedge pressure) is 12–13 mm Hg or less in most laboratories. Systolic hypertension is variably defined by a systolic blood pressure above 145–160 mm Hg, but 180 mm Hg is distinctly hypertensive. A normal pulmonary artery systolic pressure measures up to 25–30 mm Hg, and 48 mm Hg is clearly in the pulmonary hypertensive range. The normal central venous pressure and mean right atrial pressure are up to 4–6 mm Hg, and a normal ejection fraction is typically greater than 50–55%. *(Cecil, Chs. 41 and 42.5, Table 41–1)*

94.(A—True; B—True; C—True; D—False; E—True) The first three choices are all classic causes of vagally mediated slowing of the sinus node—one of the reasons why atropine is such a common preoperative medication. A decreased pulse pressure, on the other hand, inhibits baroreceptors, leading to a decreased discharge rate and an acceleration in heart rate. Facial immersion in water produces a "diving" reflex associated with an intense vagal discharge, slowing of the heart rate, and lowering of the blood pressure. *(Cecil, Ch. 41)*

95.(A—True; B—False; C—True; D—True; E—False) The normal mean central venous pressure is no more than 2–3 cm above the sternal angle. This, in turn, is about 5 cm above the midright atrium, an arbitary zero reference point. Therefore, the top normal mean central venous pressure is 7–8 cm H_2O. In normals, particularly young patients with a resting sinus bradycardia, the dominant X descent (or systolic collapse) of the venous pulse is frequently the most easily detected bedside event. Normal venous pulsations are typically visible but not palpable (owing to the very low underlying pressure). They may, however, become palpable when the pressure is increased. The venous pressure normally falls with inspiration owing to the concomitant fall in intrathoracic pressure. While the external jugular veins are more likely to be elevated independent of the mean right atrial pressure because of their more superficial location, etc., the estimated central venous pressure is normally equal in the internal and external jugular systems. *(Cecil, Ch. 39; Vanden Belt et al, pp. 8–14; Braunwald, Ch. 2)*

96.(A—True; B—True; C—False; D—True; E—False) Preload refers to the diastolic loading conditions of the heart and is described by the relationship between diastolic volume and pressure in the ventricle. Administering intravenous fluids increases the volume loading (or preload) of the ventricle. Similarly, the administration of nitroglycerin primarily causes venodilatation and diminishes preload. Digoxin exerts its cardiovascular effects primarily by increasing inotropy (although there may be some concomitant venoconstriction), while isotonic exercise increases contractility and, more importantly, the heart rate. Preload changes during upright exercise at submaximal levels are not particularly important in modifying cardiac output, but augmenting ventricular filling by inspiring against a closed glottis (the Mueller maneuver) can increase cardiac output. *(Cecil, Ch. 41)*

97.(A—True; B—True; C—True; D—True; E—False) All but the last statement accurately portray the risks of cardiac catheterization. The risk is obviously higher in patients who are potentially unstable or have such severe underlying heart disease as critical aortic stenosis, marked congestive heart failure, and unstable angina. The two most common major complications are myocardial infarction and stroke, but in experienced laboratories the risk approaches acceptable minimal levels and may be even further decreased by the use of heparin, although many laboratories do not use heparin routinely. A prior history of allergic reaction to iodinated contrast media does not prevent angiography; pretreatment with an intravenous H_2 antagonist and steroids typically prevents any clinically significant recurrence. *(Cecil, Ch. 42.5)*

98.(A—True; B—False; C—False; D—False; E—True) Although the performance characteristics of both technologies are dependent on the population to which the tests are applied, in a cohort of patients being catheterized for chest pain, the sensitivity of radionuclide angiography for the detection of CAD is approximately 85%, as compared to 70% for treadmill exercise testing. Both echocardiography and gated cardiac CT have been used to acquire resting and exercise cardiac images and, thereby, measurements of ejection fraction and wall motion. The specificity of rest/exercise radionuclide angiography (specificity being defined as the likelihood of a negative test to truly identify patients without the disease in question—true negatives divided by the sum of true negatives and false positives) is inferior to a negative treadmill exercise test (as low as 50% versus 90%, respectively). Although initially touted as a sensitive index of myocardial ischemia, a 5% or greater drop in ejection fraction is notoriously nonspecific. A very high percentage of women without underlying coronary artery disease will drop their exercise ejection fraction by 5% or more, and patients with a variety of valvular and myocardial diseases may also experience a drop in ejection fraction in response to exercise stress in the absence of concomitant CAD. In expert hands, the sensitivity and predictive accuracy characteristics of thallium perfusion imaging versus rest/exercise radionuclide angiography for the evaluation of suspected CAD are comparable, although the specificity of perfusion imaging would appear to be much higher than for radionuclide angiography (approximately 90% versus as low as 50%). *(Cecil, Ch. 42.4; Braunwald, Ch. 39; Froelicher, pp. 78–85, 100–102, 160, 168–171)*

99.(A—True; B—True; C—True; D—False; E—True) Digoxin toxicity is defined by a variety of effects of the drug on various organ systems. Although the risk of digoxin toxicity increases as the serum level rises, it is not defined by any given serum level per se. A hypokalemic patient with a serum digoxin level of less than 2.0 ng/ml may have cardiac toxicity with arrhythmias, while a patient with a level higher than 2.0 ng/ml may have no toxicity. The remaining statements are all true. The textbook space devoted to digitalis may relate to a historical perspective wherein it was once one of the few pharmacologically active and effective drugs that physicians had at their disposal. Although it continues to have a time-honored role in the treatment of atrial fibrillation, we are learning that it is frequently insufficient as the only therapy and that other drugs may be equally efficacious. It also continues to have a role in the treatment of heart failure, but there is increasing evidence that heart failure may be more favorably affected by such alternative therapies as vasodilatation. The addition of quinidine therapy is a classic cause of doubling the digoxin level in some patients, presumably by displacement of digoxin from serum binding sites by the quinidine. The majority of digoxin excretion is via the kidneys, and the serum level is very much affected by renal function. Algorithms for adjusting the dose according to renal function have proven quite valuable in decreasing the incidence of digoxin toxicity. Digoxin antibody fragments are a valuable therapeutic modality for the treatment of life-threatening digoxin toxic arrhythmias. More benign arrhythmias such as type I second-degree AV block, ectopic atrial tachycardia with block, and monofocal ventricular ectopy can be treated by discontinuing the digitalis preparation and correcting any concomitant hypokalemia, preferably under continuous ECG monitoring. *(Cecil, Ch. 43; Braunwald, Ch. 17)*

100.(A—False; B—True; C—True; D—True; E—False) A QRS duration of 0.10 to 0.11 second may also be used as a criterion for left ventricular hypertrophy, but a QRS duration of greater than 0.11 second usually identifies bundle branch block and cannot be used as a criterion. A variety of voltage criteria have been proposed for the diagnosis of left ventricular hypertrophy, but according to Romhilt et al, an R wave of greater than 3.0 mV in V_5 or V_6 is one such voltage criterion for left ventricular hypertrophy. Similarly, left axis deviation (an axis more negative than minus 30 degrees) and ST-T wave depression/inversion in leads I, aVL, and V_4–V_6 are also typical of (but not exclusive to) left ventricular hypertrophy. The P-R interval has no important diagnostic relation to left ventricular hypertrophy. *(Cecil, Ch. 42.2, Fig. 42–20; Romhilt et al; Braunwald, Ch. 7)*

101.(A—False; B—True; C—False; D—False; E—True) Peripheral arteriolar vasoconstriction, although serving to maintain blood pressure, is frequently a deleterious compensatory mechanism because of the increase in ventricular afterload. Peripheral venoconstriction promotes the transfer of blood to the central venous reservoir, thereby aiding preload. Similarly, salt and water retention and the resulting expansion of circulating blood volume also contribute to increasing ventricular end-diastolic volume and, thereby, ventricular performance. The redistribution of organ blood flow does not affect preload, and increased circulating levels of atrial natriuretic hormone (released from specific granules in atrial cells) in response to a variety of stimuli (including atrial stretch) can cause arteriolar vasodilation, diuresis, and/or natriuresis but does not produce changes in cardiac output via a primary effect on preload. *(Cecil, Ch. 43; Bates et al)*

102.(A—False; B—True; C—True; D—True; E—False) Necessary measurements for estimating a valve area include the mean (not peak) pressure difference between the chambers on either side of the stenotic valve and the cardiac output. Knowing the time per heart beat that blood flows across the obstruction (e.g., in aortic stenosis, the systolic ejection time) and multiplying that time by the heart rate gives the time per second that blood flow is contributing to the gradient. These relationships are defined by the Gorlin formula:

$$\text{Valve Area} = \frac{\text{Blood flow/second}}{\text{K} \times \text{mean gradient}}$$

Where:

$$\text{Blood flow/second} = \frac{\text{C.O. (cc/min.)}}{\underset{\text{(beats/min)}}{\text{HR}} \times \underset{\text{(sec/beat)}}{\text{Time of blood flow}}}$$

and

K = a constant or correction factor

Measuring dP/dT is not necessary for estimating the valve area. *(Cecil, Ch. 42.5)*

103. (All are True) These are all commonly found in patients with accelerated or malignant hypertension. *(Cecil, Ch. 47)*

104. (A—True; B—False; C—True; D—True; E—False) While there is no question that the effects of hypertension on certain target organs (e.g., left ventricular hypertrophy, retinopathy, cerebral vascular accident) can be reduced by antihypertensive therapy in this subgroup, there is no convincing evidence that the complications due to ischemic heart disease (i.e., angina, myocardial infarction, sudden death) can be reduced. Indeed, there is concern that diuretic treatment in certain subgroups of patients with mild hypertension may actually increase the risks of complications due to ischemic heart disease. Since the subgroups were determined retrospectively, however, the relationship between diuretics and potentiation of ischemic heart disease remains an important but unproven possibility. *(Cecil, Ch. 47; The Joint National Committee on Detection, Evaluation and Treatment of High Blood Pressure; Multiple Risk Factor Intervention Trial Research Group; Kuller et al)*

105. (A—False; B—True; C—False; D—True; E—False) Reduction of body weight and/or the maintenance of ideal body weight along with significant sodium restriction can either lower blood pressure or prevent its development/progression. Avoiding stress or even just reducing it in our society remains an impractical goal for many patients. Techniques such as stress relaxation/management also remain controversial in the long-term treatment of hypertension. A high potassium intake may help marginally in patients whose sodium is unrestricted, but it has not prevented the advent of hypertension or its progression. Isometric exercise raises the blood pressure (sometimes dramatically) and isotonic exercise, although reportedly helpful in uncontrolled trials, awaits further testing as a primary treatment modality. *(Cecil, Ch. 47)*

106. (A—True; B—False; C—True; D—True; E—False) A blood pressure of less than 140/85 is defined as normal. Blood pressure is a continuous variable, however, and the lower the blood pressure without syncope, the better the long-term prognosis. Systolic blood pressures in the 140–159 mm Hg range (with a normal diastolic blood pressure of less than 85 mm Hg) are defined as borderline isolated systolic hypertension, while diastolic blood pressures in the 85–89 mm Hg range have been reclassified as "high normal." Diastolic blood pressures of 90–104 mm Hg define mild diastolic hypertension. *(The Joint National Committee on Detection, Evaluation and Treatment of High Blood Pressure)*

107. (A—False; B—True; C—False; D—True; E—False) The 1984 Joint National Committee recommended that either a thiazide diuretic or a beta blocker be used as initial therapy in mild to moderate hypertension. Considerable controversy persists, however, concerning this recommendation because of questions surrounding the long-term effects of thiazides on the incidence of subsequent coronary artery disease. The controversy has been fueled by the known potential deleterious effects of diuretics, including hypomagnesemia, hypokalemia, hypercholesterolemia, and hyperglycemia. Hypokalemia is a well-recognized potentiating factor in ventricular arrhythmias, but a cause-effect relationship between diuretic therapy in mild to moderate hypertension and an increased risk of ischemic heart disease remains unproven. It would seem judicious, however, if electing to use diuretics as initial therapy, to use as low a dose as possible (e.g., 12.5 mg of hydrochlorothiazide or its equivalent) and to avoid going beyond the equivalent dosage of 25 mg of hydrochlorothiazide per day. *(The Joint National Committee on Detection, Evaluation and Treatment of High Blood Pressure; Kuller et al)*

108. (All are True) Obesity, COPD due to his cigarette smoking, and deconditioning are the most likely explanations for the shortness of breath. An alcoholic cardiomyopathy or a "silent" prior myocardial infarction, although possible, are less likely explanations, particularly given the normal apex impulse and absence of gallop sounds.

109. (A—True; B—True; C—True; D—True; E—False) With the exception of hyperuricemia, these are all major risk factors for coronary artery disease, are known or likely to be present in this patient, and, with patient cooperation, can be corrected. *(Cecil, Ch. 47)*

110. (All are True) The physical examination excludes coarctation and Cushing's syndrome. The clinical picture, including age, excludes all the adrenal hyperplasia syndromes. The absence of abdominal masses and hematuria excludes polycystic kidneys, and the normal electrolytes exclude primary hyperaldosteronism. *(Cecil, Chs. 47, 74, and 230.7)*

111. (All are True) These are all prudent measures for this patient. Accomplishing these goals may be difficult, however, as many fall in the general area of behavior modification, a difficult task at best. Even without hypertension, the alcohol intake is excessive and he is heading for health complications related to this alone. In this particular case, alcohol is also probably contributing to the hypertension. Similarly, the sodium-retaining properties of ibuprofen, a nonsteroidal anti-inflammatory agent, may also be contributing to the hypertension; it should be discontinued if possible. Weight loss and therapy with aspirin/acetaminophen are likely to be as helpful for the low back pain. With regard to his diet, the American Heart Association recommends that no more than 30% of total daily calories be in the form of fat. Furthermore, the substitution of polyunsaturated fats for the saturated variety wherever possible is also recommended. (The average American citizen, until recently, consumed 40% or more of his/her total calories in the form of primarily saturated fat.) Regular exercise can have several beneficial effects in patients such as this, including an enhanced sense of well-being, an adjunct to dietary weight reduction, an increase in the HDL cholesterol fraction, and active involvement of the patient in his own care. The best-tolerated form of exercise, particularly for previously sedentary patients, is walking. With this patient, who has a number of very potent risk factors for ischemic heart disease, participation in a supervised exercise rehabilitation program may be safer and more likely to enhance compliance while initiating the therapy. *(Cecil, Ch. 47)*

112. (A—True; B—False; C—True; D—False; E—True) In the supine position, preload is increased and the resting cardiac output may be increased 0.5 liter per minute or more in comparison to the upright position. The systemic veins are a large reservoir for blood volume and their constriction markedly augments preload. Similarly, isoproterenol, by its potent $beta_1$ cardiac effects (increased heart rate, increased contractility) in association with its $beta_2$ vascular effects (vasodilatation), markedly augments cardiac output. A simple increase in heart rate alone via pacing will not result in an increase in cardiac output. During the initial strain phase of a Valsalva maneuver, there is a brief increase in left-sided cardiac output that rapidly falls during the continued strain phase. *(Cecil, Chs. 41 and 44)*

113.(A—True; B—False; C—False; D—False; E—False) Digoxin, a smooth-muscle stimulant, may cause both venous and arteriolar vasoconstriction. This may account for the occasional deterioration in hemodynamics in some patients who receive intravenous digoxin. Its primary beneficial effect in congestive heart failure is to enhance ventricular contractility. The resulting improvement in heart failure results in a diminution in catecholamine levels and a slowing of the heart rate. Digoxin may have direct natriuretic effects on the kidney, but these are not usually clinically important. *(Cecil, Ch. 43)*

114.(A—True; B—True; C—True; D—False; E—False) The *initial* treatment in this situation involves choices A, B, and C. In the absence of atrial fibrillation, the use of digitalis may not be necessary. Vasodilator therapy continues to be recommended for patients not responsive to conventional therapy. Patients with cardiomyopathies seem to be more sensitive to digitalis, and the drug should be used cautiously in this clinical situation. *(Cecil, Ch. 43)*

115.(A—True; B—False; C—True; D—True; E—False) The nonsmoking patient has only hypertension as a risk factor, whereas the second patient smokes, has an elevated cholesterol, and has abnormal glucose metabolism, all of which interact to place him at a markedly elevated risk, despite his much lower systolic blood pressure. Although patients with extremes of blood pressure elevation are at highest risk for death, their numbers are small in comparison with the vast number of patients with more modest blood pressure elevations; most deaths occur in the latter group. This 10-fold risk ratio difference for stroke, with a 20 mm Hg difference in diastolic blood pressure, dramatically emphasizes the importance of widespread and accurate screening for hypertension. Since most hypertensive patients have no hypertension-related symptoms, it may be difficult to convince them to take their medications and return for adequate follow-up. *(Cecil, Ch. 47)*

116.(A—False; B—True; C—False; D—True; E—True) Although systolic hypertension in the elderly does constitute a risk factor for vascular complications, it is not clear whether it is simply a marker for already existent vascular disease; there are no convincing data that treatment alters the prognosis. A single estimate of the urinary VMA misses about one out of five patients with subsequently documented pheochromocytoma. In patients taking monoamine oxidase inhibitors, the ingestion of foods containing high levels of tyramine results in elevated tyramine blood levels, which in turn cause the release of accumulated norepinephrine from adrenergic nerve endings and striking hypertension. Out-of-hospital mild hypertension is rarely due to renovascular disease and it therefore is not cost-effective to screen such patients for this entity. In other populations, e.g., patients under age 40 with more severe hypertension, a renovascular etiology may be more frequent. When due to fibromuscular hyperplasia of the renal arteries, the hypertension may respond nicely to balloon angioplasty (dilatation). *(Cecil, Ch. 47)*

117.(A—False; B—False; C—False; D—False; E—True) The prognosis for patients without a pericardium depends on the degree of residual cardiac dysfunction. No increased likelihood of right heart failure due to "overdistention" of the right ventricle has been documented. Although a 10 mm Hg or greater inspiratory drop in the arterial blood pressure is a feature of tamponade, it may also be seen in hemorrhagic shock, obesity, and obstructive pulmonary disease. Many of the conditions associated with postpericardiotomy syndrome are associated with blood in the pericardium, but such a sequence is by no means universal or necessary. Patients with large pericardial effusions of diverse etiology frequently continue to have pericardial friction rubs. Kussmaul's sign is typical of constrictive pericarditis but is not pathognomonic; it may be seen in restrictive myocardial disease also. *(Cecil, Ch. 54)*

118.(A—True; B—False; C—False; D–False; E—False) Surgical repair of a *ruptured* aortic abdominal aneurysm probably carries a mortality rate greater than 50%. Abdominal aortic aneurysms in symptomatic patients should be repaired, regardless of size, as long as there are no other contraindications. The more remote the primary infection, the less the sensitivity of the VDRL test in identifying prior syphilis; a fluorescent treponemal antibody absorption test (FTA-ABS) is more accurate and sensitive. Although the physician should search assiduously for pulse inequalities in patients suspected of dissection, pulse equality is the rule. *(Cecil, Ch. 56)*

119.(A—True; B—False; C—True; D—True; E—False) When arterial obstruction is severe, the drop in perfusion associated with raising the leg may cause striking foot pallor. Vasodilator drug therapy is of no proven benefit in randomized double-blind controlled series and may cause harm by its greater vasodilative effect in less severely affected vessels, creating a "steal" syndrome. With critical arterial obstruction and exercise-induced arterial vasodilation, the blood pressure in the affected leg may drop precipitously. In an occasional patient, pain in an embolized extremity may be minimal and overshadowed by ischemic paralysis, wrongly suggesting that the primary problem is neurologic. In a patient with rest pain, the situation is critical; careful evaluation for surgical therapy is indicated. An exercise program is virtually impossible to initiate unless the rest pain can be controlled. *(Cecil, Ch. 57)*

120.(A—True; B—False; C—True; D—True; E—False) The immobility, venous stasis, and frequent hypercoagulable state associated with the postoperative condition are important risk factors for thrombophlebitis in surgical patients, particularly in those undergoing hip replacement and prostatectomy. Such patients are frequently asymptomatic until pulmonary embolism occurs. The most sensitive and predictive test for the diagnosis of thrombophlebitis is venous angiography. Unfortunately, it is invasive and carries a small but significant risk of inducing the disease it is evaluating. A number of anticoagulant schemes have failed to decrease the incidence of postoperative thrombophlebitis; aspirin is no exception. *(Cecil, Ch. 57)*

121.(C); 122.(B); 123.(A); 124.(E); 125.(D) 121. The physical examination of this patient is consistent with a ventricular septal defect, with the right and left ventricular enlargement and prominent pulmonary arteries on chest roentgenogram suggesting a left to right shunt. The cardiac output and pulmonary artery oxygen content would be elevated, as might the pulmonary capillary wedge pressure. The A-V_{O_2} difference in patients with left to right shunting is diminished. **122.** This patient presents with a severe urinary tract infection and possible sepsis. In a patient without other organic heart disease, the pulmonary capillary wedge pressure and the systemic vascular resistance should be decreased. The cardiac output may be increased owing to an increased heart rate accompanying fever as well as the decrease in afterload. Systemic shunting may result in an increased mixed venous oxygen content and an accompanying decreased A-Vo_2 difference. **123.** This patient presents with a history compatible with an acute myocardial infarction with accompanying congestive heart failure. In this clinical setting, the cardiac output and mixed venous oxygen concentration may be depressed. The pulmonary capillary wedge pressure, A-Vo_2 difference, and systemic vascular resistance would be elevated. **124.** This patient presents with marked chest pain, nausea, jugular venous distention, and clinical evidence of shock, suggestive of a myocardial infarction. Intermittent A waves at a pulse rate of 50 per minute suggest the possibility of complete heart block. ST elevation in the right precordial leads is also suggestive of a right ventricular infarction, in which the right atrial pressure may be equal to or exceed the pulmonary capillary wedge pressure. Because of inadequate left ventricular filling, the cardiac output is diminished. The A-Vo_2 content difference and the systemic vascular resistance may be significantly elevated. **125.** This patient presents with findings of gastrointestinal blood loss resulting in a decreased intravascular volume. Because of the decrease in intravascular volume, the cardiac output and ventricular filling pressures are diminished. As a compensatory mechanism, the systemic vascular resistance is significantly increased. The A-Vo_2 difference and mixed venous oxygen content may also be abnormal. *(Braunwald, Chs. 19, 30, 31, and 38)*

126.(C); 127.(A); 128.(B); 129.(E); 130.(D) 126. Norepinephrine results in a significant increase in systemic vascular resistance owing to direct alpha-adrenergic stimulation. This may result in a reflex decrease in heart rate, although a direct chronotropic action on the heart may be observed. With the increase in systemic vascular resistance, the blood pressure increases, as may the pulmonary capillary wedge pressure. **127.** Dobutamine, a synthetic sympathomimetic agent, is a direct $beta_1$ stimulant that produces an increase in cardiac output. Unlike dopamine, dobutamine has much less alpha-vasoconstricting activity but possesses equal positive inotropic effects. Thus, in equal inotropic doses, dobutamine tends to lower the pulmonary capillary wedge pressure while dopamine tends to increase it. Dobutamine is also reported to have a lower incidence of untoward cardiac arrhythmias and may have less effect on heart rate than dopamine. **128.** Sodium nitroprusside may have a direct effect on both arterial and venous beds, resulting in a decrease in both preload and afterload. The latter results in a decrease in systemic vascular resistance and potentially in blood pressure, although blood pressure may actually increase with an accompanying increment in cardiac output. Because of this effect, the pulmonary capillary wedge pressure is typically reduced, and the heart rate may be increased. **129.** Dopamine at doses of 1–3 mcg/kg/min may result in an increase in renal blood flow. It directly increases myocardial contractility at doses of 4–8 mcg/kg/min and may produce systemic vascular constriction through a direct alpha effect at doses in excess of 10 mcg/kg/min. The use of this agent may also be accompanied by an increased vulnerability to arrhythmias. **130.** Isoproterenol acts primarily on vascular $beta_2$ receptors, causing vasodilatation, with an accompanying decrease in systemic vascular resistance and potentially in blood pressure. It also has direct chronotropic and inotropic effects via myocardial $beta_1$ receptors. This stimulation results in an increase in cardiac output and heart rate. The major vasodilator action of isoproterenol is in the skeletal muscle beds. *(Cecil, Ch. 44)*

131.(B); 132.(A); 133.(C); 134.(E); 135.(D) All antiarrhythmics show a variety of untoward side effects. In addition to GI side effects such as nausea and diarrhea, quinidine may produce thrombocytopenia. Digoxin at toxic levels may produce Mobitz type I second-degree AV block, junctional tachycardias, and PAT with block. Procainamide therapy results in the development of antinuclear antibodies in more than 75% of patients, while only approximately one third of these will develop a lupus-like syndrome. Amiodarone therapy may be accompanied by abnormalities of liver function, thyroid hormone abnormalities, and a bluish or slate-gray skin discoloration, as well as interstitial lung disease or fibrosing alveolitis. *(Cecil, Ch. 45; Braunwald, Ch. 21)*

136.(D); 137.(A); 138.(C); 139.(D); 140.(B) Patients with atrial-septal defect may have prominent A and V waves with an intervening "X" descent, while giant A waves with a slow "Y" descent are characteristic of tricuspid stenosis. In contrast, patients with tricuspid regurgitation show prominent "C-V" waves. The right atrial pressure tracing of patients with constrictive pericarditis typically show the "M or W" shape along with the sharp "Y" descent corresponding to the early diastolic dip to the earlier rapid filling of the ventricle. Kussmaul's sign, manifested by an inspiratory increase in the jugular venous pressure, may also be observed with the constrictive pericarditis. *(Cecil, Chs. 49 and 54; Braunwald, Chs. 33 and 44)*

141.(B); 142.(B); 143.(A); 144.(E); 145.(B); 146.(D) 141. In this patient, the possibility of endocarditis is great; echocardiography can provide early identification of an intracardiac mass lesion suggestive of a vegetation. In addition, with acute aortic regurgitation, premature mitral valve closure may be an early indicator of severe aortic regurgitation and the need for aggressive surgical intervention. **142.** Although the chest roentgenogram can show a large cardiac silhouette, echocardiography allows determination of whether the enlargement is myocardial or pericardial in etiology; if myocardial, it can quantify the chamber and/or valvular involvement. **143.** Although echocardiography in adults can exclude significant aortic stenosis if leaflet mobility is normal, the absence of normal leaflet mobility does not document aortic stenosis. Similarly, left ventricular hypertrophy may be due to previous systemic hypertension. Doppler echocardiography is the only laboratory technique that allows a rough quantification of the degree of stenosis in adults. It is not without its technical limitations, however. **144.** Although echocardiography is capable of detecting thickening, fibrosis, and/or calcification of cardiac structures, it is not reliable in differentiating these entities. Chest fluoroscopy is the procedure of choice. **145.** Although the physical examination can be virtually diagnostic of hypertrophic cardiomyopathy, two-dimensional echocardiography best documents the distribution of hypertrophy and the characteristic dynamics of mitral valve motion. **146.** In some patients with aortic regurgitation, irreversible myocardial dysfunction may develop despite a well-maintained clinical status. Although echocardiography and rest/exercise radionuclide angiography have reportedly helped in the evaluation of this difficult situation, the derived measurements obtained cannot yet be used in isolation to decide on surgical intervention in a totally asymptomatic patient. Progressive left ventricular dilatation and/or a fall in exercise ejection fraction are certainly causes for concern and follow-up; chest roentgenography is helpful, and there are also electrographic correlates of progressive left ventricular dilatation. Such patients are best followed with careful history-taking and physical examination, a chest roentgenogram, and an electrocardiogram, the least invasive and expensive tests. In patients with clinically severe aortic regurgitation and/or evidence of left ventricular dilatation, it is best to obtain a baseline rest/exercise radionuclide evaluation. With evidence of systolic dysfunction, patients should be followed closely; for those who initially have normal systolic function, the physician must be guided by clinical status, the electrocardiogram, and the chest roentgenogram in determining when to repeat the exercise evaluation. *(Cecil, Chs. 42.1, 42.3, 47, 49, 50, 52, and 53; Braunwald, Chs. 3, 5, 33, and 42; Fioretti et al; Pearlman et al; Rahimtoola)*

147.(C); 148.(B); 149.(E); 150(A) 147. This patient has an atrial tachycardia with AV block, nausea, and a low serum potassium level; all are conducive to, or are highly suggestive of, digitalis toxicity. Further digoxin therapy should be withheld, the serum level checked, and potassium supplementation given. **148.** This patient shows a continuing rapid response to atrial fibrillation with a subtherapeutic digoxin level. A reasonable initial alternative is to increase the dose of digoxin and reassess the patient's clinical status once therapeutic levels are achieved. **149.** This patient has continuing atrial fibrillation with a rapid ventricular response despite a digoxin level that is slightly above the therapeutic range. It would be reasonable to add a beta blocker or verapamil to the regimen in order to obtain synergistic blocking effects at the AV node and slow the ventricular response. Even in the setting of left ventricular dysfunction, small doses of beta blockers may be well tolerated. **150.** This patient has atrial fibrillation with a well-controlled ventricular response, both at rest and with modest activity. The digoxin level is therapeutic, and there is little to be gained by increasing the digoxin dose. Further therapy for the heart failure, if any, should be directed toward optimizing the diuretic dose and/or assessing whether or not the patient is a candidate for vasodilator therapy. *(Cecil, Chs. 43 and 45)*

151.(B); 152.(C); 153.(C); 154.(C); 155.(B) Atrial septal defects (both primum and secundum) have predominant left to right shunts with increased pulmonary vascularity. Physiologically, partial anomalous pulmonary venous return is the same, the left to right shunt occurring either at the atrial or systemic venous level. Ebstein's anomaly, particularly if associated with an atrial septal defect and an ineffective right ventricle, shows diminished pulmonary vascularity, as seen in patients with tetralogy of Fallot and tricuspid atresia. *(Cecil, Ch. 49)*

156.(A); 157.(C); 158.(A); 159.(C); 160.(B) 156. Even though asymptomatic, this patient has critical aortic stenosis; because of the increased risk of sudden death, he is a candidate for surgery. Valvulotomy, if possible, is the procedure of choice; it may achieve significant palliation for a number of years. **157.** This patient has critical aortic stenosis and is a candidate for surgical intervention. The calcification of the aortic valve precludes an attempt at commissurotomy; prosthetic valve replacement is indicated. Both the likelihood of greater durability of a mechanical prosthesis (compared with a tissue valve) and the patient's young age favor selection of a mechanical prosthesis. **158.** This patient has critical mitral stenosis with appropriate symptoms. Since there is no mitral regurgitation or valvular calcification, she is a candidate for commissurotomy; the ultimate decision (commissurotomy vs. mitral valve replacement) will rest with the surgeon at the time of operation. **159.** This patient has rheumatic heart disease with mitral regurgitation and longstanding atrial fibrillation. Despite adequate control of ventricular response, the symptoms have progressed. Cardiac catheterization shows mildly abnormal left ventricular function and a widened A-V_{O_2} difference, identifying a reduced cardiac output. Prosthetic mitral valve replacement is indicated. It is likely that the atrial fibrillation will persist postoperatively, and chronic anticoagulant therapy may be necessary. A mechanical prosthesis is likely to be of superior durability. **160.** This patient has severe aortic regurgitation, pulmonary venous congestion, impaired left ventricular function, and reduced cardiac output; he is a candidate for surgical intervention. Although use of a porcine valve might be favored because of the patient's age, the gastrointestinal bleeding is a contraindication to anticoagulation, and selection of a tissue valve is mandatory. *(Cecil, Chs. 45, 49, and 52)*

161.(D); 162.(A); 163.(B); 164.(C) 161. With mitral regurgitation the volume overload enlarges and laterally displaces the left ventricular impulse, while the enhanced diastolic rapid filling associated with severe mitral regurgitation typically produces a palpable diastolic impulse and an audible third heart sound. The late systolic impulse at the lower left sternal edge is due to mitral regurgitation expanding the left atrium and pulmonary veins, thrusting the heart anteriorly, and causing the right ventricle to produce a late systolic impulse at the lower left sternal edge. **162.** With aortic regurgitation, the volume-loaded left ventricle is inferolaterally displaced and enlarged; a drop in peripheral vascular resistance usually coexists. The combination of an increased stroke volume being ejected into a dilated arterial tree causes a hyperdynamic, nonsustained apical impulse. **163.** With isolated mitral stenosis, the left ventricle is typically small and uninvolved. If the apex is palpable, it is discrete and brief. With more severe degrees of mitral stenosis, the dilated right ventricle may displace the apex away from the chest wall and prevent its being palpated. The resulting pulmonary venous and pulmonary arterial hypertension produce right ventricular hypertrophy, causing a sustained impulse at the lower left sternal edge. **164.** Aortic stenosis produces concentric left ventricular hypertrophy; with well-maintained left ventricular function, the apical impulse is typically enlarged and sustained, not laterally displaced. The decreased left ventricular compliance results in enhanced left atrial systole, which in turn produces a palpable presystolic impulse. *(Cecil, Ch. 52; Braunwald, Ch. 33)*

165.(D); 166.(F); 167.(B); 168.(C); 169.(E) In patients with an elastic arterial tree, a high peripheral vascular resistance, and a decreased cardiac output, a dicrotic arterial pulse is very typical. These physiologic circumstances are common in congestive cardiomyopathy in the younger patient. A dicrotic pulse is a variety of bifid arterial pulse, with the second peak in diastole reflecting an accentuated dicrotic wave. Another bifid arterial pulse is the bisferious pulse, with both peaks in systole and roughly of equal height. It classically occurs in association with a large volume pulse showing a wide pulse pressure and a brisk upstroke. The classic valvular cause for this is aortic regurgitation of at least moderately severe degree with or without associated aortic stenosis. A bisferious arterial pulse should be differentiated from the spike and dome arterial pulse of hypertrophic obstructive cardiomyopathy, in which the pulse volume is typically normal, the upstroke is brisk, and the second, more rounded (dome) part of the pulse is more difficult to feel. Fixed left ventricular outflow tract obstruction (e.g., valvular aortic stenosis, supravalvular aortic stenosis, or even subvalvular membranous aortic stenosis) is a classic cause for a small pulse volume with a slow rising contour. Typically with valvular aortic stenosis, there is an associated thrill or shudder. This is the classic pulsus parvus et tardus (small and late). A pericardial effusion that has achieved hemodynamic significance (tamponade) is classically associated with a high venous pressure and a drop in arterial blood pressure with inspiration of more than 10 mm Hg. *(Cecil, Ch. 39; Vanden Belt et al, pp. 15–20)*

170.(B); 171.(D); 172.(A); 173.(E); 174.(C) *(Cecil, Chs. 42.2 and 45; Braunwald, Ch. 7, Fig. 7–13)*

175.(A); 176.(E); 177.(D); 178.(B); 179.(D); 180.(C) For patients with daily arrhythmia symptoms (assuming that the arrhythmia is not captured during a 12-lead electrocardiogram), a single 24-hour period of ambulatory ECG monitoring is usually sufficient to characterize the arrhythmia. For patients with very infrequent symptoms, on the other hand, prolonged monitoring is necessary. The expense of frequent 24-hour ambulatory ECG's, however, is prohibitive. Telephone telemetry techniques, on the other hand, can be used to place an inexpensive monitoring capability in the patient's home, work, and/or leisure environment. With symptoms, monitoring is initiated using a small hand-held device applied either directly to the chest or via wrist electrodes. The ECG can be transmitted directly via a telephone to a base station or captured in the device's solid state memory for subsequent telephone transmission. In a patient with right bundle branch block and left anterior hemiblock and syncope, a higher degree AV block as a cause for the syncope deserves urgent consideration. Some might argue that a pacemaker should be placed regardless of the circumstances, but syncope is notoriously multifactorial, and this patient's AV block could be in the AV node and due to digitalis. The case for pacing would be strengthened considerably if the site of block could be localized to the His bundle or below. His bundle electrocardiography, therefore, is the procedure of choice for obtaining this measurement. For a patient with a narrow QRS tachycardia at 150 per minute, the differential diagnosis resides primarily between AV junctional re-entry (node versus accessory pathway) and atrial flutter with 2:1 AV block. Identification of atrial activity via esophageal electrocardiography should resolve the dilemma. For a patient with a wide ARS tachycardia in which this is a known 1:1 AV (or VA) relationship, further delineation of atrial activity via esophageal monitoring would not be particularly helpful. His bundle electrocardiography, on the other hand, by defining whether or not a His bundle spike precedes the QRS, could resolve whether the tachycardia is ventricular or supraventricular with aberration. For a patient with WPW, paroxysmal tachycardia, and syncope, a potentially life-threatening arrhythmia may be occurring, and aggressive evaluation and management are indicated. Electrophysiologic stimulation using intracardiac catheter techniques can localize the site of the accessory pathway, determine its conducting characteristics, precipitate the arrhythmia under laboratory conditions, and acutely test the efficacy of drugs in treating the patient's arrhythmia. *(Cecil, Chs. 42.2 and 42.5)*

181.(D); 182.(F); 183.(B); 184.(E); 185.(A) Impotence is more common with the thiazides than with beta blockers, and it must be recognized early and therapy altered in order to enhance compliance and follow-up. The side effects of captopril that were reported in the initial trials of patients with moderate to severe hypertension (proteinuria, rash, agranulocytosis, and loss of a sense of taste) all appear to be much less frequent when this agent is used in treating patients with milder degrees of hypertension. In a patient with pre-existent bronchospasm, even cardioselective beta blockers should probably be avoided because, in the dosage used to treat hypertension, even so-called $beta_1$ selective agents produce a high degree of $beta_2$ blockade. The lupus-like reaction produced by hydralazine can be minimized by keeping the dose under 200 mg per day and is more frequent in slow acetylators. The venular dilatation of nifedipine commonly causes edema. *(Cecil, Ch. 47)*

186.(B); 187.(E); 188.(D); 189.(A); 190.(C) In **A**, a large echo-free space (PE) is seen posteriorly (see below). In other views it was seen anteriorly as well. Although heart sounds may be surprisingly well preserved, one typical clinical presentation of pericardial effusion is for them to be somewhat soft. **B** (p. 36) shows findings typical of mitral valve prolapse with systolic movement of the posterior leaflet (arrow) significantly into an enlarged left atrium (LA). At the bedside, in addition to a non-ejection click, a high-frequency, mid to late systolic crescendo murmur is typical of this entity. **C** (p. 36) shows an enlarged left ventricle (LV) that is diffusely and poorly contractile, typical of congestive cardiomyopathy. Atrial and ventricular gallops along with mitral regurgitation due to mitral valve apparatus dysfunction are common findings with this entity. **D** (p. 37) shows a heavily calcified, immobile aortic valve (arrowheads) typical of valvular aortic stenosis, and transmission of the harsh, midsystolic murmur to the apex is

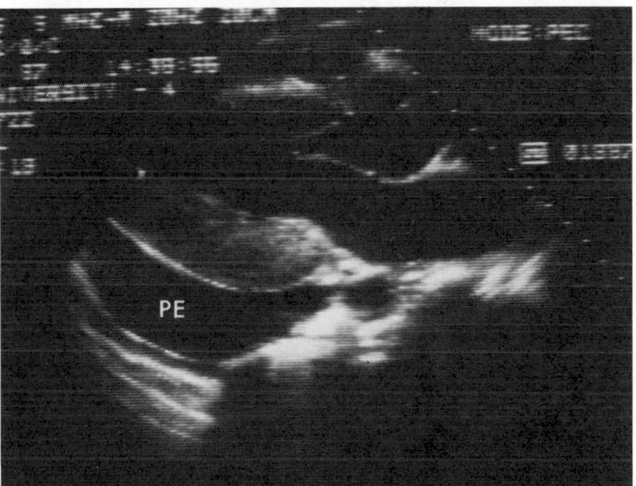

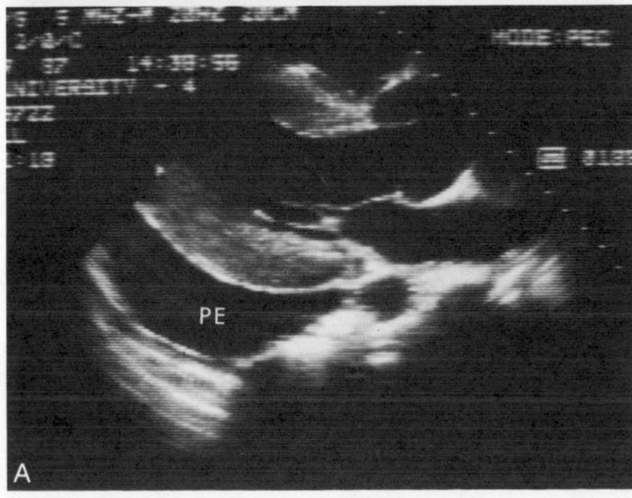

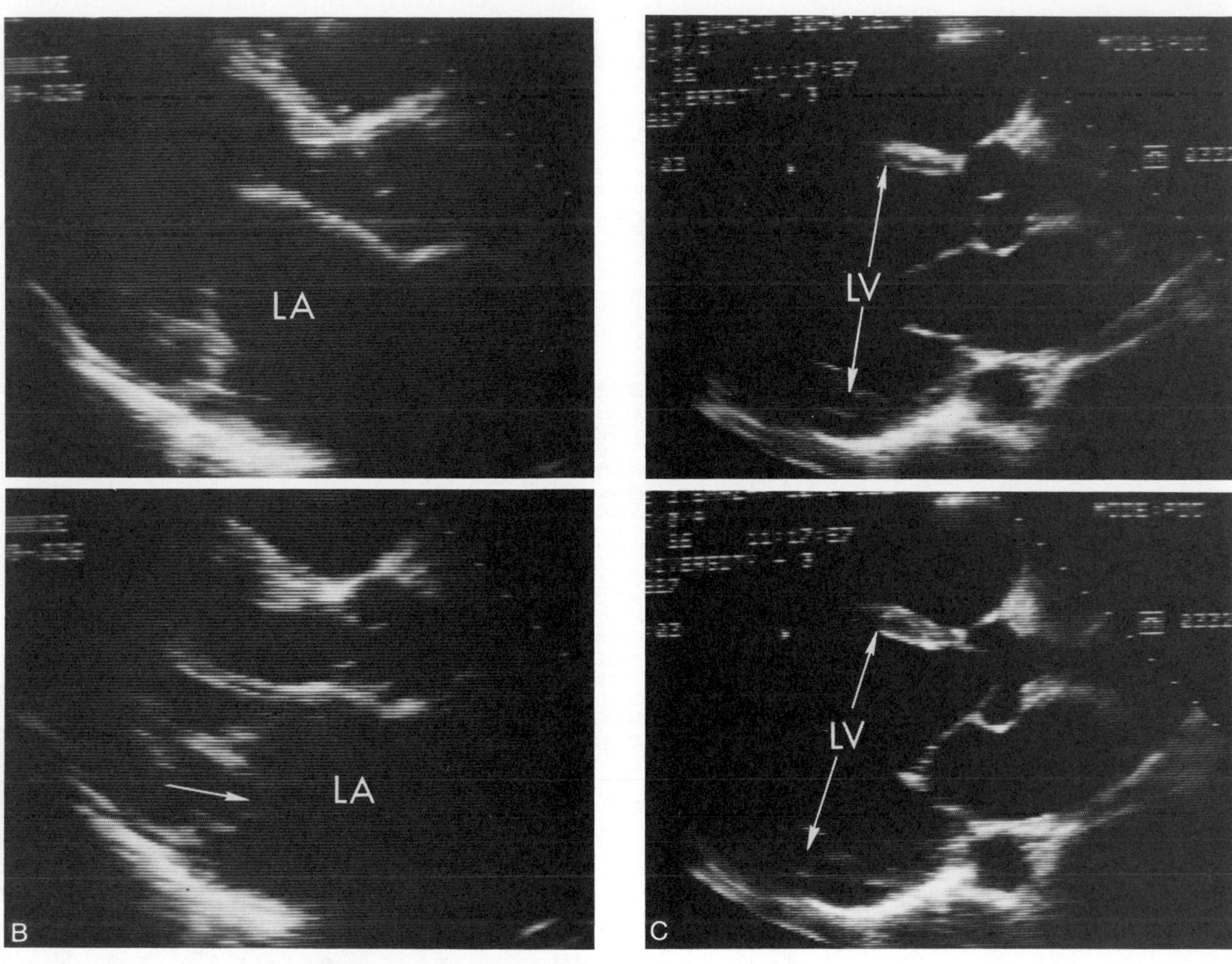
LA
LA
B
LV
LV
C

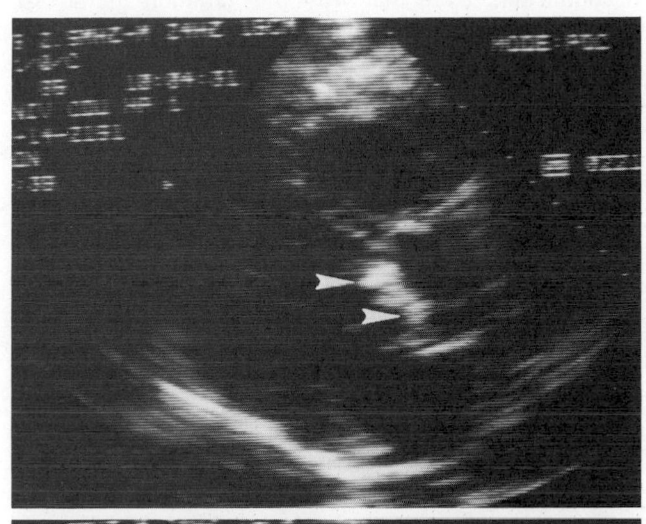

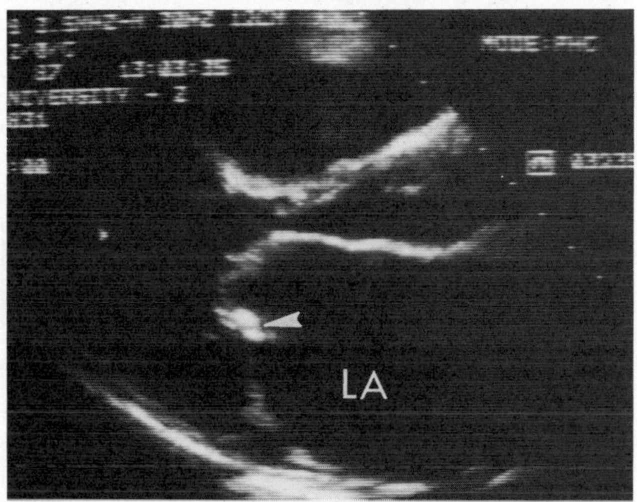
LA

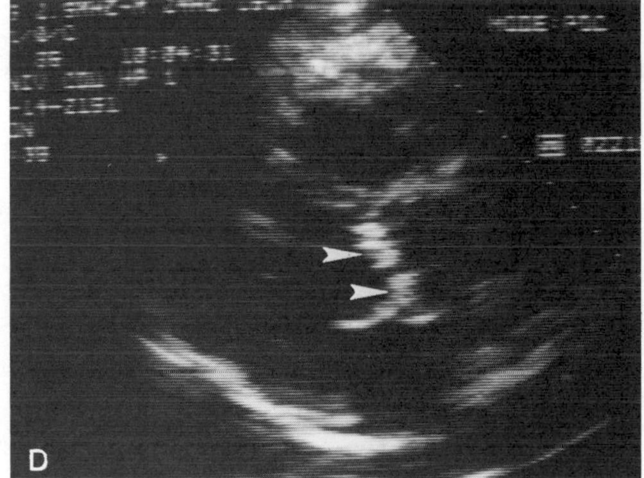
D

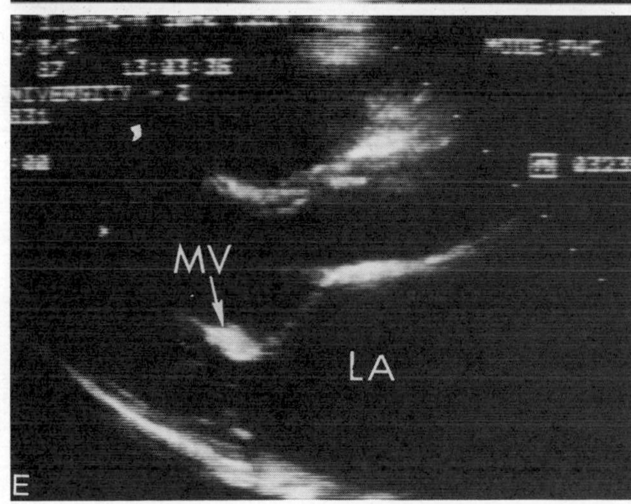
MV
LA
E

also typical. **E** (p. 37) shows classic features of rheumatic mitral valve disease with mitral valve (MV) thickening, central tethering of the leaflet tips (arrowhead) in diastole, and left atrial enlargement (LA). The corresponding classic physical finding, in addition to a loud first heart sound and an opening snap, is an apical diastolic rumble. *(Cecil, Chs. 52 and 54; Braunwald, Chs. 5 and 7)*

191.(C); 192.(E); 193.(D); 194.(A); 195.(B) (see below) **A** shows third-degree AV block with a slow, wide QRS escape rhythm. Note the constant R-R intervals with variable P-R intervals identifying AV dissociation. Numerous P waves that should have conducted (arrowheads) but did not (i.e., after the prior T wave and 0.21 second before a QRS) are present. This dysrhythmia occurred in the setting of an anterior myocardial infarction and was treated with temporary and, subsequently, permanent pacing. **B** shows sinus rhythm with slowing of the sinus pacemaker and the emergence of atrial bigeminy. Note the change in the T wave morphology in the right-hand portion of the strip due to the superimposed P waves (arrows). Since these P waves are premature and occur within the T wave of the prior beat, no pathologic evidence of AV block is present. **C** shows fixed 2:1 AV block, and the type cannot be determined. In order to "type" second-degree AV block, there must be variability in the interval from the last conducted QRS complex to the next conducted P wave. When this R-P interval varies and the subsequent P-R interval is fixed, type II second-degree AV block is defined. When the P-R interval varies reciprocally with the prior R-P interval, type I second-degree AV block is present. As in the question strip, however, when the R-P interval is constant, the P-R interval will also be constant and, therefore, the block cannot be "typed." **C** shows the same patient at a different point in time when there is variation in conduction. Note that with the variation in the R-P interval, when 1:1 AV conduction resumes, the subsequent P-R interval increases (compare the P-R following R-P No. 1 to the P-R following R-P No. 2). This identifies type I second-degree AV block and implies an AV nodal location. **D** shows sinus rhythm with three dropped P waves (arrowheads). Note that the P-R intervals neither before nor

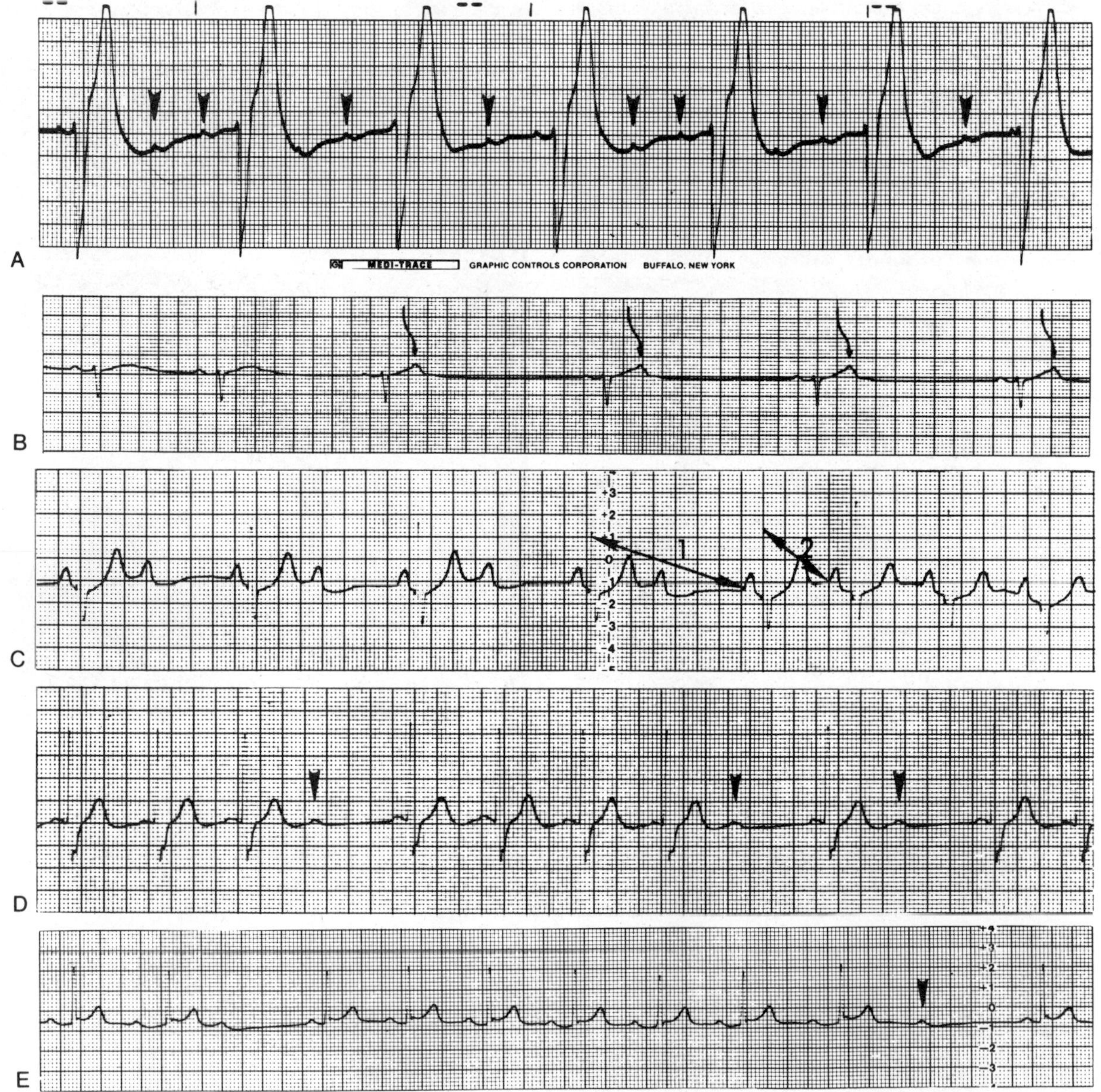

following the dropped P waves show any variability. Thus, the R-P interval varies while the P-R interval is fixed, defining type II second-degree AV block. The left-hand portion of **E** shows a relatively regular P-R interval, a progressively increasing P-R interval, and a nonconducted, on-time P wave followed by a resumption of the cycle. This inverse or reciprocal relationship between the R-P and the P-R intervals defines type I second-degree AV block. In the second episode of second-degree AV block in the right-hand portion of the strip, the P-P interval lengthens and causes an increase in the R-P, but there is a concomitant increase in the P-R interval just before the dropped P wave (arrowhead). This implies that a change in autonomic balance (increased vagal tone) is occurring coincident with the type I second-degree AV block sequence. *(Cecil, Ch. 45)*

BIBLIOGRAPHY

Bates ER, Shenker Y, Grekin RJ: The relationship between plasma levels of immunoreactive atrial natriuretic hormone and hemodynamic function in man. Circulation 73:1155–1161, 1986.

Braunwald E (ed): Heart Disease: A Textbook of Cardiovascular Disease. 3rd ed. Philadelphia, W.B. Saunders Company, 1988.

Cecil Textbook of Medicine. 18th ed. Wyngaarden JB, Smith LH Jr (eds). Philadelphia, W.B. Saunders Company, 1988.

Chesebro JH, Knatterud G, Roberts G, et al: Thrombolysis in myocardial infarction (TIMI) trial, phase I: A comparison between intravenous tissue plasminogen activator and intravenous streptokinase. Circulation 76:142, 1987.

Feigenbaum H: Echocardiography. 4th ed. Philadelphia, Lea and Febiger, 1986.

Fioretti P, Roelandt J, Box RJ, et al: Echocardiography in chronic aortic insufficiency. Circulation 67:216, 1983.

Frank S, Johnson A, Ross J Jr: Natural history of valvular aortic stenosis. Br Heart J 35:41, 1973.

Froelicher VF: Exercise Testing and Training. Chicago, Year Book Medical Publishers, 1983.

Gulamhusein S, Ko P, Carruthers SG, Klein GJ: Acceleration of the ventricular response during atrial fibrillation in the Wolff-Parkinson-White syndrome after verapamil. Circulation 65:348, 1982.

Henry WL, Bonow RO, Rosina DR, Epstein SE: Observations on the optimum time for operative intervention for aortic regurgitation. II. Serial echocardiographic evaluation of asymptomatic patients. Circulation 61:484, 1980.

Hurst JW (ed): The Heart. New York, McGraw-Hill Book Company, 1986.

The Joint National Committee on Detection, Evaluation and Treatment of High Blood Pressure: The 1984 report of the Joint National Committee on Detection, Evaluation and Treatment of High Blood Pressure. Arch Intern Med 144:1045, 1984.

Kennedy JW, Ritchie JL, David KB, et al: The western Washington randomized trial of intracoronary streptokinase in acute myocardial infarction: A 12 month follow-up report. N Engl J Med 312:1073, 1985.

Kuller LH, Hulley SB, Cohen JD, Neaton J: Unexpected effects of treating hypertension in men with electrocardiographic abnormalities: A critical analysis. Circulation 73:114, 1986.

Lee G, Amsterdam EA, Low R, et al: Efficacy of percutaneous transluminal coronary recanalization utilizing streptokinase thrombolysis in patients with acute myocardial infarction. Am Heart J 102:1159, 1981.

Lipid Research Clinics Program: The lipid research clinics coronary primary prevention trial results. 1. Reduction in incidence of coronary heart disease. JAMA 251:351, 1984.

Morganroth J, Anderson JL, Gentzkow GD: Classification by type of ventricular arrhythmia predicts frequency of adverse cardiac events from flecainide. J Am Coll Cardiol 8:697, 1986.

McNeer JR, Margolis JR, Lee KL, et al: The role of the exercise test in the evaluation of patients for ischemic heart disease. Circulation 57:64, 1978.

The Multiple Risk Factor Intervention Trial Research Group: Multiple risk factor intervention trial. Risk factor changes and mortality results. JAMA 248(12):1465, 1982.

Pearlman AS, Scoblianko DP, Saal KA: Assessment of valvular heart disease by Doppler echocardiography. Clin Cardiol 6:573, 1983.

Rahimtoola SH: Valve replacement should not be performed in all asymptomatic patients with severe aortic incompetence. J Thorac Cardiovasc Surg 79:163, 1980.

Roden DM, Woolsey RL: Flecainide drug therapy. N Engl J Med 315:36, 1986.

Rogers WJ, Mantle JA, Hood WP, et al: Prospective randomized trial of intravenous and intracoronary streptokinase in acute myocardial infarction. Circulation 68:1051, 1983.

Romhilt D, Bove KE, Norris RJ: A critical appraisal of the electrocardiographic criteria for the diagnosis of left ventricular hypertrophy. Circulation 40:185, 1969.

Vanden Belt RJ, Ronan JA, Bedynek JL: Cardiology: A Clinical Approach. Chicago, Year Book Medical Publishers, 1979.

Wellens HGG, Bar FWHM, Lie KI: The value of the electrocardiogram in the differential diagnosis of a tachycardia with a widened QRS complex. Am J Cardiol 64:27, 1978.

PART 2

RESPIRATORY DISEASE

JAMES K. BROWN

DIRECTIONS: For questions 1 to 42, choose the ONE BEST answer to each question.

QUESTIONS 1–4

A 30-year-old black woman develops fatigue, low-grade fever, 10-pound weight loss, and painful nodules on the anterior surfaces of her lower legs. Chest roentgenogram is shown below.

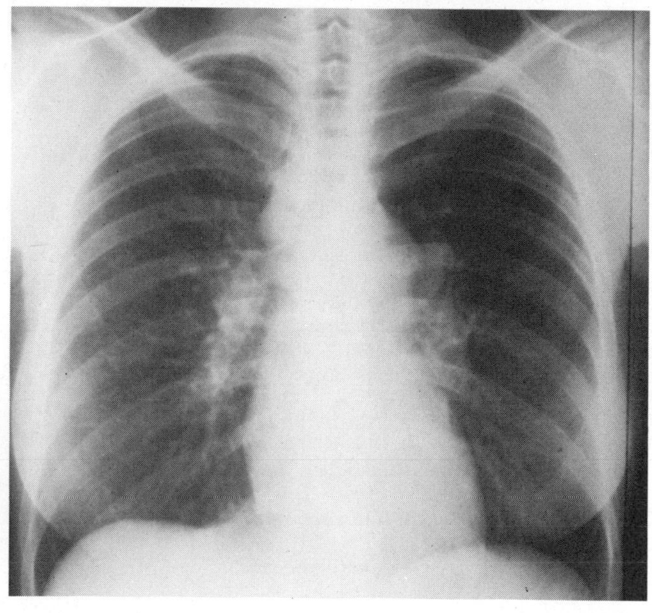

1. The single most likely diagnosis is

   A. Hodgkin's disease
   B. primary tuberculosis
   C. sarcoidosis
   D. Kaposi's sarcoma
   E. coccidioidomycosis

2. To establish the diagnosis, the most appropriate diagnostic approach or procedure in this patient is

   A. gallium scanning of the lung
   B. fiberoptic bronchoscopy or mediastinoscopy
   C. liver or conjunctival biopsy
   D. biopsy of skin lesions on lower legs
   E. careful follow-up at monthly intervals

3. The patient is at increased risk for all of the following extrapulmonary complications EXCEPT

   A. meningitis
   B. pancytopenia
   C. nephrolithiasis
   D. diabetes mellitus
   E. first-degree atrioventricular conduction block

4. The most likely outcome of this patient's illness is

   A. complete remission without treatment
   B. complete remission after appropriate radiotherapy and chemotherapy
   C. remission followed by recurrence within five years
   D. disabling dyspnea from pulmonary fibrosis
   E. death within two years

5. The single major reason for early use of heparin in patients with pulmonary thromboembolism is to

   A. dilate pulmonary vasculature
   B. eliminate the source of further emboli
   C. reverse bronchoconstriction induced by platelet-derived mediators
   D. lyse existing clot in the pulmonary circulation
   E. prevent growth of existing clot

6. In the evaluation of a patient with chronic obstructive pulmonary disease (COPD), each of the following laboratory abnormalities will help to distinguish the emphysematous from the bronchitic types EXCEPT

   A. diffusing capacity for carbon monoxide: 15 units (65% predicted)
   B. residual volume: 4.2 liters (198% predicted)
   C. arterial P_{CO_2}: 52 mm Hg
   D. transpulmonary pressure at total lung capacity: 7 cm H_2O (normal: 30–35)
   E. marked enlargement of central pulmonary arteries on chest roentgenogram

7. A 69-year-old man has pain, numbness, and weakness of the right arm that began three months ago after coronary artery bypass surgery. Since the surgery, the patient has lost 15 pounds. He has smoked two packs of cigarettes a day for 50 years. Chest roentgenogram is shown on page 41. Which of the following is the most likely cause of the current findings in this patient?

   A. Mesothelioma
   B. Pancoast's tumor

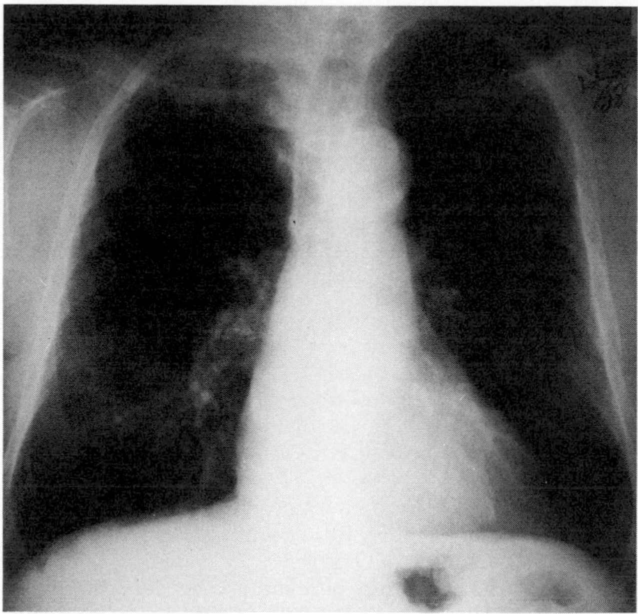

C. Pulmonary tuberculosis
D. Small-cell carcinoma of the lung
E. Intraoperative compression of the brachial plexus

QUESTIONS 8–10

8. A 65-year-old alcoholic man with cirrhosis reports that he is "coughing blood." Past history is notable for substantial cigarette use and for pulmonary tuberculosis in the 1960's that was "treated with pills for a year." Over the past five years, the patient has had cough productive of one-half cup of thick sputum daily. For the past three days, he has noted flecks of blood or clots in the sputum. Chest roentgenogram shows extensive biapical and right lower lobe scarring that is unchanged from a previous film. The most likely cause of this patient's coughing blood is

A. broncholithiasis
B. bronchogenic carcinoma
C. active tuberculous infection
D. post-tuberculous bronchiectasis
E. hematemesis confused with hemoptysis

9. The patient returns to your office six months later. He has noted no further blood in the sputum until two days ago, when he began coughing 2–3 tablespoons of clots or fresh blood every few hours. Repeat chest roentgenogram shows a new cavitary density in the right upper lobe; it is otherwise unchanged. A tomogram of the density is shown above, right. The evaluation and management of this patient's hemoptysis now should include each of the following EXCEPT

A. spirometry
B. fiberoptic bronchoscopy
C. measurement of *Aspergillus* precipitins in serum
D. sputum examination by cytology and bacteriology laboratories
E. intravenous administration of amphotericin

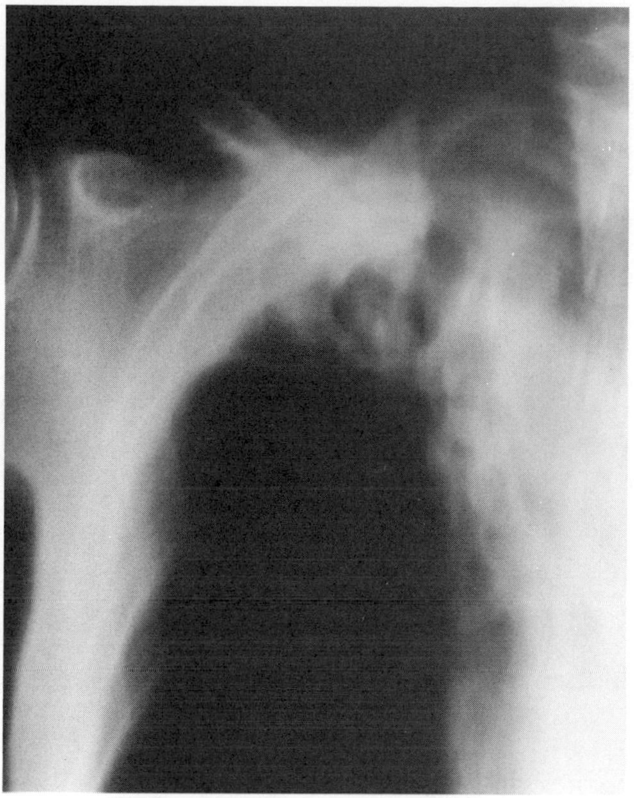

10. Although the patient's hemoptysis again subsides spontaneously, two months later you are called to the emergency room to evaluate him. He has just coughed up 600 ml of fresh blood over the previous eight hours. The initial evaluation and management now should include each of the following EXCEPT

A. notification of a thoracic surgeon
B. placement of a suction apparatus at the bedside
C. immediate bronchoscopic examination of the airways
D. placement of the patient in the decubitus position with the right side down
E. administration of high-dose morphine or codeine until the recently increased cough has been suppressed

11. A 32-year-old black man is brought to the hospital with cough and dyspnea that have increased progressively over the past two months. Routine laboratory studies show a total white blood cell count of 12,300, with 16% eosinophils and an erythrocyte sedimentation rate of 110 mm/hr; they are otherwise normal. The chest roentgenogram shown on page 42 was obtained upon admission. Three days after the patient received prednisone (60 mg orally daily), a repeat chest roentgenogram showed complete resolution of the abnormalities. The most likely diagnosis is

A. sarcoidosis
B. eosinophilic granuloma
C. chronic eosinophilic pneumonia
D. lymphocytic interstitial pneumonitis
E. allergic bronchopulmonary aspergillosis

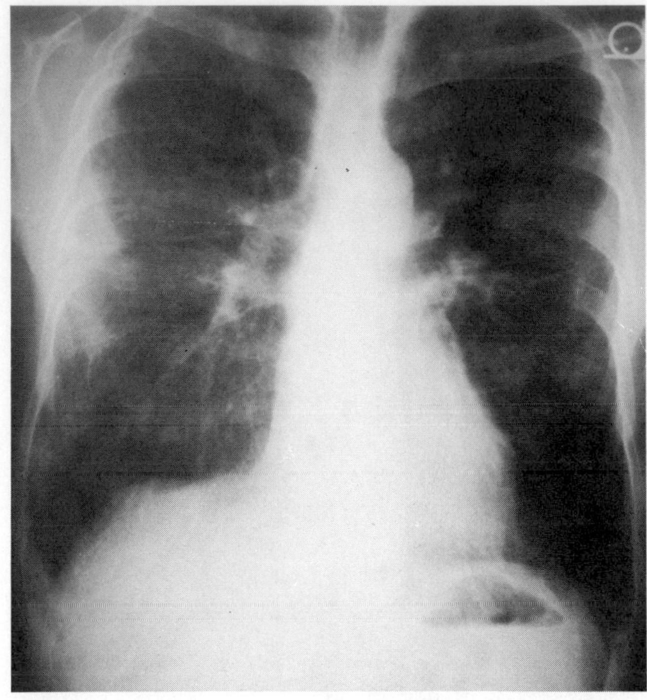

QUESTIONS 12–13

A 68-year-old man visits your office for a routine physical examination. He reports recent weight loss and a three-week history of cough productive of thick, foul-smelling sputum. Past medical history is notable only for a motor vehicle accident eight years ago and resulting grand mal seizures that have been controlled with phenytoin. Chest roentgenogram, which he obtained three days prior to his appointment with you, shows a cavity with an air-fluid level in the superior segment of the right lower lobe.

12. In your evaluation of this patient's history, which of the following questions would be most likely to help in establishing the cause of this patient's condition?

A. Has he coughed up blood?
B. Has he noted pleuritic chest pain?
C. When was the most recent grand mal seizure?
D. Has he traveled outside the U.S. recently?
E. Is there a history of tuberculosis in any member of his family?

13. In your evaluation of this patient's physical examination, which of the following findings would be the strongest indication for fiberoptic bronchoscopy?

A. Oral temperature is 103°F
B. Blood pressure is 92/64 mm Hg with the patient supine, falling to 78/58 mm Hg with patient seated
C. The patient is edentulous; examination of the head is otherwise normal
D. There are amphoric breath sounds over the right chest posteriorly
E. There are diffuse wheezes over the lungs during forced expiratory maneuver

14. Each of the following will cause increased slope of phase III in the closing volume maneuver EXCEPT

A. asthmatic bronchospasm
B. mild chronic bronchitis
C. obstruction of a mainstem bronchus unilaterally
D. obstruction of the trachea just above the carina
E. diffuse interstitial lung disease secondary to asbestos exposure

15. Which of the following statements about the relationship between cigarette smoking and lung disease is FALSE?

A. Passive inhalation of cigarette smoke increases the risk of lung cancer
B. Relationships between lung cancer risk and cigarette smoking are dose-dependent
C. In a given segment of the population, there is a 20-year lag phase between an increase in cigarette use and increased risk for lung cancer
D. Between 80 and 90% of cigarette smokers develop clinically significant chronic obstructive pulmonary disease (COPD)
E. Use of cigarettes accelerates the decline in lung function in patients with alpha$_1$-antitrypsin deficiency

16. In which of the following comatose or obtunded patients would the use of a *pressure-cycled* machine be appropriate for mechanical ventilation of the lungs?

A. A 10-year-old boy recovering from accidental barbiturate overdose
B. A 28-year-old woman who aspirated massively during obstetric anesthesia
C. A 32-year-old woman with status asthmaticus treated by general anesthesia
D. A 60-year-old man with multiple rib fractures and lung contusion after a motor vehicle accident
E. A 78-year-old man with adult respiratory distress syndrome after urosepsis

17. In the evaluation of a 55-year-old man with diffuse pulmonary infiltrates, which finding does NOT raise the likelihood that the patient has underlying acquired immunodeficiency syndrome?

A. He has hemophilia
B. He underwent surgical correction of an abdominal aortic aneurysm four years ago and required transfusions
C. He has a history of multiple contacts with female prostitutes in New York City
D. His brother, who was homosexual, died of *Pneumocystis carinii* pneumonia
E. Fresh and old needle tracks are present in the antecubital fossae

18. A 48-year-old woman has double vision, difficulty in swallowing, and weakness when attempting to rise from the sitting position. Chest roentgenograms are shown on page 43. The most likely cause of the chest roentgenographic abnormality is

A. aortic aneurysm
B. substernal thyroid
C. thymoma
D. lipoma
E. hernia

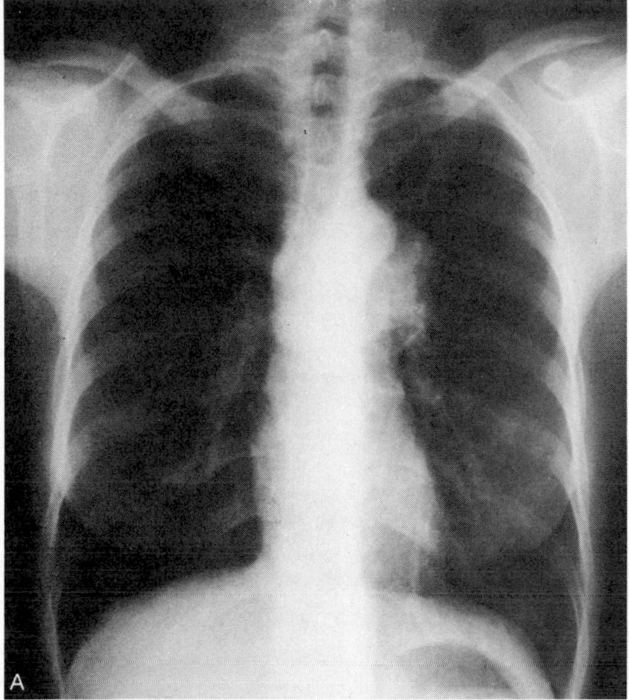

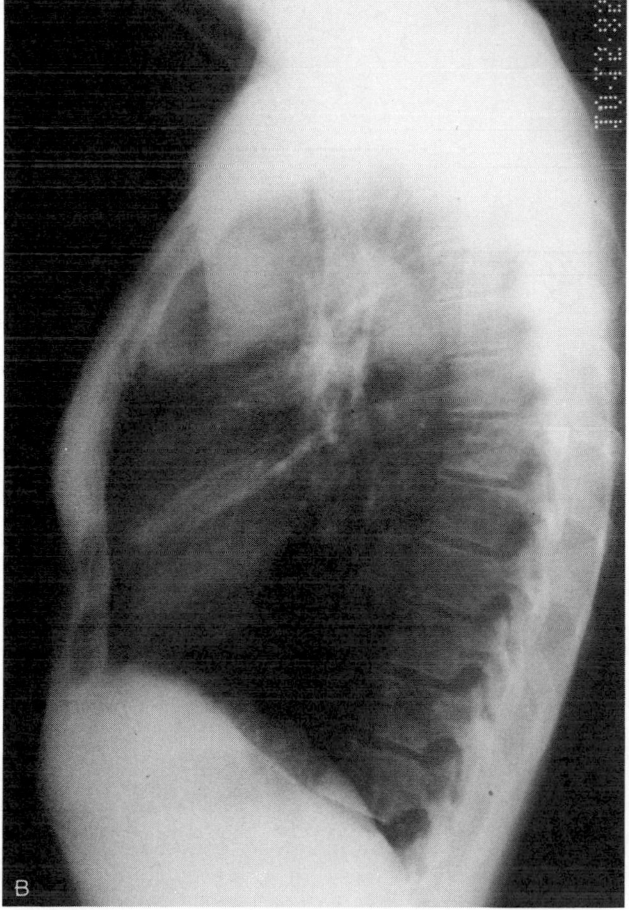

19. A 64-year-old man has had fever, weight loss, and left-sided chest pain for 3–4 weeks. Initial evaluation shows that intermediate-strength PPD skin test is positive, and the patient recalls that the same test was negative two years ago. Past medical history is notable only for an episode of third-degree heart block three years ago, requiring insertion of a pacemaker. Chest roentgenogram is shown below.

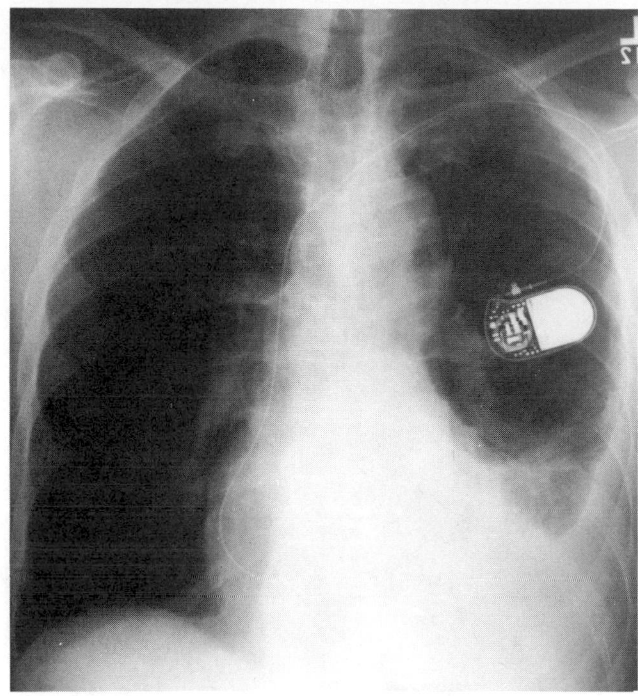

Which of the following is the most important diagnostic test for evaluating this patient's condition?

A. Sputum cytology
B. Computed tomography (CT) scan of the chest
C. Fiberoptic bronchoscopy
D. Pleuroscopy
E. Thoracentesis and pleural biopsy

20. A 50-year-old male miner with a 40 pack-year smoking history is found to have a well-differentiated epidermoid tumor occluding 95% of the lumen of the bronchus intermedius. No hilar, mediastinal, or distant metastases can be detected. Pulmonary function tests reveal that vital capacity, forced expiratory volume in one second (FEV_1), and maximal voluntary ventilation are approximately 40% of the predicted and do not improve with bronchodilator therapy. Which one of the following would you do now?

A. Recommend right pneumonectomy
B. Recommend radiotherapy
C. Offer no treatment at present, but treat any metastatic lesions with radiotherapy as they appear
D. Recommend palliative resection of a portion of the tumor via the bronchoscope to restore ventilation to the right lower lobe
E. Initiate an exercise training program and repeat pulmonary function tests in 6–10 weeks.

21. Which of the following patients would be at the LEAST risk for developing pulmonary thromboembolism?

A. An 18-year-old man with congenital deficiency of antithrombin III
B. A 19-year-old white man with mental retardation, ectopia lentis, and osteoporosis
C. A 22-year-old woman with superficial thrombophlebitis of the left arm occurring after an intravenous pyelogram

D. A 36-year-old woman with non-Hodgkin's lymphoma and compression with invasion of the left femoral vein by malignant lymph nodes
E. A 45-year-old woman who underwent a hysterectomy two days ago

22. A 40-year-old woman has bloody nasal discharge, cough, and shortness of breath of two months' duration. Urinalysis shows red blood cell casts and 4+ protein. Chest roentgenogram is shown below.

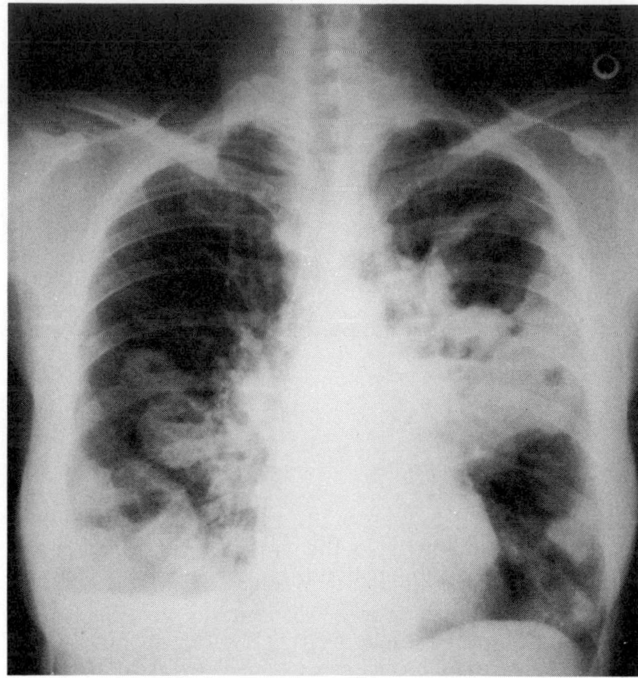

Which of the following therapeutic agents is most likely to improve this patient's condition?

A. Isoniazid
B. Prednisone
C. Methicillin
D. Amphotericin
E. Cyclophosphamide

23. Before chronic oxygen therapy is begun in a patient with end-stage chronic obstructive pulmonary disease (COPD), it is most important to check that

A. hematocrit is over 55%
B. the symptoms improve with oxygen therapy
C. arterial blood gases show a Po_2 under 55 mm Hg even after aggressive treatment
D. Pco_2 will not exceed 45 mm Hg while oxygen is being used
E. the patient is encouraged to use as little oxygen as necessary, to avoid possible dependence

24. With advances in surgery, radiation therapy, and chemotherapy, the overall five-year survival rate for all patients with bronchogenic carcinoma for the past 20 years has been about

A. 2%
B. 10%
C. 20%
D. 30%
E. 50%

25. Clinical features suggesting potential reversibility of airflow obstruction in chronic obstructive pulmonary disease (COPD) are suggested by each of the following EXCEPT

A. history of hay fever
B. nasal polyps
C. arterial hypoxemia
D. eosinophilia of the blood or sputum
E. nomal pulmonary diffusing capacity measurement (DL_{CO})

26. A 19-year-old man has "noisy breathing" and shortness of breath while jogging. He has had some recent difficulty swallowing solids; he feels otherwise healthy. Flow-volume curve is shown below.

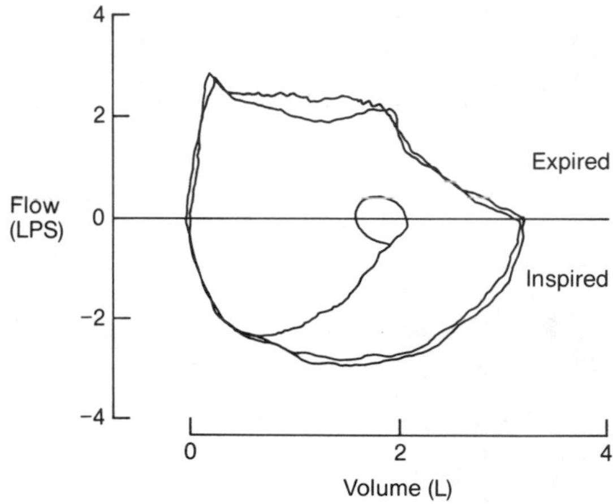

The most likely cause of this patient's condition is

A. vascular ring anomaly
B. bilateral vocal cord paralysis
C. marked enlargement of the adenoids
D. asthma with exercise-induced bronchospasm
E. congenital stenosis (fixed) of the intrathoracic trachea

27. The bacteria present in the highest concentrations in post-aspiration lung abscesses are

A. *Nocardia asteroides*
B. *Klebsiella pneumonia*
C. *Fusobacterium nucleatum* and *Bacteroides* species
D. *Staphylococcus aureus*
E. *Streptococcus pneumoniae*

28. Median survival in chronic obstructive pulmonary disease (COPD) is adversely affected by each of the following EXCEPT

A. cor pulmonale
B. resting tachycardia
C. forced expiratory volume in one second (FEV_1) under one liter
D. history of frequent bouts of purulent sputum
E. residence at an altitude of 4000 feet

29. In patients with bronchopulmonary sequestration, which of the following statements is NOT true?

A. Abnormal budding of the embryonic tracheobronchial tree is the cause
B. Chest roentgenogram usually shows a round opacity at the base of one lung

C. Systemic vascular supply is usually via a normal bronchial artery
D. Air-containing cysts develop when communication with an adjacent bronchus occurs
E. Definitive therapy is surgical removal

QUESTIONS 30–33

A 52-year-old man reports that he has shortness of breath after minimal exertion and nonproductive cough. These symptoms began shortly after a "cold" three months ago, but the patient has not suffered from fever, weight loss, or other symptoms. Physical examination reveals bibasilar rales and clubbing of the fingers. Chest roentgenogram is shown below.

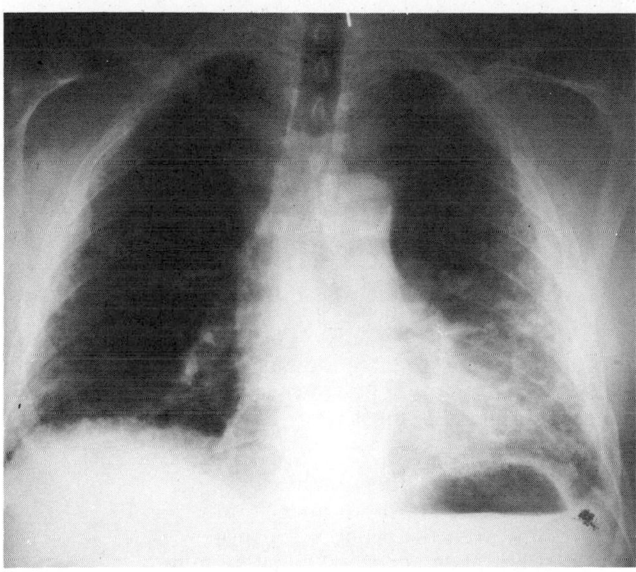

30. Given the information available, the single most likely diagnosis is

A. hypersensitivity pneumonitis
B. idiopathic pulmonary fibrosis
C. idiopathic pulmonary hemosiderosis
D. acquired immunodeficiency syndrome
E. interstitial lung disease following mycoplasmal infection

31. Each of the following arterial blood gas and pulmonary function test abnormalities is typical of those seen in this disorder EXCEPT

A. resting arterial P_{CO_2} of 52 mm Hg
B. arterial P_{O_2} of 58 mm Hg, falling to 42 with minimal exercise
C. FEV_1/FVC ratio of 89% (predicted: 72%)
D. total lung capacity of 4.9 liters (predicted: 6.4 liters)
E. diffusing capacity of 16 units (predicted: 25 units)

32. After an open lung biopsy has been performed, glucocorticoid therapy is begun. Which of the following is true in this setting?

A. Most experts recommend beginning with a low dose of prednisone and then increasing the dose until a response is observed
B. The likelihood of a beneficial response is somewhat better than in pulmonary sarcoidosis
C. The likelihood of a beneficial response is directly proportional to the extent of the fibrosis in lung parenchyma
D. Evaluation of therapeutic effects is usually possible by serial observations of symptoms, chest roentgenograms, and pulmonary function tests
E. The long-term efficacy of this therapy in prolonging survival is fairly well established

33. Three months after his initial presentation, the patient develops difficulty rising from a low chair, inability to swallow large pieces of meat, and a lilac rash on the upper eyelids. The most likely diagnosis is

A. scleroderma
B. dermatomyositis
C. polymyalgia rheumatica
D. steroid-induced myopathy
E. mixed connective tissue disease

34. A 62-year-old woman has cough and intermittent hemoptysis of six months' duration. She has also noted tenderness over both legs anteriorly below the knees. Roentgenogram of the long bones in a lower leg is shown below.

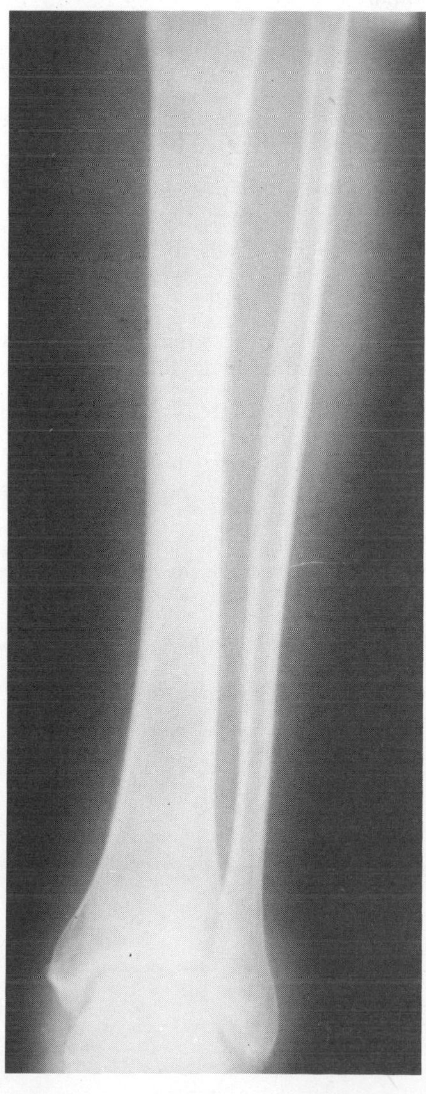

Which of the following is the most likely primary diagnosis?

A. Sarcoidosis
B. Tuberculosis
C. Rheumatoid arthritis
D. Small-cell carcinoma of the lung
E. Non–small-cell carcinoma of the lung

35. In patients with massive pulmonary thromboembolism, the most likely origin of the emboli is the

A. axillary veins
B. inferior vena cava
C. deep veins of the thigh or pelvis
D. deep veins of the legs below the knee
E. superficial veins of the lower extremities

36. In which of the following clinical settings should low-dose subcutaneous heparin NOT be administered for prevention of thromboembolism?

A. During recovery from acute myocardial infarction
B. After a laparotomy revealing unresectable colonic carcinoma
C. In an obese man who is bedridden with severe congestive heart failure
D. After emergency appendectomy in a young woman who has a previous history of deep venous thrombosis
E. After surgical extraction of a cataract in an elderly man

37. The presence of a small, unilateral pleural effusion is NOT likely to be associated with

A. *Pneumocystis carinii* pneumonia
B. *Mycoplasma pneumoniae* pneumonia
C. *Streptococcus pneumoniae* pneumonia
D. *Coccidioides immitis* pneumonia
E. pulmonary infarction

38. Which of the following statements about patients with recent pulmonary thromboemboli is correct?

A. The presence of infarction in the lung substantially worsens prognosis
B. When death occurs shortly after an untreated pulmonary embolus, the usual cause is a second pulmonary embolus
C. About 80% of all such patients will die in 2–3 weeks if they receive no therapy
D. Even when treated appropriately, patients with large pulmonary emboli usually will be left with chronic persistent dyspnea
E. Thrombolytic therapy with streptokinase or urokinase causes a substantial increment in survival compared to conventional anticoagulant therapy alone

39. Heroin addiction is associated with each of the following pulmonary complications EXCEPT

A. septic emboli
B. pulmonary edema
C. aspiration pneumonia
D. pulmonary hypertension
E. pulmonary veno-occlusive disease

40. In the presence of pulmonary emboli, vena caval interruption would NOT be appropriate in a patient who

A. recently underwent excision of a glioblastoma
B. gave birth by vaginal delivery to a term infant three days ago
C. has severe pulmonary hypertension from recurrent pulmonary emboli
D. is receiving warfarin, has prothrombin time of 24 seconds, and shows angiographic proof of recurrence
E. shows multiple peripheral cavitary infiltrates on chest roentgenogram and has a recently diagnosed tubo-ovarian abscess

41. On the chest roentgenogram of a patient with lung cancer, which of the following would suggest squamous cell carcinoma as the most likely histologic type?

A. Pleural effusion
B. Mediastinal adenopathy
C. Cavitation of the primary tumor
D. Post-obstructive lobar collapse
E. Contralateral parenchymal nodules

42. A solitary nodule noted on a routine chest roentgenogram is NOT likely to be due to malignancy if

A. the patient is younger than 30 years of age
B. the nodule is less than 2 cm in diameter
C. a coccidioidin skin test is positive
D. sputum cytologic examinations of three adequate specimens are negative
E. a roentgenogram taken three months ago shows that the nodule was less than one third of its present size

DIRECTIONS: For questions 43 to 86, you are to decide whether EACH choice is true or false. Any combination of answers, from all true to all false, may occur. Mark the answer sheet "T" or "F" in the space provided.

43. The anteroposterior and lateral chest roentgenograms shown below are often seen in patients with which of the following disorders?

A. Emphysema
B. Tracheal stenosis
C. Swyer-James syndrome
D. Acute exacerbation of asthma
E. Bilateral diaphragmatic paralysis

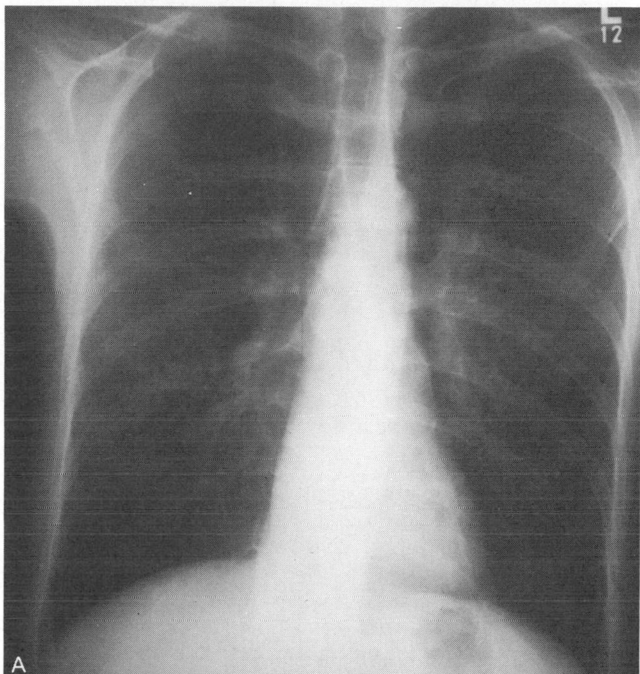

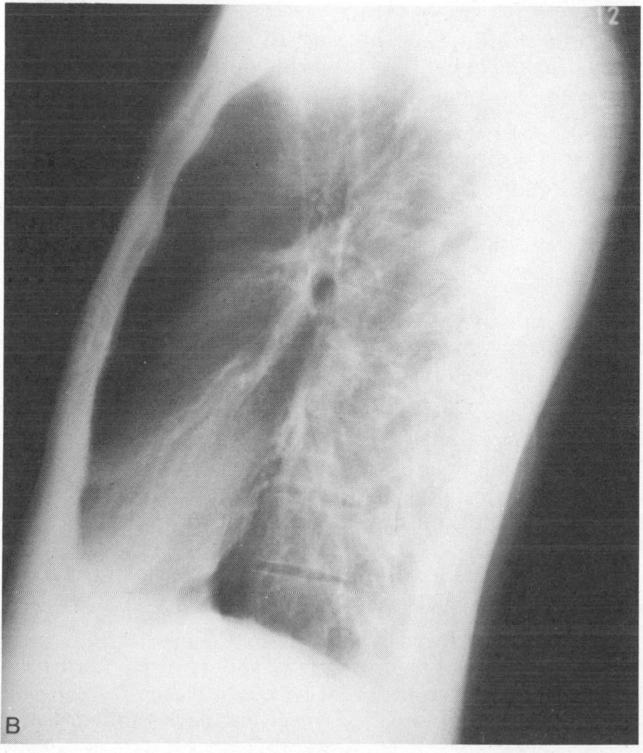

44. In a patient with mediastinal and/or hilar adenopathy on chest roentgenogram, which of the following associated features suggest(s) sarcoidosis as the cause, rather than infection or neoplasm?

A. Pleural effusion
B. Bilaterality of hilar adenopathy
C. Appearance of lung parenchymal infiltrate prior to mediastinal or hilar adenopathy
D. Isolated right paratracheal adenopathy without hilar adenopathy
E. Bronchial compression and distal lobar collapse

45. Elevation of the base of the fingernails is likely to be related to the primary disease in which of the following patients?

A. A 22-year-old man with recurrent pneumonia, chronic productive cough, infertility, and intestinal malabsorption
B. A 28-year-old woman with recurrent bouts of bronchospasm and persistent peripheral eosinophilia
C. A 32-year-old woman with chronic cough productive of copious, sometimes foul-smelling sputum for several years
D. A 44-year-old woman with intense pruritus for three months and painless jaundice for the past month
E. A 52-year-old man with a heavy smoking history and recent onset of cough with trace hemoptysis

46. A 59-year-old man has had cough for the past eight months. The cough is exacerbated by exercise or by forced expiratory maneuvers. His only previous medical problem has been mild glaucoma, which is controlled by timolol maleate ophthalmic solution. Chest roentgenogram and spirometry are normal. Which of the following is/are reasonable to include in the initial evaluation of this patient?

A. Echocardiography
B. Fiberoptic bronchoscopy
C. Gallium scanning of the lung
D. Bronchoprovocation testing with methacholine
E. Empiric trial of inhaled beta-adrenergic agonists

QUESTIONS 47–49

A 19-year-old male student with a lifelong history of asthma developed increasing dyspnea, wheezing, and a cough productive of yellowish sputum 10 days ago, shortly after contracting a "cold." Despite regular use of aminophylline tablets and increasingly frequent use of the isoproterenol cannister, symptoms have worsened to the point that he now has trouble finishing sentences without stopping to inhale. On examination the patient appears apprehensive, diaphoretic, and fatigued. Respirations are 28 per minute, with prolonged expiration and audible wheezing. Blood pressure is 140–115/90 mm Hg; pulse rate is 135 per minute. Examination of the chest reveals poor inspiratory expansion and diffuse, high-pitched wheezing. FEV_1/FVC is 500/1100 ml. Arterial blood studies show P_{O_2}

58 mm Hg, P_{CO_2} 42 mm Hg, and pH 7.38; the chest film shows overinflation with no lung infiltrate. Gram's stain of sputum shows scattered flora.

47. Appropriate therapy includes which of the following?

A. Aminophylline, 500 mg infused intravenously over 30 minutes, followed by continuous infusion of 0.7 mg/kg/hour
B. Methylprednisolone, 50–100 mg intravenously
C. Diazepam, 5–10 mg orally
D. Aerosolized isoproterenol, terbutaline, or metaproterenol
E. Supplemental oxygen by face mask

48. Appropriate therapy is begun. After initial slight improvement, the patient fails to improve further over the next 48 hours. Probable reasons for the failure to improve include

A. inspissation of mucus in the airway lumen
B. abnormally prolonged theophylline half-life owing to undetected liver disease
C. edema and cellular infiltration of the bronchial mucosa
D. the airway obstruction being in part due to coexistent pulmonary emphysema
E. untreated bacterial bronchitis

49. Three weeks later, the patient is at home, and the dyspnea and wheezing have improved markedly. However, to control these symptoms, the patient requires prednisone, 40 mg by mouth each day, as well as metaproterenol by metered dose inhaler and aminophylline tablets. If the dose of prednisone is reduced to less than 30 mg daily, the symptoms recur. The patient has gained 18 pounds and he has suffered from insomnia.

In order to help this patient reduce the dose of oral prednisone required to control the asthmatic symptoms, which of the following alternatives should be considered?

A. Make certain that the patient is using the inhaled metaproterenol optimally
B. Begin administration of metaproterenol by oral tablets
C. Attempt to administer the oral prednisone by an alternate-day regimen
D. Begin administration of inhaled glucocorticoids
E. Initiate therapy with inhaled disodium cromoglycate

50. In workers exposed to asbestos fibers, which of the following about pleural plaques is/are true?

A. They are often bilateral
B. They often cause functional impairment
C. They indicate underlying parenchymal asbestosis
D. They occur *only* after heavy, prolonged exposure
E. They indicate a greater likelihood of mesothelioma than in similarly exposed workers without plaques

51. For which of the following patients is isoniazid chemoprophylaxis indicated?

A. A 6-year-old boy whose father was recently discovered to have active tuberculosis, and who has an 18-mm reactive intermediate-strength PPD skin test and blunting of the left costophrenic sinus
B. A 15-year-old boy, a recent immigrant from Israel, who is discovered on a school survey to have a 10-mm reactive intermediate-strength PPD skin test and a characteristic scar of a previous BCG vaccination on the shoulder
C. A 42-year-old man with alcoholism who has a 12-mm reactive intermediate-strength PPD skin test and who recently underwent hemigastrectomy for peptic ulcer disease
D. A 47-year-old man, discovered on employment examination to have an 8-mm reactive intermediate-strength PPD skin test and a normal chest roentgenogram
E. A 58-year-old woman with a 12-mm reactive intermediate-strength PPD skin test and normal chest roentgenogram who must undergo radiotherapy of the left anterior chest wall for locally recurrent breast carcinoma

52. A 59-year-old man who has smoked two packs of cigarettes daily for 40 years has had swelling in both legs increasing over the past two months. He currently takes no medications. Physical examination shows an obese man with plethoric facies, faint high-pitched expiratory wheezes, distant heart sounds, and pitting edema of both lower extremities. Laboratory data include:

Hematocrit	56%
Arterial blood gases	
pH	7.36
P_{CO_2}	52 mm Hg
P_{O_2}	59 mm Hg
FEV_1/FVC	1.0L/2.8L

Echocardiogram shows right ventricular enlargement and normal left ventricular size and function. Which of the following should be included in the evaluation of this patient's condition?

A. Pulmonary angiography
B. Venography in lower extremities
C. Determination of erythropoietin concentrations in blood and urine
D. Overnight ear oximetry to monitor arterial oxygen saturation during sleep
E. Repeat arterial blood gas determinations after initiating aggressive bronchodilator therapy

53. In a healthy, nonsmoking adult, bronchoalveolar lavage (BAL) is likely to yield fluid containing which of the following?

A. More than 90% macrophages
B. Less than 20% lymphocytes
C. More than 5% polymorphonuclear leukocytes
D. Immunoglobulins IgG, IgM, and IgA in the same proportion as in serum
E. Elastase

54. In patients with obstructive sleep apnea, which of the following factors is likely to worsen the severity of the nocturnal apneic episodes?

A. Weight loss
B. Allergic rhinitis
C. Theophylline administration
D. Nocturnal oxygen administration
E. Alcohol consumption before bedtime

55. An increased value of diffusing capacity for carbon monoxide may be observed in which of these patients?

A. A 19-year-old woman with a heart murmur since birth. Electrocardiogram shows atrial fibrillation and rsR′ in the right precordial leads
B. An asymptomatic 21-year-old black woman. Chest

roentgenogram shows bilateral hilar adenopathy and reticulonodular infiltrates

C. A 29-year-old woman with Raynaud's phenomenon. Chest roentgenogram shows enlargement of the right ventricle and central pulmonary arteries bilaterally

D. A 59-year-old man with glomerulonephritis and hemoptysis. Chest roentgenogram shows diffuse alveolar infiltrates

E. A 65-year-old man recovering from hand surgery. He inadvertently receives 12 liters of intravenous saline over a two-day period

QUESTIONS 56–57

A 49-year-old man has had difficulty swallowing solids and liquids for the past year and has regurgitated undigested food for the past two months. Barium swallow shows dilation of the esophagus with smooth tapering to a distal "beak-like" obstruction. Three days after the barium swallow, the patient develops fever and cough productive of thick, foul-smelling sputum. Chest roentgenogram is shown below.

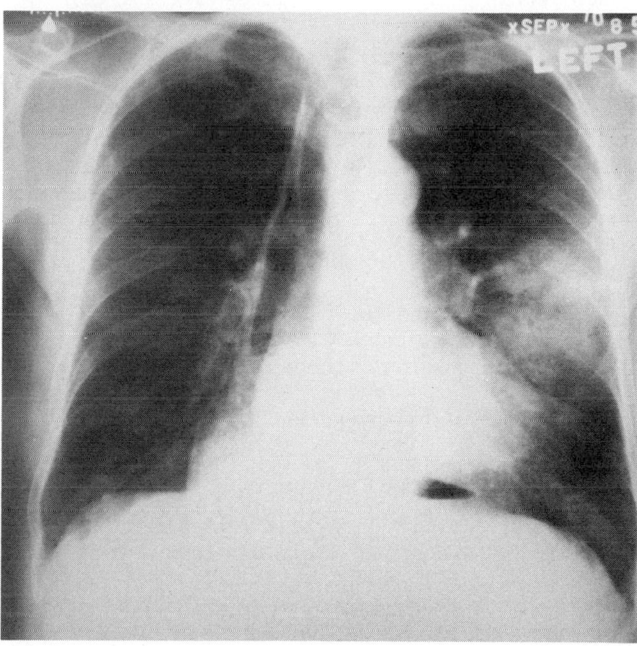

56. Immediate management of this patient's condition should include

A. antibiotics
B. glucocorticoids
C. avoidance of narcotic sedatives
D. elevation of the head of the bed during sleep
E. surgical section of the lower esophageal sphincter (Heller procedure)

57. This patient is at increased risk for the development of which of the following other pulmonary problems?

A. Empyema
B. Lung abscess
C. Nocturnal asthma
D. Acute respiratory failure
E. Chronic interstitial lung disease

58. Which of the following statements is/are applicable to patients with cystic fibrosis?

A. About 10% of patients live to age 20
B. Genetic transmission is autosomal recessive
C. Family members who carry the gene are at risk for developing mild chronic bronchitis
D. *Pseudomonas cepacia* is the organism most frequently isolated from sputum
E. Nearly all adolescent or adult patients have associated pancreatic insufficiency

QUESTIONS 59–61

A 65-year-old woman is released from the hospital two weeks after a cholecystectomy; recovery was uneventful. On the way home from the hospital, she has shortness of breath and right pleuritic chest pain, and her family drives her to the emergency room, where you are called to evaluate the problem. On physical examination, the patient is apprehensive. Respiratory rate is 22 per minute and pulse rate is 108 per minute; vital signs are otherwise normal. The surgical scar is clean, and the chest, heart, and extremities are all normal on examination. Laboratory studies include:

Hematocrit	36%
White blood cell count	11,200 (normal differential)
Arterial blood gases	
pH	7.47
P_{CO_2}	28 mm Hg
P_{O_2}	81 mm Hg

Electrocardiogram shows sinus tachycardia but is otherwise normal. Chest roentgenogram is normal.

59. Which of the following steps should be taken next?

A. Begin empiric heparin therapy
B. Perform pulmonary angiography
C. Perform impedance plethysmography
D. Perform lower extremity venography
E. Obtain ventilation and perfusion lung scans

60. As part of her initial evaluation, you choose to send the patient for ventilation and perfusion lung scans. The scans show a reduction in perfusion to a segment of the right lower lobe; ventilation is reduced in the same area. Which steps should be taken next?

A. Administer pulmonary vasodilators
B. Perform pulmonary angiography
C. Administer inhaled beta-adrenergic agonists
D. Perform pulmonary function tests
E. Continue heparin and monitor the patient's coagulation parameters carefully

61. The diagnostic study or studies selected by you in the previous question is/are completely normal. However, during the two-hour period during which these procedures have been performed, the patient's clinical status has changed. She now has right pleuritic chest pain and cough productive of purulent sputum; temperature has increased to 103°F. Which of the following steps should be taken now?

A. Admit the patient to the hospital
B. Perform fiberoptic bronchoscopy
C. Obtain blood cultures
D. Prepare to begin streptokinase
E. Obtain a specimen of sputum for Gram's stain

62. In which of the following settings is amphotericin therapy indicated, either alone or in combination with another drug or procedure?

A. Coccidioidal meningitis
B. Chronic cavitary histoplasmosis
C. Cryptococci shown on biopsy of a solitary pulmonary nodule in an asymptomatic patient
D. Disseminated candidiasis in a patient who has recently undergone aortic valve replacement
E. Aspergillosis of the lung in a patient undergoing chemotherapy for acute myelocytic leukemia

63. Arterial blood studies showing Po_2 of 65 mm Hg, Pco_2 of 32 mm Hg, and pH of 7.48 would be expected in which of the following patients?

A. An 18-year-old woman with an acute exacerbation of chronic asthma
B. A 19-year-old male student who reports sudden onset of dyspnea, circumoral numbness, and paresthesias on the eve of a final examination
C. A 22-year-old woman who has dyspnea 48 hours after normal delivery of healthy twins
D. A 45-year-old woman with chronic rheumatoid arthritis and diffuse increase in interstitial markings on chest roentgenogram
E. A 49-year-old man with recent myocardial infarction and basilar rales

64. Which of the following statements regarding the treatment of sputum-positive active tuberculosis is/are true?

A. Treatment with isoniazid and ethambutol for nine months is appropriate
B. At least three effective antituberculous drugs should be used pending results of sensitivity studies
C. The patient should be kept in hospital isolation on chemotherapy until sputum smears become negative
D. Annual chest roentgenograms should be obtained for at least 10 years after completion of chemotherapy
E. Household contacts should be treated with isoniazid only if their tuberculin skin tests are positive

65. Which of the following statements is/are likely to characterize the disorder of the patient whose chest roentgenogram is shown above right.

A. The condition, commonly of congenital origin, is often detected in childhood
B. An association with cigarette smoking, chronic bronchitis, and emphysema is frequently noted
C. Serum concentrations of trypsin inhibitory capacity are markedly depressed
D. Total lung capacity, measured by plethysmography, is 12.5 liters, but by inert gas dilution only 5.0 liters
E. Surgical resection may benefit the patient by relieving compression of the lung parenchyma at the bases

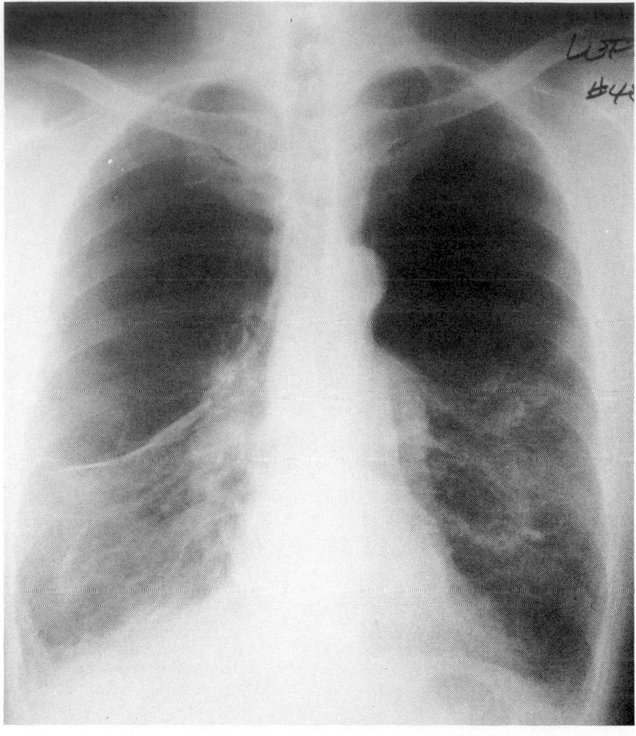

66. A 45-year-old man has dyspnea on exertion. During exercise on a bicycle ergometer, the patient's arterial Po_2, measured via an indwelling radial arterial line, decreases from 68 mm Hg at rest to 46 mm Hg at maximal exercise. Which of the following disorders is/are consistent with these findings?

A. Bronchiectasis
B. Chronic bronchitis
C. Recurrent pulmonary emboli
D. Pulmonary arteriovenous fistulae
E. Chronic use of intravenous heroin with associated pulmonary hypertension

67. The flow-volume curve pictured below would be expected in which of the following patients?

A. A 21-year-old woman with a three-month history of joint pains, hematuria, and recurrent pleuritic chest pain
B. A 28-year-old man with episodic wheezing and dyspnea
C. A 36-year-old woman with loss of vascular markings over both bases of chest roentgenogram and

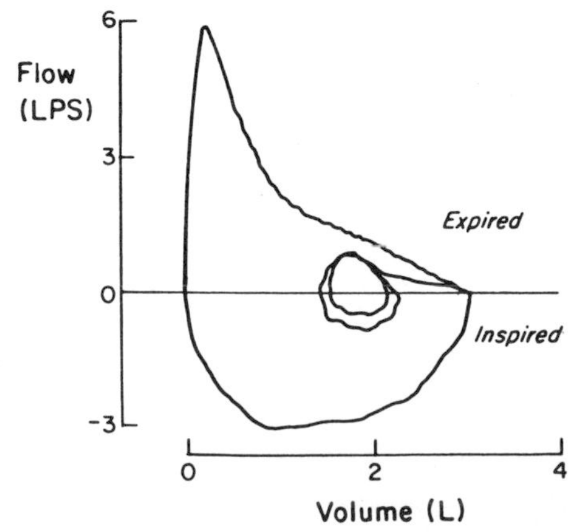

low $alpha_1$-globulin peaks on serum protein electrophoresis
D. A 38-year-old male laborer with episodic chest pain and recent onset of dyspnea two weeks after sustaining soft tissue injury of the right thigh
E. A 58-year-old foundry worker with a 50 pack-year smoking history who has dyspnea on exertion and a chronic productive cough

68. A 42-year-old woman who has smoked a pack of cigarettes daily for 20 years has a cough productive of mucoid sputum on awakening each morning. When the patient has viral upper respiratory infections, the sputum increases in volume and appears purulent. Which of the following statements is/are true?

A. Culture of sputum obtained by transtracheal aspiration probably would *not* yield bacterial organism on culture
B. Bronchography would probably reveal enlarged mucous gland ducts
C. Daily use of a broad-spectrum antibiotic is likely to reduce the frequency of bouts of purulent sputum
D. Cough and sputum production will probably improve if the patient stops smoking
E. Progressive respiratory insufficiency is likely to develop if the patient continues smoking

69. The half-life of theophylline is prolonged by which of the following?

A. Cimetidine
B. Corticosteroids
C. Oral contraceptive agents
D. Oral beta-adrenergic agents
E. Cigarette smoking

70. Which of the following laboratory abnormalities is/are likely to be found in patients with sarcoidosis?

A. Depressed serum 1,25-dihydroxy vitamin D_3
B. Elevated serum angiotensin-converting enzyme activity
C. Elevated urinary calcium
D. Elevated serum gamma globulin
E. Elevated serum acid phosphatase

71. Which of the following patients is/are likely to develop bronchiectasis?

A. A 19-year-old woman with a chloride concentration of 100 mEq/liter in sweat
B. A 30-year-old homosexual man with diffuse pulmonary infiltrates that resolve after a 14-day course of trimethoprim-sulfamethoxazole
C. A 32-year-old man with fever, chills, dense left lower consolidation on chest roentgenogram, and paired bullet-shaped gram-positive cocci in sputum
D. A 42-year-old asthmatic woman with a dual response to an *Aspergillus* skin test and recurrent episodes of wheezing associated with localized pulmonary infiltrates
E. A 62-year-old man with encasement and narrowing of the bronchus intermedius by calcified lymph nodes

72. Increasing the fraction of inspired air that is oxygen (FIO_2) to 0.40 would be expected to correct the hypoxemia of which of the following?

A. Far-advanced pulmonary emphysema
B. Large intrapulmonary arteriovenous malformation
C. Pulmonary hypertension in an adult with an uncorrected atrial septal defect
D. Acute respiratory failure occurring two days after severe trauma with multiple fractures
E. Acute exacerbation of chronic bronchitis and cor pulmonale following a viral upper respiratory infection

73. Which of the following tests will help in distinguishing a restrictive from an obstructive ventilatory defect?

A. Total lung capacity
B. FEV_1/FVC ratio
C. Slope of phase III in the closing volume maneuver
D. Vital capacity
E. Residual volume

74. A 19-year-old man develops acute appendicitis. Past medical history is notable for repeated episodes of wheezing when petting dogs or cats. Which of the following may precipitate bronchospasm in this patient during and after appendectomy?

A. Endotracheal intubation
B. Maintenance of general anesthesia with halothane
C. Administration of neostigmine to reverse paralysis induced by pancuronium
D. Humidification of the airways with nebulized distilled water
E. Postoperative orotracheal suctioning

75. A 28-year-old woman with a history of nasal polyps has episodes of dyspnea, chest tightness, and shortness of breath that have recently begun to occur whenever she takes aspirin. She should be advised to avoid the use of medications containing

A. codeine
B. indomethacin
C. sodium salicylate
D. acetaminophen
E. H_2-receptor–blocking antihistamines (e.g., cimetidine)

76. Which of the following disorders is/are suggestive of a pulmonary complication of rheumatoid arthritis?

A. Scattered parenchymal nodules
B. Interstitial pulmonary fibrosis
C. Recurrent wheezing, dyspnea, and chest tightness
D. Severe irreversible airway obstruction with hyperinflation
E. Inspiratory stridor following a viral upper respiratory infection

77. A 22-year-old white man visits your office because of the recent onset of recurrent episodes of wheezing. You decide to begin the patient on metaproterenol administered by a metered-dose inhaler. In discussing this medication with the patient, you should

A. ask the patient to have the pharmacist show him the proper technique for using the metered-dose inhaler
B. describe possible side effects, including skeletal muscle tremor and palpitations

C. tell him that the likelihood of these side effects is about the same when metaproterenol is taken by mouth or by inhalation
D. point out that metaproterenol is preferred over albuterol because of its greater $beta_2$-adrenergic selectivity
E. point out that use of the inhaled medication may be stopped or reduced if the patient ever receives a course of corticosteroids for treatment of an exacerbation of the asthma

78. In the evaluation of a patient with sudden onset of dyspnea, which of the following findings would suggest that pulmonary thromboembolism is NOT the cause?

A. Remission of dyspnea within 15–20 minutes
B. Acute onset of diffuse expiratory wheezes
C. Complete lack of other symptoms; normal physical examination
D. Two-week history of right-sided pleuritic chest pain, increasing progressively, prior to onset of dyspnea
E. Acute increase in Pco_2 and reciprocal decrease in Po_2 since prior arterial blood gas determination

79. Which of the following is/are included among signs of unusual severity in an asthmatic attack?

A. Sputum eosinophilia
B. Pco_2 of 40 mm Hg
C. FEV_1 under 1.0 liter
D. Pulsus paradoxicus of 40 mm Hg
E. Observed residual volume 200% of predicted

80. Which of the following factors INCREASE the risk of severe hemorrhage in patients treated with heparin for pulmonary thromboembolism?

A. Use of a "bolus" of heparin to initiate its anticoagulant effect
B. Concurrent administration of warfarin
C. Maintenance of activated partial thromboplastin time at four times control
D. Maintenance of anticoagulation by intermittent administration every six hours
E. Treatment of pain with nonsteroidal anti-inflammatory agents

QUESTIONS 81–84

A confused 55-year-old woman is brought by ambulance to the emergency room. Her husband tells you that she has a 50 pack-year smoking history, a chronic cough, and a four-year history of progressive dyspnea on exertion, especially after upper respiratory infections. She recently complained to her husband of a 10-pound weight gain over her usual weight of 150 pounds. She contracted a "cold" one week ago and has had progressive cough, dyspnea, and headache. When she entered the ambulance one hour ago, she was oriented and responsive.

The patient appears flushed and disoriented. Blood pressure is 160/85 mm Hg; pulse rate is 106 per minute and bounding; respirations are 14 per minute. She is afebrile. Funduscopic examination reveals mild papilledema; chest expansion is poor, and there are scattered rhonchi on inspiration with a prolonged expiratory phase. Neck veins are distended to the jaw; there is a left parasternal lift but no cardiac murmurs or gallops. The liver is enlarged, and there is pitting ankle edema. Laboratory data include:

Hemoglobin	16.0 g/dl
Hematocrit	55%
White blood cell count	12,800 cells/mm^3
Serum sodium	134 mEq/L
Serum chloride	81 mEq/L
Serum potassium	6.1 mEq/L
Serum bicarbonate	34 mEq/L
Arterial blood gases:	
Po_2	105 mm Hg
Pco_2	95 mm Hg
pH	7.25

Electrocardiogram shows an axis of 115 degrees with a persistent S wave in V_5–V_6. The chest roentgenogram shows enlargement of the main pulmonary arteries bilaterally. Gram's stain of sputum shows numerous PMN's and mixed bacterial flora.

81. The arterial blood gases indicate

A. that the patient should be immediately switched to breathing room air, so that the hypoxic drive to breathe will be restored
B. that the patient was given supplemental oxygen in the ambulance
C. that carbonic anhydrase should be given to eliminate excess bicarbonate
D. alveolar hypoventilation of more than 3–5 days' duration
E. probable lactic acidosis

82. Initial therapy should include

A. a loading dose of 500 mg of aminophylline followed by a constant infusion of 70 mg/hour
B. digoxin, 0.5 mg intravenously
C. an oral cation-exchange resin to correct hyperkalemia
D. administration of a nebulized bronchodilator aerosol (metaproterenol, terbutaline)
E. sedation and bed rest

83. The abnormal appearance of the pulmonary artery on the chest roentgenogram and the right axis deviation on the electrocardiogram should be treated with

A. heparin, until perfusion lung scan, angiogram, or both exclude acute pulmonary embolization
B. morphine sulfate to reduce cardiac preload
C. hydralazine or diazoxide to reduce pulmonary vascular resistance
D. phlebotomy of 2 units or more to reduce the hematocrit to less than 50%
E. measures to increase alveolar ventilation and to maintain arterial Po_2 over 55 mm Hg

84. Despite appropriate management, the patient's condition deteriorates to the point that mechanical ventilatory assistance is initiated. Ventilatory treatment should include

A. 10–15 cm of positive end-expiratory pressure (PEEP)
B. an FIo_2 adequate to maintain arterial oxygen saturation in the range of 90–95%
C. careful avoidance of overinflation of the tube's cuff
D. adjusting tidal volume and rate to maintain arterial Pco_2 at approximately 50–55 mm Hg
E. sterility of all gas delivery circuits

85. Interstitial lung disease (ILD) due to an underlying systemic collagen vascular disease can be distinguished from idiopathic ILD by which of the following?

A. Involvement of extrapulmonary organs
B. The presence of circulating immune complexes
C. The presence of antinuclear antibody in the serum
D. The lack of uptake of gallium-67 by the lung parenchyma
E. The predominance of lymphocytes and macrophages in the cellular infiltrate of alveolar tissue on open lung biopsy

86. In a patient with suspected lung cancer, the presence of which of the following would favor small-cell carcinoma rather than other histologic types?

A. Horner's syndrome
B. Eaton-Lambert syndrome
C. Superior vena cava syndrome
D. Favorable response to chemotherapy
E. Inappropriate secretion of antidiuretic hormone

DIRECTIONS: Questions 87 to 139 are matching questions. For each numbered item, choose the most likely associated lettered item from those provided. Use each lettered item ONLY ONCE.

QUESTIONS 87–91

For each description of dyspnea below, select the most likely general pathophysiologic mechanism of the disorder (A–E).

A. Bronchospasm
B. Psychogenic cause
C. Diaphragmatic paralysis
D. Increased left atrial pressure
E. Inflammatory infiltration of the interstitium of the lung

87. Occurs immediately after lying down

88. Occurs 60–120 minutes after onset of sleep

89. Occurs five minutes after cessation of exercise

90. Improves or remains unchanged during exercise

91. Worsens in the late afternoon or evening and improves over the weekend

QUESTIONS 92–96

For each patient described below, select the most likely form of bronchogenic carcinoma (A–E).

A. Adenocarcinoma
B. Small-cell carcinoma
C. Large-cell carcinoma
D. Squamous cell carcinoma
E. Bronchioloalveolar cell carcinoma

92. A 58-year-old man with a heavy smoking history who has hemoptysis, a 4-cm mass in the superior segment of the right lower lobe, and ipsilateral hilar adenopathy

93. A 61-year-old man with a heavy smoking history who has a large right hilar mass, mediastinal widening, anemia, and abnormal liver function tests

94. A 66-year-old woman who has progressive systemic sclerosis, diffuse interstitial fibrosis, and multiple enlarging infiltrates through both lung fields

95. A 66-year-old woman with recent development of grand mal seizures who has a 2.5-cm nodule in the periphery of the left upper lobe

96. A 68-year-old man with a heavy smoking history who has a 4-cm wide, bulky mass in the periphery of the left lower lobe

QUESTIONS 97–101

For each patient described below, select the most appropriate pleural fluid analysis (A–E).

	WBC's (cells/mm^3)	Protein (g/dl)	Amylase (units/dl)	Glucose (mg/dl)	Triglycerides (mg/dl)
A.	1,200	4.2	150	5	18
B.	15,000	6.8	1258	25	25
C.	550	2.2	125	110	16
D.	62,000	5.9	115	36	59
E.	10,100	3.2	96	122	225

97. A 32-year-old woman with non-Hodgkin's lymphoma, progressively increasing mediastinal adenopathy, and large left pleural effusion

98. A 32-year-old alcoholic woman with fever, weight loss, vague right-sided chest pain, and large right pleural effusion

99. A 45-year-old alcoholic man with epigastric pain, fever, and large left pleural effusion two hours after esophageal sclerotherapy for variceal bleeding

100. A 62-year-old man with longstanding rheumatoid arthritis and a large right pleural effusion

101. A 68-year-old man with longstanding hypertension, cardiomegaly, and bilateral pleural effusions

QUESTIONS 102–106

Match each of the following laboratory abnormalities (A–E) with the form of interstitial lung disease with which it is associated.

A. Positive Shirmer test
B. Iron-deficiency anemia
C. Langerhans' cells in bronchoalveolar lavage
D. Anti-alveolar basement membrane antibodies in serum
E. Elevated concentrations of triglycerides in pleural fluid

102. Goodpasture's syndrome

103. Eosinophilic granuloma

104. Lymphangioleiomyomatosis

105. Idiopathic pulmonary hemosiderosis

106. Lymphocytic interstitial pneumonitis

QUESTIONS 107–111

For each description below, select the most appropriate antiasthmatic medication (A–E).

A. Epinephrine
B. Methylxanthines
C. Glucocorticoids
D. Ipratropium bromide
E. Disodium cromoglycate

107. Onset of effect may require six hours

108. Use should never be initiated during an acute attack

109. Use should be avoided in patients with severe systemic hypertension

110. Use should be avoided in patients with glaucoma or benign prostatic hypertrophy

111. Standard maintenance should be reduced in patients with congestive heart failure

QUESTIONS 112–116

For each patient described in the following questions, select the most appropriate arterial blood gas values (A–E).

	pH	P_{CO_2} (mm Hg)	P_{O_2} (mm Hg)
A.	7.21	53	74
B.	7.36	55	64
C.	7.41	32	65
D.	7.48	32	100
E.	7.61	29	80

112. A 28-year-old man who reports dyspnea after mild exertion. Since sustaining a femural fracture one year ago, he has noted episodes of transient dyspnea associated with palpitations and light-headedness. Perfusion lung scan shows multiple segmental defects.

113. A 29-year-old male medical student who consents to having a radial arterial puncture performed by another student for practice. Five attempts are required before an arterial sample is obtained.

114. A 39-year-old woman who is brought to the emergency room after ingestion of 30 capsules of phenobarbital. The patient is obtunded and has infrequent respiratory movements.

115. A 40-year-old man, a 255-pound chronic smoker, reports mild shortness of breath that has gradually worsened over the past 10 days in association with an upper respiratory tract infection. Forced expiratory volume in one second is 750 ml.

116. The same patient described in Question 115 continues to deteriorate; endotracheal intubation and mechanical ventilation of the lungs are required. Initial ventilator settings are: tidal volume—1250 ml; respiratory rate—32.

QUESTIONS 117–121

For each patient described below, select the most likely form of chronic obstructive pulmonary disease (A–E).

A. Cystic fibrosis
B. Extrinsic asthma
C. Chronic bronchitis
D. Immotile cilia syndrome
E. $Alpha_1$-antitrypsin deficiency

117. A 22-year-old man with mild diabetes mellitus, who has daily cough productive of one-half cup thick sputum

118. A 25-year-old woman with recurrent episodes of shortness of breath and cough shortly after moving into a new apartment

119. A 26-year-old man with chronic productive cough for 10 years, recurrent sinusitis, and infertility

120. A 42-year-old male cigarette smoker with dyspnea and nonproductive cough associated with a history of recurrent pneumothoraces and chronic hepatitis

121. A 56-year-old nonsmoking male miner with a daily chronic productive cough during the winter months for the past four years

QUESTIONS 122–126

For each of the patients described below, select the most likely cutaneous or mucosal lesion (A–E).

A. Multiple petechiae in both axillae
B. Draining sinus on lateral chest wall
C. Purplish submucosal lesion on the hard palate
D. Exuberant violaceous nodules over the nose and malar areas
E. Black pigmented nodules along folds of skin in axillary and perineal areas

122. A 24-year-old homosexual man with fever, weight loss, and diffuse alveolar infiltrates on chest roentgenogram

123. A 31-year-old man with confusion and dyspnea 24 hours after fracturing his femur at a ski resort

124. A 52-year-old black woman with hypercalcemia and interstitial fibrosis of the lung

125. A 69-year-old man with confusion, fever, dense consolidation with cavitation in the right lower lobe

126. A 74-year-old man with hemoptysis and a right hilar mass on chest roentgenogram

QUESTIONS 127–130

For each toxic manifestation described, select the drug (A–D) most likely to be responsible.

A. Streptomycin
B. Isoniazid
C. Rifampin
D. Ethambutol

127. Dizziness, nausea, and hearing impairment

128. Petechial rash over both lower extremities

129. Loss of visual acuity

130. SGOT elevation

QUESTIONS 131–135

For each of the conditions described below, select the drug (A–E) most likely to be responsible.

A. Busulfan
B. Prednisone
C. Hydralazine
D. Methysergide
E. Nitrofurantoin

131. Mediastinal widening

132. Parenchymal and pleural fibrosis

133. Fever, pleuritic pain, pleural effusion

134. Fever, cough, pulmonary infiltrates, eosinophilia

135. Fever, dyspnea, diffuse pulmonary infiltrates, type II cell hyperplasia

QUESTIONS 136–139

For each of the following extrapulmonary manifestations, select the associated pulmonary neoplasm (A–D).

A. Adenocarcinoma
B. Squamous cell carcinoma
C. Small-cell carcinoma
D. Large-cell anaplastic carcinoma

136. Hypokalemia

137. Gynecomastia

138. Hypercalcemia

139. Marantic endocarditis

PART 2

RESPIRATORY DISEASE

ANSWERS

1.(C) The chest roentgenogram shows bilateral hilar and right paratracheal adenopathy. These findings, in a young black patient with erythema nodosum, indicate that the single most likely diagnosis is sarcoidosis. *(Cecil, Ch. 69)*

2.(B) Although the chest roentgenographic findings and erythema nodosum are suggestive of the diagnosis of sarcoidosis, the fever and weight loss raise the possibility of other diagnoses, such as Hodgkin's disease or tuberculosis. Thus, it is important in such a patient to obtain biopsies of tissue to look for noncaseating granulomas and to exclude lymphoma or infections. In general, one should select sites for biopsy which appear most obviously involved. In this patient, therefore, fiberoptic bronchoscopy or mediastinoscopy would be the preferred diagnostic approach. Liver or conjunctival biopsy should be performed only when those organs clearly are involved clinically. The use of "blind" biopsy procedures should be discouraged. The skin lesion, erythema nodosum, should not be biopsied, because the histopathology of this lesion is a nonspecific vasculitis. Gallium scanning is not useful as a diagnostic procedure in patients with suspected sarcoidosis but may be helpful in following the course of the disease. *(Cecil, Ch. 69)*

3.(D) Sarcoidosis is a systemic disease. Thus, although the lungs are the organ involved most frequently, patients with pulmonary sarcoidosis may develop a variety of extrapulmonary abnormalities. These include nephrolithiasis, conduction abnormalities of the heart, pancytopenia from enlargement of the spleen, and chronic meningitis. For unclear reasons, the pancreas is spared in sarcoidosis, and diabetes mellitus is not a recognized complication of the disease. *(Cecil, Ch. 69)*

4.(A) Approximately 80% of patients with stage I pulmonary sarcoidosis (i.e., with hilar and paratracheal adenopathy only on chest roentgenogram) will experience complete remission within two years. Radiotherapy is not appropriate treatment for sarcoidosis. Fibrosis of the lung occurs in only 5–10% of patients with pulmonary sarcoidosis. *(Cecil, Ch. 69)*

5.(E) The major reason for the early use of heparin in patients with pulmonary thromboemboli is to prevent growth of clot that already is present in the circulation. By preventing further development of clot in the pulmonary circulation, heparin also *may* prevent the subsequent release of bronchoactive mediators; however, this potential effect is not the major reason for heparin's use. Heparin does not lyse existing clot, dilate pulmonary vasculature, or eliminate the source of further emboli. *(Cecil, Ch. 67; Raskob and Hull)*

6.(B) Diffusing capacity for carbon monoxide will be reduced in the emphysematous, but not the bronchitic, type of COPD. Residual volume will be increased in either type, and therefore the increased value shown is not a helpful distinguishing feature. The bronchitic type is much more commonly associated with increased arterial P_{CO_2} and enlarged pulmonary arteries than the emphysematous type. A markedly reduced transpulmonary pressure at total lung capacity indicates the loss of elastic recoil of the lung. This abnormality is characteristic of the emphysematous, but not the bronchitic, type of COPD. *(Cecil, Ch. 61)*

7.(B) The history and chest roentgenogram are typical of a superior sulcus, or Pancoast's, tumor of the right lung. These tumors commonly invade the brachial plexus, resulting in a C7–T2 neuropathy in the arm. In small-cell carcinoma of the lung, the primary tumor usually is a central pulmonary mass, not a peripheral or pleural mass. The apical lesions of pulmonary tuberculosis almost never cause brachial neuropathy. Brachial plexus injury is not a common complication of coronary artery bypass surgery. Mesotheliomas usually are located on the lateral or diaphragmatic pleura. *(Cecil, Ch. 70)*

8.(D) Among all patients with hemoptysis, bronchiectasis is the cause in 20–30%. In a patient with hemoptysis associated with scarring of the lung from old tuberculosis and with longstanding chronic sputum production, by far the most likely cause of the hemoptysis is post-tuberculous bronchiectasis. Although such a patient should be evaluated carefully for active tuberculous infection and for bronchogenic carcinoma, these diagnoses are somewhat less likely. The fact that the expectorated blood is mixed with sputum makes an upper gastrointestinal source of the blood unlikely, although this site as well as the nose always should be considered as source of "coughed blood." Like bronchiectasis, broncholithiasis is a sequela of pulmonary tuberculosis which may cause hemoptysis. However, broncholithiasis is much less common than bronchiectasis in this setting. *(Cecil, Chs. 58 and 66)*

9.(E) The tomogram shows a round intracavitary mass, and its appearance is typical of an aspergilloma. Aspergillomas develop when the fungus *Aspergillus* colonizes preexisting cavities in the lung. These cavities usually have been caused by tuberculosis, sarcoidosis, or bullous emphysema. The finding of elevated *Aspergillus* precipitins in serum, which occurs in all patients with aspergilloma, will help to establish the diagnosis. Hemoptysis occurs in 60–70% of patients with aspergilloma and usually subsides spontaneously. Because an occasional patient with aspergilloma progresses to develop massive, life-threatening hemoptysis, spirometry should be obtained in this patient in order to assess the pulmonary reserve for possible future lung resection. He should be re-evaluated at this point for bronchogenic carcinoma and for active tuberculosis by fiberoptic bronchoscopy and sputum examinations. The bronchoscopy should be performed shortly after the patient's presentation to be certain that the site of current bleeding conforms to the location of the new abnormality on chest roentgenogram. Although intracavitary administration of amphotericin occasionally lyses aspergillomas, intravenous administration of this toxic drug does *not* help. *(Cecil, Chs. 58 and 376)*

10.(E) In a patient with massive hemoptysis, the most pressing danger is drowning from spread of blood throughout the lungs. Therefore, immediate measures should be directed toward helping the patient to clear the blood from the affected site and to protect the unaffected lung. Because the most likely site of bleeding in the patient described is the right upper lobe, the patient should be placed in the decubitus position with the right side down to minimize spillage into the left side. Suctioning the oropharynx and trachea may help the patient clear the blood from the airways when bleeding is especially brisk. High-dose sedatives should be avoided because they may suppress the patient's ability to cough. In the setting of massive hemoptysis, bronchoscopic examination of the airways always should be performed to establish the site, or at least the side, of the blood's origin. Even this magnitude of hemoptysis frequently will subside spontaneously. However, a thoracic surgeon always should be part of the management team from the beginning because lung resection may be necessary. *(Cecil, Ch. 58)*

11.(C) The findings on the initial chest roentgenogram are diffuse interstitial infiltrates that are most pronounced in the peripheral lung fields. These findings, as well as their very rapid resolution after administration of corticosteroids, are characteristic of chronic eosinophilic pneumonia. Eosinophilia and pulmonary infiltrates may occur in allergic bronchopulmonary aspergillosis, but symptoms of asthmatic bronchospasm are predominant in this disorder, and the roentgenographic infiltrates are central in location rather than peripheral. Very rapid responses to corticosteroids are unusual in lymphocytic interstitial pneumonitis, pulmonary sarcoidosis, and eosinophilic granuloma. *(Cecil, Ch. 63; Lynch and Flint)*

12.(C) Both the history of a seizure disorder and the chest roentgenographic finding of a cavitary lesion make the most likely diagnosis post-aspiration bacterial lung abscess. Lung abscesses often occur after an episode of aspiration of gastric contents. Such an episode presumably impairs normal defense mechanisms in the lung and allows for the development of a superimposed bacterial infection. Factors predisposing to aspiration include seizures, drug abuse, alcoholism, esophageal or gastric disorders, and neurologic disorders that impair normal mechanisms of swallowing. Thus, in the patient described, the finding that he had experienced a grand mal seizure in recent weeks would add greatly to the likelihood that the roentgenographic abnormality is lung abscess developing after an episode of aspiration. Although tuberculosis may cause an isolated cavity in the lung, this roentgenographic abnormality is not the most common one in pulmonary tuberculosis. Eliciting a history of recent foreign travel may be important, because parasites such as *Entamoeba histolytica* may cause isolated cavities in the lung. However, parasitic diseases are rare causes of lung abscess in the United States. Hemoptysis and pleuritic chest pain are noted occasionally by patients with lung abscess, but the presence of these symptoms is nonspecific and does not help in establishing the cause of the abscess. *(Cecil, Ch. 64)*

13.(C) In patients with post-aspiration bacterial lung abscess, the origins of the bacteria in the abscess are the periodontal crevices. These bacteria, when aspirated into the lung, are the inoculum. For this reason post-aspiration bacterial lung abscess is uncommon in an edentulous patient. Lung abscess in an edentulous elderly man is more likely related to an underlying bronchial obstruction, such as endobronchial neoplasm, than to aspiration. Examination of the airways by fiberoptic bronchoscopy is therefore appropriate in this setting. All the other physical findings described—fever, orthostatic changes in blood pressure, amphoric breath sounds, and diffuse wheezing—may occur in patients with lung abscess of any etiology. None of these findings, however, is an indication for bronchoscopic examination of the airways. *(Cecil, Ch. 64)*

14.(D) The slope of phase III in the closing volume maneuver is an exceedingly sensitive test of the distribution of ventilation. Whenever a disease process involves the lung parenchyma or airways diffusely or when the mainstem bronchi are involved unevenly, abnormalities of distribution of ventilation will occur. Thus the slope of phase III will be abnormal in unilateral obstruction of a mainstem bronchus, in asthmatic bronchospasm, in mild chronic bronchitis, or in asbestosis. In tracheal obstruction, uniformity of the distribution of ventilation is preserved, and the slope of phase III will be normal. *(Cecil, Ch. 59)*

15.(D) Only a minority of cigarette smokers develop clinically significant COPD. Recent evidence has established that passive inhalation of cigarette smoke clearly increases the risk for lung cancer. The fact that large numbers of women began smoking in the 1950's and that the prevalence of lung cancer in women increased markedly in the late 1970's is an example of the 20-year lag that apparently exists between onset of heavy cigarette use and increased risk of lung cancer. The risk of lung cancer in cigarette smokers clearly is "dose-dependent"; hence, in evaluating a pulmonary condition in a cigarette smoker, it is important to establish what number of packs were smoked for what number of years. The use of cigarettes accelerates the decline of lung function in alpha$_1$-antitrypsin deficiency, probably by further reducing antiprotease defense mechanisms in the lung. *(Cecil, Chs. 61 and 70)*

16.(A) In pressure-cycled ventilators, the changeover from the inspiratory to the expiratory phase occurs when inspiratory pressure reaches a set value. The disadvantage of these ventilators is that the delivered minute volume of ventilation will change if resistance or compliance in the respiratory system changes. In general, therefore, pressure-cycled ventilators should not be used in patients who have profound abnormalities of the airways or lungs. By contrast, in patients with neurogenic respiratory failure, in whom the airways and lungs are relatively normal, it is reasonable to use pressure-cycled ventilators. For these reasons, volume-cycled ventilators are used most commonly. *(Cecil, Ch. 73)*

17.(D) The risk of acquired immunodeficiency syndrome (AIDS) is increased in any patient receiving blood products, as in patients requiring transfusions during surgery or in hemophiliacs. Risk is also increased in intravenous drug users, as well as in those with multiple sexual contacts with female prostitutes in New York City. At the present time, the presence of AIDS in a family member is not known to increase risk. *(Cecil, Ch. 346)*

18.(C) The described symptoms are characteristic of myasthenia gravis, and the chest roentgenogram shows an anterior mediastinal mass. In this setting, the most likely cause of the mass is thymoma. *(Cecil, Chs. 71 and 518)*

19.(E) In patients with unilateral pleural effusions and positive PPD skin tests, it is imperative to evaluate the possibility of pleural tuberculosis. The most effective way of establishing the diagnosis is by thoracentesis and pleural biopsy. Culture of the fluid or biopsy specimen or histologic examination of the biopsy will yield bacteriologic or histologic evidence of pleural tuberculosis in 80–90% of those who eventually are established to have the diagnosis. *(Cecil, Ch. 71; Light)*

20. (A) In assessing the probable effects of pulmonary resection on pulmonary function, it is important to consider whether the tumor is significantly impairing function preoperatively. In this case, the nearly complete obstruction of the bronchus intermedius prevents the participation of the right lower lobe in the FEV_1, vital capacity, and maximal voluntary ventilation. Removal of this nonfunctioning lung should not greatly impair postoperative pulmonary function. *(Cecil, Ch. 70)*

21. (C) The three general categories of disorders that predispose to pulmonary thromboembolism are stasis or slowing of blood flow in the venous system; damage to blood vessels, particularly their intimal linings; and alterations in blood coagulation mechanisms. The postoperative state causes stasis and increases the risk of thromboembolism primarily on that basis. Compression and invasion of veins by lymphomatous nodes cause both stasis and intimal damage. Congenital deficiency of antithrombin III alters blood coagulation mechanisms. Homocystinuria is associated with recurrent thromboembolism. In this disorder, the mechanism by which the biochemical deficiency (in cystathionine beta-synthase) causes thromboembolism is not known. Superficial thrombophlebitis of the arm would not increase the risk for developing pulmonary thromboembolism. *(Cecil, Chs. 67 and 194; Bell and Simon)*

22. (E) The association of nasal discharge, cavitary lesions on chest roentgenogram, and glomerulonephritis is characteristic of Wegener's granulomatosis. The single therapeutic agent that is most likely to benefit patients with the disease is cyclophosphamide, although prednisone also should be included in the initial regimen. *(Cecil, Chs. 63 and 441)*

23. (C) In patients with COPD and persistent arterial hypoxemia (Po_2 less than 55 mm Hg), both the quality of life and longevity are improved with continuous administration of low-flow oxygen. These benefits of therapy accrue even to patients without polycythemia, pulmonary hypertension, or right heart failure; the benefits are most likely with *continuous* therapy. This therapy may be used even in patients whose Pco_2 rises and stabilizes with an increase in FIo_2. Chronic hypercapnia is well tolerated so long as adequate oxygen levels are maintained. *(Cecil, Ch. 61; Anthonisen)*

24. (B) Advances in the diagnosis and treatment of lung cancer have been in the development of transthoracic and transbronchial methods for biopsy of suspicious lesions, in earlier detection of metastatic disease so that patients can be spared unnecessary thoracotomy, and in the use of radiation and chemotherapy for small-cell carcinoma. So far, neither these methods nor aggressive programs for early detection have had any impact on five-year survival rates of lung cancer, which remain at about 9%. *(Cecil, Ch. 70)*

25. (C) Features that suggest potential reversibility of COPD, indicating that a trial of steroids may be worthwhile, include a 20% or greater improvement in FEV_1 after bronchodilator treatment, a history of fluctuation in the severity of symptoms, a wheezy or noisy chest on physical examination, a chest roentgenogram that shows overinflation but is otherwise normal, eosinophilia of the blood or sputum, evidence of atopy, and a normal diffusing capacity for carbon monoxide. Hypoxemia may be equally severe in reversible and irreversible COPD. *(Cecil, Chs. 60 and 61)*

26. (A) The abnormality on this flow-volume curve is characteristic of a variable intrathoracic tracheal abnormality. This type of abnormality occurs because of softening of cartilages in the intrathoracic portion of the trachea. During expiration, the positive pleural pressure will exceed intratracheal pressure; flow limitation, as shown by the plateau on the expiratory portion of the flow-volume curve, will occur. During inspiration, pleural pressure will be more negative than intratracheal pressure; the affected region of the trachea will dilate rather than narrow, and inspiratory flow will be normal. Vascular ring anomaly is a congenital abnormality of the great vessels such that vascular compression of the trachea and esophagus occurs. The result in the trachea is failure of the cartilages to develop normally in the compressed area. Fixed stenosis of the intrathoracic trachea will cause limitation of flow during both inspiration and expiration. Asthma may cause expiratory flow limitation, but the contour of the expiratory curve usually is concave rather than a plateau. Enlargement of the adenoids or bilateral vocal cord paralysis may cause localized airway obstruction, but the flow limitation is either fixed (with approximately equal limitation of inspiratory and expiratory flow) or "variably extrathoracic" (with limitation predominantly of inspiratory flow). *(Cecil, Ch. 61; Shuford)*

27. (C) The anerobic bacteria normally present in the periodontal crevices are present in highest concentrations in post-aspiration lung abscesses. These include *Fusobacterium nucleatum*, *Bacteroides* species, peptostreptococcus, and others. *(Cecil, Ch. 64)*

28. (D) Although there is considerable variability, median survival in COPD is shorter in patients with a low FEV_1, rapid heart rate, cor pulmonale, or severe blood gas abnormalities. Longevity is also reduced in patients residing at altitudes above 3500 feet. Respiratory infections may cause acute, severe respiratory deterioration but have surprisingly little influence on the overall course of the disease. *(Cecil, Ch. 61)*

29. (C) In bronchopulmonary sequestration, the systemic vascular supply is via an abnormal vessel that arises either from the adjacent thoracic aorta or from the abdominal aorta. Thus, demonstration of such an abnormal vessel by aortography is the optimal way to establish that a lower lung field opacity is a bronchopulmonary sequestration. *(Cecil, Ch. 62)*

30. (B) The case description and chest roentgenogram are most consistent with the diagnosis of idiopathic pulmonary fibrosis. Patients with hypersensitivity pneumonitis usually have recurrent episodes of fever, cough, and dyspnea shortly after exposure to the offending antigen; rarely, these patients develop chronic symptoms without a recognized prior period of acute episodes. Pulmonary infiltrates in patients with acquired immunodeficiency syndrome usually occur after prodromal fever and weight loss. Idiopathic pulmonary hemosiderosis most commonly develops in patients younger than 20 years of age. Chronic interstitial lung disease may develop after an episode of mycoplasmal pneumonia, but only when the pneumonia has been extensive and protracted. *(Cecil, Ch. 63)*

31. (A) Patients with interstitial lung disease of mild to moderate severity usually have chronic alveolar hyperventilation. Thus the arterial P_{CO_2} usually will be lower than normal. Hypoxemia that worsens with exercise is characteristic of patients with interstitial lung disease, as are increased FEV_1/FVC ratio, reduced total lung capacity, and reduced diffusing capacity. *(Cecil, Ch. 63)*

32. (D) Only 10–20% of patients with idiopathic pulmonary fibrosis will derive substantial improvement from glucocorticoid therapy, and this proportion is less than in patients with pulmonary sarcoidosis. Most experts recommend initiating glucocorticoid therapy with a large single daily dose and then reducing the dose after 4–6 weeks. The greater the amount of fibrosis on open lung biopsy, the less likely it is that glucocorticoid therapy will benefit the patient. The hypothesis that glucocorticoids prolong the survival of patients with idiopathic pulmonary fibrosis has never been tested in a large-scale controlled fashion; their long-term efficacy has thus not been established. *(Cecil, Ch. 63)*

33. (B) Symptoms of proximal muscle weakness, dysphagia, and a lilac or heliotrope rash on the upper eyelids are characteristic manifestations of dermatomyositis. In most connective tissue disorders associated with interstitial lung disease, systemic extrapulmonary manifestations of the disease develop well before pulmonary manifestations. However, in polymyositis and dermatomyositis associated with interstitial lung disease, cough and dyspnea precede systemic signs of the disease about 50% of the time. *(Cecil, Chs. 63 and 443)*

34. (E) The roentgenogram shows periosteal elevation consistent with the diagnosis of hypertrophic pulmonary osteoarthropathy. This paraneoplastic syndrome occurs much more commonly in association with non–small-cell carcinoma of the lung than with small-cell carcinoma. *(Cecil, Ch. 70)*

35. (C) A number of studies have confirmed that the majority of pulmonary thromboemboli originate in the deep veins of the thigh or pelvis. For unclear reasons, deep veins below the knee much less commonly harbor thrombi that embolize and produce clinically significant problems. *(Cecil, Ch. 67; Moser and LeMoine)*

36. (E) The use of low-dose heparin (5000 units administered twice daily) will reduce the risk of venous thromboembolism in an appreciable number of hospitalized patients who require bed rest. These include those with a prior history of venous thromboembolism, severe congestive heart failure, the presence of some malignancies (particularly adenocarcinomas), and those recovering from acute myocardial infarction. If even minor bleeding would result in serious morbidity, such as in patients undergoing surgery of the eye, brain, or spinal cord, anticoagulant therapy should not be used. In such a setting, the risk of venous thromboembolism may be reduced by other measures, such as leg elevation and compression and early postoperative ambulation. *(Cecil, Ch. 67; Coon)*

37. (A) *Pneumocystis* organisms typically proliferate in the alveolar spaces, causing an inflammatory response with alveolar filling by a foamy, proteinaceous material containing clumps of both trophozoites and cysts. The association of a pleural reaction with *Pneumocystis* pneumonia is so unusual that even with proof of *Pneumocystis* infection by biopsy, an additional, coincident infection is likely. By contrast, pleural effusion is frequently associated with *S. pneumoniae* pneumonia and pulmonary infarction and is occasionally noted with *C. immitis* and *M. pneumoniae* pneumonia. *(Cecil, Chs. 264, 370, and 386)*

38. (B) In patients with diagnosed pulmonary thromboembolism, approximately 30%, not 80%, will die if they receive no anticoagulant therapy; the usual cause of death is a second embolus. The prognosis and mortality are not altered substantially by the presence of infarction in the lung or by the use of thrombolytic therapy. Interestingly, even large pulmonary emboli usually lyse or are recanalized; chronic persistent dyspnea is an unusual sequela. *(Cecil, Ch. 67)*

39. (E) Foreign materials such as talc crystals or cotton fibers may be injected with heroin into peripheral veins and are filtered from the circulation by precapillary pulmonary vessels. A fibrotic inflammatory response in vascular or perivascular tissues obliterates the vascular bed and causes eventual pulmonary hypertension. Septic emboli may result from direct injection of contaminated material or from embolization of valvular vegetations from right-sided endocarditis. Pulmonary edema often complicates heroin overdose and is presumed to be due to a transient change in permeability of the alveolar-capillary membrane. Aspiration may result from drug-induced impairment of consciousness or from misguided attempts to resuscitate an unconscious drug user by pouring milk or other material into the mouth and throat. Veno-occlusive disease is a disorder of unknown etiology; it develops in postcapillary vessels, which are protected from the effects of intravenous injection of foreign matter by the filtering action of pulmonary arteries, arterioles, and capillaries. *(Cecil, Ch. 16)*

40. (B) Anticoagulation is effective treatment for pulmonary emboli, and the accepted indications for interruption of the vena cava are few. They include an absolute contraindication to anticoagulation, such as recent brain surgery or major bleeding, recurrence of embolism on effective anticoagulation, recurrent pulmonary emboli leading to pulmonary hypertension, and septic emboli from an infected focus. Anticoagulation is usually well tolerated in the postpartum period, and the hemorrhagic complications that may occur can ordinarily be managed without severe morbidity or mortality. *(Cecil, Ch. 67)*

41. (C) For unclear reasons, cavitation of the primary tumor occurs much more commonly in squamous cell carcinoma of the lung than in other histologic types. Other roentgenographic features are nonspecific. *(Cecil, Ch. 70)*

42. (A) Because the prospects for long-term survival are so good after resection of bronchogenic carcinoma presenting as a small solitary nodule, the presence of any nodule must be investigated. Malignancies presenting as solitary nodules grow (doubling time between 15 days and 24 months), are at some point under 2 cm in diameter, and often do not communicate with an airway lumen (sputum cytology is generally not positive). A previous case of coccidioidomycosis is common in the American Southwest and does not confer immunity against malignancy. Bronchogenic carcinoma is very rare in patients under 35 years of age, but the patient should still be followed with roentgenograms and the nodule resected if growth is noted and no specific diagnosis has been made. *(Cecil, Ch. 70)*

43. (A—True; B—False; C—False; D—True; E—False) The chest roentgenograms show increased lung volumes and depressed diaphragms bilaterally with a loss of normal upward diaphragmatic curvature. The findings are characteristic of the hyperinflation of the lungs which occurs in patients with diffuse obstruction of the airways seen during exacerbations of asthma or in emphysema. In Swyer-James syndrome, diminished vascular markings in one lung cause unilateral hyperlucency. In tracheal stenosis, the lung volumes are normal. In bilateral diaphragmatic paralysis, some loss of diaphragmatic curvature may occur, but the diaphragms are elevated rather than depressed. *(Cecil, Ch. 61)*

44. (A—False; B—True; C—False; D—False; E—False) Bilaterality of the hilar adenopathy favors the diagnosis of sarcoidosis rather than infection or neoplasm. However, pleural effusion, the appearance of lung parenchymal infiltrates prior to the development of mediastinal or hilar adenopathy, isolated right paratracheal adenopathy without hilar adenopathy, and bronchial compression are all distinctly unusual in patients with sarcoidosis. Thus, these features should prompt a careful evaluation of the patient for infection or neoplasm. *(Cecil, Ch. 69)*

45. (A—True; B—False; C—True; D—True; E—True) Clubbing is not specific for diseases of the respiratory system. It occurs in patients with ascending cholangitis (D) as well as in patients with bronchiectasis, lung cancer, or cystic fibrosis (C, E, and A). Clubbing is not associated with asthma. *(Cecil, Ch. 70; Smith)*

46. (A—False; B—False; C—False; D—True; E—True) Of adults with unexplained chronic cough, one third to one half will turn out to have mild asthma that was not recognized previously. Exacerbation by exercise or forced expiratory maneuvers is typical of cough associated with asthma. In asthmatic patients, cough may be brought on or exacerbated by any form of therapy with beta-adrenergic antagonists, including ophthalmic application of agents such as timolol maleate. Therefore, the initial evaluation of the patient described could include either methacholine bronchoprovocation testing, which always will be abnormal if the patient has asthma, and/or an empiric trial of inhaled beta-adrenergic agonists, which will relieve cough associated with asthma in most instances. Fiberoptic bronchoscopy (to look for localized endobronchial lesions), gallium scanning of the lung (to look for subradiographic interstitial lung disease), and echocardiography (to evaluate cardiac function) are all reasonable procedures to use for evaluation of cough. However, in the clinical setting described, these tests should be ordered only after the patient has been evaluated for asthma. *(Cecil, Ch. 58; Irwin et al)*

47. (A—False; B—True; C—False; D—True; E—True) A loading dose of aminophylline should not be given in a patient who has been using it chronically. Maintenance intravenous therapy, methylprednisolone, and inhaled adrenergic aerosols are appropriate for initial therapy for a patient who has worsened despite outpatient use of full doses of bronchodilators. Sedation should be avoided in an already fatigued asthmatic patient, as it may reduce respiratory drive. Unlike some patients with chronic obstructive bronchitis, asthmatics do not depend on the hypoxic drive to breathe, and oxygen should be given if the PO_2 is less than 60 mm Hg. *(Cecil, Ch. 60)*

48. (A—True; B—False; C—True; D—False; E—True) Bronchial obstruction is due not only to constriction of smooth muscle but also to inspissation of mucus and to edema and cellular infiltration of the mucosa, which may be worsened by coexistent bronchitis. Prolonging the half-life of theophylline would be expected to increase, not decrease, its effectiveness. Pulmonary emphysema is unlikely in a 19-year-old patient. *(Cecil, Ch. 60)*

49. (A—True; B—False; C—True; D—True; E—True) In the asthmatic patient who requires a large dose of oral prednisone to control symptoms, a number of approaches may be attempted to reduce the requirement for the large dose or to reduce the attendant side effects such as weight gain and insomnia. Administering the glucocorticoids by an alternate-day oral regimen, by inhalation, or by initiating therapy with inhaled cromoglycate are all reasonable approaches to try. Because many asthmatic patients use metered-dose inhalers improperly, it is important to review the proper technique with them frequently. Often this maneuver alone will permit them to reduce the dose of oral prednisone. Switching the mode of administration of metaproterenol from a metered-dose inhaler to oral tablets usually results in the development of intolerable systemic manifestations of catecholamine excess. *(Cecil, Ch. 60)*

50. (A—True; B—False; C—False; D—False; E—False) Pleural plaques occur in 10–20% of asbestos workers. Even though they are often bilateral, they rarely cause functional impairment and are not associated with any greater risk of pulmonary fibrosis (asbestosis) or mesothelioma than seen in similarly exposed workers without plaques. Pleural plaques may develop after only minimal exposure to asbestos fibers. *(Cecil, Ch. 536)*

51. (A—False; B—False; C—True; D—False; E—True) The child must be considered to have active tuberculosis and requires complete two- or three-drug therapy; one-drug therapy would be inadequate. For the immigrant, presumably with previous BCG vaccination, a modest PPD reaction is anticipated and no treatment is indicated. Patients with gastrectomy represent a group at greater risk than is acceptable for developing active tuberculosis, and chemoprophylaxis with one drug is indicated. There is no real advantage in using chemoprophylaxis in healthy patients over 35 years of age who have a positive skin test, because they have fewer remaining years to be at risk for developing active disease and have a greater risk of INH liver toxicity. In patients with a positive tuberculin reaction, radiation therapy to the chest is associated with an increased risk of active tuberculosis in the next five years; this risk is minimized by isoniazid chemoprophylaxis. *(Cecil, Ch. 302)*

52. (A—False; B—False; C—False; D—True; E—True) In patients with severe chronic obstructive pulmonary disease (COPD), hypoxemia is the most likely cause of right ventricular enlargement, bilateral pedal edema, and polycythemia; it should therefore not be necessary to obtain erythropoietin values, pulmonary angiograms, or venograms. In the patient described, it would be important to initiate aggressive bronchodilator therapy to determine if arterial blood gas values improve substantially such that right ventricular size, pedal edema, and hematocrit values diminish after this intervention alone. In patients with COPD, severe hypoxemia may occur episodically during sleep or exercise. Episodic hypoxemia during sleep is especially common in obese patients with the bronchitic (type B) form of COPD. Therefore, in the patient described, overnight ear oximetry should be performed. *(Cecil, Ch. 61; Anthonisen)*

53. (A—True; B—True; C—False; D—False; E—False) Analysis of BAL fluid permits assessment of the number, type, and state of activation of the effector cells making up the alveolitis in patients with interstitial lung disease. In healthy, nonsmoking adults, the cells in BAL fluid consist largely (90% or more) of macrophages; the remainder are lymphocytes, mostly T cells. Polymorphonuclear leukocytes are rare. Immunoglobulins are present in the lower respiratory tract, with IgG exceeding IgA and both greatly exceeding IgM. Elastase is not normally identifiable. *(Cecil, Ch. 63)*

54.(A—False; B—True; C—False; D—True; E—True) In patients with obstructive sleep apnea, the oropharynx intermittently occludes during normal inspiration. Factors that may worsen the obstruction include alcohol consumption and oxygen therapy, presumably because these factors are associated with dampening of the neural mechanisms that normally preserve oropharyngeal patency. Allergic rhinitis may also be a factor, because increased nasal resistance leads to the generation of more negative pressures in the oropharynx during inspiration and therefore to a greater tendency for inspiratory oropharyngeal collapse. Weight loss and theophylline usually ameliorate obstructive sleep apnea. *(Cecil, Ch. 458; Sullivan and Issa)*

55.(A—True; B—False; C—False; D—True; E—True) An important determinant of the diffusing capacity for carbon monoxide is the pulmonary capillary blood volume, and factors that increase this volume will increase diffusing capacity. These factors include increased intravascular blood volume, as in the patient with iatrogenic fluid overload (E), and increased pulmonary blood flow, as in the patient with atrial septal defect (A). Diffusing capacity also may be increased in patients with Goodpasture's syndrome and alveolar hemorrhage (D), because the amount of hemoglobin available for taking up the carbon monoxide is increased by alveolar hemorrhage. Decreased diffusing capacity is common in patients with sarcoidosis (B), in which the alveolar-capillary membrane is thickened, and with primary pulmonary hypertension (C), in which small pulmonary arteries are obliterated. *(Cecil, Chs. 48, 49, 59, and 61)*

56.(A—True; B—False; C—True; D—True; E—False) The symptoms and findings on barium swallow suggest the diagnosis of achalasia. Chest roentgenogram shows a dilated esophagus with an esophageal air-fluid level to the right of the mediastinum and an infiltrate in the left lung. The association of these roentgenographic findings with fever and a cough productive of thick sputum indicates the presence of "aspiration pneumonitis," a bacterial pneumonitis developing secondarily after aspiration of esophageal contents. Appropriate management should include antibiotics. To minimize the chance of massive aspiration, the patient should avoid sedatives and elevate the head of the bed. Glucocorticoids should not be administered, because their use increases the likelihood of bacterial sepsis. Definitive therapy of the achalasia by bougie dilatation or by surgery should be postponed until after the active pulmonary infection has been treated. *(Cecil, Chs. 98 and 537; Wolfe et al)*

57.(All are True) Aspiration of esophageal or gastric contents may produce a variety of pulmonary problems. Recurrent aspiration during sleep may cause wheezing because of irritation of the airways. Sudden massive aspiration, such as may occur during induction of general anesthesia, may cause acute respiratory failure. Infectious complications include both lung abscess and empyema. Recurrent episodes of aspiration-induced injury of the lung may cause chronic interstitial lung disease. *(Cecil, Ch. 537; Little)*

58.(A—False; B—True; C—False; D—False; E—True) Cystic fibrosis is an autosomal recessive disorder, and carriers of the gene are not at increased risk for pulmonary disease. In the 1980's, nearly 50% of patients with cystic fibrosis live to age 20 years or beyond. Pulmonary infections in patients with cystic fibrosis are most commonly related to infection with *Pseudomonas aeruginosa* and *Staphylococcus aureus*. *Pseudomonas cepacia* occurs in the sputum in only 5–10% of cases. By adolescence or adulthood, virtually all patients with cystic fibrosis have pancreatic insufficiency. *(Cecil, Ch. 66)*

59.(A—True; B—False; C—False; D—False; E—True) The most likely diagnosis in this setting is pulmonary thromboembolism. Therefore, ventilation and perfusion lung scans are the most appropriate tests to order. Segmental defects on perfusion scan with preservation of ventilation to the same area of lung would make the likelihood of the diagnosis very high. A totally normal perfusion scan would virtually exclude the diagnosis. Thus, the results of these scans should be obtained before doing more invasive tests, such as pulmonary angiography. Impedance plethysmography and lower extremity venography may establish the site of origin of a pulmonary embolus, but they are less direct diagnostic tests for pulmonary thromboembolism than scans or pulmonary angiography. Therapy with heparin should be started empirically because the likelihood of pulmonary emboli is relatively great in this clinical setting. *(Cecil, Ch. 67)*

60.(A—False; B—True; C—False; D—False; E—True) Because results of the ventilation and perfusion lung scans are equivocal, the patient next should undergo pulmonary angiography, and heparin should be continued. *(Cecil, Ch. 67)*

61.(A—True; B—False; C—True; D—False; E—True) The finding of a normal pulmonary angiogram virtually excludes the diagnosis of pulmonary embolism. Thrombolytic therapy with streptokinase certainly should not be initiated in the absence of a diagnosis of pulmonary emboli confirmed by angiography, and heparin should be discontinued. The development of fever in this setting warrants both admission of the patient to the hospital and evaluation for infectious processes. The most likely diagnosis is bacterial pneumonia. *(Cecil, Ch. 67)*

62.(All are True) Untreated *Candida* endocarditis is a lethal disease, and amphotericin therapy must be combined with removal of a probably infected prosthesis. There is no other effective therapy for invasive aspergillosis. The demonstration of cryptococci in a pulmonary nodule requires treatment for the foci, which may not be clinically evident but certainly exist and which cause trouble in nearly 20% of cases. When truly progressive granulomatous disease exists, cavitary histoplasmosis is a fatal disease unless treated with amphotericin B. Coccidioidomycosis is the most resistant of diseases that respond to amphotericin B, but no other drug has been proven as effective. *(Cecil, Chs. 369, 373, and 375)*

63.(A—True, B—False; C—True; D—False; E—True) The arterial blood gases show acute, uncompensated respiratory alkalosis with an abnormally great alveolar-arterial oxygen difference. Acute pulmonary embolism (C), asthma (A), and congestive heart failure (E) are associated with an abnormal drive to ventilation (causing the P_{CO_2} to fall) and with hypoxemia. Diffuse alveolar fibrosis (D) is associated with hyperventilation, but because the disorder is chronic, renal excretion of bicarbonate should have normalized the pH. In a patient with normal lungs (B), acute hyperventilation *increases* arterial Po_2. *(Cecil, Ch. 59)*

64. (All are False) Effective antituberculous therapy reduces infectivity so rapidly that isolation (or even hospitalization) of patients with uncomplicated pulmonary tuberculosis is no longer considered necessary. After completion of a course of chemotherapy, the chances of reactivation are so remote as to make prolonged follow-up unnecessary. Primary isoniazid resistance is unusual in the United States, so that treatment with isoniazid and ethambutol is usually adequate; a third antituberculous drug is not needed to cover the remote possibility that a resistant strain is present, except in recent immigrants. A nine-month course of therapy is effective only if two bactericidal drugs (e.g., isoniazid and rifampin) are used. All household contacts of a new active case should be treated, regardless of their skin-test status. *(Cecil, Ch. 302)*

65. (A—False; B—True; C—False; D—True; E—True) The chest roentgenogram shows typical bullae in the upper lung fields bilaterally. This abnormality most commonly occurs in association with cigarette smoking, chronic bronchitis, and emphysema. Unlike bronchogenic cysts, bullae are not usually of congenital origin and are not usually detected until adulthood. Bullae do not communicate with the airways in most instances. Therefore, total lung capacity by gas dilution, which measures only the volume of gas in the chest communicating with the airways, will be substantially less than total lung capacity by plethysmography, which measures all compressible gas in the chest. The chest roentgenographic findings are not characteristic of $alpha_1$-antitrypsin deficiency, in which the destruction of lung is more severe at the bases of the lung than at the apices. If the compressed lung parenchyma is relatively normal, the patient may benefit from surgical resection of the apical bullae. *(Cecil, Ch. 62)*

66. (A—False; B—False; C—True; D—True; E—True) Worsening hypoxemia during exercise implies that the cause of the hypoxemia is either impaired diffusion or right to left shunting of blood. Impaired diffusion commonly occurs in patients with chronic intravenous drug use or in those with recurrent pulmonary emboli. A right to left shunt occurs in patients with pulmonary arteriovenous fistulae. In bronchiectasis or chronic bronchitis, the most likely cause of hypoxemia is ventilation-perfusion mismatching, and the hypoxemia usually does not worsen with exercise. *(Cecil, Ch. 59)*

67. (A—False; B—True; C—True; D—False; E—True) The flow-volume curve is concave, suggesting a reduction in maximal expiratory flow at mid and low lung volumes; this pattern results from loss of lung recoil, as in emphysema (C) or from an increase in airway resistance, as in asthma or chronic obstructive bronchitis (B and E). The interstitial diseases associated with collagen vascular diseases increase lung recoil, causing abnormally high flow rates (A). Recurrent pulmonary emboli (D) obliterate pulmonary vessels, reducing diffusing capacity, but do not affect lung recoil or airway resistance. *(Cecil, Ch. 59)*

68. (A—False; B—True; C—False; D—True; E—False) Simple chronic bronchitis is diagnosed when productive cough is present on most days for at least three months of the year. Cough and mucous gland hypertrophy (detected as abnormally enlarged ducts on bronchography) develop in response to chronic irritation, usually by cigarette smoke, and improve when the irritant is removed. The effect of cigarette smoking on airway function seems to be independent of its effect on mucus secretion, as smokers with productive cough do not have a greater decline in lung function than asymptomatic smokers. Regular use of an antibiotic would reduce the duration and severity of exacerbations, which are due to overgrowth of bacteria that have colonized the respiratory tract, but would not reduce the frequency of exacerbations. *(Cecil, Ch. 61; Sackner)*

69. (A—True; B—False; C—True; D—False; E—False) Theophylline is metabolized in the liver; both oral contraceptive agents and cimetidine inhibit hepatic metabolism of theophylline and prolong its half-life. Cigarette smokers metabolize theophylline more rapidly and need larger doses than nonsmokers. Neither beta-adrenergic agents nor corticosteroids affect theophylline metabolism. *(Cecil, Ch. 61; Bukowskyj et al.)*

70. (A—False; B—True; C—True; D—True; E—False) Serum 1,25-dihydroxy vitamin D_3 concentrations tend to be elevated, rather than depressed, in sarcoidosis. Hypercalciuria ocurs in 30–50% of sarcoid patients. Serum angiotensin-converting enzyme is elevated in 80–90% of patients with active disease. About one third have elevated serum gamma globulin. Serum *alkaline* phosphatase is increased in about 20% of cases, but acid phosphatase is normal. *(Cecil, Ch. 69)*

71. (A—True; B—False; C—False; D—True; E—True) The development of bronchiectasis requires partial destruction of the airway wall. It is not commonly observed after a pneumonitis that is primarily intra-alveolar, such as *Pneumocystis carinii* pneumonia (B). Also, bronchiectasis does not commonly occur after acute bacterial pneumonia (C), in part because of the current availability of appropriate antibiotic therapy. Factors that impair mucociliary clearance and lead to chronic bronchial infections commonly cause bronchiectasis. These include localized bronchial obstruction (E) by any mechanism and inspissation of secretions from cystic fibrosis (A). In allergic bronchopulmonary aspergillosis (D), bronchiectasis occurs commonly. The reasons are immune-mediated damage to the airway wall and inspissation of bronchial secretions causing impaired mucociliary clearance. *(Cecil, Ch. 65)*

72. (A—True; B—False; C—False; D—False; E—True) Increasing alveolar Po_2 will not correct hypoxia due to shunting of blood through an intracardiac defect (C), through fluid-filled alveoli (as in post-traumatic adult respiratory distress syndrome—D), or through an arteriovenous malformation. Hypoxia due to mismatching of ventilation and perfusion (A and E) is distinguished by its correction on administration of supplemental oxygen. *(Cecil, Ch. 59; West)*

73. (A—True; B—True; C—False; D—False; E—True) Total lung capacity will be reduced by definition in all patients with a restrictive ventilatory defect but normal or increased in obstruction. In many patients with a restrictive defect, the FEV_1/FVC ratio will be increased because of increased elastic recoil of the lung; in obstruction, the FEV_1/FVC ratio usually is decreased. Residual volume often increases in patients with obstructive ventilatory defects; in patients with a restrictive defect, residual volume is normal or decreased. Because of the increased residual volume in obstructive ventilatory defects, vital capacity will decrease. Vital capacity also may decrease in restrictive defects, and therefore this test is not helpful in distinguishing the two types of abnormalities. Abnormalities of the slope of phase III of the closing volume maneuver are extremely sensitive to diffuse abnormalities of the lung parenchyma or airways, but they do not permit one to distinguish restrictive from obstructive ventilatory defects. *(Cecil, Ch. 59)*

74. (A—True; B—False; C—True; D—True; E—True) In patients with asthma and wheezing associated with exposure to specific allergens, a variety of nonallergenic stimuli also may induce bronchospasm. In the perioperative setting, these nonallergenic stimuli may include any mechanical manipulation of the airways, such as endotracheal intubation and postoperative orotracheal suctioning. For humidification of the airways in an intubated patient, one always should use iso-osmotic solutions because hypo-osmotic (e.g., distilled water) or hyperosmotic solutions may induce bronchospasm in asthmatic patients. Most general anesthetics, including halothane, are potent bronchodilators and therefore do not provoke bronchospasm. Neostigmine bromide, an agent often used to reverse the skeletal muscular paralytic effects of pancuronium bromide, is an inhibitor of acetylcholinesterases. Therefore, administration of neostigmine may provoke bronchospasm by vagal mechanisms in asthmatic patients. *(Cecil, Ch. 60; Geiger and Hedley-Whyte)*

75. (A—False; B—True; C—False; D—False; E—False) About 10% of asthmatic patients have a peculiar triad of bronchospasm, nasal polyps, and sensitivity to aspirin. The mechanism is unknown but may have to do with drug-induced alteration in prostaglandin metabolism. Indomethacin, aminopyrine, and yellow food dyes (e.g., tartrazine yellow) may also trigger attacks of severe bronchospasm, urticaria, and even hypotension. These patients do not react to sodium salicylate, further suggesting that the condition is not immunologically mediated. *(Cecil, Ch. 60)*

76. (A—True; B—True; C—False; D—True; E—True) Rheumatoid arthritis may adversely affect the lungs and airways in several ways. Involvement of the cricoarytenoid joints may produce upper airway obstruction (E). Obliterative bronchiolitis (D), interstitial fibrosis, and pulmonary parenchymal rheumatoid nodules all have been associated with rheumatoid arthritis, but asthma (C) has not. *(Cecil, Chs. 63–65)*

77. (A—False; B—True; C—False; D—False; E—False) The selectivity of metaproterenol and albuterol as $beta_2$-adrenergic agonists is approximately the same. Undesirable side effects include skeletal muscle tremor and palpitations, but these side effects are much less likely to occur when the agents are administered by inhalation rather than taken by mouth. It is important for the *physician* to show the patient the proper technique for using metered-dose inhalers, because a large proportion of asthmatic patients use these devices improperly. During an exacerbation of the asthma, the inhaled $beta_2$-adrenergic agonists always should be continued, even when systemic corticosteroids are administered. *(Cecil, Ch. 60)*

78. (A—False; B—True; C—False; D—True; E—True) Dyspnea is the most common symptom of pulmonary thromboemboli, but certain associated findings in a dyspneic patient suggest other causes. Pleuritic chest pain occurs in approximately 80% of patients with pulmonary thromboemboli; however, onset of pleurisy *prior* to onset of dyspnea is exceedingly uncommon in patients with this problem. Although *localized* wheezes may be found in patients with pulmonary thromboembolism, an association of dyspnea with diffuse wheezes suggests alternative diagnoses. Because pulmonary emboli increase physiologic dead space in the lung, arterial Pco_2 usually decreases. The finding of acute increases in Pco_2 raises the possibility of other diagnoses. Rapid resolution of dyspnea and lack of other symptoms with a normal physical examination occur commonly in patients with pulmonary thromboembolism. *(Cecil, Ch. 67; Moser)*

79. (A—False; B—True; C—True; D—True; E—False) Sputum eosinophilia and a doubling of residual volume may be found in asthmatic patients whose signs and symptoms of asthma have disappeared. Ventilatory drive is increased in asthmatic attacks, so hypocapnia is typical except with very severe airflow obstruction. Pulsus paradoxicus reflects the wide swings in pleural pressure which occur with severe airflow obstruction. *(Cecil, Ch. 60)*

80. (A—False; B—False; C—True; D—True; E—True) Occasional side effects of heparin therapy include thrombocytopenia, osteopenia, and hypoaldosteronism. However, the most serious side effect is major bleeding, which occurs in 5–10% of patients treated with full doses of heparin. Anticoagulation with heparin always should be initiated by bolus injection, and the use of a bolus does not increase the risk of bleeding. Maintenance of anticoagulation by constant intravenous infusion of heparin causes less risk of bleeding than when it is administered intermittently. The activated partial thromboplastin time should be maintained at 1.5–2.0 times control; a greater degree of anticoagulation increases risk of bleeding. Heparin and warfarin should be administered concurrently during a period of changeover from one drug to the other, and the risk of bleeding is not increased during this period. Nonsteroidal anti-inflammatory agents should not be administered concurrently with heparin, because their use markedly increases the risk of gastric hemorrhage. *(Cecil, Ch. 67)*

81. (A—False; B—True; C—False; D—True; E—False) Mean alveolar oxygen tension (PAo_2) can be estimated from the formula $PAo_2 = PIo_2 - 1.25 \times Paco_2$, where PIo_2 is partial pressure of oxygen in inspired gas and $Paco_2$ is partial pressure of carbon dioxide in arterial blood. Breathing room air at sea level, this patient would have a calculated PAo_2 of 32 mm Hg. As it is impossible for arterial Po_2 to be *greater* than alveolar Po_2, the PIo_2 must have been greater than 150 mm Hg, implying that supplemental oxygen was given. Switching the patient to room air would mean that unless alveolar ventilation improved, alveolar Po_2 would be 32 mm Hg—a dangerously low value. One cannot count on the respiratory system responding rapidly enough to avoid a precipitous fall in arterial Po_2. The increase in arterial Pco_2 largely reflects alveolar hypoventilation. The high bicarbonate excludes superimposed metabolic acidosis and implies chronic respiratory insufficiency. With uncompensated respiratory acidosis of this severity, pH would be about 7.15. Carbonic anhydrase should not be used in an unstable patient already acidotic from respiratory failure. *(Cecil, Chs. 72 and 73)*

82. (A—True; B—False; C—False; D—True; E—False) The hyperkalemia reflects acute acidosis and will improve as alveolar ventilation is increased. No additional therapy is required. The right-sided heart failure evident on physical examination will improve as gas exchange is improved and pulmonary vascular resistance decreases. Digoxin is unnecessary and carries the risk of toxicity with the shifts in potassium ion that will follow correction of the respiratory acidosis. A normal loading dose of aminophylline should be given if the patient has been taking no theophylline-containing medications. Because the drug is metabolized in the liver, half the usual maintenance dose should be used in the presence of right-sided heart failure with hepatic congestion. Aerosolized bronchodilators are safe and effective in reducing bronchospasm and in increasing mucociliary clearance. Sedation is contraindicated in a patient already on the verge of CO_2 narcosis. *(Cecil, Ch. 72)*

83.(A—False; B—False; C—False; D—False; E—True) Pulmonary embolism need not be invoked to account for pulmonary hypertension and right ventricular strain in a hypoxic, hypercapnic patient with chronic obstructive lung disease. Hypoxia and hypercapnic acidosis are responsible for contraction of vascular smooth muscle; pulmonary hypertension will resolve as gas exchange is improved. Phlebotomy is not necessary for polycythemia with a hematocrit of less than 60%. At higher levels, an increase in blood viscosity significantly impedes blood flow in small vessels. Morphine sulfate would further depress the respiratory center and is contraindicated. Intravenous aminophylline and methylprednisolone, aerosolized adrenergic agents, verbal stimulation, and judicious use of supplemental oxygen are all appropriate. *(Cecil, Ch. 72)*

84.(A—False; B—True; C—True; D—True; E—True) PEEP is indicated for increasing lung volume and for stabilizing alveolar units in conditions in which intra-alveolar exudation of fluid and loss of surfactant reduce lung compliance and lead to closure of peripheral airways. In chronic bronchitis, lung compliance is normal or increased, and therefore PEEP ordinarily should not be used during mechanical ventilation. Inflation pressures in the cuff of the endotracheal tube should be checked frequently to avoid tracheal mucosal damage from overinflation. Because the serum bicarbonate level is elevated, reducing arterial P_{CO_2} to the normal range of 40 ± 1.5 mm Hg would cause severe alkalosis; adjusting arterial P_{CO_2} to approximately 50–55 mm Hg would be an appropriate first goal for this patient. Adequate saturation of hemoglobin is achieved at an arterial P_{O_2} of 60 mm Hg. The F_{IO_2} should be kept no higher than necessary to avoid oxygen toxicity. With oxygen saturation less than 90%, there is potential danger of ischemic damage to tissues supplied by partially obstructed vessels. All gas delivery circuits that communicate with the airways should be kept sterile. *(Cecil, Chs. 72 and 73)*

85.(A—True; B—False; C—False; D—False; E—False) Idiopathic ILD is sometimes associated with circulating immune complexes and antinuclear antibody. Although the idiopathic form of ILD is sometimes associated with a predominantly neutrophil-macrophage alveolitis, a lymphocyte-macrophage alveolitis is often found, as is also true of the alveolitis of collagen vascular disease. Gallium-67 uptake is believed to reflect the activity of alveolitis but does not distinguish its underlying cause. Because ILD may precede other clinical evidence of collagen vascular disease, the telltale involvement of skin, kidney, joints, or other organs may not be apparent for as long as two years. *(Cecil, Ch. 63)*

86.(A—False; B—True; C—False; D—True; E—True) Eaton-Lambert syndrome, ectopic hormone syndromes, and a favorable response to chemotherapy all occur much more commonly in small-cell carcinoma of the lung than in non–small-cell pulmonary malignancy. Manifestations that relate to local compression or invasion of the tumor are nonspecific and do not necessarily favor the diagnosis of small-cell carcinoma; the latter include superior vena cava and Horner's syndrome. *(Cecil, Ch. 70)*

87.(C); 88.(D); 89.(A); 90.(B); 91.(E) In the evaluation of a patient with dyspnea, defining the precise timing of the dyspnea often helps to establish its cause. In patients with interstitial lung disease from hypersensitivity pneumonitis, exposure to an offending antigen often induces inflammation of the lung by type III immunologic mechanisms that require 6–8 hours to develop after the exposure. Thus, if the patient's exposure begins in the early morning when he or she begins work, the dyspnea may not occur until late afternoon or evening. Improvement in symptoms over the weekend also suggests the possibility of hypersensitivity pneumonitis from an occupational exposure. In dyspnea from almost any organic cause, it is unlikely that the symptoms will improve or remain unchanged during exercise. Thus, when a patient describes this timing of the dyspnea, a psychogenic cause may be present. Onset of shortness of breath 60–120 minutes after the onset of sleep is characteristic of paroxysmal nocturnal dyspnea from increased left atrial pressure. Onset of dyspnea immediately after lying down occurs in patients with diaphragmatic paralysis, because abdominal contents displace the flaccid diaphragm upward into the thorax. Dyspnea occurring 5 minutes after cessation of exercise is characteristic of exercise-induced bronchospasm. *(Cecil, Ch. 58; Clausen)*

92.(D); 93.(B); 94.(E); 95.(A); 96.(C) Bronchioloalveolar cell carcinoma often appears multicentric in its origin and occurs with increased frequency in patients with progressive systemic sclerosis. Squamous cell carcinoma is more common in men and often appears as a perihilar mass; it typically spreads first to local draining nodes. Small-cell carcinoma often causes mediastinal widening and spreads hematogenously, seeding the bone marrow, liver, brain, adrenals, and other sites early in its course. Adenocarcinoma, now the most common of bronchogenic carcinomas, occurs more often in women than other histologic types and often presents as a peripheral nodule; it has a tendency to metastasize early to the brain. Large-cell carcinoma often presents as a bulky mass in the lung periphery. *(Cecil, Ch. 70)*

97.(E); 98.(D); 99.(B); 100.(A); 101.(C) Lymphomas are the most common cause of chylous pleural effusions, which are characterized by their milky appearance and their high triglyceride concentration. Transudative effusions in patients with congestive heart failure are characterized by low cellular and protein concentrations. Pleural effusions occurring because of esophageal rupture characteristically are exudates with very high concentrations of amylase, which is of salivary origin. Pleural effusions associated with rheumatoid arthritis are exudates and often contain very low glucose concentrations. Anaerobic empyemas, which are exudates with very high concentrations of white blood cells and moderately low glucose concentrations, usually develop after an episode of aspiration, as may occur frequently in alcoholic patients. *(Cecil, Ch. 71; Light)*

102.(D); 103.(C); 104.(E); 105.(B); 106.(A) Lymphocytic interstitial pneumonitis occurs most commonly in association with Sjögren's syndrome, in which the Shirmer test for dry eyes will be positive. Goodpasture's syndrome is characterized by diffuse pulmonary hemorrhage, glomerulonephritis, and circulating antialveolar and antiglomerular basement membrane antibodies. Eosinophilic granuloma causes a chronic interstitial pneumonitis affecting the upper and middle zones of the lung. In this disorder, the diagnosis is established by demonstration of Langerhans' cells in bronchoalveolar lavage. Lymphangioleiomyomatosis is a disorder of young women characterized by interstitial lung disease and pleural effusions that are chylous (and therefore contain elevated concentrations of triglycerides). Idiopathic pulmonary hemosiderosis is characterized by recurrent episodes of alveolar hemorrhage such that iron-deficiency anemia occurs. *(Cecil, Ch. 63)*

107.(C); 108.(E); 109.(A); 110.(D); 111.(B) Glucocorticoids may require 6–12 hours for onset of their effect in treating asthmatic patients in exacerbation. Ipratropium bromide is an anticholinergic agent and may cause increased intraocular pressure in patients with glaucoma or urinary retention in patients with enlargement of the prostate. Epinephrine, a mixed alpha- and beta-adrenergic agonist, elevates systemic blood pressure by its alpha-adrenergic effects on vascular smooth muscle, and its use as an antiasthmatic agent should be avoided in patients with severe hypertension. The half-life of methylxanthines in the circulation is prolonged in patients with congestive heart failure, and therefore the maintenance dose should be reduced in these patients. The use of disodium cromoglycate should be reserved for patients with chronic stable asthma, and its use should never be initiated during acute attacks. *(Cecil, Ch. 60)*

112.(C); 113.(D); 114.(A); 115.(B); 116.(E) During acute changes in alveolar ventilation, for every 1 mm Hg change in PCO_2, the pH changes by 0.075 unit in the opposite direction. Thus, in the patient with mild acute hyperventilation associated with the pain of an arterial puncture **(113)**, the pH is slightly alkalotic. Similarly, in relatively acute hypoventilation associated with drug overdose **(114)**, the pH is significantly acidotic. After 1–2 days of hyper- or hypoventilation, renal compensation occurs, and the pH returns toward normal. Thus, in a 10-day episode of worsening respiratory failure in the setting of underlying chronic obstructive pulmonary disease **(115)**, the pH is relatively normal despite significant hypercarbia. Similarly, in chronic hyperventilation associated with pulmonary vascular disease (pulmonary emboli, **112**), the pH is normal despite significant hypocarbia. The renal compensation for chronic hypoventilation is retention of bicarbonate. Therefore, when patient 115 undergoes endotracheal intubation and the lungs are ventilated at an inappropriately rapid rate **(116)**, the pH rises precipitously. This iatrogenic form of alkalosis may cause arrhythmias, hypotension, and seizures. *(Cecil, Ch. 73)*

117.(A); 118.(B); 119.(D); 120.(E); 121.(C) Although there are a variety of different types of "chronic obstructive pulmonary disease," in the individual patient certain historical features of the illness often will suggest a specific type. The association of diabetes mellitus with a chronic productive cough in a young adult suggests the diagnosis of cystic fibrosis. Productive cough on most days for at least three months annually during two or more successive years is, by definition, simple chronic bronchitis. The association of obstructive lung disease with recurrent pneumothoraces and chronic hepatitis suggests the diagnosis of $alpha_1$-antitrypsin deficiency. Recurrent sinusitis and infertility in a young adult male are characteristic of immotile cilia syndrome. A recent change in residence associated with the onset of recurrent episodes of shortness of breath and cough is characteristic of extrinsic asthma. *(Cecil, Chs. 60, 61, 65, and 66)*

122.(C); 123.(A); 124.(D); 125.(B); 126.(E) Patients with disorders of the lung frequently have characteristic skin lesions. Acanthosis nigricans (E) occurs in patients with cancer of the lung as well as of the gastrointestinal tract. The appearance of showers of petechiae over the axillae or over other sites on the upper half of the body is characteristic of fat embolism syndrome occurring in a patient with a recent traumatic fracture. Purplish submucosal lesions on the hard palate strongly suggest the diagnosis of Kaposi's sarcoma and acquired immunodeficiency syndrome. A draining sinus on the lateral chest wall in a patient with a cavitating pneumonitis is consistent with the diagnosis of actinomycosis. Violaceous nodules over the nose and malar areas are characteristic of lupus pernio, a cutaneous manifestation of chronic sarcoidosis. *(Cecil, Chs. 68, 69, 70, and 297; Katz and Beerman)*

127.(A); 128.(C); 129.(D); 130.(B) Streptomycin's major toxicity is vestibular, but it may also cause hearing impairment. Isoniazid frequently causes modest elevation in SGOT. Experience shows that these usually resolve spontaneously with continued therapy. Rifampin has been reported to cause thrombocytopenia, especially when it is given intermittently, owing to the production of antiplatelet antibody. Ethambutol may cause optic neuritis when given at a dose of 25 mg/kg, but this effect is rare at the customary dose of 15 mg/kg. *(Cecil, Ch. 302)*

131.(B); 132.(D); 133.(C); 134.(E); 135.(A) A vast number of drugs are associated with pulmonary toxicity. Hydralazine may produce a lupus-like condition with acute pleurisy. Nitrofurantoin may cause slowly progressive diffuse infiltrative disease if taken chronically for suppression of bacterial urinary tract infections; it may also produce an acute syndrome with fever, cough, pulmonary infiltrates, and eosinophilia. Methysergide may provoke fibrosis of the lung parenchyma and pleura. Diffuse pulmonary infiltration, cough, fever, and dyspnea may appear long after the initiation of treatment with busulfan. The changes in type II alveolar cells may be mistaken for malignancy. Corticosteroids can lead to an increase in mediastinal fat, causing mediastinal widening on the chest radiograph. *(Cecil, Ch. 63)*

136.(C); 137.(D); 138.(B); 139.(A) Hypokalemic metabolic alkalosis is a prominent manifestation of the ectopic production of ACTH; this systemic manifestation of lung cancer occurs most commonly in association with small-cell carcinoma of the lung. Hypercalcemia in patients with primary pulmonary malignancy is most commonly associated with squamous cell carcinoma and is related to increased osteolysis caused most frequently by the synthesis and secretion of humoral hypercalcemic factors by the tumor. Gynecomastia tends to occur in association with large-cell anaplastic carcinomas of the lung. Adenocarcinoma is the most common pulmonary neoplasm that is associated with marantic endocarditis. *(Cecil, Chs. 70 and 173; Smith)*

BIBLIOGRAPHY

Anthonisen NR: Long-term oxygen therapy. Ann Intern Med 99:519, 1983.

Bell WR, Simon TL: Current status of pulmonary thromboembolic disease: Pathophysiology, diagnosis, prevention and treatment. Am Heart J 103:239, 1982.

Bukowskyj M, Nakatsu K, Munt PW: Theophylline reassessed. Ann Intern Med 101:63, 1984.

Cecil Textbook of Medicine. 18th ed. Wyngaarden JB, Smith LH Jr (eds). Philadelphia, W. B. Saunders Company, 1988.

Clausen JL: Finding the cause of shortness of breath. A practical approach to a complicated differential. J Respir Dis 3:11, 1982.

Coon WW: Venous thromboembolism: Prevalence, risk factors, and prevention. Clin Chest Med 5:391, 1984.

Geiger K, Hedley-Whyte J: Preoperative and postoperative considerations. *In* Weiss EB, Segal MS, Stein M (eds): Bronchial Asthma: Mechanisms and Therapeutics. Boston, Little, Brown and Company, 1985, p. 892.

Irwin RS, Corrao WM, Pratter MR: Chronic persistent cough in the adult: The spectrum and frequency of causes and successful outcome of specific therapy. Am Rev Respir Dis 123:413, 1981.

Katz AS, Beerman H: Pulmonary-cutaneous disorders. *In* Fishman AP (ed): Pulmonary Diseases and Disorders. New York, McGraw-Hill Book Company, 1980, p. 29.

Light RW (ed): Symposium on pleural diseases. Clin Chest Med 6:1, 1985.

Little JW: Pulmonary aspiration. Medical Staff Conference, University of California, San Francisco. West J Med 131:122, 1979.

Lynch JP, Flint A: Sorting out the pulmonary eosinophilic syndromes. J Respir Dis 5:61, 1984.

Moser KM: Pulmonary embolism. Am Rev Respir Dis 115:829, 1977.

Moser KM, LeMoine JR: Is embolic risk conditioned by location of deep venous thrombosis? Ann Intern Med 94:439, 1981.

Raskob GE, Hull RD: Venous thromboembolism confirmed: What next? J Respir Dis 7:79, 1986.

Sackner MA (ed): Recent advances in the management of obstructive airways disease. Chest 88:75S, 1985.

Shuford WH: The Aortic Arch and Its Malformations. Springfield, IL, Charles C Thomas, Publisher, 1974.

Smith LH: Systemic manifestations of carcinoma of the lung. *In* Murray JF, Nadel JA (eds): Textbook of Respiratory Medicine. Philadelphia, W. B. Saunders Company, 1988.

Sullivan CE, Issa FG: Obstructive sleep apnea. Clin Chest Med 6:633, 1985.

West JB: Assessing pulmonary gas exchange. N Engl J Med 316:1336, 1987.

Wolfe JE, Bone RC, Ruth WE: Effect of corticosteroids in the treatment of patients with gastric aspiration. Am J Med 63:719, 1977.

PART 3

RENAL DISEASE

ALLAN S. POLLOCK and DAVID G. WARNOCK

DIRECTIONS: For questions 1 to 36, choose the ONE BEST answer to each question.

QUESTIONS 1–3

A 67-year-old man is brought to the emergency room with fever, nausea, and vomiting. For the past 10 days he has taken ampicillin for an upper respiratory infection. Temperature is 100.6°F. Blood pressure is 125/70 mm Hg (supine) and 90/56 mm Hg (standing). Pulse rate is 92 per minute (supine) and 122 per minute (standing). Physical findings include rare basilar rales and wheezes, a faint macular rash on the trunk and legs, and a moderately enlarged prostate. Roentgenogram of the chest shows a faint right lower lobe infiltrate. Urinalysis shows 1+ proteinuria, 10–20 WBC's/hpf, 20–30 RBC's/hpf, and several white cell casts. A Wright's stain of spun urinary sediment reveals many eosinophils. Laboratory data include:

Serum electrolytes	
Sodium	134 mEq/L
Potassium	5.8 mEq/L
Chloride	110 mEq/L
Bicarbonate	14 mEq/L
Blood urea nitrogen	88 mg/dl
Serum creatinine	2.8 mg/dl
White blood cell count (WBC)	13,200/mm^3
Eosinophils	12%
Polymorphonuclear leukocytes (PMN's)	68%
Lymphocytes	12%
Monocytes	8%
Arterial pH	7.24
Urine	
Sodium	58 mEq/L
Chloride	34 mEq/L
Potassium	17 mEq/L
pH	5.7

1. Which of the following is the most likely cause of this clinical syndrome?

A. Obstructive uropathy at the level of the prostate
B. Acute glomerulonephritis
C. Tubulointerstitial nephritis
D. Volume depletion
E. Mild chronic renal insufficiency

2. Which of the following is LEAST likely to contribute to hypotension in this patient?

A. Vomiting
B. Decreased glomerular filtration rate (GFR)
C. Salt-losing nephropathy
D. Pneumonia
E. Fever

3. Which of the following is most likely to contribute to systemic acidosis in this patient?

A. Distal tubular dysfunction
B. Type II renal tubular acidosis with bicarbonate wasting
C. Vomiting
D. Decreased GFR
E. Lactic acidosis

QUESTIONS 4–5

A 59-year-old male truck driver comes to the emergency room because of lethargy, nausea, and vomiting over the preceding five days and markedly decreased urinary volume. He has a history of mild hypertension treated with dietary salt restriction. For the past several months he has had urinary hesitancy and nocturia. Blood pressure is 105/60 mm Hg; pulse rate is 125 per minute. There is a 20 mm Hg orthostatic drop in blood pressure. Physical examination shows prostatic enlargement. The patient is unable to produce a urine specimen. The bladder is not distended by percussion. Plain film of the abdomen shows two renal outlines of normal size. Ultrasound examination of the kidneys shows normal renal size; there is no dilatation of the renal pelvis or ureters. Laboratory studies show:

Serum electrolytes	
Sodium	132 mEq/L
Potassium	5.2 mEq/L
Chloride	90 mEq/L
Bicarbonate	22 mEq/L
Blood urea nitrogen	110 mg/dl
Serum creatinine	13 mg/dl
Calcium	8.1 mg/dl
Phosphate	6.2 mg/dl
Hemoglobin	13.5 g/dl

After rehydration with 5 liters of normal saline, the patient remains anuric. The next morning, repeat ultrasound examination of the kidneys shows bilateral distention of the renal pelvis. Placement of a bladder catheter yields 2000 ml of clear urine, and urine production continues at 1000 ml per hour over the next five hours.

4. Which of the following is most likely to explain the abnormalities of renal function seen in this patient?

A. Chronic renal failure
B. High circulating levels of vasopressin
C. Obstructive uropathy at the level of the prostate
D. Renal artery stenosis
E. A toxic nephropathy

5. Which of the following best explains the initially normal ultrasound examination?

A. Improper interpretation of the examination
B. Extracellular fluid depletion
C. Acute glomerulonephritis
D. Bilateral ureteral obstruction
E. Uric acid nephropathy

6. A 28-year-old man has sudden onset of shortness of breath and right-sided pleuritic chest pain. He has had the nephrotic syndrome for two years, and biopsy-proven membranous glomerulonephritis that failed to respond to prednisone. On physical examination he is tachypneic and in moderate distress. He has 3+ pitting edema of the lower extremities. Roentgenogram of the chest is normal. Arterial blood gases include a P_{O_2} of 62 mm Hg and a P_{CO_2} of 22 mm Hg. Electrolytes are normal. Which one of the following would be appropriate to perform at this time?

A. Excretory urogram
B. Renal venography
C. Biopsy of the lung
D. Repeat kidney biopsy
E. None of the above

7. For which of the following causes of metabolic alkalosis is determination of urine chloride concentration significant?

A. Bartter's syndrome
B. Diuretic abuse
C. Surreptitious vomiting
D. Primary hyperaldosteronism
E. Cushing's syndrome

QUESTIONS 8–9

A 72-year-old woman comes to the hospital with a productive cough, shortness of breath, and fever. She has had two episodes of pneumococcal pneumonia within the past six months, has had fatigue over the past several months, and has noted the recent onset of lower back pain. On physical examination she is pale. Temperature is 101°F. There are no clinical signs of volume depletion. Chest roentgenogram shows a left lower lobe infiltrate. Renal ultrasound examination shows two 11-cm kidneys without signs of obstruction. Laboratory data include:

Serum electrolytes	
Sodium	144 mEq/L
Potassium	5.1 mEq/L
Chloride	117 mEq/L
Bicarbonate	17 mEq/L
Blood urea nitrogen	42 mg/dl
Serum creatinine	2.3 mg/dl
Calcium	11.4 mg/dl
Hemoglobin	9 g/dl
Arterial blood studies	
P_{O_2}	62 mm Hg
P_{CO_2}	32 mm Hg
pH	7.34

Urinalysis shows a specific gravity of 1.008, pH 6.6, 1–2 RBC's/hpf, and a trace-positive dipstick examination for protein. The urine sulfosalicylic acid reaction is strongly positive for protein.

8. Which of the following best explains the patient's condition?

A. Amyloidosis
B. Multiple myeloma
C. Immune-complex glomerulonephritis
D. Chronic renal insufficiency with superimposed pneumonia
E. None of the above

9. If the patient described above had a positive dipstick examination for protein and a measured 15-g/24-hour protein excretion rate, which diagnosis would be most likely?

A. Amyloidosis
B. Multiple myeloma
C. Immune-complex glomerulonephritis
D. Chronic renal insufficiency with superimposed pneumonia
E. None of the above

QUESTIONS 10–11

A 28-year-old woman with a 15-year history of insulin-dependent diabetes is brought to the emergency room in a disoriented state. She has a two-day history of upper respiratory infection and has been vomiting for the past day. Laboratory tests include:

Serum electrolytes	
Sodium	100 mEq/L
Potassium	6.0 mEq/L
Chloride	74 mEq/L
Bicarbonate	6 mEq/L
Serum glucose	540 mg/dl
Blood urea nitrogen	88 mg/dl
Serum creatinine	3.8 mg/dl
Plasma osmolality	368 mOsm/kg
Plasma ketones	positive at a 1:32 dilution

The laboratory notes that the patient's plasma is lipemic.

Arterial blood studies	
P_{CO_2}	21 mm Hg
pH	7.04
Urine	
Sodium	55 mEq/L
Glucose	4+
pH	4.9

10. What is the major mechanism contributing to this patient's hyponatremia?

A. Osmotic diuresis
B. Impaired free water clearance
C. Increased distal delivery of an impermeant anion
D. Laboratory artifact in the measurement of serum sodium
E. ADH effect based on a physiologic nonosmotic stimulus

11. Which mechanism best explains the measured level of urine sodium?

A. Osmotic diuresis
B. Salt-losing nephropathy
C. Impaired free water clearance
D. Increased distal delivery of an impermeant anion
E. ADH effect based on a physiologic nonosmotic stimulus

QUESTIONS 12–13

A 66-year-old man with recently diagnosed oat cell carcinoma of the lung, without apparent central nervous system metastases, comes to the hospital with confusion. There is no history of vomiting and he takes no medicine. Physical examination reveals obtundation without any localizing findings. There is no clinical evidence of extracellular fluid (ECF) depletion. Laboratory tests include:

Serum electrolytes	
Sodium	108 mEq/L
Potassium	4.4 mEq/L
Chloride	82 mEq/L
Bicarbonate	20 mEq/L
Blood urea nitrogen	6 mg/dl
Serum creatinine	0.7 mg/dl
Serum uric acid	3.8 mg/dl
Urine	
Sodium	50 mEq/L
Potassium	12 mEq/L
pH	5.0
Osmolality	860 mOsm/kg

12. What is the major mechanism contributing to this patient's hyponatremia?

A. Osmotic diuresis
B. Impaired free water clearance
C. Laboratory artifact in the measurement of serum sodium
D. ADH effect based on a physiologic nonosmotic stimulus
E. Decreased total body water with a larger decrease in total body sodium

13. Which mechanism explains the measured level of urine sodium?

A. Osmotic diuresis
B. Salt-losing nephropathy
C. Impaired free water clearance
D. Increased distal delivery of an impermeant anion
E. The patient is in sodium balance and the extracellular fluid compartment is not depleted

QUESTIONS 14–15

A 68-year-old man has increasing hypertension three weeks after an aortic angiogram and subsequent repair of an abdominal aortic aneurysm. In the hospital he received brief courses of several drugs, including cephalosporin, cimetidine, and heparin. He is currently receiving aspirin and dipyridamole. Physical examination now shows a blood pressure of 170/110 mm Hg. Bruits are heard in both femoral arteries. There is some mottling of the lower extremities and subungual petechiae on a lower extremity nail bed. Laboratory data include:

Serum electrolytes	
Sodium	142 mEq/L
Potassium	5.1 mEq/L
Chloride	104 mEq/L
Bicarbonate	20 mEq/L
Blood urea nitrogen	60 mg/dl
Serum creatinine	3.2 mg/dl
Complete blood count	
Hematocrit	35%
White blood cell count	10,500/mm^3
Polymorphonuclear leukocytes	80%
Lymphocytes	12%
Eosinophils	8%

Urinalysis shows pH 5.0, 2+ protein, 1–3 WBC's/hpf, and 10–15 RBC's/hpf.

14. Choose the diagnosis most likely to explain the azotemia and hypertension in this patient.

A. Nephrosclerosis
B. Atheroembolic disease
C. Drug-induced interstitial nephritis
D. Radiocontrast-induced renal disease
E. Postoperative acute tubular necrosis

15. Which is the most likely prognosis for the renal disease?

A. Complete recovery in 2–3 days
B. Complete recovery in 10–14 days
C. Stabilization of the renal function at the current level
D. Progressive deterioration of renal function over months
E. The disorder has no characteristic course

QUESTIONS 16–17

A 49-year-old woman with known polycystic renal disease and a serum creatinine of 3.0 mg/dl comes to the emergency room because of abdominal and flank pain. She states that she noted some blood-tinged urine the preceding day. Physical examination shows blood pressure of 180/105 mm Hg, pulse of 92 per minute, and temperature of 38°C. There is no orthostasis. Large bilateral upper quadrant masses are palpated; the right is somewhat tender. Bowel sounds are normal. A plain film of the abdomen reveals large upper quadrant masses bilaterally. An abdominal sonogram shows large polycystic kidneys with multiple overlapping echoes. A few areas in the upper pole of the right kidney have complex echoes. No solid masses are seen. Urinalysis shows 1+ protein, RBC's >100/hpf, and WBC's 5–10/hpf.

16. Which of the following is the most likely cause of the patient's condition?

A. Renal infarction
B. Urinary infection
C. Renal cell carcinoma
D. Hemorrhage into a renal cyst
E. Arteriovenous malformation of the kidney

17. Which procedure is most reasonably indicated at this time?

A. Observation
B. Surgical exploration
C. Renal angiography
D. Intravenous pyelogram
E. Computed tomography (CT) scan of the abdomen

18. A 45-year-old man who has a 10-year history of insulin-dependent diabetes comes to the emergency room because of fever, chills, and flank pain radiating to the right lower quadrant. He reports mild feverishness for about one day, with the sudden onset of the flank and abdominal pain over the last two hours. He believes he passed some solid material in the urine earlier in the day but did not collect it. Physical examination shows an ill-appearing man; temperature is 39°C. There is right costovertebral angle tenderness as well as deep right upper quadrant tenderness. Laboratory studies show:

Electrolytes	normal
Blood urea nitrogen	34 mg/dl
Serum creatinine	1.0 mg/dl

White blood cells 13,500/mm³
Hematocrit 41%
Urinalysis shows pH 6.0, >100 WBC's/hpf, and 50 RBC's/hpf; some white blood cell clumps are seen, along with a large amount of debris.

A renal ultrasound suggests mild dilatation of the right renal pelvis and upper right ureter. The kidney size is 12 cm bilaterally. A radiograph of the kidney, ureter, and bladder (KUB) shows a nonspecific gas pattern and a radiopaque mass at the right ureteropelvic junction. Which of the following is the most likely diagnosis?

A. Renal abscess
B. Uncomplicated pyelonephritis
C. A uric acid stone with infection
D. A calcium oxalate stone with infection
E. Renal papillary necrosis with infection

QUESTIONS 19–22

A 68-year-old woman is followed as an outpatient for hypertension that has become difficult to control. She has a long history of cigarette smoking. She is taking furosemide, potassium chloride, metoprolol, and clonidine, all of which have recently been increased. Blood pressure is 177/114 mm Hg; pulse rate is 58 per minute. The optic fundi show grade II KW changes. The lungs are clear and there is an S_4 gallop heard. The abdomen is not tender, and abdominal bruits are heard. There is no edema. A renal sonogram shows 9.5- and 7.7-cm kidneys with some increase in echogenicity. Laboratory studies show:

Serum electrolytes	
Sodium	136 mEq/L
Potassium	3.2 mEq/L
Chloride	90 mEq/L
Bicarbonate	32 mEq/L
Blood urea nitrogen	31 mg/dl
Serum creatinine	1.8 mg/dl

The complete blood count and urinalysis are normal.

The dose of furosemide is increased and captopril, 12.5 mg three times daily, is begun. One week later the patient returns to the emergency room because of weakness. Blood pressure is now 115/66 mm Hg, and pulse rate is 62 per minute. Physical examination shows an ill-appearing woman. There is no jugular venous distention. The lungs are clear. Cardiac examination is unchanged from the patient's initial visit. Some pedal edema is present. Electrocardiogram is unchanged from past tracings. Laboratory studies now show:

Serum electrolytes	
Sodium	132 mEq/L
Potassium	5.3 mEq/L
Chloride	100 mEq/L
Bicarbonate	21 mEq/L
Blood urea nitrogen	84 mg/dl
Serum creatinine	4.1 mg/dl

Urinalysis shows pH 5.0, trace protein, and no cells; a rare hyaline cast is noted.

19. What is the most likely cause of the deterioration in the clinical status of this patient?

A. Excessive diuresis
B. Renal embolization
C. Acute tubular necrosis
D. Drug-induced interstitial nephritis
E. Renal artery stenosis with decreased renal function caused by captopril

20. Which measure is most reasonably indicated at the time of presentation?

A. Acute hemodialysis
B. Renal arteriography
C. Percutaneous renal biopsy
D. CT scan of the abdomen
E. Hydration and observation

21. Discontinuation of which one of the following medicines is most likely to improve the clinical picture?

A. Captopril
B. Clonidine
C. Metoprolol
D. Furosemide
E. Potassium chloride

22. Once the renal function is stabilized, which diagnostic procedure should be undertaken?

A. Repeat sonogram
B. Plasma renin activity
C. CT scan with contrast
D. Rapid-sequence intravenous pyelogram
E. Digital subtraction angiogram of both renal arteries

QUESTIONS 23–24

A 26-year-old woman has an eight-year history of systemic lupus erythematosus, marked by polyserositis and arthralgias. She also has mild essential hypertension that has been treated with two dyazide capsules per day, and she was last seen six months before. Seven days ago she developed pleuritic chest pain, low-grade fever, and nonproductive cough. Chest roentgenogram showed mild blunting of both costovertebral angles. The rest of the examination was unremarkable; there was no evidence of thrombophlebitis. Ibuprofen administration was begun. The patient now returns because of weakness and lethargy. Blood pressure now is 90/60 mm Hg, and pulse rate is 110 per minute. Skin turgor is poor. Current laboratory results include:

Serum electrolytes	
Sodium	130 mEq/L
Potassium	5.7 mEq/L
Chloride	105 mEq/L
Bicarbonate	22 mEq/L
Blood urea nitrogen	40 mg/dl
Serum creatinine	3.7 mg/dl

Urinalysis shows 1+ protein, 2–4 WBC's/hpf, and no casts.

23. Which of the following is the most likely cause of the deterioration of renal function in this patient?

A. Pyelonephritis
B. Lupus nephritis
C. Excessive diuresis
D. Acute renal failure
E. Urinary obstruction due to triamterene stones

24. Which one of the following should be ordered now?

A. Renal biopsy
B. Stop all medications
C. Volume repletion (2 liters/day normal saline)
D. Start methylprednisolone, 1 g daily for three days
E. Abdominal CT scan with contrast

QUESTIONS 25–26

A 40-year-old woman was evaluated for edema of some months' duration and was found to have the nephrotic syndrome. The 24-hour urinary protein excretion was 11 g. Serum creatinine was 0.9 mg/dl, and creatinine clearance was 88 ml/min. A percutaneous renal biopsy revealed four glomeruli with a normal light microscopic pattern. Immunofluorescence was negative, and electron microscopy revealed fusion of the glomerular foot processes without evidence of immune deposits.

After an eight-week course of prednisone, 60 mg daily, the edema was slightly improved, although the patient noted cushingoid appearance. The 24-hour urinary protein excretion was 5 g. Prednisone was discontinued and she was managed with diuretics and sodium restriction with an improvement of the edema.

Two years later, the patient is found to have persistent edema and a serum creatinine of 3.7 mg/dl, with 14 g of protein in a 24-hour collection of urine.

25. If a renal biopsy were to be performed now, the most likely histologic diagnosis would be

A. IgA nephropathy
B. minimal change disease
C. membranous glomerulonephritis
D. focal sclerosing glomerulonephritis
E. membranoproliferative glomerulonephritis

26. Which of the following should be used to treat the recurrent nephrotic syndrome in this patient?

A. Aspirin plus dipyridamole
B. Prednisone, 60 mg orally daily
C. Prednisone plus cyclophosphamide
D. Methylprednisolone, 1 g daily for three days
E. None of the above

27. A 32-year-old woman underwent successful renal transplantation for therapy of idiopathic focal sclerosing glomerulonephritis four months ago and is now seen in a renal clinic for follow-up. She has received prednisone and cyclosporine as immunosuppressive agents and has not had an episode of acute renal allograft rejection thus far in the course. On this visit the patient reports mild distress over recent headaches. Physical examination shows hypertension (160/105 mm Hg) for the first time since the transplant; the examination is otherwise normal. Serum creatinine is 2.1 mg/dl, after having been 1.2–1.3 mg/dl for the past three months. The complete blood count and urinalysis are normal.

A percutaneous renal biopsy of the transplanted kidney is performed. Light microscopy of this biopsy specimen is reported to be normal. The most likely cause for this clinical presentation is

A. acute allograft rejection
B. chronic allograft rejection
C. cyclosporine nephrotoxicity
D. de novo renal disease in an allograft
E. recurrent focal sclerosis in a transplanted kidney

28. Which of the following is often seen in cyclosporine nephrotoxicity?

A. Hypertension
B. Hyperkalemia
C. Nephrotic-range proteinuria
D. Hyperchloremic metabolic acidosis
E. Pyuria and casts in the urinary sediment

QUESTIONS 29–30

A 78-year-old man is brought to the emergency room by a neighbor who was alarmed after not hearing from him for three days. The patient is barely conscious and has an obvious left hemiparesis. Blood pressure is 90/60 mm Hg with a pulse rate of 120 per minute. He is afebrile. The mucous membranes are dry, and there is tenting of the skin over the forehead. There is early skin breakdown on the left hip. The remainder of the physical examination is consistent with dehydration and a cerebrovascular accident. There is no sign of heart failure or pulmonary infiltrates. Weight is 70 kg. Laboratory studies show:

Serum electrolytes	
Sodium	162 mEq/L
Potassium	5.0 mEq/L
Chloride	120 mEq/L
Bicarbonate	24 mEq/L
Serum glucose	181 mg/dl

29. What is the calculated free water deficit in this patient?

A. 1 liter
B. 2 liters
C. 4 liters
D. 6 liters
E. 10 liters

30. In planning fluid therapy, which of the following is appropriate?

A. Half of the calculated water deficit should be administered as hypotonic fluid immediately and the remainder over 8–12 hours
B. Initial extracellular volume (ECV) repletion should be made with isotonic saline, and the free water deficit should be repaired with hypotonic fluids over 48 hours
C. Furosemide should be administered and the measured urinary sodium loss should be replaced with hypotonic saline
D. The calculated free water deficit should be administered as half-normal saline over the next 24 hours
E. The calculated free water deficit should be administered as half-normal saline over the next 48 hours

QUESTIONS 31–32

A 78-year-old woman is evaluated in the emergency room because of a four-day history of vomiting, muscle cramps, and low-grade fever. She has been unable to eat anything and has drunk only tea, water, and 7-Up. The previous history is unremarkable.

31. Which of the following would be the most likely electrolyte disturbance?

A. Hyponatremia
B. Hyperkalemia
C. Hypokalemia
D. Anion gap acidosis
E. Hyperchloremic metabolic acidosis

32. The most likely urinary electrolyte findings would be

A. urine sodium = 30 mEq/L; urine potassium = 60 mEq/L
B. urine sodium = 30 mEq/L; urine chloride = 90 mEq/L

C. urine sodium = 30 mEq/L; urine chloride = 30 mEq/L
D. urine sodium = 3 mEq/L; urine potassium = 20 mEq/L
E. urine sodium = 3 mEq/L; urine chloride = 50 mEq/L

QUESTIONS 33–34

A 60-year-old man is seen in the emergency room because of muscle cramps and paresthesias. He has a history of recurrent squamous cell carcinoma of the head and neck and finished a course of *cis*-platinum three weeks before admission to the emergency room. Local radiation therapy is planned for the immediate future. He has also noted frequent watery diarrhea over the past month and has not been able to eat or drink well. Physical examination does not show significant volume depletion. There is a positive Chvostek's sign, serum calcium of 5.8 mg/dl, and serum magnesium of 0.7 mEq/L. The urinary magnesium concentration on a random urine sample is 20 mEq/L.

33. Which factor is LEAST likely to have contributed to the hypomagnesemia in this patient?

A. Diarrhea
B. Hypocalcemia
C. Poor oral intake
D. *Cis*-platinum therapy
E. A paraneoplastic syndrome from a squamous cell carcinoma

34. Which factor is most likely to have contributed to the hypocalcemia?

A. Diarrhea
B. Hypomagnesemia
C. Poor oral intake
D. *Cis*-platinum therapy
E. A paraneoplastic syndrome from a squamous cell carcinoma

35. A 19-year-old man is brought to the emergency room from a small community hospital in a rugged region of the state. He was fighting a fire in a mountainous region five days before and was injured when a tree fell on his right leg. There was no extensive blood loss or hypotension; a femoral fracture was stabilized with traction. The major reason for transfer is the development of acute renal failure attributed to rhabdomyolysis and the need for acute hemodialysis. On arrival the morning after a five-hour ambulance ride, the patient appears ill. He is slightly obtunded and reports breathlessness and chest discomfort. Blood pressure is 90/70 mm Hg; pulse rate is 130 per minute. There is jugular venous distention; the lungs are clear. The heart sounds are distant and difficult to evaluate in the emergency room. The rest of the physical findings are consistent with the injury. Laboratory studies show:

Serum potassium	6.9 mEq/L
Serum bicarbonate	13 mEq/L
Blood urea nitrogen	168 mg/dl
Serum creatinine	14.7 mg/dl
Calcium	7.7 mg/dl
Phosphate	8.8 mg/dl
Hemoglobin	11 g/dl
Hematocrit	33%
White blood cell count	11,000/mm^3

A supine chest film with suboptimal technique reveals an enlarged cardiac silhouette with clear lung fields. An electrocardiogram shows a tachycardia and peaked T waves, but generally low voltage. Although arrangements were made for immediate hemodialysis, the patient became increasingly hypotensive.

The most likely reason for the clinical deterioration after transfer is

A. hyperkalemia
B. uremic acidosis
C. volume overload
D. acute pericarditis
E. the general effects of acute renal failure

36. Each of the following statements regarding radiocontrast-induced renal failure is correct EXCEPT

A. it is more likely to occur in volume-depleted patients
B. it usually occurs 24–48 hours after radiocontrast administration
C. it is initially associated with a low urinary sodium concentration
D. it develops more frequently in patients with underlying renal disease
E. when it occurs in a diabetic patient, recovery of renal function is uncommon

DIRECTIONS: For questions 37 to 73, you are to decide whether EACH choice is true or false. Any combination of answers, from all true to all false, may occur. Mark the answer sheet "T" or "F" in the space provided.

37. Which of the following statements regarding post-streptococcal glomerulonephritis is/are true?

A. Both sexes are equally affected
B. All age groups are equally affected
C. All age groups have a similar prognosis
D. Nephrotic-range proteinuria is common
E. Renal biopsy is necessary for management

38. Which of the following is/are true about anti–glomerular basement membrane (anti-GBM) disease?

A. The presence of linear deposits of immunoglobulin along the glomerular capillary basement membrane is specific for the diagnosis of anti-GBM disease
B. The presence of both linear deposits of immunoglobulin along the glomerular capillary basement membrane and anti-GBM antibodies in the serum is required for diagnosis
C. It is always rapidly progressive
D. It is characteristically marked by the presence of azotemia, an abnormal urinary sediment, and pulmonary hemorrhage
E. Treatment with plasmapheresis is indicated

39. Which of the following is/are true about IgA nephropathy?

A. It is commonly associated with the nephrotic syndrome
B. Immunofluorescent studies of renal biopsy will establish the diagnosis
C. Gross hematuria is common
D. Its recurrence in renal allografts usually leads to graft failure
E. The prognosis is favorable in a majority of patients

40. Which of the following is/are true regarding membranous glomerulonephritis?

A. Spontaneous remission is rare
B. The nephrotic syndrome is usually present at diagnosis
C. Electron microscopy of renal biopsy specimens shows granular electron-dense subepithelial deposits and spikes of basement membrane
D. Corticosteroids have been shown to slow progression of renal insufficiency
E. Hypocomplementemia is common

41. Which of the following is/are true of the nephrotic syndrome?

A. Plasma volume is usually increased
B. It is usually associated with renal sodium wasting
C. It occurs with either diffuse or focal forms of glomerulonephritis
D. The rate of infection is increased
E. Albumin infusions are of significant benefit for treatment of hypoalbuminemia and edema

42. Which of the following characteristics occur(s) in acute, but rarely in chronic, renal failure?

A. Minimal or mild anemia
B. Radiographic signs of renal osteodystrophy
C. Bilaterally small kidneys
D. Dilute urine with a high urine sodium
E. Hypertension

43. Which of the following characteristics occur(s) in acute tubular necrosis but rarely in acute prerenal or postrenal failure?

A. Total anuria
B. Marked day-to-day variation in urine output
C. Fractional excretion of sodium of 5%
D. Urine-to-plasma creatinine ratio of 14:1
E. Cellular and pigmented casts on microscopic examination of the urine

44. Which of the following is/are characteristic of analgesic-associated nephropathy?

A. Equal sex distribution
B. Normal-sized kidneys
C. Anemia out of proportion to azotemia
D. Sterile pyuria
E. Papillary necrosis

45. Which of the following is/are true of toxemia of pregnancy?

A. It occurs most commonly in young primiparous and older multiparous women
B. It is associated with glomerular endothelial swelling and fibrin deposition
C. It is frequently associated with azotemia
D. All patient groups have a high incidence of developing hypertension in later life
C. Blood pressure usually returns to normal within two weeks after delivery

46. A 47-year-old man has an excretory urogram for investigation of microscopic hematuria discovered on a routine urinalysis. He is apparently healthy and entirely without complaints. Kidneys are of normal size, with calcification of and collection of dye in dilated medullary structures. Serum electrolytes, BUN, creatinine, calcium, phosphorus, and uric acid are normal. Creatinine clearance is 103 ml per minute. Urinalysis reveals rare red blood cells and no protein. Which of the following is/are true of this patient?

A. There is a significant chance that he will develop symptomatic renal stones
B. There is a significant chance that he has hypercalciuria
C. He is likely to have impaired maximal urine concentration
D. His condition is likely to progress gradually to chronic end-stage renal disease
E. His children each have a 1-in-2 chance of developing the same condition

47. Which of the following statements about renal cell carcinoma is/are true?

A. Its presence in both kidneys indicates the occurrence of metastatic disease
B. Erythrocytosis is the most commonly associated hematologic abnormality

C. If the entire tumor is surgically removable, tumor extension into the renal vein does *not* compromise the prognosis
D. Hypercalcemia is found in only a minority of patients
E. A five-year apparent cure rate of 60–70% is to be anticipated in patients with surgically resectable lesions

48. Which of the following is/are true regarding light chain nephropathy?

A. It is a marker of amyloidosis
B. It is a cause of the nephrotic syndrome
C. It is always a consequence of multiple myeloma
D. It is sometimes associated with abnormalities of urinary acidification
E. Its development is primarily a function of the degree of light chain excretion

QUESTIONS 49–50

A 19-year-old man has a four-year history of type I diabetes mellitus; the disease is well controlled on split-dose NPH insulin. The patient is clinically well. Weight is 70 kg. On a routine evaluation, urinalysis shows pH 5.0, no protein, and no cells. Findings of 24-hour urine collection show:

Total volume	1950 ml
Total creatinine	1610 mg
Urine protein	375 mg

The serum creatinine was 0.7 mg/dl, and the calculated creatinine clearance was 160 ml/min.

49. The results of the 24-hour urine collection

A. are consistent with the clinical history
B. are normal for the patient's age and size
C. represent a 48-hour collection due to patient error
D. reflect creatinine secretion that falsely raises the creatinine clearance rate
E. represent a laboratory error in blood creatinine determination

50. Twelve years later, the same patient is found to have proliferative retinopathy. Renal function evaluation shows a 24-hour protein excretion of 4 g, and a creatinine clearance of 84 ml/min. Which of the following is/are correct?

A. Despite the proteinuria, renal function is normal
B. It is very likely that the patient will develop end-stage renal disease within the next five years
C. A renal biopsy should be performed to establish the diagnosis of diabetic nephropathy
D. Microalbuminuria (375 mg/24 hr) at the first evaluation is an indication that the patient will develop diabetic nephropathy
E. Regular insulin should be added so that "tight" control will prevent deterioration of renal function

51. Which of the following is/are true of diabetic nephropathy?

A. It is associated with the nephrotic syndrome
B. It develops only in insulin-requiring diabetics
C. It may arise at any time during the course of the disease
D. Its development may be avoided by careful diabetic control
E. It is more likely to be present in patients with other microvascular diabetic complications

QUESTIONS 52–53

A 67-year-old man is referred to you by a dermatologist because of edema. He has a 25-year history of severe chronic neurodermatitis. Repeated skin biopsies have excluded more serious pathology. The patient reports that edema has been slowly developing over a few months. He also notes malaise.

Blood pressure is 168/108 mm Hg; pulse rate is 88 per minute. Physical examination shows an ill-appearing man; his appearance is remarkable for numerous linear atrophic skin lesions on the trunk and extremities. Several recent excoriations of various ages are also noted. The optic fundi show grade I arteriolar narrowing. There is mild jugular venous distention. The lungs are clear. The heart is somewhat enlarged, with distant heart sounds. The abdomen is obese. There is 3+ pitting edema of the lower extremities. Some distal sensory neuropathy is also noted. Laboratory studies show:

Serum electrolytes	
Sodium	144 mEq/L
Potassium	5.0 mEq/L
Chloride	101 mEq/L
Bicarbonate	18 mEq/L
Blood glucose	122 mg/dl
Blood urea nitrogen	86 mg/dl
Serum creatinine	6.4 mg/dl

A 24-hour creatinine clearance is 14 ml/min. The 24-hour urinary protein excretion is 16.2 g; 85% of it is albumin.

Renal sonogram reveals 14-cm kidneys bilaterally, with no signs of obstruction.

52. Which of the following renal diagnoses is/are likely to be associated with this degree of proteinuria?

A. Amyloidosis
B. Diabetic nephropathy
C. Hypertensive nephrosclerosis
D. Membranous glomerulonephritis
E. Immune complex glomerulonephritis

53. Which of the following is/are associated with relatively large kidneys despite advanced renal insufficiency?

A. Amyloidosis
B. Nephrosclerosis
C. Polycystic disease
D. Diabetic nephropathy
E. Membranous nephropathy

QUESTIONS 54–55

A 72-year-old woman, hospitalized for hip replacement, has a decrease in renal function 12 days after surgery. She has a history of hypertension and very mild congestive heart failure treated with digitalis and diuretics. These have been continued in hospital along with cimetidine. Four days after surgery, parenteral analgesics were stopped and replaced by ibuprofen. Ten days after surgery, pyuria was noted. The patient was afebrile. The Foley catheter was removed and a course of tobramycin was begun. On the twelfth day after surgery, the patient was noted to have presacral and pedal edema. Serum creatinine had risen to 2.7 mg/dl, from 1.1 mg/dl preoperatively. You are asked to see the patient on the twelfth day after surgery.

The patient is an elderly woman in bed who is alert. Blood pressure is 170/98 mm Hg; pulse rate is 90 per minute. Physical examination shows mild jugular venous distention. The lungs have a few rales at the bases which clear with deep breathing. There is a soft S_3 gallop, as well as presacral and lower extremity edema. Laboratory studies show:

Serum electrolytes	
Sodium	134 mEq/L
Potassium	5.7 mEq/L
Chloride	100 mEq/L
Bicarbonate	21 mEq/L
Blood urea nitrogen	46 mg/dl
Serum creatinine	2.7 mg/dl
Creatinine clearance	23 ml/min
Urine	
Sodium	35 mEq/L
Potassium	5 mEq/L

Urinalysis shows pH 6.5 and 1+ protein; many white blood cells are seen, with a few cellular casts and eosinophils. The 24-hour volume is 650 ml.

54. Which of the following causes of deterioration in renal function is/are likely?

A. Pyelonephritis
B. Excessive diuresis
C. Aminoglycoside-induced renal failure
D. Ibuprofen-induced interstitial nephritis
E. Cimetidine-induced elevation in creatinine

55. Which of the following measures is/are appropriate at this time?

A. Renal biopsy
B. Stop all medications
C. Start methylprednisolone, 1 g daily for three days
D. Volume repletion (2 liters/day normal saline)
E. Abdominal CT scan with contrast

QUESTIONS 56–58

A 42-year-old woman is hospitalized for treatment of gram-negative osteomyelitis thought to be a consequence of intravenous drug use. After six weeks of therapy with an aminoglycoside and a cephalosporin, the patient reports progressive muscle weakness. A consultation is requested.

The patient is a thin woman lying in bed. Blood pressure is 108/68 mm Hg; pulse rate is 98 per minute. The patient is afebrile. Physical examination shows that the lungs, heart, and abdomen are normal. There is demonstrable weakness of the shoulder and quadriceps muscle groups. There is a positive Chvostek's sign. Laboratory studies show:

Serum electrolytes	
Sodium	142 mEq/L
Potassium	2.0 mEq/L
Chloride	109 mEq/L
Bicarbonate	23 mEq/L
Blood urea nitrogen	19 mg/dl
Serum creatinine	0.9 mg/dl
Calcium	6.8 mg/dl
Phosphate	4.1 mg/dl
Magnesium	0.6 mEq/L

Over the next 24 hours the patient receives potassium chloride, 200 mEq orally and intravenously, as well as intravenous calcium gluconate. The symptoms and electrolyte abnormalities persist.

56. Which of the following treatments is/are indicated at this time?

A. Vitamin D therapy
B. Oral calcium carbonate
C. A potassium-sparing diuretic
D. Intramuscular magnesium sulfate
E. Continued administration of potassium chloride

57. Which of the following mechanisms is/are likely to be operative in this patient?

A. Hypomagnesemia has led to inappropriate renal potassium wasting
B. Aminoglycoside administration has resulted in aminoglycoside-induced acute tubular necrosis
C. Long-term aminoglycoside administration has produced primary renal magnesium wasting, potassium wasting, and calcium wasting
D. Long-term aminoglycoside administration has produced hyperaldosteronism, which subsequently results in hypomagnesemia and hypokalemia
E. Long-term aminoglycoside administration has produced primary renal potassium wasting, which subsequently results in hypomagnesemia and hypocalcemia

58. Which of the following is/are true concerning the hypokalemia in this patient?

A. Oral rather than intravenous potassium replacement therapy is indicated
B. It is likely that the total-body potassium deficit is at least 500 mEq
C. The potassium deficit cannot be fully replaced until the magnesium deficit is corrected
D. Respiratory alkalosis can explain a serum potassium of 2.0 mEq/L by a shift of potassium into cells
E. Renal potassium wasting would be diagnosed if the 24-hour urinary potassium excretion rate were 45 mEq when the serum potassium was 2.0 mEq/L

59. A 32-year-old man has a 15-year history of diabetes; serum creatinine is 2.3 mg/dl. A diagnosis of diabetic nephropathy is established by renal biopsy. Which of the following is/are true of this patient?

A. He should never be subjected to a radiocontrast study
B. He has a less than 30% chance of having hypertension at this time
C. He has a 50% chance of having the nephrotic syndrome at this time
D. Because of his age, nephropathy is likely to be his only major organ system diabetic complication to date
E. He is likely to develop end-stage renal disease requiring dialysis within the next four years

60. Which of the following is/are true of hypertensive nephrosclerosis culminating in significant chronic renal failure?

A. It is associated with heavy proteinuria and hematuria
B. It is often a consequence of mild hypertension sustained over many years
C. Aggressive control of blood pressure may prevent or ameliorate further deterioration

D. Renal histopathology shows sclerosis and obsolescence of glomeruli as well as arteriolar sclerosis
E. Aggressive control of blood pressure may be associated with a transient worsening of renal function

QUESTIONS 61–62

A 57-year-old woman comes to the emergency room because of malaise and edema. She has been previously healthy and takes no medicines. A comprehensive physical examination, including routine laboratory tests, was performed three months ago and was entirely normal. The patient reports these symptoms for a few weeks. She has noted no change in her urine volume but does note nocturia. Physical examination shows a mildly ill woman with hypertension and pedal edema. No other remarkable physical findings were noted. Laboratory studies show:

Serum electrolytes	
Sodium	138 mEq/L
Potassium	5.3 mEq/L
Chloride	100 mEq/L
Bicarbonate	18 mEq/L
Blood urea nitrogen	62 mg/dl
Serum creatinine	4.8 mg/dl
Hematocrit	31%
White blood cell count	9,700/mm^3
Erythrocyte sedimentation rate	40 mm/hr

Urinalysis shows pH 5.5, 2+ protein, 10–20 RBC's/hpf, and rare red blood cell casts.
Antinuclear antibodies, complement (CH_{50}), antistreptolysin-O(ASO) titer, and rheumatoid antibodies were normal.

A percutaneous renal biopsy is performed. Light microscopy reveals that about 80% of the glomeruli seen are affected with proliferating epithelial crescents. Immunofluorescence shows nonspecific trapping of low levels of IgG and IgA, complement, and fibrin.

61. Which of the following renal syndromes is/are likely to appear with this clinical and histologic picture?

A. IgA nephropathy
B. Polyarteritis nodosa
C. Wegener's granulomatosis
D. Post-streptococcal glomerulonephritis
E. Idiopathic rapidly progressive glomerulonephritis

62. Which of the following therapies is/are appropriate at this time?

A. Hemodialysis
B. Plasmapheresis
C. Cyclophosphamide
D. Intravenous methylprednisolone
E. Warfarin and dipyridamole

63. Which of the following is/are true of uremic acidosis?

A. Urine pH is usually greater than 6.0
B. Hypokalemia worsens the acidosis by suppressing ammonia production
C. Anion gap acidosis develops only when the GFR falls below 20 ml/min
D. Renal ammonia production and excretion are low, considering the degree of acidosis
E. Bicarbonate wasting is observed when isotonic bicarbonate is infused to restore the serum bicarbonate to normal levels

QUESTIONS 64–65

A 67-year-old man is referred to a nephrologist for evaluation for hemodialysis. The patient has a long history of hypertension; past medical history is otherwise unremarkable. Over the past year, the creatinine clearance has fallen to 12 ml/min and symptoms of uremia have developed, including malaise, decreased appetite, pruritus, and some mild sensory impairment. The blood pressure had required three drugs (a diuretic, a beta blocker, and clonidine) with only fair control; recently, increasing hypertension required increases in antihypertensive medicine dosage and the addition of minoxidil. An abdominal CT scan, performed three months previously for other reasons, showed kidney sizes of 7.3 and 9.2 cm. An electrocardiogram is consistent with left ventricular hypertrophy. Blood pressure now is 170/112 mm Hg. The optic fundi demonstrate grade II changes with arteriovenous nicking. There are no signs of heart failure, and examination shows left ventricular hypertrophy. Abdominal and femoral bruits are heard. There is no edema. Laboratory studies show:

Serum potassium	3.6 mEq/L
Serum bicarbonate	19 mEq/L
Blood urea nitrogen	99 mg/dl
Serum creatinine	6.8 mg/dl
Calcium	7.8 mg/dl
Phosphate	6.2 mg/dl
Hemoglobin	7.5 g/dl
Hematocrit	22%

Urinalysis shows trace proteins, no cells.

A renal ultrasound confirms the kidney size noted on the CT scan and does not demonstrate obstruction.

64. Which of the following is/are indicated at this time?

A. Renal angiography
B. Retrograde pyelography
C. Excretory urogram
D. Phosphate binders and calcium supplements
E. Placement of a hemodialysis vascular access

65. Which of the following is/are true concerning the hypertension in this patient?

A. It is unlikely that better control will be achieved
B. Volume overload plays a major role in the hypertension
C. Converting enzyme inhibitors should be used in this patient
D. Severe renal artery and aortic atherosclerosis is likely to be present
E. Renal artery revascularization should be undertaken to preserve renal function

QUESTIONS 66–67

A 50-year-old man with polycystic kidney disease has received chronic hemodialysis for three years. He is now noted to have persistent hypercalcemia of 11.1 mg/dl. Serum phosphate is controlled at 3.2 mg/dl. He takes 0.5 g calcium carbonate daily, aluminum hydroxide phosphate binders, but no vitamin D supplements. Radiographs of the hands show subperiosteal reabsorption of the distal phalangeal tufts. A high-resolution ultrasound examination of the neck shows four enlarged parathyroid glands measuring from 1.2 to 2.8 cm in diameter. An immunoassay determination of parathyroid hormone is about 500 times normal for that assay.

66. Which of the following is/are true of the parathyroid abnormalities in this patient?

A. Subtotal parathyroidectomy, leaving a small portion of one gland, should be performed
B. Removal of the largest parathyroid gland should be performed to control the hyperparathyroidism
C. Therapy with vitamin D analogues should be begun to reverse the hyperparathyroidism
D. Better control of serum phosphate is likely to reverse the excessive parathyroid hormone secretion
E. Control of serum phosphate early in the course of renal disease might have prevented the development of these abnormalities

67. Which of the following is/are direct consequences of secondary hyperthyroidism in this patient?

A. Metastatic soft tissue calcifications
B. Hyperchloremic metabolic alkalosis
C. Hypercalcemia due to enhanced reabsorption of bone calcium
D. Hypercalcemia due to enhanced gastrointestinal absorption of calcium
E. Pathologic fractures due to cystic lesions in bones (brown tumors)

68. Which of the following statements regarding aminoglycoside-induced renal failure is/are true?

A. It is more likely to occur in elderly patients
B. It is associated with a low urinary sodium concentration
C. It normally starts to develop after several days of therapy
D. It usually resolves within two weeks after the initial recovery begins
E. It develops more frequently in patients with underlying renal disease

69. Which of the following diuretics is/are associated with metabolic acidosis?

A. Thiazide
B. Amiloride
C. Furosemide
D. Acetazolamide
E. Ethacrynic acid

70. Which of the following diuretics is/are associated with hypokalemia?

A. Thiazide
B. Amiloride
C. Furosemide
D. Acetazolamide
E. Ethacrynic acid

71. Which of the following diuretics is/are useful in treating patients with calcium-containing kidney stones?

A. Thiazide
B. Amiloride
C. Furosemide
D. Acetazolamide
E. Ethacrynic acid

72. A 60-year-old man is being evaluated for progressive renal insufficiency. One kidney was lost at age 20 owing to trauma. Other pertinent medical history includes gout and recent symptoms of nocturia and hesitancy. Serum creatinine is 6.4 mg/dl, and blood urea nitrogen is 80 mg/dl. Ultrasound examination shows a single kidney with marked hydronephrosis and a thinned renal cortex. Which of the following is/are true concerning this case of obstructive uropathy?

A. Renal damage is permanent at this point
B. Hemodialysis must be instituted at this time
C. Hyperchloremic metabolic acidosis with hyperkalemia is often seen in this setting
D. A uricosuric agent (e.g., probenecid) should be started in view of the gout history
E. Further urologic evaluation is *not* warranted

73. Which of the following statements is/are true of analgesic nephropathy?

A. Pyuria is a frequent finding
B. Nephrotic-range proteinuria is common
C. There is an increased incidence of transitional cell carcinoma
D. The renal function can be stabilized if the patient stops abusing analgesics
E. Massive renal potassium wasting and sodium chloride wasting are often observed

DIRECTIONS: Questions 74 to 85 are matching questions. For each numbered item, choose the most likely associated lettered item from those provided. Each numbered item has ONLY ONE answer. Within each set of questions, each lettered item may be the answer to one, more than one, or none of the numbered items.

QUESTIONS 74–80

For each of the therapeutic agents listed below, select the most likely associated complication.

A. Impaired free water excretion
B. Nephrogenic diabetes insipidus
C. Secondary nephrotic syndrome
D. Hypokalemia
E. Hyperkalemia

74. Gold

75. Chlorpropamide

76. Lithium

77. Carbenicillin

78. Succinylcholine

79. D-Penicillamine

80. Spironolactone

QUESTIONS 81–85

For each of the following clinical diagnoses, select the appropriate serum electrolyte determinations.

	A	B	C (mEq/L)	D	E
Sodium	142	138	138	138	122
Potassium	5.7	2.2	4.2	5.7	5.7
Chloride	100	112	112	112	76
Bicarbonate	16	16	16	16	16

81. Diabetic ketoacidosis

82. Type IV renal tubular acidosis (RTA)

83. Distal (type I) RTA

84. Proximal (type II) RTA

85. Uremic acidosis—not usually hyponatremic

PART 3

RENAL DISEASE

ANSWERS

1.(C); 2.(B); 3.(A) The most likely diagnosis is acute tubulointerstitial nephritis. The presence of fever, rash, and eosinophilia is highly suggestive of but not essential to the diagnosis. Pyuria with eosinophiluria is very common in this disorder. Although most commonly associated with methicillin, it may occur as a consequence of other penicillin derivatives as well as many other drugs. Tubulointerstitial nephritis is often associated with mild proteinuria and renal tubular dysfunction out of proportion to the decrement in the GFR. These defects often include hyperchloremic acidosis with a normal anion gap, hyperkalemia, inappropriate renal salt loss, and inability to form a concentrated urine. *(Cecil, Ch. 82; Brenner and Rector, Chs. 20 and 25)*

4.(C); 5.(B) The most likely diagnosis is obstructive uropathy. The well-preserved hemoglobin concentration and only slightly depressed calcium concentration suggest that the renal failure is of recent onset. The history of urinary hesitancy suggests that the patient has prostatism. The ultrasound examination that was normal initially, then showed signs of obstruction the next day, was caused by severe volume depletion resulting in inadequate urine flow and inadequate pressure to distend the renal pelvis. In the presence of anuria, bladder catheterization must be performed to eliminate lower urinary tract obstruction, a potentially reversible cause of acute renal failure. *(Cecil, Ch. 83; Brenner and Rector, Chs. 19 and 33)*

6.(B) The patient's condition is consistent with pulmonary thromboembolism. Renal vein thrombosis and thromboembolic events occur in an unusually large proportion of patients with the nephrotic syndrome, particularly when caused by membranous glomerulonephritis. When evaluating a patient with this condition, particular attention should be paid to the presence of thrombus in the renal veins. Chronic renal vein thrombosis does not usually produce a decrement in renal function. *(Cecil, Chs. 81 and 87; Brenner and Rector, Ch. 21)*

7.(C) Surreptitious vomiting, in which the primary defect is loss of HCl, is the only one of these causes of metabolic alkalosis in which the urine chloride is low, and in which chloride (saline) replacement will repair the defect. In Bartter's syndrome and diuretic abuse, there is an increased delivery of chloride to the distal nephron. In mineralocorticoid excess, alkalosis is maintained by continued generation of bicarbonate by the distal nephron. ECF is expanded and there is no chloride depletion. *(Cecil, Ch. 77; Brenner and Rector, Ch. 13)*

8.(B); 9.(A) The patient has a history consistent with multiple myeloma. The presence of a negative dipstick for protein but a positive sulfosalicylic acid reaction for protein is characteristic of Bence Jones proteinuria. This patient also has hypercalcemia and a normal anion gap metabolic acidosis. Plasma cell dyscrasias are associated with renal involvement in over 50% of cases. Acute renal failure may result from hypercalcemia, dehydration, or progressive renal insufficiency characterized by isosthenuria and dysfunction of proximal and distal tubules. The degree of renal dysfunction may reflect the intensity of Bence Jones proteinuria. The nephrotic syndrome or nephrotic-range proteinuria is not characteristic of multiple myeloma per se. When encountered in a plasma cell dyscrasia, it should suggest the development of secondary amyloidosis, which may occur in 10% of patients with multiple myeloma. These patients may have very heavy proteinuria and normal or large kidneys coexisting with azotemia. *(Cecil, Ch. 163; Brenner and Rector, Chs. 23 and 25)*

10.(D); 11.(A) The patient has ketoacidosis. Typically, a significant degree of extracellular volume depletion is present in this disorder. However, the measured serum sodium must be corrected for the appearance of elevated concentrations of glucose in the ECF. Even when this is done, there is a significant difference between measured and calculated plasma osmolality. This suggests the presence of either an unmeasured osmotically active substance in the plasma or artifactual hyponatremia. In the presence of diabetic ketoacidosis with lipemic plasma, hyperlipemia is the likely cause of artifactual hyponatremia. In a volume-depleted state, the urine sodium is expected to be low. It is not low in this patient, because of an osmotic diuresis (glycosuria). *(Cecil, Ch. 77; Brenner and Rector, Ch. 13)*

12.(B); 13.(E) The patient's clinical and laboratory data are highly suggestive of the syndrome of inappropriate antidiuretic hormone (SIADH), a common consequence of oat cell carcinoma of the lung. He has hyponatremia with a high urine osmolality. To make the diagnosis of SIADH, there must be no evidence of ECF concentration. Associated findings that support the notion of ECF *expansion* are a low BUN and serum creatinine and uric acid. The ADH elaborated by the tumor represents a nonphysiologic stimulus for continued urinary concentration in the face of hypo-osmolality. Thus, the patient has an impaired free water clearance and continues to retain free water despite hyponatremia. The presence of a high urine sodium concentration despite hyponatremia and hypo-osmolality underscores the fact that in SIADH there is *expansion* of the ECF. Therefore, the major physiologic stimulus to sodium retention—ECF volume depletion—is not present. In SIADH, sodium excretion reflects sodium intake and not plasma osmolality. *(Cecil, Ch. 77; Brenner and Rector, Ch. 11)*

14.(B); 15.(D) The patient has renal atheroembolic disease. In this disorder, cholesterol microemboli from ragged atherosclerotic plaques in the major vessels are showered distally. They lodge in the kidney as well as other organs, where their effects may be silent or may produce cutaneous lesions, pancreatitis, or CNS manifestations. In the kidney, cholesterol crystals may lodge in the small arterioles and produce an inflammatory perivascular reaction that ultimately leads to sclerosis of the blood vessel. This sclerosis, accompanied by varying degree of inflammation, is often accompanied by the pathologic hallmark of the disease—

the cholesterol cleft, a cleft-like area that was occupied by the cholesterol crystal. These clefts may be found in many organs. The precipitating events for cholesterol embolization may be major trauma, major vessel angiography, or vascular surgery; it may occasionally occur spontaneously. The renal manifestations include hypertension, eosinophilia, and progressive renal impairment developing over weeks to months after the precipitating event. The azotemia is usually not reversible (although exceptions have been reported). Although not treatable, this disorder should be considered as an explanation for progressive azotemia and hypertension that develop weeks to months after an aortic angiogram or aortic surgery. *(Cecil, Ch. 87; Brenner and Rector, Ch. 26)*

16.(D); 17.(A) In polycystic kidney disease the kidneys are massively enlarged with tubular cysts—dilatations of tubules which continue to enlarge over years. Among the complications of this disorder are bleeding and infection of the cysts. The typical presentation of cyst bleeding is flank or abdominal pain and hematuria, although blood loss is not usually severe and stops spontaneously. Since bacteriuria and urinary infection are also very common in polycystic kidney disease, the index of suspicion for urinary tract infection should be high. Renal ultrasound examination of polycystic kidneys usually shows masses of large overlapping cysts. The presence of cysts with complex echoes in this case is consistent with bleeding into a cyst. However, since there may be an increased incidence of renal cell carcinoma in polycystic renal disease, and bleeding or complex sonographic echoes may be a manifestation of this, a CT scan with contrast may be useful in ruling out renal cell carcinoma. *(Cecil, Ch. 91; Brenner and Rector, Ch. 30)*

18.(E) The patient's clinical presentation is suggestive of renal colic. The ultrasound suggests obstruction; the fever and urinary findings are suggestive of infection. The passage of tissue-like material and the fact that this patient is diabetic should strongly suggest papillary necrosis, a condition to which diabetics are particularly susceptible. Diabetes accounts for about 50% of all cases of papillary necrosis. It is thought that because of impaired microcirculation, diabetic papillae are particularly susceptible to infarction and necrosis. It is often, although not always, associated with urinary infection, although the entire process may be asymptomatic if there is no infection or obstruction. *(Cecil, Chs. 83, 85, and 90; Brenner and Rector, Chs. 24, 31, and 33)*

19.(E); 20.(E); 21.(A); 22.(E) The patient has renal artery stenosis exacerbating the hypertension. The small kidney is probably nonfunctional. The acute deterioration in blood pressure with the institution of small doses of captopril, along with the history of severe hypertension and disparate kidney size, strongly suggests that renal renin production by the kidney with the stenotic artery was partly responsible for the hypertension. When the renin-angiotensin pathway is interrupted by an angiotensin-converting enzyme inhibitor, both hypotension and a decrease in renal function result. Captopril is most likely to decrease renal function in states in which renal perfusion is critically dependent on renal renin production, e.g., bilateral renal artery stenosis (or stenosis in the renal artery of a single functioning kidney), or in markedly prerenal states. Although unequal renal size on sonogram, intravenous pyelogram, or CT scan suggests the diagnosis of renal artery stenosis, the only definitive diagnostic procedure is a renal angiogram. With discontinuation of captopril, renal function is expected to improve to the baseline value. *(Cecil, Ch. 87; Brenner and Rector, Ch. 27)*

23.(D); 24.(B) This patient probably has underlying lupus nephritis that is not clinically evident. The addition of ibuprofen has resulted in acute hemodynamically mediated renal failure. In addition to the nonsteroidal anti-inflammatory drug (NSAID), there are reports that triamterene in combination with a number of drugs, including NSAID's and captopril, can produce acute renal failure in patients with underlying renal disease. Prudence suggests discontinuation of both the combination diuretic and the NSAID. *(Cecil, Chs. 78 and 82; Brenner and Rector, Chs. 25 and 34)*

25.(D); 26.(E) This is an example of focal sclerosing glomerulonephritis that was initially diagnosed as minimal change disease—an occurrence that is not uncommon. The initial renal biopsy diagnosis was minimal change or nil disease based on the absence of any specific light microscopic and immunofluorescence findings along with the absence of any electron microscopic findings other than fusion of the glomerular epithelial foot processes. The treatment, prednisone, was appropriate for this diagnosis. However, the development of azotemia is not characteristic of minimal change disease. Focal sclerosing glomerulonephritis is a common cause of nephrotic syndrome. It is most often idiopathic, although it can be associated with heroin abuse as well as long-term vesicoureteral reflux. It begins with the juxtamedullary nephrons and causes focal and segmental sclerosis of the glomerular tuft without immune deposits. It is therefore not uncommon to miss this diagnosis on an intimal renal biopsy and to diagnose minimal change disease—a diagnosis of exclusion. Focal sclerosing glomerulonephritis is not generally believed to be responsive to steroid therapy. *(Cecil, Ch. 81; Brenner and Rector, Chs. 20–22)*

27.(C); 28.(A) Several diagnoses must be considered in a renal transplant recipient with a recent increase in creatinine concentration. These include acute rejection, often associated with fever, leukocytosis, hypertension, and allograft tenderness; and surgical or urologic causes of graft dysfunction. The immunosuppressive drug cyclosporine has dramatically improved the results of renal (as well as cardiac and liver) transplantation. However, it has two major and several minor toxicities: renal, in which it can cause reversible azotemia and hypertension, and central nervous system, in which it may cause headache, paresthesias, tremors, and seizures. In evaluating a renal transplant recipient taking cyclosporine who experiences an increase in creatinine concentration, percutaneous renal biopsy is often performed to differentiate between acute rejection, which is associated with an acute interstitial cellular infiltrate, and cyclosporine toxicity, in which the histology is for the most part normal. *(Cecil, Ch. 80; Brenner and Rector, Ch. 45)*

29.(D); 30.(B) The patient's presentation is not unusual. Hypernatremia in adults, with rare exceptions of hypothalamic function, is a serious disorder with considerable mortality, precisely because in order to become hypernatremic considerable other pathology must be present. Although there may be an impairment of thirst sensation in the elderly, the urge to drink when plasma sodium is elevated is strong. It is usually the patient with significant sensory impairment and inability to seek water who becomes hypernatremic. This patient's free water deficit is about 6 liters. In addition, there are signs suggestive of ECV depletion. Isotonic saline is needed to repair the ECV depletion and free water to repair the water deficit. In treating hypernatremia it is important to consider that the brain is a major target of disorders of water metabolism. In hypernatremia, in order to avoid brain shrinkage, the brain generates intracellular solute, often termed "idiogenic osmoles," to offset plasma hyperosmolality. These osmotically active substances are generated in hypernatremia after several hours. Rapid reduction of plasma sodium will result in swelling of a brain in which intracellular solute has been generated. Therefore, correction of hypernatremia of more than a few hours' duration should be undertaken slowly. It has been suggested that the plasma sodium be decreased no more than about 2 mEq/hr. This generally translates to correction over about 48 hours. Seizures are the clinical manifestation of cerebral edema in over-rapid correction of hypernatremia. *(Cecil, Ch. 77; Brenner and Rector, Ch. 11)*

31.(A); 32.(D) This patient is losing gastric contents—sodium, chloride, and acid—and replacing them with fluids that are essentially free water. Although a normal individual will excrete free water to maintain plasma osmolality, volume depletion (as well as pain) is a potent nonosmotic stimulus to the release of antidiuretic hormone (ADH). ADH impairs free water clearance by preventing the formation of dilute urine. The final result in this patient will be loss of NaCl and HCl and retention of free water, producing hyponatremia and metabolic alkalosis. ECV depletion will cause renin and aldosterone production. This favors avid distal sodium reabsorption as well as potassium and proton secretion by the distal tubule. In addition, the incremental elevation of plasma bicarbonate after each episode of vomiting may obligate further potassium loss. Hypokalemia and metabolic alkalosis will eventually result as well. *(Cecil, Ch. 77; Brenner and Rector, Ch. 13)*

33.(D); 34.(B) The two major routes of magnesium loss are the urine and gastrointestinal tract. A normal individual placed on a magnesium-free diet will rapidly lower urinary magnesium losses to an almost negligible level. Hypomagnesemia will ensue because of persistent GI losses. Renal magnesium wasting is seen in a variety of disorders, including diuretic use, Bartter's syndrome, hyperparathyroidism, hyperaldosteronism, and hyperthyroidism, and as a result of toxic injury by a variety of drugs, including aminoglycosides and *cis*-platinum. Although the magnesium loss of *cis*-platinum may be profound, it probably abates within 1–2 months. The patient in question has hypomagnesemia because of continued diarrheal GI loss with poor oral intake. The contribution of *cis*-platinum–induced renal magnesium wasting is highlighted by the elevated urinary magnesium concentration. When extrarenal magnesium loss is present, the normal renal response is avid magnesium conservation; 24-hour urinary magnesium excretion falls to a few milliequivalents per day within one week of extrarenal hypomagnesemia. Pure hypomagnesemia can cause hypocalcemia by impairment of parathyroid hormone release and action. *(Cecil, Ch. 82; Brenner and Rector, Ch. 15)*

35.(D) This case illustrates one of the severe complications associated with renal failure: pericarditis with tamponade. This complication of uremia has been described for over 100 years. It is thought to be related to the uremic state rather than a viral pericarditis (as in that seen in chronic dialysis patients), in that it often reverses with dialytic therapy. Pathologically and echocardiographically, pericarditis and pericardial effusion are demonstrable in a large proportion of patients with acute and chronic renal failure. When presenting without symptomatic tamponade, pericarditis is one of the classic indications for dialysis in acute or chronic renal failure. With tamponade, pericardiocentesis, intensive dialysis, and, occasionally, surgical pericardiotomy are needed. *(Cecil, Ch. 78; Brenner and Rector, Chs. 19 and 37)*

36.(E) Radiocontrast-induced renal failure is a common entity. Its etiology is unclear, although both a direct toxic effect of the hyperosmolar contrast substance and intratubular deposition of protein debris have been postulated as causes. The renal failure associated with radiocontrast agents occurs 24–48 hours after contrast administration. It is often associated with an initially low urine sodium concentration and is usually oliguric rather than high-output. Advanced age, volume depletion, and pre-existing renal disease seem to be risk factors. It is uncommon in otherwise normal individuals. Patients with diabetic renal disease seem to be at increased risk. Indeed, diabetic patients with significantly elevated creatinine concentrations (>4–5 mg/dl) often develop irreversible renal failure. This, however, is not the rule in most patients, who recover renal function after radiocontrast-induced renal failure. *(Cecil, Chs. 78 and 82; Brenner and Rector, Chs. 19 and 34)*

37.(All are False) Post-streptococcal glomerulonephritis most commonly affects children and young adults, although it has been reported to occur in older adults. There is a male predominance of approximately 2 to 1. Although proteinuria is almost universal, the nephrotic syndrome is uncommon. The prognosis in children is generally thought to be very good, clinical recovery being very common. The prognosis in adults is less certain, and several investigators note persistent urinary abnormalities, hypertension, and azotemia. In an uncomplicated case of post-streptococcal glomerulonephritis, in which the history of antecedent streptococcal infection, serology, and clinical course are typical, renal biopsy is probably unnecessary. *(Cecil, Ch. 81; Brenner and Rector, Ch. 22)*

38.(A—False; B—True; C—False; D—False; E—True) The diagnosis of anti-GBM disease is warranted *only* when anti–glomerular basement membrane antibodies are present in both the serum and glomeruli, where a characteristic linear immunofluorescent pattern is present. Although rapid progression to end-stage renal disease is common, more chronic forms are recognized. The clinical syndrome of pulmonary hemorrhage and glomerulonephritis (Goodpasture's syndrome) is not always associated with anti–glomerular basement membrane antibody. Preliminary therapeutic trials with plasmapheresis have been promising but not conclusive. *(Cecil, Ch. 81; Brenner and Rector, Ch. 23)*

39.(A—False; B—True; C—True; D—False; E—True) IgA nephropathy is pathologically characterized by IgA deposits in mesangial areas of glomeruli. The clinical presentation is often preceded by an upper respiratory infection. Gross hematuria often follows, and its presence does not necessarily indicate a poor prognosis. The disease usually has a benign course, although up to 25% of adults with this disease may have a gradual progression to renal failure. Although IgA deposits may appear in the transplanted kidney, graft failure has not been attributed to recurrence of this disease. *(Cecil, Ch. 81; Brenner and Rector, Ch. 22)*

40.(A—False; B—True; C—True; D—True; E—False) Membranous glomerulonephritis is characterized by a 25% spontaneous remission rate. The nephrotic syndrome is present at diagnosis 85% of the time, but this may represent selection bias. Electron microscopic examination of renal biopsy specimens reveals granular electron-dense deposits, often surrounded by spikes of basement membrane. Hypocomplementemia is distinctly uncommon. A recent collaborative study suggests that corticosteroids slow the progression of renal insufficiency. *(Cecil, Ch. 81; Brenner and Rector, Ch. 22)*

41. (A—False; B—False; C—True; D—True; E—False) The nephrotic syndrome—heavy proteinuria, edema, and hypoalbuminemia—is a common consequence of a variety of glomerular diseases of both focal and diffuse pathology. It is characterized by an often decreased plasma volume and avid sodium retention. Management of nephrotic edema includes salt restriction and diuretics. Although albumin infusions are of transient benefit, the added albumin is rapidly lost from the circulation. There is an increased infection rate in the nephrotic syndrome, a finding attributed to loss of circulating immunoglobulins. *(Cecil, Ch. 81; Brenner and Rector, Ch. 21)*

42. (A—True; B—False; C—False; D—False; E—False) Anemia may be present in both acute and chronic renal failure, but it is usually more pronounced in the chronic form. Patients with polycystic renal disease may have only mild anemia when they reach end-stage renal disease. Although hypocalcemia, hyperphosphatemia, and disorders of parathyroid hormone are present in both acute and chronic renal failure, radiographic signs of osteodystrophy are present only in established renal disease. Bilaterally small kidneys are a characteristic of the chronic disease. Hypertension may occur in either form. A dilute urine with a high urine sodium does not distinguish acute from chronic renal disease. *(Cecil, Chs. 78 and 79; Brenner and Rector, Chs. 37 and 38)*

43. (A—False; B—False; C—False; D—False; E—True) Total anuria and marked variations in urine output are most characteristic of postrenal failure. In acute tubular necrosis, an elevated fractional excretion of sodium and a urine-to-plasma creatinine concentration ratio of <20:1 are common. In prerenal failure, the fractional excretion of sodium is low (<1%) and the urine-to-plasma creatinine ratio is high. In the early phases of postrenal failure, the urinary findings may resemble those in prerenal failure; after 24 hours, however, fractional excretion of sodium rises and the urine-to-plasma creatinine ratio falls. Thus, the fractional excretion of sodium is useful in distinguishing oliguria of prerenal causes from that caused by acute tubular necrosis. It may not distinguish between obstruction and nonoliguric forms of intrinsic renal failure. Cellular and "brown" casts are typical of acute tubular necrosis, whereas fine granular or hyaline casts are more characteristic of prerenal azotemia. *(Cecil, Ch. 78; Brenner and Rector, Chs. 19 and 33)*

44. (A—False; B—False; C—True; D—True; E—True) The diagnosis of analgesic-associated nephropathy, which is often difficult to establish, has been made with increasing frequency in this country. It has been estimated to account for at least 20% of cases of chronic interstitial nephropathy. It is believed to arise from toxic effects of analgesics or their metabolites on the deep renal interstitium. Although phenacetin has been suggested as the most nephropathic analgesic compound, there is strong indication that aspirin, especially in combination with phenacetin, is also significant. The incidence is predominantly in women. There is usually a history of consumption of >1 kg of analgesic, although this history is characteristically difficult to elicit. In the late stages, excretory urography usually shows small kidneys with cortical scarring and evidence of papillary necrosis. Anemia out of proportion to the degree of azotemia is common and is attributed to chronic gastrointestinal blood loss. *(Cecil, Ch. 82; Brenner and Rector, Ch. 34)*

45. (A—True; B—True; C—False; D—False; E—True) Toxemia of pregnancy, a disorder characterized by hypertension, edema, and proteinuria, occurs in the last trimester of pregnancy. It affects 5–10% of pregnancies and occurs most commonly in young primiparous women and in multiparous women over 35 years of age. The incidence of toxemia is increased in the presence of pre-existing renal disease. In a primiparous woman, the occurrence of toxemia does not necessarily presage later hypertension, although in the older multiparous woman it often does. Despite the presence of abnormal renal histology, azotemia or renal failure is not common in toxemia. *(Cecil Ch. 88; Brenner and Rector, Ch. 28)*

46. (A—True; B—True; C—True; D—False; E—False) Medullary sponge kidney is a disorder characterized by ectasia and calcification of medullary collecting tubules. It is most often diagnosed by its characteristic appearance on excretory urogram in an asymptomatic patient. It is probably a congenital rather than a hereditary disorder, although it occurs in several systemic diseases including the Ehlers-Danlos syndrome. Renal calculi, hypercalciuria, and urinary tract infection are common. A decreased urine concentrating ability is frequent, but other tubular abnormalities and renal insufficiency are not. *(Cecil, Ch. 91; Brenner and Rector, Ch. 30)*

47. (A—False; B—False; C—True; D—True; E—True) Although usually arising in one kidney, renal cell carcinoma may arise in both kidneys without indicating metastatic disease. Erythrocytosis is among the many paraneoplastic syndromes associated with renal cell carcinoma, but it is rare; anemia is the most common hematologic abnormality. Hypercalcemia, sometimes responsive to prostaglandin synthesis inhibitors, is present in only 5–10% of patients. Direct tumor extension into the renal vein or vena cava or the presence of a "tumor thrombus" in the venous circulation does not adversely influence the surgical cure rate of renal cell carcinoma, as long as the tumor is surgically approachable and resectable. When the tumor is resectable, the five-year apparent cure rate in renal cell carcinoma is 60–70%. However, the metastatic disease can occur many years after an initial surgical "cure." *(Cecil, Chs. 93 and 247; Brenner and Rector, Ch. 35)*

48. (A—False; B—False; C—False; D—True; E—False) Light chain nephropathy is a disorder in which the overproduction and urinary excretion of immunoglobin light chains are associated with renal dysfunction, including renal tubular acidosis, impaired urinary concentrating ability, and azotemia. Although most commonly associated with multiple myeloma, it may occur in nonmalignant plasma cell dyscrasias and lymphomas, etc. There are probably two mechanisms by which light chains cause renal dysfunction. This first includes precipitation of proteins in the concentrated, acidic medullary tubules, producing obstruction. The second is less clear but probably relates to the direct toxic effects of some light chains on tubular function. It is noteworthy that the light chains that seem to be the most toxic in vivo and in vitro are those with relatively basic isoelectric points. Thus, some patients with large amounts of urinary light chains have no renal dysfunction, whereas others with a lesser excretion of basic light chains may have significant renal dysfunction. There is some evidence that reducing the light chain load, either by plasmapheresis or by treatment of the underlying disease, may improve the renal prognosis. Light chain nephropathy does not cause nephrotic syndrome, nor is it a cause or result of amyloidosis per se. *(Cecil, Ch. 82; Brenner and Rector, Chs. 23 and 25)*

49. (A—True; B—True; C—False; D—False; E—False)
50. (A—False; B—True; C—False; D—True; E—False)
51. (A—True; B—False; C—False; D—False; E—False) Early type I diabetes is often accompanied by an elevation in creatinine clearance which represents true hyperfiltration. Often the patients with the most marked elevation in GFR early in their course go on to develop diabetic nephropathy. These patients often have microalbuminuria—levels of albumin excretion below that ordinarily detected with dipstick methods. In evaluating the results of a 24-hour urinary collection and creatinine clearance, a suspiciously high or low result is often found. Although laboratory error and a failure of the patient to correctly collect the specimen should always be considered, a rough check on the adequacy of the collection can be made by calculating the creatinine index, i.e., the 24-hour excretion of creatinine per kilogram of body weight. For a normally muscled male it is in the range of 18–23 mg/kg/24 hr. Thus, although this patient's creatinine clearance of 160 ml/min is certainly high, his creatinine index is normal, and this represents an accurate estimate of creatinine clearance. Although it is known that a small part of urinary creatinine excretion is due to creatinine secretion, in normal individuals this represents only a small part of the calculated creatinine clearance. However, in a variety of renal diseases, creatinine secretion can falsely and significantly raise the measured creatine clearance over the true GFR.

Diabetic nephropathy is increasingly common with prolonged survival of insulin-dependent diabetics; it is a major cause of end-stage renal disease. It usually arises in patients with 10–15 years of insulin-dependent diabetes, although a few patients develop it without a marked insulin requirement. It is virtually always associated with the nephrotic syndrome and evidence of other microvascular disease, especially some stage of diabetic retinopathy. There is currently considerable interest in the pathogenesis of this disease, as well as measures that may prevent the development of this devastating complication of diabetes. At present, however, there is no clear evidence that good diabetic control will prevent this complication. *(Cecil, Ch. 85; Brenner and Rector, Ch. 31)*

52. (A—True; B—True; C—False; D—True; E—False)
53. (A—True; B—False; C—True; D—True; E—False) Nephrotic syndrome may be the result of a variety of primary and secondary renal diseases. Chronic glomerulonephritides such as diabetes, membranous nephropathy, focal glomerulosclerosis, amyloidosis, IgA nephropathy, and membranoproliferative glomerulonephritis may cause the nephrotic syndrome. Nephrotic proteinuria tends to decrease with advancing renal dysfunction and decreases in GFR. In patients with nephrotic syndrome and very heavy proteinuria in the face of advanced azotemia, two causes of the nephrotic syndrome must be particularly considered: diabetes mellitus and amyloidosis. In diabetes, the kidney size is often remarkably preserved and is often large, despite advanced renal insufficiency. Although this is not the rule in amyloidosis, it can also be observed in this condition. This patient presumably had secondary amyloidosis as a result of decades of chronic skin infections. The prognosis for patients with renal insufficiency from amyloidosis is very poor. *(Cecil, Chs. 74 and 81; Brenner and Rector, Chs. 21 and 23).*

54. (A—False; B—False; C—False; D—True; E—False)
55. (A—True; B—True; C—False; D—False; E—False) Although this patient's course was punctuated by several events that may be associated with renal dysfunction, the one most likely cause based on the information presented is the administration of nonsteroidal anti-inflammatory agents. This is based on the time course after beginning various medicines: Two days is too soon for the development of aminoglycoside-induced renal dysfunction. NSAID-induced renal dysfunction appears in several forms. In patients with pre-existing renal disease and especially in patients who are functionally prerenal (e.g., dehydration, congestive heart failure, cirrhosis with ascites), NSAID's can produce a reversible decrease in GFR. This is thought to occur on the basis of an impairment of intrarenal hemodynamics caused by prostaglandin synthesis inhibition. In addition, NSAID's can cause acute interstitial nephritis—characterized by pyuria and eosinophiluria, acute renal failure, and, in rare instances, nephrotic syndrome. In this patient the presence of pyuria and eosinophiluria suggests interstitial nephritis, as does hyperkalemia in the presence of a low urine potassium—a manifestation of impaired tubular function.

Renal biopsy is needed to ascertain the diagnosis of acute interstitial nephritis. In many settings, a high index of clinical suspicion will lead to the discontinuation of possibly offending drugs without a biopsy. Steroid therapy is usually effective in reversing the renal dysfunction associated with acute interstitial nephritis; however, it is not clear that steroids affect the ultimate resolution of the disease. Some clinicians use steroids empirically in this setting. However, in a patient at some risk for steroid-associated complications, it is prudent to document the presence of interstitial nephritis with renal biopsy before deciding on steroid treatment. *(Cecil, Ch. 82; Brenner and Rector, Ch. 34)*

56. (A—False; B—False; C—False; D—True; E—True)
57. (A—True; B—False; C—True; D—False; E—False)
58. (A—False; B—True; C—True; D—False; E—True) Long-term aminoglycoside therapy, such as that employed in the treatment of endocarditis, deep visceral abscess, and osteomyelitis, may be associated with primary renal magnesium wasting, potassium wasting, and calcium wasting in the absence of classic aminoglycoside-induced renal failure. The mechanism is unknown. Profound hypomagnesemia is associated with renal potassium wasting, which can be severe and relatively resistant to large doses of potassium. Hypocalcemia is a well-known consequence of hypomagnesemia and reflects an impairment of the release and effect of parathyroid hormone. Repair of the magnesium deficit is necessary for the restoration of normal calcium homeostasis. A serum potassium as low as 2.0 mEq/L indicates severe total body potassium depletion of 500–1000 mEq. *(Cecil, Ch. 82; Brenner and Rector, Chs. 15 and 34)*

59. (A—False; B—False; C—False; D—False; E—True) Diabetic nephropathy presenting with azotemia and heavy proteinuria is generally observed to progress to end-stage renal disease at a predictable and inexorable rate. Virtually all patients with this diagnosis have nephrotic proteinuria, hypertension, and retinal vascular disease. The absence of these concomitant features should draw the diagnosis of diabetic nephropathy into question. Radiocontrast-induced renal failure is a particular risk in azotemic diabetic patients. The incidence of dye-induced renal failure increases with increasing creatinine concentration; in patients with creatinine concentrations >4–5 mg/dl, it can produce irreversible renal failure. However, if necessary, a dye study can be performed in this patient with careful prestudy hydration and observation. *(Cecil, Ch. 85; Brenner and Rector, Ch. 31)*

60.(A—False; B—False; C—True; D—True; E—True) Hypertensive nephrosclerosis is usually the result of severe sustained hypertension or malignant or accelerated hypertension. It is associated with minimal proteinuria and hematuria. The renal histopathology demonstrates the changes of small vessel arteriolar sclerosis and obsolescence of glomeruli. Hypertension is a risk factor for deterioration in all chronic renal diseases. The rate of deterioration can be diminished with hypertensive control. In azotemia associated with malignant hypertension, renal function can be improved with blood pressure control. In patients with advanced azotemia from hypertensive nephrosclerosis, marked reductions in blood pressure to the normal range can be associated with transient worsening of renal function. *(Cecil, Chs. 79, 81, and 87; Brenner and Rector, Ch. 27)*

61.(A—False; B—False; C—False; D—False; E—True)
62.(A—False; B—True; C—False; D—True; E—False) Rapidly progressive glomerulonephritis is a diagnosis that includes a heterogeneous group of disorders characterized by a rapid deterioration of renal function and proliferation of epithelial crescents affecting more than 80% of glomeruli. Etiologic disorders include Goodpasture's syndrome, Henoch-Schönlein purpura—an extreme in the spectrum of IgA nephropathy, post-streptococcal glomerulonephritis, a variety of immune complex diseases, and idiopathic rapidly progressive glomerulonephritis. Post-streptococcal glomerulonephritis usually appears with a recent history of a streptococcal infection and an elevated ASO titer. IgA nephropathy is associated with prominent deposition of IgA in glomeruli. Since it is relatively uncommon, there are few large studies on treatment. Plasmapheresis, pulse steroids, and low-dose heparin have proven effective in some patients, primarily those with significant immune deposits visible on immunofluorescent staining of renal biopsy tissue. Goodpasture's syndrome appears to be responsive to the removal of anti–glomerular basement antibodies with plasmapheresis and immunosuppression. The prognosis for this disorder is variable. Patients with oliguria and serum creatinine concentrations greater than 5 mg/dl at the time of presentation appear to do poorly, while patients with rapidly progressive glomerulonephritis as a result of post-streptococcal glomerulonephritis often recover. *(Cecil, Chs. 78 and 81; Brenner and Rector, Chs. 19, 21, 22, and 23)*

63.(A—False; B—False; C—True; D—True; E—True) The acidosis of advanced uremia is a state in which renal compensatory mechanisms are inadequate to maintain external acid-base balance. Even before acidosis appears in uremia, careful balance studies indicate that there is net positive acid balance; i.e., acid is buffered by body tissues, including bone. The normal renal compensatory mechanisms in acidosis include an increase in renal ammoniagenesis; ammonia is the major urinary buffer responsible for the increment in acid excretion. In addition, there is an increased fractional proximal reabsorption of bicarbonate. When uremic acidosis supervenes, the reduction in renal mass prevents an appropriate increment in urinary ammonia. When GFR is below about 20–25% of normal, there is an absolute retention of organic and inorganic acid anions, leading to an increased anion gap. At this point, although the urine is normally acid, a bicarbonate load cannot be adequately reabsorbed and bicarbonaturia on alkali loading will result. Hyperkalemia inhibits and hypokalemia stimulates renal ammoniagenesis. *(Cecil, Chs. 77 and 79; Brenner and Rector, Ch. 13)*

64.(A—True; B—False; C—False; D—True; E—True)
65.(A—False; B—False; C—False; D—True; E—True) This patient has symptoms and laboratory findings of uremia after a long history of hypertension that has become increasingly difficult to control. Since there are already indications for the initiation of dialysis, provisions for vascular access would be prudent at this time. The findings of hypocalcemia and hyperphosphatemia require treatment with phosphate binders and calcium. The more challenging issue, which should be addressed in all patients approaching end-stage renal disease, is whether there are reversible features of the renal disease. This patient displays severe and worsening hypertension, disparate kidney sizes (the larger being almost normal), and evidence of large-vessel atherosclerosis, all of which should raise the possibility of atherosclerotic major renal artery disease. Renal artery stenosis of a single functioning kidney can cause both refractory hypertension and a decrement in kidney function. Although most patients with this degree of renal dysfunction would have a volume-mediated component to their hypertension, further diuresis in this patient might actually worsen the hypertension by adding a further stimulus to renal renin production. Although the clinical situation is suggestive, a renal angiogram is needed to confirm the diagnosis. In a series of patients with similar presentation, renal revascularization has improved renal function in some cases and blood pressure control in a significant number. The use of angiotensin-converting enzyme inhibitors in this setting would be likely to produce hypotension and a marked decrease in renal function. *(Cecil, Chs. 79, 81, and 87; Brenner and Rector, Chs. 27, 37, and 39)*

66.(A—True; B—False; C—False; D—False; E—True)
67.(A—True; B—False; C—True; D—False; E—True) This patient has significant complications of the syndrome of uremic osteodystrophy, along with the disorders of parathyroid function which are often present in patients with end-stage renal disease. Although still a subject of debate and active investigation, it is believed that progressive phosphate retention in renal disease produces subtle hypocalcemia that results in increased parathyroid hormone (PTH) secretion. PTH subsequently causes phosphaturia and increased 1,25-hydroxyvitamin D synthesis by the kidney. Vitamin D increases gut calcium and phosphate absorption and may directly inhibit PTH secretion. Therefore it is believed that aggressive control of calcium and phosphate *early* in renal failure may prevent later development of hyperparathyroidism. Measures to accomplish this may include phosphate binders, calcium supplements, and vitamin D analogues. Later in renal disease, when the reduction in renal mass further impairs both phosphate excretion and 1,25-hydroxyvitamin D synthesis, progressive parathyroid hypertrophy ensues—the parathyroid glands may enlarge from pea-sized organs to palpable masses. At this time, both the threshold for calcium inhibition of PTH secretion and the basal rate of PTH secretion are altered. Bone reabsorption becomes the major route of homeostasis of plasma calcium concentration. Loss of bone

mineral content as well, metastatic calcifications, and a number of other features of uremic osteodystrophy may follow.

This patient manifests hypercalcemia in the face of a well-controlled serum phosphate and radiographic evidence of increased bone reabsorption. Since renal vitamin D production is impaired, hypercalcemia is maintained through bone reabsorption. Although PTH can cause metabolic acidosis in states of primary hyperparathyroidism by decreasing renal bicarbonate reabsorption, in this case the kidneys contribute little to acid-base balance. In this case subtotal parathyroidectomy (three glands, plus the greater portion of the fourth) is indicated. Subsequent control of calcium and phosphate and administration of vitamin D may be required. *(Cecil, Ch. 79; Brenner and Rector, Ch. 39)*

68. (A—True; B—False; C—True; D—False; E—True) Aminoglycoside-induced renal failure is a common clinical entity resulting from the effects of these intrinsically nephrotoxic drugs. It is associated with elevated levels of aminoglycosides. Since these drugs are eliminated almost exclusively by the kidney, a subtle and unnoticed decrease in renal function during the course of therapy may lead to accumulation of the drug and potentiate nephrotoxicity. Because of the renal elimination, pre-existing renal disease is a risk factor, as is advanced age. However, with careful monitoring of drug levels and dosage adjustment, they can be given safely to almost any patient. Even with doses that are too large at the outset, renal dysfunction usually does not become evident before 4–6 days of treatment. Renal failure from aminoglycosides is typically nonoliguric; with a relatively fixed urine output typically in the range of 1–2 liters/day with a high sodium concentration. Even though the serum creatinine may begin to fall within a few weeks of cessation of aminoglycoside therapy, full recovery of premorbid renal function may actually take months. *(Cecil, Ch. 82; Brenner and Rector, Ch. 34)*

69. (A—False; B—True; C—False; D—True; E—False) Both acetazolamide and amiloride inhibit specific renal processes dealing with acid secretion or bicarbonate reabsorption. Acetazolamide, a carbonic anhydrase inhibitor, inhibits a significant proportion of proximal tubule bicarbonate reabsorption, simulating type II renal tubular acidosis (RTA). Amiloride acts as a specific inhibitor of the conductive sodium channel in the collecting duct and may simulate the defect seen in type IV RTA. Other diuretics that primarily promote sodium chloride loss and cause volume depletion are more likely to produce the picture of metabolic alkalosis. *(Cecil, Chs. 77 and 84; Brenner and Rector, Ch. 12)*

70. (A—True; B—False; C—True; D—True; E—True) Each of the diuretics mentioned, with the exception of amiloride, can and does cause hypokalemia. Thiazides and the loop diuretics furosemide and ethacrynic acid increase sodium delivery to the collecting duct and produce volume depletion. The secondary hyperaldosteronism enhances sodium reabsorption and potassium secretion in the distal nephron. The increased delivery of sodium to a distal nephron stimulated by aldosterone enhances potassium secretion. Acetazolamide may produce bicarbonaturia. The presence of the poorly reabsorbable bicarbonate anion in the distal tubule obligates the secretion of an accompanying cation to maintain electroneutrality. Potassium is the cation secreted in great quantity. Amiloride inhibits one of the aldosterone-induced transport systems—the conductive sodium channel—and interdicts the process of distal sodium reabsorption and, secondarily, potassium secretion. *(Cecil, Chs. 77 and 84; Brenner and Rector, Ch. 12)*

71. (A—True; B—False; C—False; D—False; E—False) Thiazide diuretics have been widely used to treat nephrolithiasis caused by hypercalciuria. They act by two mechanisms to reduce urinary calcium excretion. First, in conjunction with a modest sodium restriction, they produce a small degree of volume depletion, which increases proximal tubular reabsorption of sodium and calcium. Secondly, in the distal convoluted tubule (the site of thiazide action) they reduce luminal entry of sodium into the distal tubular cell and lower intracellular sodium. This results in an increase in sodium-calcium exchange at the basolateral membrane of the distal tubular cell, effecting a net increase in calcium reabsorption by this segment, thereby lowering urinary calcium excretion. The loop diuretics, furosemide and ethacrynic acid, in combination with a high sodium intake, can actually increase urinary calcium—hence their use in the acute treatment of hypercalcemia. *(Cecil, Ch. 90; Brenner and Rector, Ch. 12)*

72. (A—True; B—False; C—True; D—False; E—False) This is a case of obstructive uropathy in a patient with a single functioning kidney. In general, the obstruction of one of two normal kidneys produces little renal dysfunction. The renal blood flow and GFR in the obstructed kidney fall rapidly. There are reported cases of relief of obstruction to a single functioning kidney with some recovery of function many weeks after the onset of obstruction. In the case of bilateral obstruction, or when there is only a single functioning kidney, obstruction of more than about one week's duration begins to produce irreversible damage. This is ultimately manifested as an absolute loss of nephron mass, evidenced on imaging by a thinned cortex, and some degree of permanent residual impairment. This patient is just entering the range of end stage renal disease. The sonographic findings of a thinned cortex indicate that recovery of renal function is unlikely to be complete. In this setting it is imperative to attempt to relieve the obstruction, because if a small improvement in renal function can be obtained, the need for dialytic therapy is obviated or at least significantly delayed. Although relief of acute obstruction is often associated with a dramatic and rapid postobstructive diuresis, no such marked diuresis is usually seen in the setting of chronic obstruction. However, after relief of obstruction, a gradual improvement in renal function may ensue over several weeks or more. Therefore, it is almost always worthwhile to seek and relieve urinary obstruction. A variety of specific disorders of renal function can be seen in obstruction, including impaired concentrating ability and acid secretory defects. *(Cecil, Ch. 83; Brenner and Rector, Ch. 33).*

73. (A—True; B—False; C—True; D—True; E—False) Analgesic nephropathy was identified as a cause of renal disease more than 30 years ago. It is the result of long-term abusive ingestion of kilogram quantities of analgesics containing phenacetin (now banned in most of the Western world) or acetaminophen—usually in a combination product. It produces chronic tubulointerstitial disease in which papillary necrosis is common. It is thought that phenacetin and its metabolite, acetaminophen, are accumulated in the papillary regions, where they overwhelm glutathione reductase–dependent detoxification mechanisms. The papillary areas of the kidney are uniformly the first to be affected, with sclerosis and necrosis of capillaries, followed by ischemic necrosis and fibrosis of the renal parenchyma. Clinically, pyuria without nephrotic-range proteinuria is common. Although all interstitial diseases produce disorders of sodium conservation, true massive salt-losing nephropathy is rare in this (and any) renal disease. There appears to be a real increase in the incidence of uroepithelial malignancy in patients with analgesic abuse. In addition, prior to the development of transitional cell malignancies, a purportedly pathognomonic finding—subepithelial microvascular sclerosis—may be found in the renal pelvis, ureters, or bladder epithelia. It is thought that analgesic abuse nephropathy accounts for a significant proportion of the chronic interstitial renal disease in the United States, and an even larger proportion in Scandinavia and Australia. *(Cecil, Ch. 82; Brenner and Rector, Ch. 34)*

74.(C); 75.(A); 76.(B); 77(D); 78(E); 79.(C); 80.(E) Impaired free water excretion is characteristic both of drugs causing true SIADH, such as vincristine, cyclophosphamide, and chlorpropamide, and of drugs with intrarenal effects, such as the thiazide diuretics. *(Cecil, Ch. 77)* Nephrogenic diabetes insipidus, unresponsive to vasopressin and leading to polyuria and pure water loss, may be a side effect of such drugs as lithium, demethylchlortetracycline, and vinblastine. *(Cecil, Chs. 77 and 82)* The nephrotic syndrome can result from the administration of heavy metals, penicillamine, and anticonvulsants. Recently the syndrome has been associated with the use of nonsteroidal anti-inflammatory agents, especially fenoprofen. *(Cecil, Ch. 81)* Hypokalemia based on renal potassium loss can result from administration of both thiazides and loop diuretics. In addition, poorly reabsorbable anions such as carbenicillin can induce renal potassium loss. *(Cecil, Ch. 77)* Hyperkalemia is a dangerous abnormality that may occur when potassium-sparing diuretics are given injudiciously. In addition, depolarizing muscle relaxants such as succinylcholine can produce sudden hyperkalemia based on rapid shifts of potassium from muscle cells to ECF. *(Cecil, Ch. 77; Brenner and Rector, Ch. 11)*

81.(E); 82.(D); 83.(B); 84.(C); 85.(A) Type IV RTA is characterized by hyperkalemia and hyperchloremic acidosis with a normal anion gap. Distal (type I) RTA is also characterized by hyperchloremic acidosis with a normal anion gap, but hypokalemia is often a feature because bicarbonate present in the distal tubule acts as a nonreabsorbable anion and can obligate continued potassium loss. Proximal (type II) RTA is again characterized by normal-anion-gap hyperchloremic acidosis. In the steady state, however, there is no bicarbonaturia and no hypokalemia. Uremic acidosis is caused both by a failure of ammoniagenesis and by renal net acid secretion (as in type IV RTA) but also by a net retention of nonmetabolizable acids, producing an elevated anion gap. Finally, in diabetic ketoacidosis, the clue is the elevated anion gap, as well as hyponatremia caused by hyperglycemia. *(Cecil, Ch. 84; Brenner and Rector, Ch. 13)*

BIBLIOGRAPHY

Brenner BM, Rector FC Jr: The Kidney. 3rd ed. Philadelphia, W. B. Saunders Company, 1986.

Cecil Textbook of Medicine. 18th ed. Wyngaarden JB, Smith LH Jr (eds). Philadelphia, W. B. Saunders Company, 1988.

PART 4

GASTROINTESTINAL DISEASE

NATHAN M. BASS, RODGER A. LIDDLE, and CHARLES E. REESE

DIRECTIONS: For questions 1 to 50 choose the ONE BEST answer to each question.

1. In alcohol-induced acute pancreatitis, which of the following conditions does NOT indicate severe disease?

   A. Blood glucose level greater than 200 mg/dl
   B. Fluid sequestration greater than 6 liters
   C. Hematocrit drop of more than 10 percentage points
   D. Serum calcium level greater than 11.5 mg/dl
   E. Arterial Po_2 less than 60 mm Hg

2. Which of the following is NOT a feature of the Zollinger-Ellison syndrome?

   A. Secretory diarrhea
   B. Fat malabsorption
   C. Vitamin B_{12} malabsorption
   D. Antral G-cell hyperplasia
   E. Large gastric folds

QUESTIONS 3–4

A 37-year-old female postgraduate student in parasitology comes to the emergency room because of fever and pain in the right upper abdominal quadrant, both first noted several days ago. The pain is always present, worsens with movement, and has become progressively more severe. The only previous gastrointestinal symptoms were a two-week illness characterized by bloody diarrhea, which occurred several months ago during a field study in Mexico; and intermittent, transient pain in the right upper abdominal quadrant after eating, of several years' duration. She has had no other medical problems and is the mother of two children. Temperature is 102°F. Physical examination shows a moderately obese white woman in some distress. There is no scleral icterus. Liver span is 15 cm in the midclavicular line, and the edge is tender to palpation. Laboratory studies include:

White blood cell count	16,500/mm³
Serum transaminase (AST)	2 times normal
Serum alkaline phosphatase	4 times normal
Serum bilirubin	0.8 mg/dl

A counterimmunoelectrophoresis for amebic infection is performed, and the results are pending.

Ultrasonography shows stones in the gallbladder, but no stones in the common duct or ductal dilatation. A transverse scan through the hepatic parenchyma is shown above, right column.

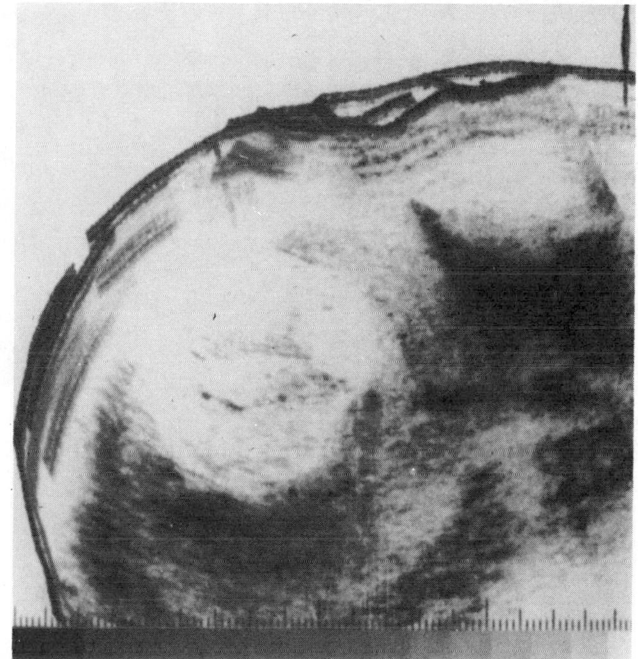

3. As consultant to the attending physician, which one of the following would you recommend next?

   A. Liver-spleen scans with technetium-^{99}m sulfur-colloid and gallium-67
   B. Alpha-fetoprotein determination
   C. Metronidazole, 750 mg three times daily for 10 days
   D. Laparotomy
   E. Computed tomography of the liver and biliary tract

4. The counterimmunoelectrophoresis returns positive the day after admission, and the attending physician now independently decides to begin therapy with metronidazole, without further diagnostic studies. However, 72 hours after therapy is begun, the patient has not improved. Temperature rises to 106°F, and the WBC count increases to 26,000/mm³. Which one of the following would you next recommend?

   A. Continue metronidazole, but add clindamycin and gentamicin in appropriate doses
   B. Switch from metronidazole to chloroquine

C. Laparotomy
D. Percutaneous aspiration of the mass with guidance by ultrasonography
E. Retrograde cholangiography

5. A 39-year-old male insurance agent is referred to you for evaluation of mid-abdominal pain radiating to the back. The pain is described as severe, gnawing, and episodic, lasting for weeks at a time. He drinks alcohol socially, averaging 1–2 drinks a week. Physical examination shows no abdominal mass or tenderness, and stool is negative for occult blood. The patient's hematocrit, serum electrolytes, liver chemistries, and serum amylase are all normal. Upper GI series and abdominal ultrasound studies are also normal. An endoscopic retrograde pancreatogram is shown below.

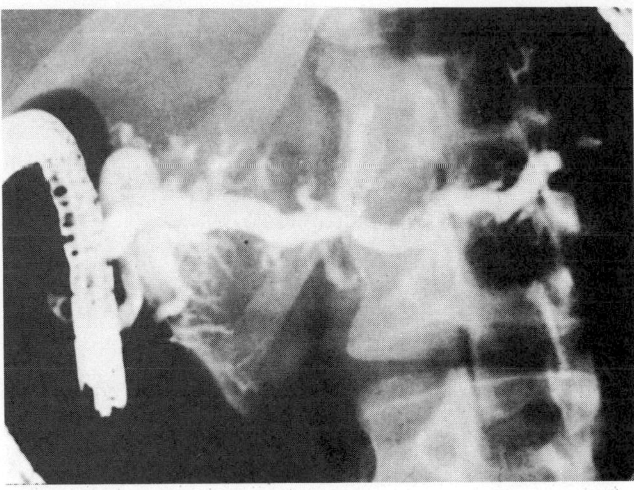

Which of the following statements is true of this patient's condition?

A. Hyperlipidemia is a common cause of the disease
B. Pancreatic calcifications are almost always present
C. Typically the abdominal pain worsens in severity
D. Diabetes mellitus is an unusual complication of this disease
E. Limited field radiation therapy may enhance survival

6. A 26-year-old homosexual male has loose stools, abdominal cramps, flatulence, and malaise of several weeks' duration. Twenty-four hours ago, the patient developed bloody diarrhea, tenesmus, and low-grade fever (101°F). Physical examination is normal except for trace guaiac-positive stool on digital rectal examination. Examination of a fresh stool specimen reveals motile trophozoites with ingested red blood cells. What is the most appropriate next step in the management of this patient?

A. Immediate indirect hemagglutination testing to establish the diagnosis of invasive amebiasis
B. Immediate flexible sigmoidoscopy and biopsy to establish the diagnosis of invasive amebiasis
C. Air-contrast barium enema to rule out a mass lesion (ameboma), as this may prompt early surgical intervention
D. Immediate treatment with metronidazole, 750 mg three times daily for 5–10 days, plus diloxanide furoate, 500 mg three times daily for 10 days
E. Treatment of this patient's asymptomatic sexual partner with diloxanide furoate, 500 mg three times daily for 10 days

7. A 57-year-old man has severe heartburn and nocturnal cough. Simple measures for the treatment of gastroesophageal reflux disease (liquid antacids, elevation of the head of the bed, nothing by mouth prior to bedtime) fail to alter the patient's symptoms. Which of the following is NOT among acceptable measures for the further treatment of this patient?

A. H_2-receptor blocking agents
B. Parasympathomimetic agents
C. Anticholinergic agents
D. Alginic acid-antacid agents
E. Antireflux surgery

8. A 56-year-old woman is referred to you for evaluation of possible cancer of the pancreas, suspected on the basis of epigastric pain radiating to the back associated with an 8-pound weight loss. Physical examination and routine blood tests, including serum amylase, are normal. The next appropriate diagnostic test to detect pancreatic cancer is

A. urine amylase
B. upper gastrointestinal series
C. ultrasonography or computerized tomography of the pancreas
D. radioisotopic pancreatic scan with ^{75}Se-selenomethionine
E. visceral angiography

9. Which of the following statements regarding the hepatitis delta virus is INCORRECT?

A. It is a defective RNA virus
B. It has been implicated as a common cause of fulminant hepatitis
C. Anti-delta IgG present in the serum confers immunity to the virus
D. Delta viral hepatitis occurs only in association with acute or chronic B viral hepatitis
E. In North America, intravenous drug addicts are the group at highest risk for delta infection

10. A 25-year-old male graduate student complains of severe epigastric abdominal pain that is relieved by food. The pain typically awakens him at night 2–3 hours after going to bed. On endoscopic examination he is found to have a 1-cm duodenal ulcer. Which of the following diets would you recommend?

A. Six small meals per day
B. Three regular meals per day plus a bedtime snack
C. Three regular meals per day without a bedtime snack
D. Low roughage, bland diet
E. Low roughage, bland diet supplemented with milk and cream

QUESTIONS 11–12

A 40-year-old woman with known alcoholic cirrhosis of the liver is admitted to the hospital because of increasing abdominal girth, fever, and diffuse, vague abdominal discomfort. Physical examination reveals a febrile (101.5°F) woman with scleral icterus. Abdominal examination shows an enlarged, tender liver (14 cm span), active bowel sounds, distention, and a positive fluid wave, but there is no rebound tenderness or guarding. Paracentesis shows white blood cell count of 535 mm^3 (76% neutrophils) with a negative Gram's stain. Serum creatinine is 1.9 mg/dl; total bililrubin is 2.4 mg/dl. Other laboratory results are within normal limits.

11. Which of the following is true about this patient's condition?

A. Despite empiric treatment with a third-generation cephalosporin, the risk of mortality in this patient exceeds 60%
B. If nontoxic blood levels of aminoglycoside are maintained, the risk of this patient's developing renal failure is low (less than 10%)
C. As aminoglycosides diffuse well into the peritoneum, therapeutic levels are easily achieved; serum levels need not be followed
D. Most organisms cultured with spontaneous bacterial peritonitis are sensitive to chloramphenicol, and it is an acceptable initial therapeutic agent
E. This patient should *not* be treated with empiric antibiotics

12. The chemical analysis of ascites complicated by bowel perforation is different from that of the ascites of spontaneous bacterial peritonitis in the concentration of all of the following EXCEPT

A. pH
B. glucose
C. lactate dehydrogenase
D. polymorphonuclear cells
E. total protein concentration

QUESTIONS 13–14

A 44-year-old man who has drunk 6 ounces of whiskey daily for many years is evaluated for intermittent episodes of epigastric pain relieved by antacids. During an attack, moderate epigastric tenderness is present. Laboratory tests show:

Hematocriti	46%
White blood cell count	10,000/mm^3
Serum creatinine	1.2 mg/dl
Serum amylase	500 IU/L (normal <110)
Urinary creatinine	120 mg/dl
Urinary amylase	50 IU/L

Examination of the stool for occult blood is positive (2+).

Upper gastrointestinal series shows duodenal bulb deformity.

13. The amylase:creatinine clearance ratio in this patient is

A. 0.001%
B. 0.1%
C. 1%
D. 10%
E. not determinable from these data

14. The most likely diagnosis is

A. acute pancreatitis with secondary spasm of duodenal bulb
B. coexistent acute pancreatitis and peptic ulcer disease
C. peptic ulcer disease and macroamylasemia
D. peptic ulcer disease with posterior penetration into the pancreas
E. alcoholic hepatitis

15. A 42-year-old woman is referred to you by her general practitioner because of a "skin rash." She states that the skin, particularly of the hands and feet, often blisters and abrades easily. Physical examination is normal except for a liver span of 14 cm in the midclavicular line. Her hands are shown below. Laboratory studies include:

Serum transaminase (AST)	Twice elevated
Urinary uroporphyrin	Tenfold elevated
Urinary coproporphyrin	Threefold elevated
Urinary porphobilinogen	Normal
Fecal protoporphyrin	Normal

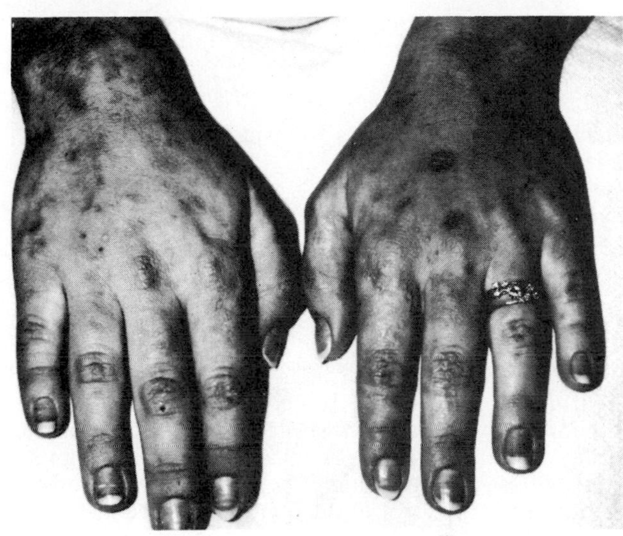

Which of the following would NOT be of diagnostic importance in evaluating this patient?

A. Use of alcohol
B. Use of barbiturates
C. Use of oral contraceptives
D. Evidence of iron overload
E. Presence of an hepatocellular carcinoma

16. Which of the following statements regarding Norwalk virus induced gastroenteritis is INCORRECT?

A. It accounts for approximately one third of epidemics of viral gastroenteritis in the United States
B. Malabsorption of fat and xylose may occur during the illness
C. Mucosal lesions are prominent in the stomach
D. The clinical illness is self-limiting within 48 hours
E. Some outbreaks have been traced to shellfish

17. Which of the following statements regarding diverticulosis of the colon is INCORRECT?

A. Half the population of Europe can expect to acquire this disease
B. Its prevalence is reduced among Westerners eating a fiber-rich diet
C. Barium enema will reveal an irregular luminal contour, with collection of barium noted inside and outside the diverticulum
D. The disorder may be associated with marked local tenderness, a palpable sigmoid loop, and some degree of large bowel obstruction
E. Severe blood loss from colonic diverticula is considered to be the most common cause of life-threatening lower gastrointestinal hemorrhage in the elderly

18. A 27-year-old black man with sickle cell disease presents with chills, fever to 103°F, jaundice, and right upper quadrant pain. The patient has previously received a total of 67 units of blood, and five weeks ago he underwent a partial exchange transfusion prior to minor surgery. Physical examination reveals an enlarged liver and tenderness in the right upper quadrant of the abdomen. Laboratory studies show:

Serum bilirubin	27 mg/dl
Serum transaminases:	
SGOT	5 times normal
SGPT	2 times normal
Serum alkaline phosphatase	13 times normal
Prothrombin time	12 seconds (control: 11)

Which of the following is the most likely cause of this patient's current illness?

A. Uncomplicated acute cholecystitis
B. Hemochromatosis
C. Hepatic infarction owing to a sludging of sickled cells in the sinusoids
D. Choledocholithiasis with cholangitis
E. Viral hepatitis

19. A 30-year-old white woman has sudden onset of right upper quadrant pain. She has been taking oral contraceptives for eight years and has suffered from mild rheumatoid arthritis for which she takes nonsteroidal anti-inflammatory drugs. Physical examination shows a tender, poorly defined mass in the right upper quadrant. A technetium-^{99}m sulfur colloid scan is shown below. Angiography reveals a hypovascular area in the right hepatic lobe. Which of the following is the most likely diagnosis?

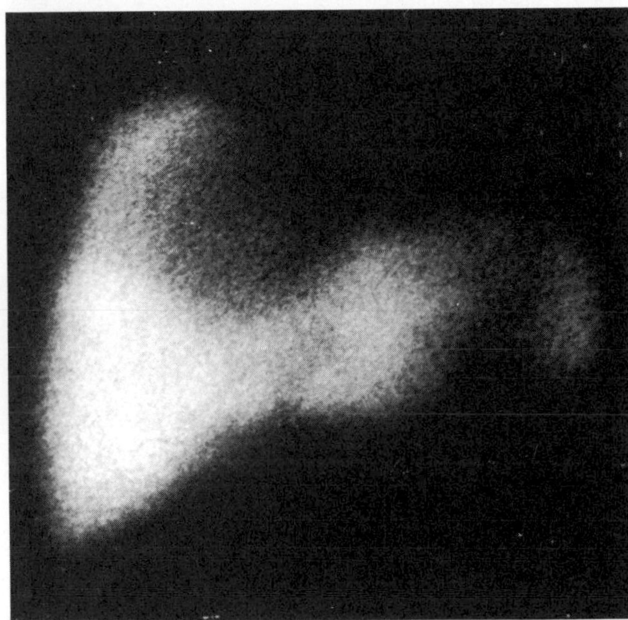

A. Hepatic adenoma
B. Cavernous hemangioma
C. Hepatocellular carcinoma
D. Nodular regenerative hyperplasia
E. Focal nodular hyperplasia of the liver

20. A 31-year-old man has had blood-streaked stools and a mucosanguineous rectal discharge for several months. Proctosigmoidoscopy reveals diffusely friable mucosa in the distal rectum that bleeds with swabbing. The more proximal rectum and distal sigmoid colon appear normal. Which one of the following would NOT cause these symptoms?

A. Lymphogranuloma venereum
B. Trauma
C. Nonspecific ulcerative proctitis
D. Granuloma inguinale
E. Radiation

21. A 32-year-old woman is admitted to the hospital because of six hours of cramping, right lower quadrant and suprapubic pains, and gross hematochezia. She had a period of intravenous drug usage 10 years ago, and an episode of hepatitis at the age of 25. Physical examination shows postural hypotension and a liver edge palpable 2 cm below the right costal margin. Sigmoidoscopy demonstrates normal mucosa to 25 cm with dark red blood clots coming down from above. Nasogastric aspiration reveals yellow fluid but no blood. A technetium scan of the abdomen is performed (see illustration).

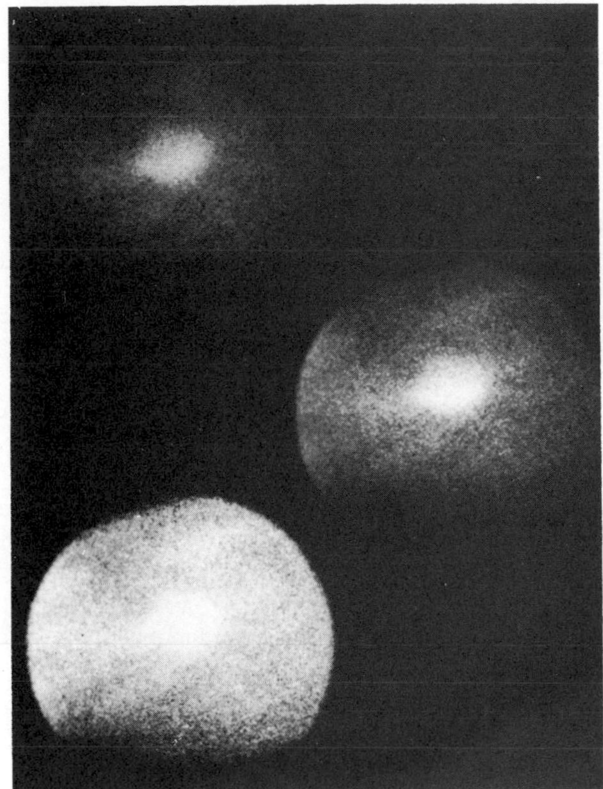

Which of the following is the most likely diagnosis?

A. Ileal varices
B. Endometriosis of the bowel
C. Ileal Crohn's disease
D. Meckel's diverticulum
E. Small bowel lymphoma

QUESTIONS 22–23

A 40-year-old asymptomatic male bank executive undergoing examination for a life insurance policy is found to have two spider angiomata on the anterior chest and a 13-cm liver span with a firm edge. The spleen tip is just palpable. He drinks 1–2 bottles of wine on a weekly basis. Ten years ago, he developed diarrhea and was told after a sigmoidoscopic examination that he had "colitis." The diarrhea lasted five months, during which he was treated with Azulfidine. Since that time, bowel movements have been normal. Laboratory studies show:

Serum alanine aminotransferase	100 units/ml
Serum aspartate aminotransferase	40 units/ml
Serum alkaline phosphatase	8 times normal
Serum bilirubin	0.7 mg/dl
Serum cholesterol	320 mg/dl

22. Which of the following is most likely to account for these findings?

A. Pericholangitis
B. Choledocholithiasis
C. Alcoholic hepatitis
D. Primary biliary cirrhosis
E. Primary sclerosing cholangitis

23. Which of the following is likely to be of greatest diagnostic use in the initial evaluation of the findings in this patient?

A. Technetium-^{99}m HIDA scan
B. Liver biopsy
C. Oral cholecystography
D. Intravenous cholangiography
E. Endoscopic retrograde cholangiography

24. A 26-year-old woman is referred to you because of a recent episode of small bowel obstruction that resolved spontaneously. Melanin deposits are seen on the buccal mucosa and palms; physical examination is otherwise normal. Stools are positive for occult blood. Family history reveals similar pigmentary changes in her mother and a maternal uncle, both of whom suffered recurrent attacks of abdominal pain and distention. Her uncle died at age 65 of an intestinal adenocarcinoma. Her mother is alive and well at the age of 68. Laboratory studies reveal a hematocrit of 34%, hemoglobin of 11.5 g/dl, white blood cell count of 8000/mm^3, normal electrolytes, and normal urinalysis. Which of the following is true of this patient?

A. She has a high risk of intestinal adenocarcinoma
B. The melanin spots were not present at birth
C. Consanguinity in the family is a likely finding
D. Histologic examination of the intestinal lesions would reveal hamartomas
E. Colectomy would be curative

QUESTIONS 25–26

A 27-year-old man with a past history of alcohol and drug abuse is admitted to the hospital in a coma. He was found in his room by a friend and no recent history is available. Physical examination reveals a jaundiced male who responds by withdrawal to deep pain, has hypoactive but symmetric muscle stretch reflexes, and has intact oculovestibular and oculocephalic reflexes. Laboratory studies include:

Serum transaminase (AST)	50 times normal
Serum bilirubin	8 mg/dl
Prothrombin time	22 seconds (control: 11)
Serum alkaline phosphatase	2 times normal

25. Which one of the following would be the LEAST likely cause of this patient's condition?

A. Acetaminophen ingestion
B. Non-A, non-B hepatitis virus infection
C. Alcoholic hepatitis
D. Acute delta infection in a patient with chronic hepatitis B virus infection
E. Hepatitis B virus infection

26. Which one of the following diagnostic studies would be LEAST important to the immediate management of this patient?

A. Serum electrolytes
B. Blood glucose level
C. Blood acetaminophen level
D. Blood urea nitrogen
E. Assessment of response to naloxone (Narcan)

27. A 73-year-old woman, previously in excellent health, reports a 20-pound weight loss over two months, intermittent diarrhea, and a waxing and waning skin rash. The rash (see photographs below) begins with an erythematous base, develops superficial central blistering, and finally crusts over. Healing is accompanied by hyperpigmentation. The process takes 7–14 days, with lesions developing in a new area while others are resolving.

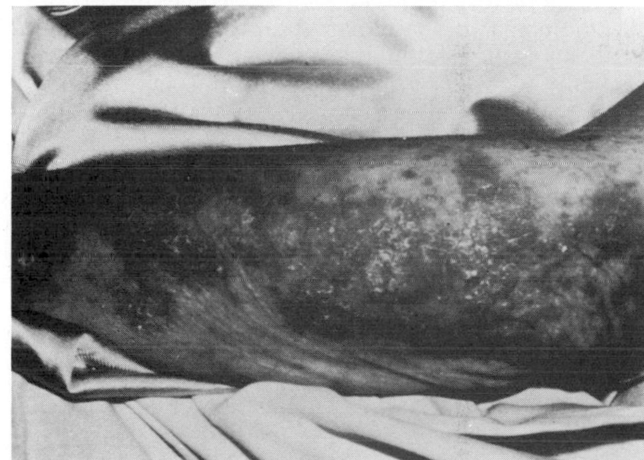

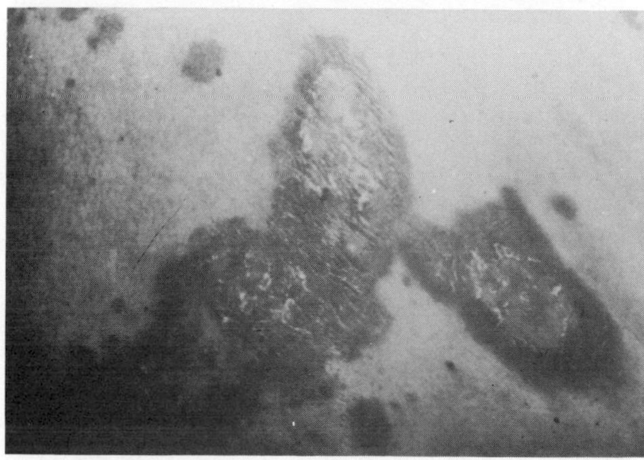

Physical examination shows the skin lesions; it is otherwise unremarkable. The lesions are primarily located on the perineum, along intertriginous zones, at the ankles to midcalf, and around the mouth and nose. Laboratory studies show hemoglobin of 10.8 g/dl and hematocrit of 29.7%; MCV and MCH are normal. All other laboratory results are within normal limits. You would expect this patient to have all the following EXCEPT

A. MEN 1 syndrome
B. metastatic disease
C. low levels of amino acids
D. glucose intolerance or frank diabetes
E. elevated levels of VIP (vasoactive intestinal polypeptide)

28. A 48-year-old woman has a history of intermittent, cramping abdominal pain and diarrhea. Physical examination shows jugular venous distention, a cardiac murmur of pulmonic stenosis, and an enlarged liver. This history and set of physical findings are most strongly suggestive of

A. Crohn's disease
B. Gardner's syndrome
C. diabetic autonomic neuropathy
D. carcinoid tumor
E. nonocclusive intestinal ischemia

QUESTIONS 29–30

A 38-year-old male restaurateur comes to your office with a one-day history of black, tarry stools. He reports having episodic epigastric pain over the past three weeks which occurs between meals and awakens him at night. The pain is usually relieved by meals or antacids. On the morning of his visit he awoke with severe abdominal pain and nausea; he vomited clear fluid. On physical examination, blood pressure is 140/90 mm Hg, pulse rate is 100 bpm, temperature is 98°F, and respirations are 16 per minute. He is anicteric, and the liver is nontender with a span of 12 cm in the midclavicular line. The abdomen is tender in the epigastrium, and bowel sounds are decreased. Stool is black and positive for occult blood. Laboratory data show:

White blood cell count	11,000/mm^3
Hemoglobin	10.5 g/dl
Hematocrit	34%
Serum alkaline phosphatase	85 IU/L (normal <71)
Serum bilirubin	1.5 mg/dl

The upper gastrointestinal series is shown below.

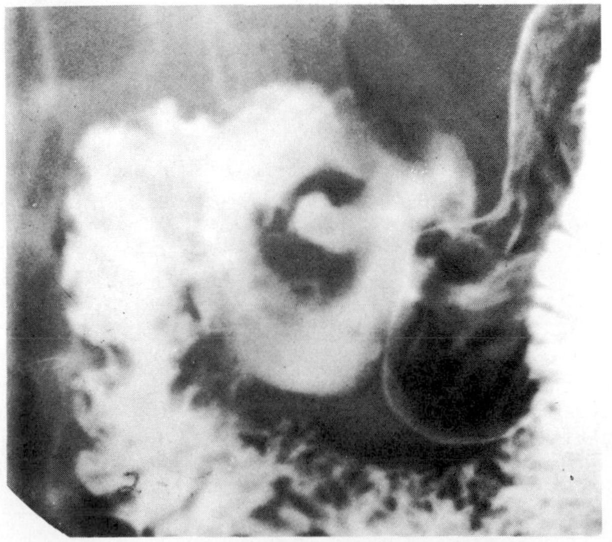

29. Which of the following diagnostic tests would be most appropriate during the initial management of this patient?

A. Ultrasound of the biliary tract and pancreas
B. Endoscopy with brushings for cytology
C. Histalog stimulation test with measurement of gastric acid
D. Measurement of serum gastrin
E. None of the above

30. Which of the following would be appropriate treatment?

A. Liquid antacids (140 mEq of buffering capacity), one and three hours after meals and at bedtime
B. Cimetidine, 400 mg after meals and at bedtime
C. Propantheline, 30 mg plus antacid tablets (20 mEq/tablet) four times daily
D. Ranitidine, 50 mg twice daily
E. None of the above

31. Bacteria are of major importance in the pathogenesis of malabsorption in each of the following EXCEPT

A. tropical sprue
B. gastrocolic fistula
C. scleroderma involving the small bowel
D. diabetic enteropathy
E. multiple jejunal diverticula

32. A 62-year-old man underwent resection of an abdominal aortic aneurysm under halothane anesthesia four days ago. The operation lasted eight hours, the patient received 12 units of blood, and he was hypotensive on several occasions during the procedure. The postoperative course has been complicated by renal failure and gram-negative sepsis. The patient has become progressively jaundiced since the operation. Liver function tests show:

Serum transaminase (SGOT)	72 IU/L
Serum alkaline phosphatase	2 times normal
Prothrombin time	12 seconds (control: 11)
Serum bilirubin	
Total	22 mg/dl
Direct	15 mg/dl

Which of the following is LEAST likely to be contributing to the patient's jaundice?

A. Increased bilirubin production
B. Sepsis
C. Halothane-induced liver injury
D. Renal failure
E. Intraoperative hypotension

QUESTIONS 33–34

A 56-year-old Chinese man reports the abrupt onset of lower abdominal cramping pain, vomiting, and temperature of 38.5°C. He had a similar episode of abdominal pain one month ago which resolved after two to three days. The patient had no emesis or fever at that time. He says that he has had no other medical problems.

On physical examination, temperature is 38.0°C, blood pressure is 120/70 mm Hg, with orthostatic change, and pulse is 120 bpm. Examination of the abdomen shows active bowel sounds and tender left upper quadrant without rebound/guarding to palpation. Liver and spleen are normal. No masses are discerned. There is gross blood on digital rectal exam. Laboratory studies show hemoglobin of 12.8 g/dl and hematocrit of 37.5%; MCV and MCH are normal.

33. In addition to flexible sigmoidoscopy, the initial management of this patient should include

A. steroids
B. antibiotics
C. sulfasalazine
D. barium enema with reflux into terminal ileum
E. angiography of the inferior mesenteric artery

34. The most common finding on endoscopic evaluation of the colon in this patient would be

A. adenocarcinoma of the rectum
B. vascular ectasias in the cecum
C. 0.5-cm sessile polyp at the splenic flexure
D. areas of submucosal hemorrhage at the splenic flexure
E. normal examination, without etiology of hemorrhage

QUESTIONS 35–36

A 38-year-old black male school teacher underwent an antrectomy and vagotomy with a Billroth II anastomosis (gastrojejunostomy) one year ago for recurrent peptic ulcer disease. Over the past two months he has developed abdominal discomfort, bloating, and occasional vomiting after eating.

35. Which of the following is LEAST likely to be the cause of this patient's symptoms?

A. Afferent loop obstruction
B. Gastric outlet obstruction
C. Bile reflux gastritis
D. Chronic pancreatitis
E. Cholelithiasis

The patient also has had chronic diarrhea with a weight loss of 15 pounds over the past year. Hematocrit is 35%, hemoglobin is 10 g/dl, and stool fat excretion is 15 g/day on a 100 g/day fat diet. Stool is negative for occult blood.

36. What is the most likely cause of anemia in this patient?

A. Vitamin B_{12} deficiency
B. Folate deficiency
C. Iron deficiency
D. Anemia of chronic disease
E. None of the above

37. A 55-year-old man with end-stage alcoholic cirrhosis is brought into the emergency room after having become progressively confused and lethargic over the previous week. That morning he was incontinent of a black, tarry stool. He has taken diazepam occasionally at night to help him sleep and takes spironolactone for ascites. Temperature is 37°C. Physical examination shows fetor hepaticus, asterixis, jaundice, vascular spiders, palmar erythema, and ascites. The patient is barely rousable to spoken commands. Laboratory studies show:

White blood count	11,000/mm^3
Hematocrit	28%
Serum sodium	128 mEq/L
Serum potassium	5.6 mEq/L
Blood urea nitrogen	26 mg/dl

A diagnostic aspiration of the ascites is performed and reveals a white blood cell count of 750/mm^3 (80% polymorphonuclear leukocytes). Which of the following is LEAST likely to have contributed to the mental status of this patient?

A. Infection
B. Sedative drugs
C. Gastrointestinal bleeding
D. Deterioration in hepatic function
E. Diuretic-induced electrolyte imbalance

38. A 19-year-old woman has intermittent bloody diarrhea of seven days' duration. Appropriate diagnostic studies establish the diagnosis of ulcerative colitis with pancolonic involvement. The patient responds to an initial course of steroids/sulfasalazine and is then maintained on the sulfasalazine alone. She has read extensively about idiopathic inflammatory bowel disease and the risk of neoplasm and discusses her conclusions with you. Each is correct EXCEPT

A. her age of onset puts her at greater risk to develop cancer
B. patients with continuously active colitis are at greater risk of developing cancer
C. the extent of macroscopic bowel inflammation correlates directly with the risk of developing cancer
D. the number of years with the disease is the best recognized risk factor in developing colon cancer
E. subtotal colectomy does *not* eliminate the risk of colon cancer in the retained rectal mucosa

39. A 76-year-old male archaeologist consults you about his upcoming two-month trip to rural Mexico. The patient reports that when he was there two years ago, he had several episodes of an acute diarrheal illness that completely disrupted his work. He states that his health has been excellent; he is troubled with low back pain that has been evaluated and found to be degenerative joint disease (L1–L4). The patient takes aspirin, 650 mg orally three or four times daily for symptomatic relief; the medication is always effective. Which of the following would you recommend?

A. Drinking noncarbonated bottled water throughout the trip
B. Administration of bismuth subsalicylate (Pepto-Bismol) liquid, 60 ml four times daily, or two 300-mg tablets four times daily, throughout the trip
C. Administration of trimethoprim, 160 mg, and sulfamethoxazole, 800 mg, daily throughout the trip
D. Administration of immune serum globulin, 2 ml intramuscularly a week before the trip
E. Hepatitis B vaccination, the first dose a month before the trip

40. A 56-year-old woman has cutaneous flushing and diarrhea. Past medical history is unremarkable. The diarrhea seems to occur with or directly after the flushing episodes; it is nonbloody and of modest volume, not associated with any abdominal discomfort. Physical examination is notable for facial telangiectasias, and during the exam the patient experiences a typical flushing episode. You observe a flush beginning on the face which spreads to the trunk and upper extremities. The facial telangiectasias become much more pronounced; they are initially red and then purple. Laboratory testing is within the normal limits, with the exception of 24-hour collection for urinary 5-hydroxyindoleacetic acid (5-HIAA), which is 12 mg/24 hr (normal <10 mg/24 hr). Which of the following is most correct about this patient's condition?

A. Blood pressure tends to increase during a flushing episode
B. False-positive urinary 5-HIAA determinations are commonly noted
C. The appendix is the most likely site of disease in this patient
D. Overproduction of serotonin is responsible for the flushing episodes in this patient
E. Left-sided endocardial fibrosis is found in more than one third of patients

QUESTIONS 41–42

A 37-year-old woman referred to you after routine screening shows a fivefold elevation of serum transaminase. The patient says she feels well except for occasional itching and is fully active while raising her three young children. Past medical history includes mild hypertension, for which she takes alpha-methyldopa, and blood transfusion for postpartum hemorrhage after the birth of her first child eight years ago. Physical examination shows a healthy-appearing woman with several vascular "spiders" on her chest and back. Liver span is approximately 15 cm in the midclavicular line, and the edge is nontender. Spleen tip is barely palpated with deep inspiration; there is no ascites. Additional laboratory studies include:

Hematocrit	37%
Platelet count	120,000/mm^3
Prothrombin time	12 seconds (control: 11)
Serum bilirubin	1.2 mg/dl
Serum alkaline phosphatase	3 times elevated
HBsAg	Negative

41. Which one of the following would be the LEAST satisfactory explanation for this patient's hepatic disorder?

A. Chronic non-A, non-B hepatitis resulting from transfusions received after the birth of her first child
B. Primary biliary cirrhosis
C. "Autoimmune-type" chronic hepatitis (lupoid hepatitis)
D. Hemochromatosis
E. Drug-induced liver disease

42. A liver biopsy reveals chronic active hepatitis with postnecrotic cirrhosis. The patient is advised to stop taking all medications, but after six months laboratory studies are unchanged. She remains asymptomatic except for mild and intermittent pruritus. The best course of action now would be to advise the patient of the findings and

A. begin prednisone
B. begin cholestyramine
C. begin prednisone plus azathioprine
D. begin symptomatic treatment with a topical emollient
E. recommend a repeat biopsy in three months if the biochemical abnormalities persist, regardless of the symptoms

43. Vasculitis of the bowel wall with perforation occurs in each of the following EXCEPT

A. polyarteritis nodosa
B. familial Mediterranean fever
C. rheumatoid arthritis
D. systemic lupus erythematosus
E. Köhlmeier-Degos disease

QUESTIONS 44–45

A 75-year-old black man is brought to the emergency room with a one-day history of rectal bleeding. Yesterday he passed four large stools containing large amounts of bright red blood within one hour. Bleeding stopped until this morning when he passed large amounts of red blood and clots three times within two hours. Five hours later he passed bright red blood twice, and because of severe weakness and dizziness he came to the emergency room. The patient has severe hypertension that is being treated with propranolol, hydralazine, and furosemide. Five years ago he underwent resection of an abdominal aortic aneurysm with placement of a Dacron graft. Ten years ago he had an anterior myocardial infarction, and he has had occasional exertional angina pectoris since then. He has had five episodes of angina at rest today, each relieved by nitroglycerin. Laboratory studies show:

Hematocrit	18%
White blood cell count	9500/mm^3
Platelet count	250,000/mm^3
Prothrombin time	11 seconds (control: 11)
Serum electrolytes	
Sodium	145 mEq/L
Potassium	3.5 mEq/L
Chloride	100 mEq/L
Bicarbonate	19 mEq/L
Liver function studies	All within normal range

The electrocardiogram shows evidence of an old anterior myocardial infarction and hypertension; it is otherwise normal. Sigmoidoscopy reveals normal mucosa with blood in the lumen. Nasogastric tube aspiration shows no blood and no bile.

44. After initial stabilization and blood replacement, which one of the following would be the most reasonable initial diagnostic test?

A. Colonoscopy
B. Barium enema
C. Upper gastrointestinal panendoscopy
D. Computerized tomography of the abdomen
E. Selective inferior mesenteric artery arteriography

45. Which of the following lesions is LEAST likely to be the cause of the patient's hematochezia?

A. Duodenal ulcer
B. Bleeding diverticula
C. Aortoduodenal fistula
D. Angiodysplasia of the colon
E. Villous adenoma of the rectum

46. A 21-year-old man has had recurrent upper abdominal pain and intermittent jaundice for one month. The patient was in a motorcycle accident six months ago. Eight weeks ago he was stabbed in the upper abdomen. Exploratory laparotomy at that time revealed lacerations of the liver and colon, which were repaired without incident. Physical examination now shows the laparotomy scar; there are no other abnormalities. The stool is repeatedly positive for occult blood. Laboratory studies include a serum bilirubin of 2 mg/dl, a serum transaminase (SGOT) twice normal, and a serum 5′-nucleotidase three times normal. Proctosigmoidoscopy, barium enema, and upper gastrointestinal films are all normal. Which of the following tests is most likely to provide a definitive diagnosis?

A. Intravenous cholangiography
B. Ultrasonography

C. Arteriography
D. Laparoscopy
E. Liver biopsy

47. A 27-year-old woman has intermittent crampy abdominal discomfort and alternating periods of constipation and diarrhea. The usual pattern of symptoms is to have several (2–4) loose bowel movements daily for 3–4 days, then 1–2 days without bowel movement. The patient reports that her appetite is excellent and her weight stable. She notes that the episodes follow particular job and life stresses. Physical examination is unremarkable; her stool is negative for WBC's. Three examinations failed to reveal fecal ova or parasites. Evaluation with flexible sigmoidoscopy, air-contrast barium enema, and upper gastrointestinal series is entirely normal. Which of the following would you recommend?

A. Glucose tolerance test
B. Lactose tolerance test
C. D-Xylose tolerance test
D. Secretin stimulation test
E. None of the above

48. Which of the following patients is LEAST likely to have Wilson's disease?

A. A 5-year-old girl who has a history of severe cholestasis since infancy and Kayser-Fleischer rings
B. A 13-year-old boy who has chronic active hepatitis, hemolysis, and a normal plasma concentration of ceruloplasmin
C. A 14-year-old girl who has fulminant hepatic failure and a normal slit-lamp examination of the eyes
D. A 28-year-old woman who has cirrhosis, aminoaciduria, glucosuria, uricosuria, hypercalciuria, and osteomalacia
E. A 42-year-old man who has cirrhosis and sunflower cataracts

49. A 62-year-old housewife is admitted with midepigastric postprandial pains occurring 30 minutes after meals. She has lost 20 pounds over the past six months. She says she has a good appetite but is afraid to eat because of the predictability of the pain. Physical examination shows obvious signs of weight loss; it is otherwise normal. An upper gastrointestinal series, endoscopy, oral cholecystogram, sigmoidoscopy, and barium enema are normal. Laboratory values show:

Hematocrit	38%
White blood cell count	8100/mm^3
Serum albumin	4.0 g/dl
Serum alkaline phosphatase	Normal
Serum bilirubin	Normal
Serum transaminase (SGOT)	Normal
Serum lactic dehydrogenase	Normal
Serum amylase	Normal

Stools are negative for occult blood on six successive days.

Which one of the following tests would most likely give the correct diagnosis?

A. Laparoscopy
B. Exploratory laparotomy
C. Mesenteric angiography
D. Computed tomography of the abdomen
E. Psychiatric evaluation

50. A 65-year-old male Chinese immigrant has progressive jaundice and pruritus. Evaluation reveals a small cholangiocarcinoma. Which of the following is most likely to be associated with this clinical setting?

A. *Ascaris lumbricoides*
B. *Fasciola hepatica*
C. *Schistosoma mansoni*
D. *Strongyloides stercoralis*
E. *Clonorchis sinensis*

DIRECTIONS: For questions 51 to 96, you are to decide whether EACH choice is true or false. Any combination of answers, from all true to all false, may occur. Mark the answer sheet "T" or "F" in the space provided.

QUESTIONS 51–52

A 75-year-old woman who has calcific/aortic stenosis and hypotensive blood pressure is admitted to the hospital because of a third episode of hematochezia within a year. She has no pain, hematemesis, nausea, melena, or weight loss, but has been taking indomethacin and aspirin for degenerative joint disease. Previous evaluations (within the past three months) have included normal air-contrast upper gastrointestinal series, normal air-contrast barium enema (no colonic diverticula), and normal flexible fiberoptic sigmoidoscopy. Physical examination on admission shows a Grade III/VI aortic stenosis murmur and dark red guaiac-positive stools; it is otherwise normal. Hematocrit is 22% (normochromic, normocytic red blood cell indices).

51. Which of the following statements concerning this patient is/are correct?

A. The prior barium enema is a sensitive means of excluding colonic diverticula
B. An acute hemorrhage is more likely than chronic intermittent blood loss
C. An upper gastrointestinal tract lesion is excluded by the clinical findings
D. The previous gastrointestinal evaluation excludes the possibility of colonic vascular ectasias
E. On the basis of the patient's evaluations, a small bowel lesion is the most likely source of hemorrhage

The patient is given 3 units of packed red blood cells and 2 liters of normal saline over 12 hours with normalization of blood pressure and pulse. She continues to pass approximately 50 ml of dark red stool every hour. Nasogastric aspirate shows "coffee grounds" and a few flecks of dark red blood. Endoscopy and sigmoidoscopy are negative. A technetium-^{99}m pertechnetate in vivo red blood cell scan is performed (see figure below). The scan shown was taken 12 hours after administration of intravenous radionuclide. Previous scans at 5 minutes, 1 hour, and 4 hours were normal.

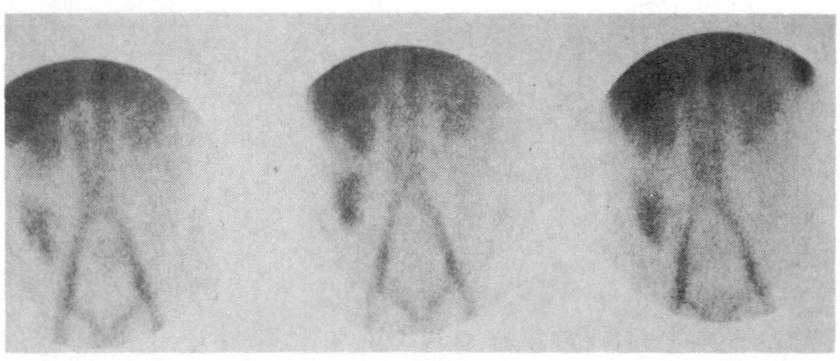

52. Which of the following statements concerning the figure shown is/are correct?

A. Bleeding from the small intestine may present with this scan pattern
B. This area would be shown best by repeat air-contrast barium radiography
C. Colonoscopy is *not* likely to show a specific lesion in this area
D. The presence of a lesion in this location may be associated with underlying heart disease in the patient
E. *Entamoeba histolytica, Mycobacterium tuberculosis,* bowel vascular ectasias, and Crohn's disease are all associated with bleeding from this location

53. You are asked to see a 33-year-old Hispanic man two weeks after gastric resection and gastroenterostomy for severe acid peptic disease (a bleeding gastric ulcer). While the patient initially tolerated a liquid diet without problem, he now has malaise, weakness, sweating, and loose bowel movements since he has been advanced to a regular diet. Which of the following is/are true about this patient?

A. His regimen should be a low-carbohydrate, solid diet
B. His regimen should be a high-carbohydrate, solid diet
C. His regimen should be changed to a full liquid, high-carbohydrate, high-protein diet
D. He should be encouraged to take all nourishment in an upright position
E. He should be encouraged to take all nourishment in a recumbent position

54. Factors associated with increased risk of pancreatic carcinoma include which of the following?

A. Hyperlipidemia
B. Pancreas divisum
C. Cigarette smoking
D. Alcoholic pancreatitis
E. Hereditary pancreatitis

55. In a 53-year-old chronic alcoholic man with a 20-year history of cigarette smoking, chest roentgenogram shows a 2-cm left upper lobe pulmonary nodule. Serum amylase level is three times normal; blood chemistry results are otherwise normal. Which of the following is/are true?

A. Amylase secretion is a feature of metastatic carcinomas originating in the lung
B. The hyperamylasemia is likely due to elevation of salivary amylase isoenzyme
C. Salivary hyperamylasemia is associated with inflammatory changes of the gland
D. A normal serum lipase level helps exclude pancreatitis as a cause of the hyperamylasemia
E. Macroamylasemia can be excluded by a low renal amylase:creatinine clearance ratio

56. Conditions associated with gastric acid hypersecretion include which of the following?

A. Pernicious anemia
B. Small intestinal resection
C. Vasoactive intestinal polypeptide (VIP)–secreting tumor
D. Systemic mastocytosis
E. Cushing's syndrome

57. Which of the following statements regarding the liver in pregnancy is/are correct?

A. Acute fatty liver of pregnancy is nearly always fatal
B. The infant of a woman with a positive HBsAg, positive anti-HBc, and positive anti-HBe has a greater than 50% chance of becoming a chronic carrier of HBsAg
C. Cholestasis of pregnancy is commonly associated with preeclampsia
D. Acute fatty liver of pregnancy is commonly associated with preeclampsia
E. Pregnancy is associated with the development of cholesterol gallstones

58. Adenocarcinoma of the large bowel is the third most common cancer in the United States. Which of the following patients is/are at an increased risk for the development of colorectal neoplasm?

A. A 22-year-old woman with Peutz-Jeghers syndrome confined to the small intestine
B. A 36-year-old man who has a 10-year history of severe ulcerative proctitis
C. A 44-year-old woman whose sister has colonic adenocarcinoma
D. A 48-year-old woman with history of breast cancer, status post–curative surgery
E. A 48-year-old man with prostatic cancer
F. An 83-year-old man in excellent health

59. Which of the following has/have been established as favorable treatment for acute pancreatitis?

A. Antibiotics
B. Anticholinergics
C. Nasogastric suction
D. Parenteral alimentation
E. Elemental diet

QUESTIONS 60–61

A 37-year-old male painter develops epigastric abdominal pain radiating to the back which gradually worsens over a six-day period. The pain is now accompanied by nausea and vomiting. He reports similar, less severe episodes over the past four years; the symptoms abated when he stopped drinking his usual half-pint of alcohol each day. Physical examination is notable for temperature of 36.9°C, a tender liver with a span of 12 cm in the midclavicular line, and moderate epigastric tenderness. Stool is negative for occult blood. Laboratory data include:

Hematocrit	52%
White blood cell count	11,500/mm^3
Serum alanine aminotransferase	50 units/L
Serum aspartate aminotransferase	75 units/L
Serum bilirubin	2.0 mg/dl
Prothrombin time	11.5 seconds (control: 11)
Serum amylase	210 IU/ml

Computed tomography (CT scan) of the abdomen is shown above, right column.

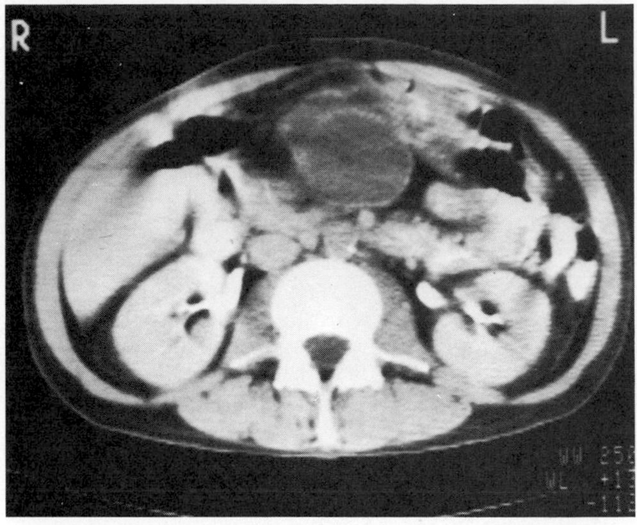

60. Initial therapy should include which of the following?

A. Broad-spectrum antibiotics
B. Parenteral nutrition
C. Exploratory laparotomy
D. Needle aspiration
E. Serial ultrasound or computed tomography (CT scans)

Eight weeks later, the patient's symptoms have not improved.

61. Which of the following should be considered now?

A. Broad-spectrum antibiotics
B. Parenteral nutrition
C. Upper gastrointestinal endoscopy
D. Surgical drainage
E. Serial ultrasound or computed tomography (CT scans)

62. Which of the following statements regarding isoniazid-associated hepatitis is/are true?

A. Isoniazid-associated hepatitis occurs most frequently in middle-aged and elderly individuals, in whom the incidence of severe liver disease may exceed 2% of those receiving the drug
B. Isoniazid produces a characteristic injury that is usually distinguishable from acute viral hepatitis and chronic active hepatitis on liver biopsy
C. In many patients, hepatotoxicity will not become evident until many months after beginning isoniazid therapy
D. Isoniazid-induced liver injury is typically accompanied by a skin rash or eosinophilia
E. Many patients will develop mild elevations of serum transaminases after beginning isoniazid therapy, but most of these do not develop severe liver disease

63. In a patient who has ulcerative colitis of 25 years' duration, which of the following concerning cancer screening is/are correct?

A. Carcinoembryonic antigen (CEA) is a sensitive reliable test for early cancer
B. When Hemoccult cards are used for home stool

screening, the patient should restrict intake of poultry, fish, and red meats
C. Dysplasia on rectal biopsy pathology is an indication for pancolonoscopy and multiple biopsies
D. Single-contrast barium enema radiography plus flexible fiberoptic sigmoidoscopy can reliably exclude the possibility of cancer
E. When Hemoccult cards are used, therapeutic doses of ferrous sulfate and ascorbic acid (vitamin C) are both likely to give false-negative stool guaiac tests

64. A 38-year-old male executive has just undergone an unusually thorough medical evaluation, including a physical examination, laboratory tests, glucose tolerance test, and roentgenograms of the chest and gastrointestinal tract. The only abnormality was an oral cholecystogram showing radiolucent gallstones, for which the patient is now referred to you. A careful history reveals no abdominal symptoms. Which of the following statements regarding this patient is/are correct?

A. There is a 75% or better chance that symptoms due to gallstones will develop in the future
B. Cancer is found more often in gallbladders with stones than in gallbladders without stones
C. There is about a 50% chance that a life-threatening complication of cholelithiasis will develop in the future
D. From a statistical standpoint, elective cholecystectomy performed now would increase this patient's lifespan
E. Percutaneous transhepatic cholangiography should be done to exclude choledocholithiasis

65. A 48-year-old man with chronic alcoholism has a two-year history of intermittent epigastric pain. Over the past year, he has had a 10-pound weight loss associated with voluminous diarrhea. Both the abdominal pain and diarrhea improve when the patient does not eat. On a 100-g fat diet, stool fat content was 18 g/day. Which of the following is/are likely to be true of this patient?

A. Absorption of calcium and iron is normal
B. Impaired oral glucose tolerance would be expected
C. Megaloblastic anemia resulting from vitamin B_{12} malabsorption would be expected
D. Flatulence and watery diarrhea after a carbohydrate meal would be expected
E. At least 90% of the exocrine secretory capacity of the pancreas has been lost

66. A 46-year-old delivery man is admitted to the hospital with nausea, vomiting, and severe abdominal pain radiating to the back. He has recently lost his job and has been on an alcoholic binge, increasing his usual daily alcohol intake from three drinks to a fifth of vodka. He has no prior history of abdominal pain or dyspepsia. Blood pressure is 100/60 mm Hg, pulse is 110 bpm, temperature is 38°C, and respirations are 22 per minute. The physical examination shows mild scleral icterus and marked epigastric tenderness. Bowel sounds are decreased. Stool is negative for occult blood. Chest roentgenogram shows a small left pleural effusion. Plain radiograph of the abdomen in normal. Laboratory data include:

Serum aspartate aminotransferase (AST)	45 units/L
Serum alkaline phosphatase	150 IU/L (normal <71)
Serum bilirubin	2.9 mg/dl
Serum amylase	4 times normal
Serum lipase	4 times normal

Which of the following statements is/are true?

A. The pleural effusion is likely to be an exudate with high lipase content
B. The elevated serum bilirubin indicates probable coincident alcoholic liver disease
C. The degree of hyperamylasemia correlates with the severity of disease
D. Adult respiratory distress syndrome is a complication of this disease
E. Development of cholangitis in this setting is an indication for emergency surgery

67. Which of the following statements regarding alpha$_1$-antitrypsin deficiency is/are true?

A. It is part of the differential diagnosis of cholestasis in infancy
B. Rounded eosinophilic cytoplasmic inclusions in periportal hepatocytes seen on liver biopsy are diagnostic of the P_iZZ phenotype
C. The majority of individuals with the homozygous P_iZZ phenotype will develop overt liver disease before the age of 15
D. Hepatocellular carcinoma is a rare occurrence in adults with cirrhosis secondary to alpha$_1$-antitrypsin deficiency
E. Patients with cryptogenic cirrhosis and chronic active hepatitis show an increased prevalence of alpha$_1$-antitrypsin heterozygous Z phenotypes

68. Which of the following statements concerning esophageal cancer is/are true?

A. Adenocarcinoma is the most common histologic type
B. It is associated with alcohol intake and tobacco smoking
C. A normal double-contrast barium esophagogram in a patient with dysphagia adequately excludes esophageal cancer
D. Methotrexate, doxorubicin, and 5-fluorouracil as single agents produce measurable tumor regression in most cases
E. Squamous cell carcinoma of the cervical esophagus is radiosensitive

69. A 48-year-old man who does not drink alcohol is admitted to the hospital because of severe periumbilical pain radiating to the back. Three weeks ago he had an episode of similar but much less severe pain, and an oral cholecystogram at that time was normal. On physical examination the patient is acutely ill with shock, respiratory distress, and diffuse abdominal tenderness with rebound. Laboratory studies show:

Hematocrit	54%
White blood cell count	22,000/mm^3
Serum amylase	1800 IU/L
Serum albumin	4.5 g/dl
Serum calcium	10.2 mg/dl
Serum glucose	360 mg/dl
Serum cholesterol	300 mg/dl
Serum triglycerides	2350 mg/dl

Which of the following might have caused this episode of severe pancreatitis?

A. Diabetic ketoacidosis
B. Hyperparathyroidism
C. Thiazide diuretics
D. Acute leukemia
E. Hyperlipoproteinemia

70. A 59-year-old white male accountant is referred to you for evaluation of a 2.5-cm gastric ulcer. Which of the following would be helpful in determining whether or not the ulcer is malignant?

A. The patient has lost 10 pounds over the past two months
B. He has had no abdominal pain associated with the ulcer
C. Gastric acid is present in the stomach
D. The ulcer is located on the lesser curvature of the stomach
E. Roentgenogram shows that gastric folds radiate from the ulcer crater

71. Which of the following treatments for bleeding esophageal varices results in lowering of pressure in the portal vein?

A. Propranolol
B. Vasopressin
C. Variceal sclerotherapy
D. Distal splenorenal shunt
E. End-to-side portacaval shunt

72. Which of the following statements regarding celiac disease is/are correct?

A. Once established in early childhood, spontaneous symptomatic remission is rare
B. It increases the risk of developing squamous carcinoma of the esophagus
C. Corticosteroids do not affect the clinical course of uncomplicated celiac sprue
D. Subacute combined degeneration of the spinal cord may occur in the absence of vitamin B_{12} deficiency
E. Mucosal lesions of celiac sprue are present in the vast majority of patients with dermatitis herpetiformis

73. Which of the following statements regarding hepatic transplantation is/are true?

A. The best results have been obtained in children with biliary atresia
B. Fulminant hepatic failure is an absolute contraindication to transplantation
C. Primary biliary cirrhosis commonly recurs in patients receiving transplants for this condition
D. Most patients surviving the first three postoperative months will live for at least three years
E. The results of transplantation for hepatocellular carcinoma have improved with the use of cyclosporine

74. A 65-year-old woman who underwent subtotal gastrectomy and Billroth II gastrojejunostomy two years ago is evaluated for a 30-pound weight loss and diarrhea. She passes four or five loose watery stools after each meal; there has been no nocturnal diarrhea. Proctoscopy is normal. Examination of the stool shows many muscle fibers and fat globules. Barium enema is illustrated. Which of the following statements is/are correct?

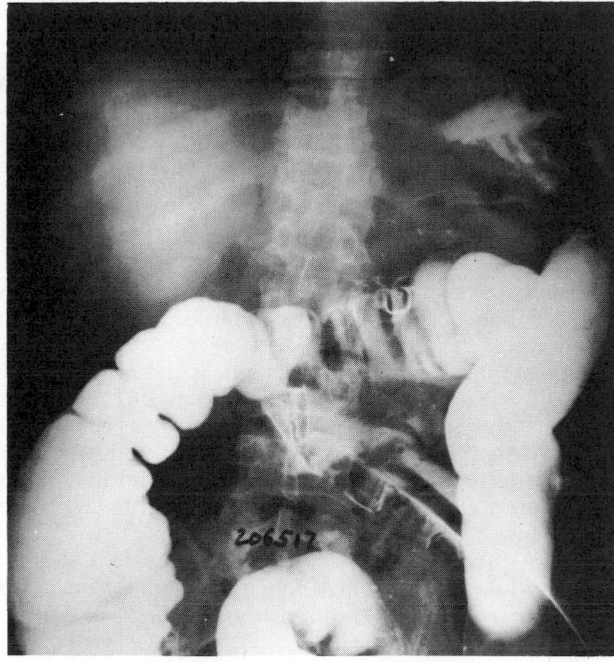

A. The patient was given a larger-than-normal volume of barium contrast material, which has refluxed to the proximal gastrointestinal tract
B. A subphrenic collection of barium suggestive of an abscess has developed from a perforating colonic carcinoma
C. The differential diagnosis includes Crohn's disease, carcinoma, and abdominal trauma
D. The diarrhea is due to fecal contamination and overgrowth of colonic flora in the upper gastrointestinal tract
E. An upper gastrointestinal series will reliably demonstrate the same findings

75. Which of the following clinical features is/are commonly found in Whipple's disease?

A. Fever
B. Lymphadenopathy
C. Hepatosplenomegaly
D. Migratory arthritis
E. Pulmonary interstitial fibrosis

76. A 33-year-old male pharmacist sees you for a second opinion regarding surgical treatment for recurrent duodenal ulcer disease. Over the past 18 months he has had three episodes of epigastric pain and discrete duodenal ulcers diagnosed by upper gastrointestinal series or endoscopy. The first ulcer was located on the posterior surface of the duodenal bulb; on the second occasion an ulcer was found on the anterior surface; and on the third occasion a postbulbar ulcer was found. On each occasion he was treated with an 8-week course of H_2-receptor antagonists and maintained on a daily bedtime dose. Episodes of pain are becoming more frequent and severe and are of longer duration. Which of the following would be appropriate to consider in the management of this patient?

A. Measurement of serum gastrin
B. Antrectomy and vagotomy
C. Vagotomy and pyloroplasty

D. Highly selective vagotomy
E. Total gastrectomy

77. In which of the following conditions may rectal biopsy be of particular value in diagnosis?

A. Traveler's diarrhea
B. Schistosomiasis
C. Ascariasis
D. Balantidiasis
E. Amyloidosis

78. Which of the following statements regarding the relationship between hepatitis B virus infection and hepatocellular carcinoma is/are true?

A. In the United States, serologic markers of hepatitis B virus infection are more common in patients with hepatocellular carcinoma than in controls
B. Hepatitis B viral DNA is frequently incorporated into the host genome of nonmalignant liver tissue surrounding the tumor in patients who are HBsAg-positive
C. A positive test of HBsAg in serum is associated with more than a 100-fold increase in the incidence of hepatocellular cancer in humans
D. Hepatitis B virus infection may be associated with hepatocellular carcinoma in the absence of cirrhosis
E. Hepatocellular carcinoma associated with hepatitis B virus infection is more common in males than in females

79. Which of the following is/are among causes of secondary chronic intestinal pseudo-obstruction?

A. Hyperthyroidism
B. Chagas' disease
C. Dermatomyositis
D. Hyperparathyroidism
E. Tricyclic antidepressants
F. Laxatives

80. For which of the following patients is colonoscopy as surveillance for colonic neoplasia an appropriate procedure?

A. A 37-year-old man with Crohn's disease of the colon, which was diagnosed at age 19
B. A 37-year-old man in excellent health whose father and older brother had adenocarcinoma of the colon
C. A 37-year-old man with severe ulcerative proctitis, who has had the disease for more than 20 years
D. A 37-year-old asymptomatic man with pancolonic ulcerative colitis, maintained on sulfasalazine, 2 g daily; he was diagnosed at age 29
E. A 57-year-old man with no gastrointestinal complaints; liver biopsy shows metastatic adenocarcinoma

81. A 31-year-old female journalist is referred to you because of epigastric pain unresponsive to treatment with antacids and H_2-receptor antagonists. She reports burning epigastric pain, fullness, nausea, bloating, and belching shortly after eating meals. She has had no vomiting, diarrhea, constipation, obstipation, fever, or severe pain. She has had no abdominal surgery. Physical examination is normal. Urinalysis, serum chemistries, complete blood count, and serum amylase are normal. Upper gastrointestinal series, esophagogastroduodenoscopy, and sonogram of the pancreas, gallbladder, and biliary tract are normal. Which of the following statements is/are true about this condition?

A. Symptoms are frequently exacerbated by fat ingestion
B. Development of a duodenal ulcer is likely
C. Development of pancreatitis is likely
D. Treatment with metoclopramide is indicated
E. Cholecystectomy may improve the patient's condition

82. A 27-year-old homosexual man has a two-month history of diarrhea, vomiting, and liver and abdominal pain. He has lost 10 pounds over the period of this illness. On physical examination, he is found to have a temperature of 38.1°C, generalized lymphadenopathy, and oral candidiasis. A small bowel biopsy is performed (see illustration).

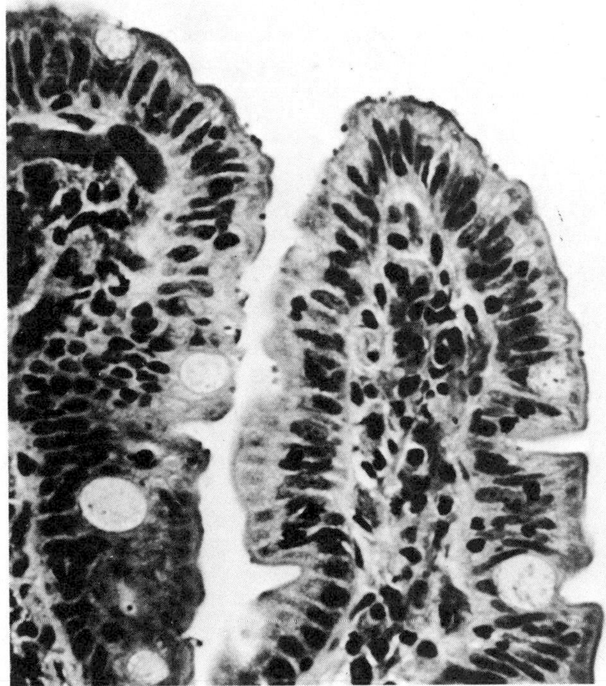

Which of the following statements is/are true regarding the infectious agent seen in the biopsy?

A. It is a cause of self-limited gastrointestinal illness in immunocompetent persons
B. It may cause obstructive lesions of the biliary tract in immunocompromised hosts
C. It causes ulcerative lesions throughout the gastrointestinal tract in immunocompromised hosts
D. Domesticated animals are a potential source of infection in humans
E. Treatment of the patient with spiramycin is likely to eradicate this organism

83. Which of the following is/are true concerning Hirschsprung's disease?

A. It occurs at a rate of 1 in 5000 live births
B. It is more common in children with Down's syndrome

C. It is 5 to 10 times more common in females than males
D. It results from dilatation of an aganglionic segment of the bowel

84. Which of the following is/are associated with increased intestinal loss of plasma protein?

A. Cholera
B. Celiac disease
C. Whipple's disease
D. Abetalipoproteinemia
E. Primary lymphangiectasia

85. Which of the following statements regarding intestinal gas production is/are true?

A. On average, about 600 ml of flatus is passed per rectum daily
B. Bacterial metabolism is the sole source of intestinal H_2 production
C. Hydrogen sulfide accounts for about 20% of the gas present in flatus
D. Patients with complaints of "gas pains" are often found to have excessive air swallowing (aerophagy)
E. Intestinal methane production is more commonly found in patients with carcinoma of the colon than in the general population

86. A 34-year-old woman who is known to have Crohn's disease, involving mainly the distal ileum and proximal ascending colon, undergoes surgical resection of 120 cm of the distal ileum and ascending colon with an ileotransverse colonic anastomosis, because of obstructive symptoms. Which of the following statements regarding this patient is/are true?

A. Diarrhea may result in part from increased colonic water and salt secretion
B. Renal oxalate stones may result from increased colonic oxalate absorption
C. The risk of this patient's developing gallstones is less than that of the general population
D. There is an increased risk of bacterial overgrowth in the lumen of the remaining small intestine
E. Because fat absorption occurs mainly in the proximal small intestine, steatorrhea is unlikely to result

87. A 39-year-old white woman seeks medical attention for pruritus. Serum alkaline phosphatase is elevated five times normal, and antimitochondrial antibodies are positive to a titer of 1:3200. A liver biopsy reveals dense lymphocytic infiltrates in the portal tracts surrounding the interlobular bile ducts, with some degeneration of bile duct epithelium. A few granulomas are seen near abnormal-appearing bile ducts. Which of the following statements is/are true?

A. Serum immunoglobulin M is probably elevated
B. Serum bile acid measurement will be helpful in confirming the diagnosis
C. Treatment with penicillamine is of established value in improving survival
D. The patient is more likely to have antithyroid antibodies than the general population
E. The patient is more likely to develop retroperitoneal fibrosis than the general population

QUESTIONS 88–89

A 33-year-old homosexual man comes to the emergency room because of severe abdominal pain and distention, fever, and bloody diarrhea of two days' duration. For the past two years he has had frequent episodes of mucous and bloody diarrhea, tenesmus, and cramps lasting up to three weeks. Admission laboratory tests include hematocrit 35%, white blood cell count 13,500/mm^3, serum sodium 142 mEq/L, serum potassium 3.2 mEq/L. A plain film of the abdomen is shown below.

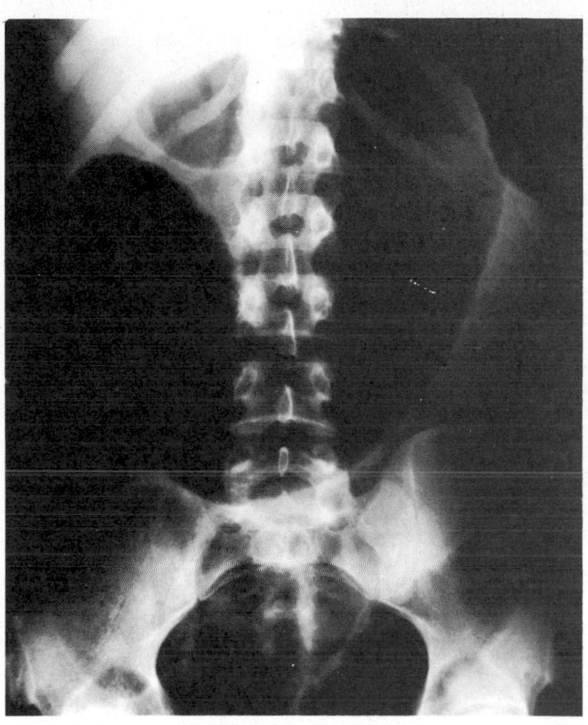

88. Which of the following would explain the patient's illness?

A. Shigellosis
B. Ulcerative colitis
C. Giardiasis
D. Crohn's colitis
E. Amebiasis

89. Stool cultures are negative, and no ova or parasites are visible on three successive stool examinations. Proctosigmoidoscopy reveals a diffusely granular friable mucosa to 15 cm. Which of the following diagnostic tests is/are indicated in this patient?

A. Barium enema
B. Serology for *Entamoeba histolytica*
C. Colonoscopy to the midtransverse colon
D. Blood cultures
E. Repeat plain film of abdomen within 24 hours

90. Which of the following is/are associated with a secretory diarrhea?

A. *Shigella*
B. Prostaglandins E_2 (PGE_2)

C. Phenolphthalein
D. Adenocarcinoma of rectum
E. Chenodeoxycholic acid

91. An 18-year-old white man reports the recent onset of "yellow eyes." He has recently been fasting in order to lose weight. He has no history of hepatitis risk factors or contacts. Physical examination shows scleral icterus; there are no other abnormal findings. Laboratory data show:

Hemoglobin	14.5 g/dl
Reticulocyte count	< 1 %
Serum bilirubin	4.0 mg/dl

All other tests on the liver panel are normal.

Which of the following statements regarding this patient is/are correct?

A. Red cell survival is often shortened in this condition
B. Urinalysis will most likely give a positive test for bilirubin
C. The condition affecting this patient is seen mainly in females
D. Nicotinic acid administration will likely exacerbate the jaundice
E. Liver biopsy is indicated in order to exclude chronic liver disease

92. As surveillance for malignancy, sequential or periodic esophagogastroduodenoscopy is indicated in patients

A. with gastric atrophy
B. with pernicious anemia
C. with biopsy-proven Barrett's epithelium
D. undergoing repeated dilations of esophageal strictures
E. with a large gastric ulcer diagnosed on upper gastrointestinal air-contrast barium series
F. with a large duodenal ulcer diagnosed on upper gastrointestinal air-contrast barium series

93. Which of the following statements is/are correct regarding post-transfusional non-A, non-B (NANB) viral hepatitis?

A. The acute manifestations of infection are characteristically mild
B. In patients with chronic infection, the development of cirrhosis is uncommon
C. Diagnosis can be established by testing for specific antibody responses to the viral agents
D. Pretransfusion immune serum globulin administration effectively reduces the risk of developing NANB viral infection
E. Chronic hepatitis is less likely to occur following a mild or anicteric acute NANB hepatitis than following a severe acute illness

94. Endoscopic retrograde cholangiopancreatography (ERCP) uses a side-viewing flexible endoscope to cannulate the duodenal papilla, instill contrast material,, and obtain radiographic imaging of the pancreatic and biliary ductal systems. The procedure is indicated in which of the following patients?

A. A 33-year-old woman who has had three episodes of midepigastric and right upper quadrant discomfort. Ultrasound shows normal anatomy. Laboratory studies show:

Serum alkaline phosphatase	120 IU/L
Total serum bilirubin	0.6 mg/dl
Serum amylase	800 IU/L

B. A 36-year-old woman with episodic midepigastric and right upper quadrant discomfort. Ultrasound shows a mass in the head of the pancreas and metastatic lesions throughout the liver. Laboratory studies show:

Serum alkaline phosphatase	289 IU/L
Total serum bilirubin	2.4 mg/dl
Serum amylase	47 IU/L

C. A 53-year-old man with a single episode of midepigastric abdominal pain, nausea, vomiting, and anorexia. Abdominal ultrasound does not show cholelithiasis or ductal dilatation. Laboratory studies show:

Serum alkaline phosphatase	100 IU/L
Total serum bilirubin	0.8 mg/dl
Serum amylase	1500 IU/L

D. A 53-year-old man with a single episode of midepigastric pain, nausea, vomiting, and anorexia. Ultrasound shows cholelithiasis. Laboratory studies show:

Serum alkaline phosphatase	100 IU/L
Total serum bilirubin	0.8 mg/dl
Serum amylase	1500 IU/L

95. Which of the following statements regarding hemochromatosis is/are correct?

A. It is among the most common genetically transmitted diseases
B. HLA typing is useful for family screening if the HLA type of the proband is known
C. The presence of a transferrin saturation less than 50% virtually excludes symptomatic hemochromatosis
D. In nonalcoholic patients, the presence of stainable iron in 50% of hepatocytes on liver biopsy establishes the diagnosis
E. In male alcoholic patients, the presence of a transferrin saturation greater than 50%, an elevated serum ferritin concentration, and stainable iron in 50% of hepatocytes establishes the diagnosis

96. Which of the following types of treatment has/have been shown to improve survival in patients with the hepatorenal syndrome?

A. Intravenous dopamine infusion
B. Peritoneovenous shunting
C. Hemodialysis
D. Hemofiltration
E. Renal transplantation

DIRECTIONS: Questions 97 to 182 are matching questions. For each numbered item, choose the most likely associated lettered item from those provided. Each numbered item has ONLY ONE answer. Within each set of questions, each lettered item may be the answer to one, more than one, or none of the numbered items, unless otherwise specified.

QUESTIONS 97–100

Each of the following patients has an hepatic abnormality related to the use of a drug. For each patient, choose the most likely drug.

A. Isoniazid
B. Phenytoin
C. Methyldopa
D. Methotrexate
E. Acetaminophen
F. Perhexilene maleate
G. Oral contraceptives
H. Erythromycin estolate

97. A 20-year-old woman with fever, lymphadenopathy, rash, hepatomegaly, and jaundice

98. A 28-year-old woman with massive ascites and hepatomegaly

99. A 45-year-old woman with asymptomatic cirrhosis and psoriasis

100. A 55-year-old man with severe right upper quadrant pain

QUESTIONS 101–106

Match each of the following clinical histories with the most appropriate liver biopsy (*A–F*, below and on p. 104). (*Note:* Use each figure only once.)

101. A 32-year-old homosexual man with fever and weight loss

102. A 36-year-old woman with documented cholelithiasis who now has fever, chills, right upper quadrant pain, and jaundice

103. A 39-year-old black woman with asymptomatic hilar adenopathy

104. A 42-year-old woman with pruritus, jaundice, hypercholesterolemia, and a positive antimitochondrial antibody test

105. A 46-year-old white man with chronic hepatitis B surface antigenemia, esophageal varices, and hepatosplenomegaly

106. A 53-year-old alcoholic man with ascites, hepatosplenomegaly, and esophageal varices

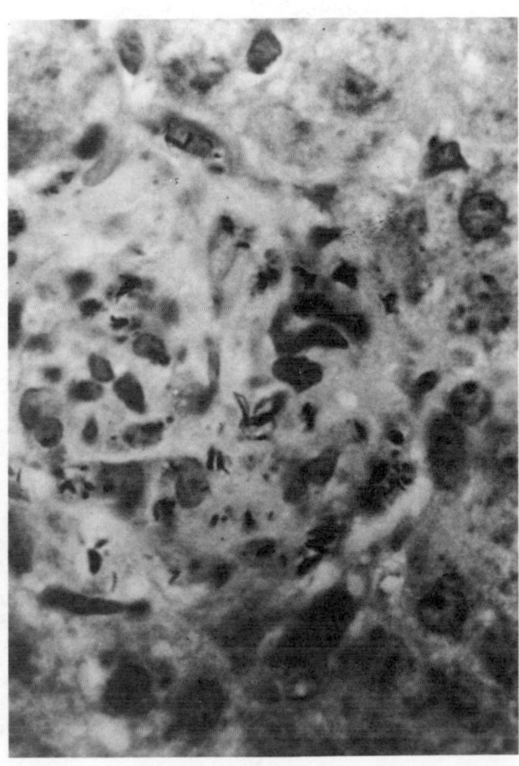

A

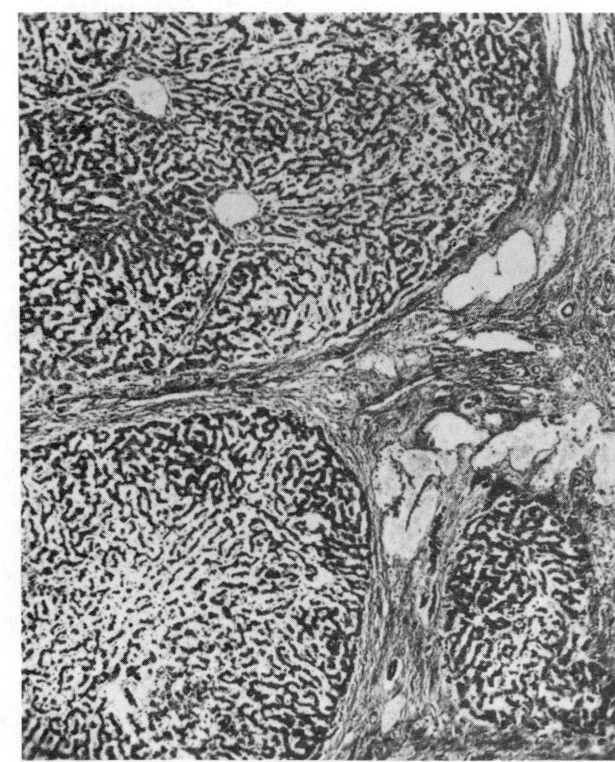

B

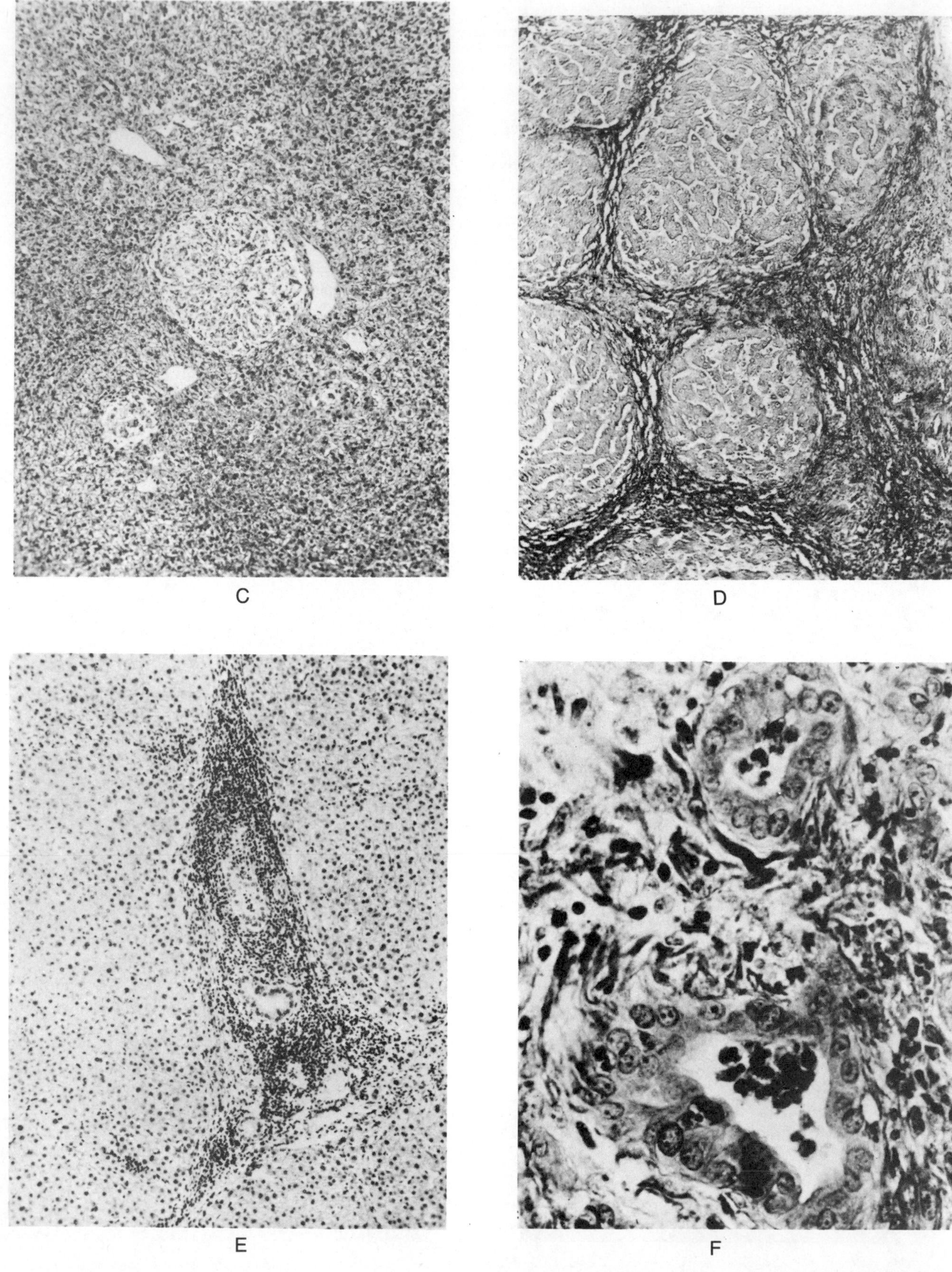
C
D
E
F

QUESTIONS 107–109

For each of the following, select the most appropriate lettered item

A. Acute pancreatitis
B. Chronic pancreatitis
C. Both A and B
D. Neither A nor B

107. Predisposes to pancreatic ascites

108. Is a cause of multiorgan fat necrosis

109. Can result from the passage of gallstones down the common bile duct

QUESTIONS 110–114

For each of the following descriptions of esophageal motility, select the most appropriate lettered answer.

A. Normal
B. Achalasia
C. Scleroderma esophagus
D. "Nutcracker" esophagus
E. Diffuse esophageal spasm
F. Nonspecific esophageal motility disorder

110. Lower esophageal sphincter pressure = 50 mm Hg
Incomplete lower esophageal sphincter relaxation
Aperistalsis in esophageal body
Simultaneous contractions on deglutition
Low-amplitude contractions (mean = 10 mm Hg)

111. Lower esophageal sphincter pressure = 25 mm Hg
Normal relaxation of the lower esophageal sphincter
Normal peristalsis in esophageal body
Prolonged contractions on deglutition
High-amplitude contractions (greater than 120 mm Hg)

112. Lower esophageal sphincter pressure = 20 mm Hg
Complete lower esophageal sphincter relaxation
Single peristaltic waves in the esophageal body
Single esophageal contractions on deglutition
Mean-amplitude contractions of 30–50 mm Hg

113. Lower esophageal sphincter pressure = 35 mm Hg
Incomplete lower esophageal sphincter relaxation
Simultaneous (nonperistaltic) contractions in the esophageal body
Repetitive contractions on deglutition
High-amplitude contractions (mean = 75–90 mm Hg)

114. Lower esophageal sphincter pressure = 10 mm Hg
No change in resting pressure with swallow
Aperistalsis in esophageal body
Aperistalsis on deglutition
Low-amplitude contractions (mean = 5 mm Hg)

QUESTIONS 115–117

For each patient described below, select the lettered procedure most appropriate to perform next. (*Note:* Use each lettered item only once.)

A. Computed tomography
B. Percutaneous transhepatic cholangiography
C. Cholescintigraphy with technetium-^{99}m HIDA
D. Oral cholecystography
E. Endoscopic retrograde cholangiography

115. A 48-year old, previously healthy male lawyer has a one-day history of increasing right upper quadrant abdominal pain. Temperature is 100°F. On abdominal examination the right upper quadrant is diffusely tender without a palpable mass. Serum bilirubin concentration is 1.2 mg/dl, alkaline phosphatase is 70 IU/L (normal <71 IU/L), SGOT is 32 IU/L (normal <26 IU/L), and prothrombin time is normal.

116. A 53-year-old woman has a three-day history of fever and jaundice. Four months ago she underwent an uncomplicated cholecystectomy for acute cholecystitis. Temperature is 101°F. On abdominal examination there is mild right upper quadrant tenderness. Serum bilirubin is 3.5 mg/dl, alkaline phosphatase is 250 IU/L (normal <71 IU/L), SGOT is 55 IU/L (normal <26 IU/L), and white blood count is 12,000 with 80% polymorphonuclear leukocytes and 5% band forms.

117. A 70-year-old retired woman is admitted for evaluation of progressive jaundice and pruritus over the past four weeks. Over the past two to three months she has lost 20 pounds and has had mild chronic abdominal pain localized to the epigastrium and right upper quadrant. Serum bilirubin is 10.5 mg/dl, alkaline phosphatase is 695 IU/L (normal <71 IU/L), SGOT is 40 IU/L (normal <26 IU/L). Ultrasound examination is of poor quality and fails to visualize the extrahepatic bile ducts; the intrahepatic bile ducts are dilated.

QUESTIONS 118–121

For each of the following, select the most appropriate lettered answer.

A. Gastrinoma (Zollinger-Ellison syndrome)
B. Vasoactive intestinal peptide (VIP)–secreting tumor
C. Both A and B
D. Neither A nor B

118. Cause of a metabolic acidosis

119. Most frequently located in the pancreas

120. Diarrhea is improved by nasogastric suction

121. Symptomatic improvement occurs with high-dose glucocorticoids

QUESTIONS 122–125

For each of the patients described below, select the most likely computed tomography (CT) radiograph (*A–E,* on p. 106)

122. A 32-year-old man with abdominal pain of three weeks' duration; physical examination notes generalized abdominal pain and fever of 102°F; stool is guaiac negative.

123. A 60-year-old woman who underwent sigmoid colectomy for Dukes' C colonic adenocarcinoma three years ago; for the past three months she has had weight loss and cramping abdominal pains; stool is guaiac positive.

124. A 65-year-old man with hematochezia of three months' duration; abdominal examination is normal; rectal examination demonstrates a large firm rectal mass and gross blood.

125. A 73-year-old woman with chronic constipation who has had fevers, chills, and cramping abdominal pains for the past week; on physical examination, generalized tenderness is noted; stool is hard, brown, and guaiac negative.

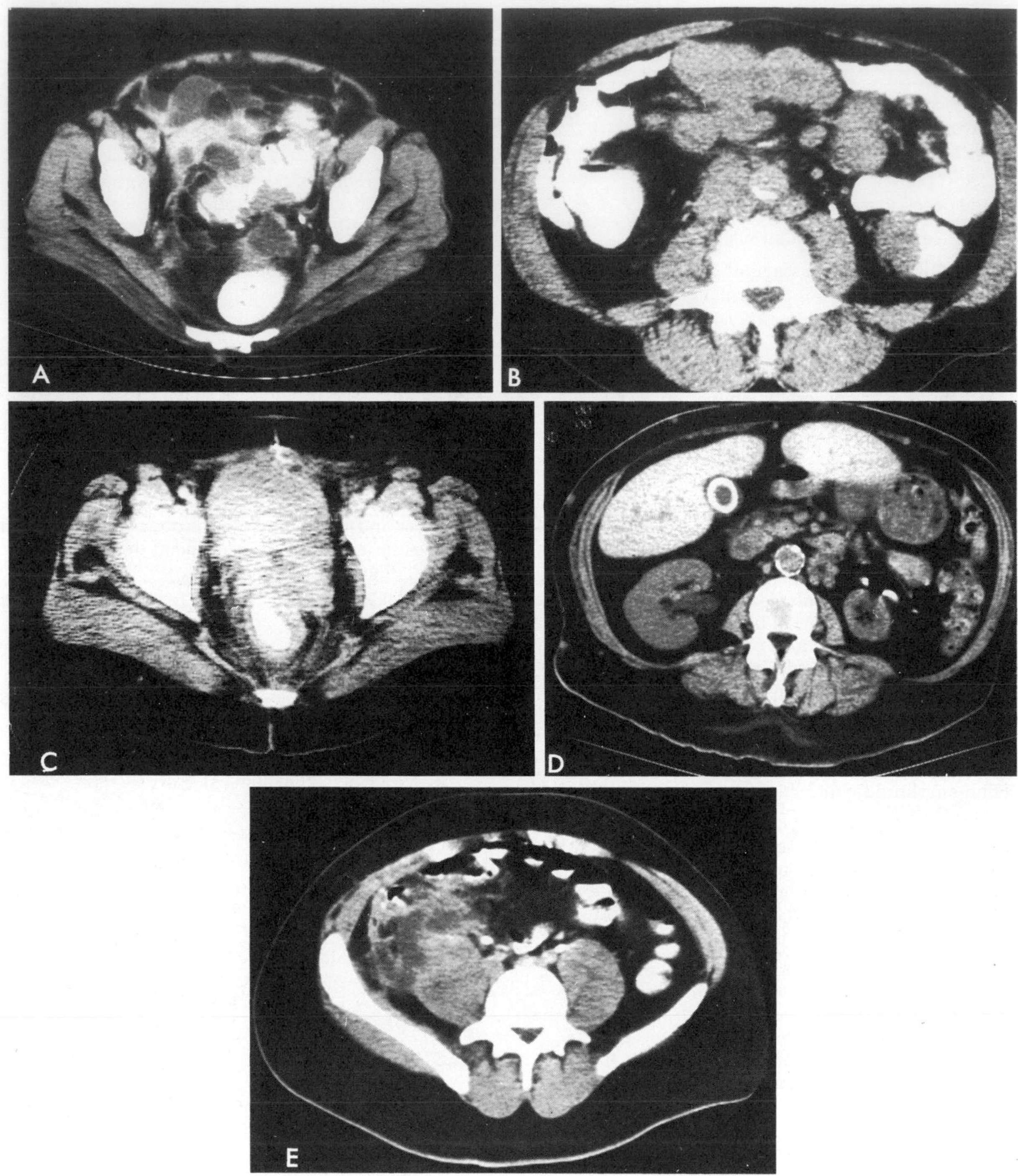

QUESTIONS 126–129

For each of the following statements select the most appropriate lettered answer.

A. Cimetidine
B. Antacids
C. Sucralfate
D. Prostaglandins
E. None of the above

126. Cause of metabolic alkalosis

127. Cause of decrease in gastrin secretion

128. Cause of increase in gastric bicarbonate production

129. Effective treatment for Zollinger-Ellison syndrome

QUESTIONS 130–135

For each description below, select the most applicable disorder. (*Note:* Use each lettered item only once.)

A. Intestinal angina
B. Colonic ischemia
C. Henoch-Schönlein purpura
D. Mesenteric arterial embolus
E. Mesenteric venous thrombosis
F. Nonocclusive intestinal infarction

130. Associated with weight loss due to fear of eating

131. Associated with congestive heart failure, shock, and anoxia

132. Sudden in onset, usually involving the superior mesenteric artery

133. Associated with portal hypertension and hypercoagulable states

134. Often responsive to general supportive care without need for angiography or surgery

135. Known to produce unusual patterns of involvement that do not correlate with the anatomic distribution of the major arteries

QUESTIONS 136–140

For each patient described below, select the most appropriate set of serologic markers. (*Note:* Use each lettered answer only once.)

	anti-HAV	anti-HAV (IgM type)	HBsAg	HBeAg	anti-HBs	anti-HBc	anti-HBc (IgM type)	anti-HBe	anti-delta
A.	+	−	−	−	+	−	−	−	−
B.	+	+	−	−	−	−	−	−	−
C.	+		+	+		+			
D.	−	−	−	−	+	−	−	−	+
E.	−	−	−	−	−	−	−	−	−
F.	−	+	+	−	−	+	−	+	−
G.	+	−	+	−	−	+	−	+	+
H.	+	+	−	+	−	−	−	−	−

136. A 4-year-old girl from an upper-middle-class American family with acute post-transfusion hepatitis following repair of a congenital heart defect

137. A 20-year-old male day-care center worker with acute hepatitis

138. A 32-year-old mother of an HBsAg-positive infant

139. A 32-year-old male intravenous drug abuser with biopsy-proven chronic hepatitis who has recently suffered an exacerbation of his disease

140. A 64-year-old healthy woman from Surinam with entirely normal liver function tests

QUESTIONS 141–145

Several cutaneous lesions are important manifestations of underlying gastrointestinal disease. For each lesion listed below, select the appropriate associated gastrointestinal condition. (*Note:* Use each lettered item only once.)

A. Carcinoid
B. Glucagonoma
C. Crohn's disease
D. Gluten enteropathy
E. Ulcerative colitis
F. Acute pancreatitis
G. Malabsorption syndrome
H. Gastric adenocarcinoma

141. Erythema nodosum

142. Pyoderma gangrenosum

143. Acanthosis nigricans

144. Nodular fat necrosis

145. Dermatitis herpetiformis

QUESTIONS 146–150

For each of the patients described below, select the most appropriate radiograph (*A–E*, below and p. 108)

146. A 40-year-old Japanese man who reports early satiety and 10-pound weight loss

147. A 60-year-old man who has iron deficiency anemia and who had previous gastric surgery for ulcer disease; stools are positive for occult blood

148. A 65-year-old woman with achlorhydria who has no clinical symptoms

149. A 68-year-old man who has chronic epigastric pain; basal acid output is 1 mEq/hour and peak acid output is 3 mEq/hour

150. A 72-year-old man with a history of gastric ulcer at age 65; he has recently noted the onset of midepigastric discomfort. He takes no medication

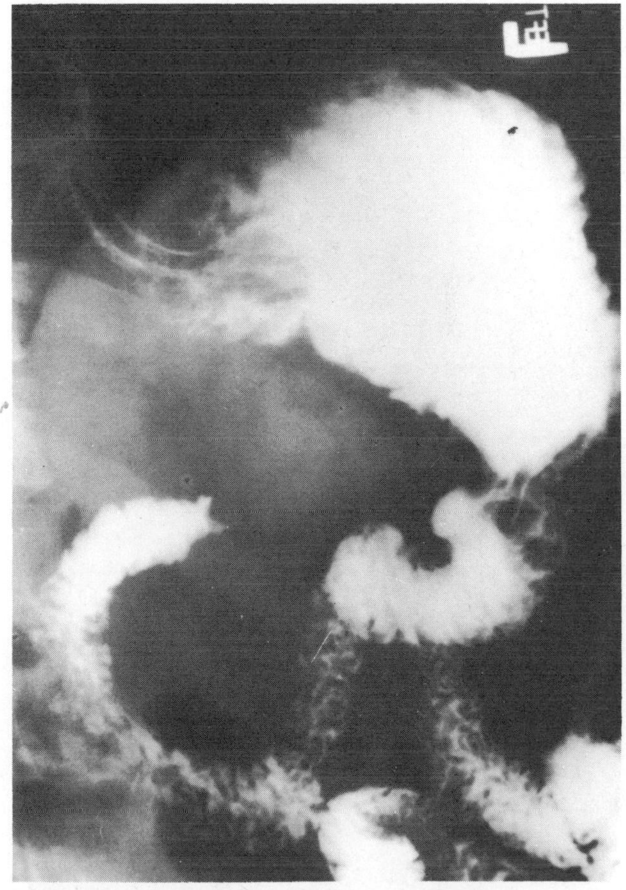

A

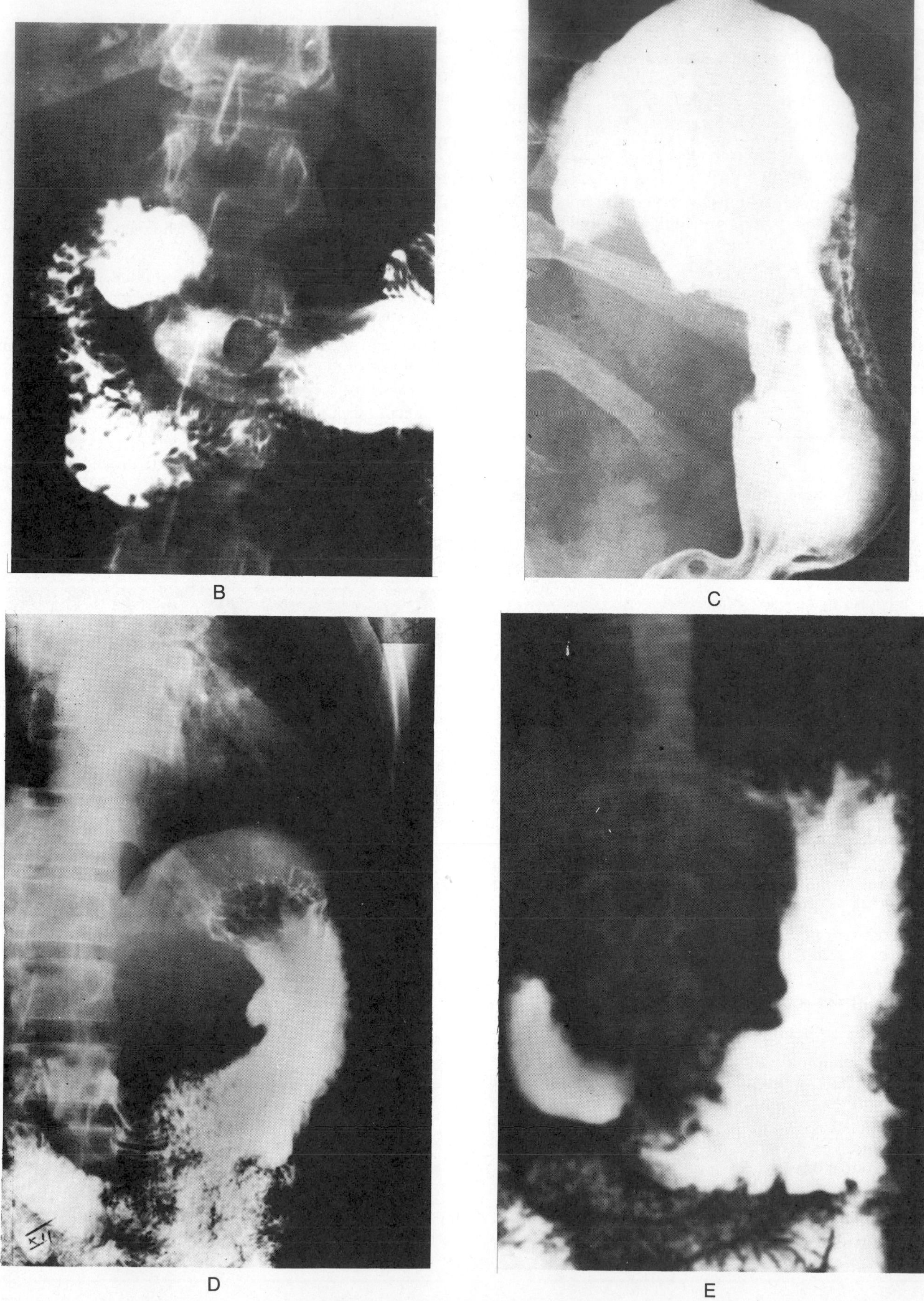
B
C
D
E

QUESTIONS 151–153

For each of the following, select the most appropriate lettered answer.

A. ^{14}C-glycine-cholate breath test

B. Hydrogen breath test

C. Both A and B

D. Neither A nor B

151. Useful in the diagnosis of small bowel bacterial overgrowth syndrome

152. Useful in the diagnosis of malabsorption due to disease of the terminal ileum

153. Useful in the diagnosis of intestinal lactase deficiency (lactose intolerance)

QUESTIONS 154–158

For each of the following patients, select the most likely associated barium enema radiograph (*A–E*, below and on page 110).

154. A 25-year-old man who has had periumbilical abdominal pains, constipation, fevers, and chills for the past 24 hours; white blood cell count is 17,500/mm^3

155. A 27-year-old woman with a six-year history of cramping abdominal pain, fever, and diarrhea with mucus and blood

156. A 30-year-old man referred for evaluation of intermittent hematochezia; several of his close relatives have developed colonic cancer before the age of 40

157. A 45-year-old Vietnamese refugee with postprandial cramping abdominal pains, constipation, and fever; roentgenogram of the chest shows apical pleural scarring

158. A 60-year-old woman with severe suprapubic cramping abdominal pains, fever, chills, and constipation

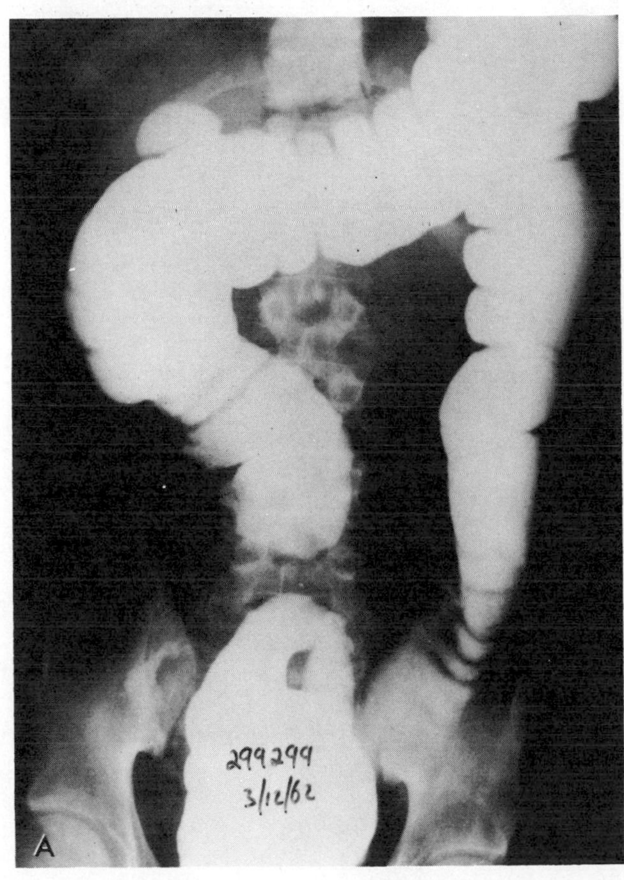

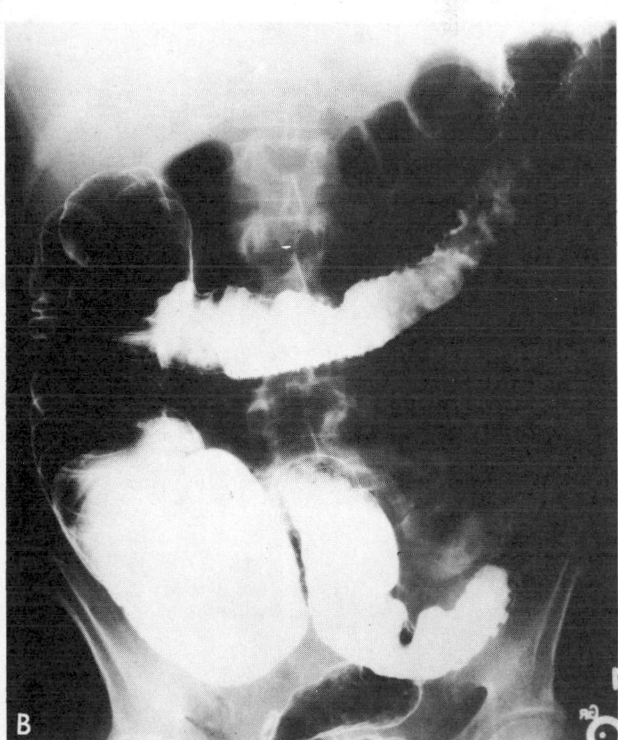

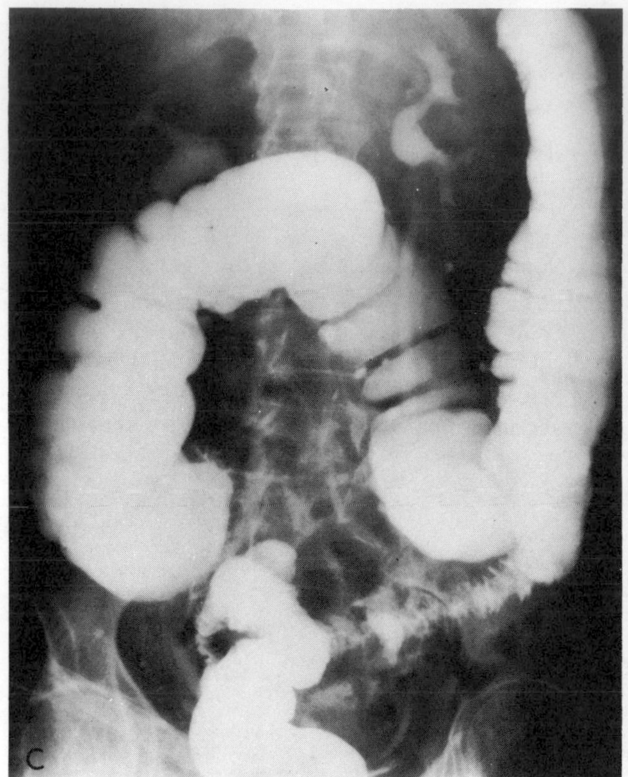
C

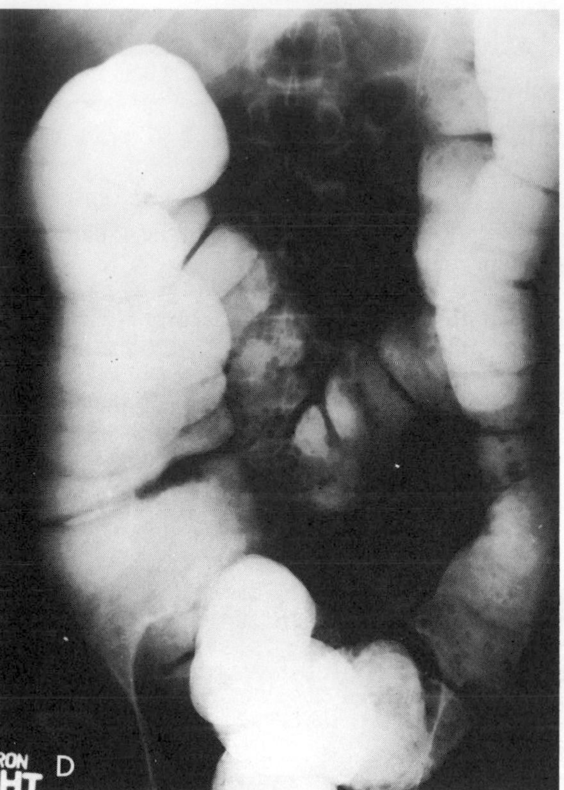
D

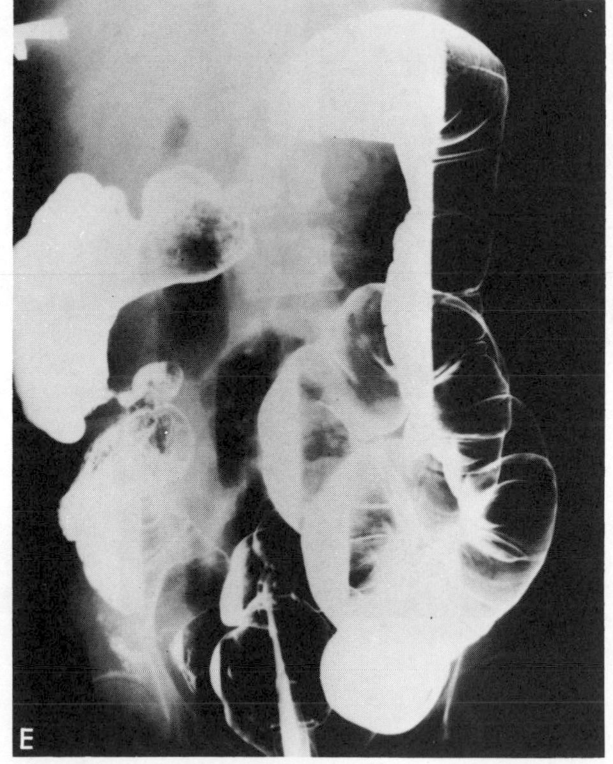
E

QUESTIONS 159–161

The two photomicrographs (below) show the jejunal histology of a patient before (*A*) and after (*B*) specific medical therapy for the bowel lesion. Each of the following patients could have had similar before-and-after small bowel histology. For each case history, select the treatment the patient is most likely to have received.

A. Quinacrine hydrochloride, 100 mg three times daily for seven days
B. Pancrease, two capsules with each meal or snack
C. Tetracycline, 250 mg four times daily and folic acid, 5 mg daily
D. Gluten-free diet
E. High-protein diet

159. A 25-year-old white man returns to the United States from a six-week trip to Nepal. He consults you because of a two-week history of anorexia, watery diarrhea, flatulence, and weight loss (5 pounds). He has abdominal cramps prior to most episodes of diarrhea, which occur between three and six times per day. There has been no fever. Laboratory data and physical examination are unremarkable except for a 24-hour fecal fat excretion of 13 g (normal <5).

160. A 45-year-old retired British Army officer who operates a bar in Singapore has had progressive weight loss (50 pounds) and fatigue over the past 18 months. He notes bulky, frequent (two to four per day) stools but states that he has had frequent stools with rare episodes of diarrhea since he moved to Singapore six years ago. He has a sore tongue, dry skin, muscle weakness, and fatigue. There has been no abdominal pain. Physical examination reveals an emaciated man with glossitis. Abdominal examination is normal except for mild abdominal distention, and the stool is negative for occult blood and ova and parasites. Hematocrit is 29%, with a mean corpuscular volume of 110 cu microns; electrolytes and liver function tests are normal. Serum calcium is 7.5 mg/dl; serum albumin is 3.0 g/dl. 24-hour fecal fat excretion is 30 g.

161. A 45-year-old reformed alcoholic man with documented cirrhosis of the liver has lost 40 pounds over the past two years. He denies any alcohol intake in the past three years and claims to eat a normal diet. He notes mild abdominal distention, excessive flatus, and one or two soft stools per day. He denies abdominal pain. Two months ago he fell down three steps and suffered a crush fracture of the second lumbar vertebra. Physical examination reveals evidence of weight loss, mild abdominal distention, an enlarged hard liver palpable 4 cm below the right costal margin, and a normal rectum. Hematocrit is 29% with a mean corpuscular volume of 78 cu microns. Electrolytes are normal. Serum calcium is 7.5 mg/dl, serum phosphorus is 1.0 mg/dl; serum alkaline phosphatase is 320 IU/L (normal <71). Serum transaminase (SGOT) is 45 IU/L (normal <37), and serum bilirubin is 1.1 mg/dl. Prothrombin time is 14 seconds (control: 11). 24-hour fecal fat excretion is 55 g. A D-xylose test shows a five-hour urinary excretion of 1.5 g (normal >4).

QUESTIONS 162–166

For each of the following, select the most appropriate option for management.

A. Portosystemic shunt surgery
B. Variceal sclerotherapy
C. Splenectomy
D. All of the above
E. None of the above

162. A 33-year-old man with repeated variceal hemorrhage secondary to portal vein thrombosis

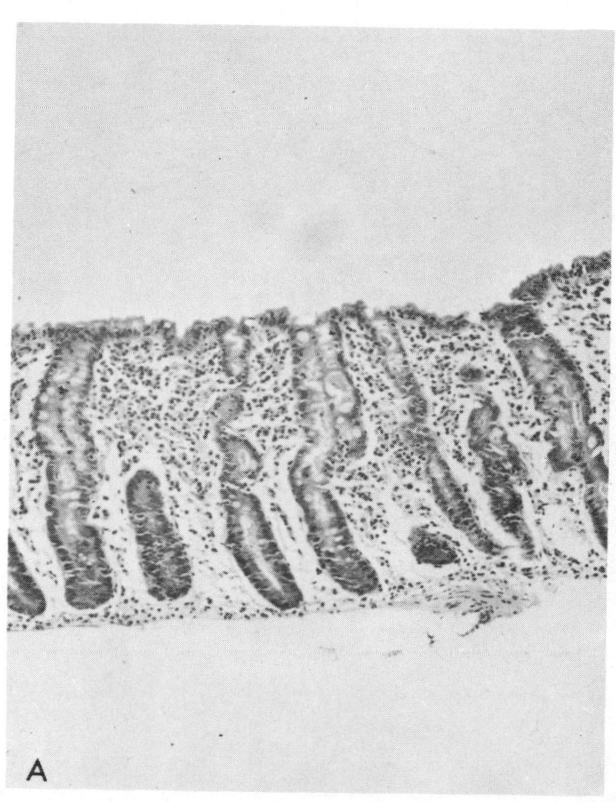

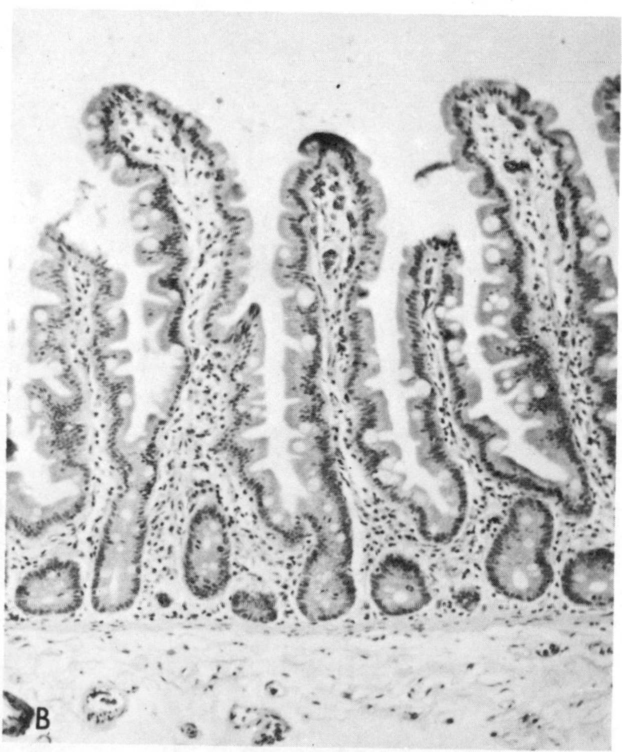

163. A 48-year-old man with hypersplenism (platelet count 50,000/mm^3) secondary to cryptogenic cirrhosis

164. A 50-year-old woman with primary biliary cirrhosis and large esophageal varices and no history of bleeding

165. A 54-year-old alcoholic man with Child's class C cirrhosis who has acute variceal hemorrhage

166. A 64-year-old man with bleeding gastric varices secondary to splenic vein thrombosis

QUESTIONS 167–172

For each of the following patients, select the most likely colonic biopsy photomicrograph (*A–F*, below and on p. 113). (*Note*: Use each figure only once.)

167. A 22-year-old man with cramping abdominal pains, mucous and bloody diarrhea, and tenesmus after returning from a one-month scientific expedition to Central America

168. A 32-year-old woman with multiple episodes of cramping right lower quadrant abdominal pains, non-bloody diarrhea, and a rectal fissure on anoscopic examination

169. A 45-year-old woman with episodes of bloody diarrhea, cramping abdominal pains, and low-grade fever; the episodes occur two to three times a year each and last about two weeks

170. A 50-year-old Egyptian man with splenomegaly and recurrent variceal hemorrhages

171. A 65-year-old man with iron deficiency anemia and weakness but no altered bowel habits

172. A 73-year-old woman who has acute onset of bloody diarrhea; three weeks ago, she received a seven-day course of ampicillin for a urinary tract infection

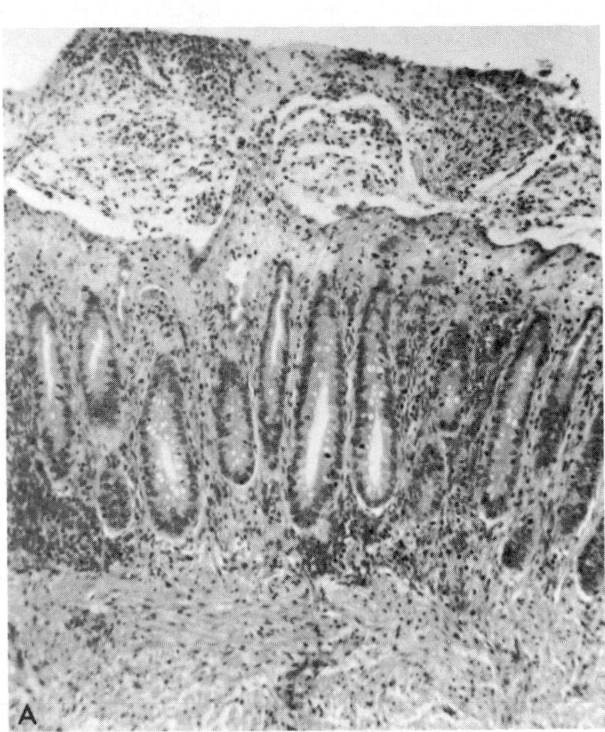
A

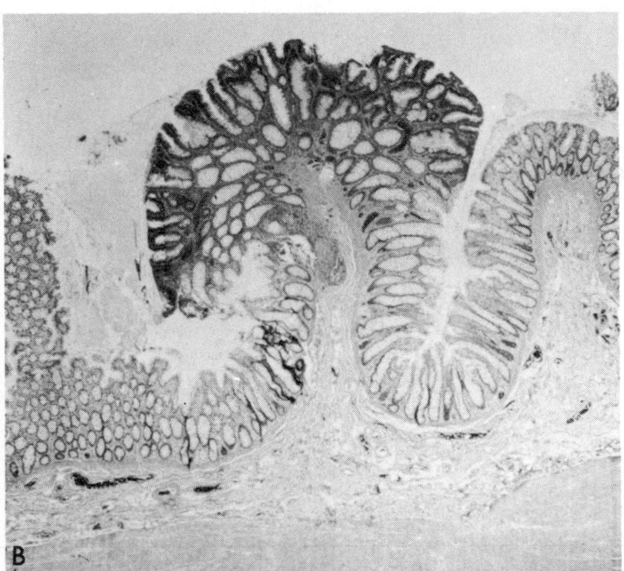
B

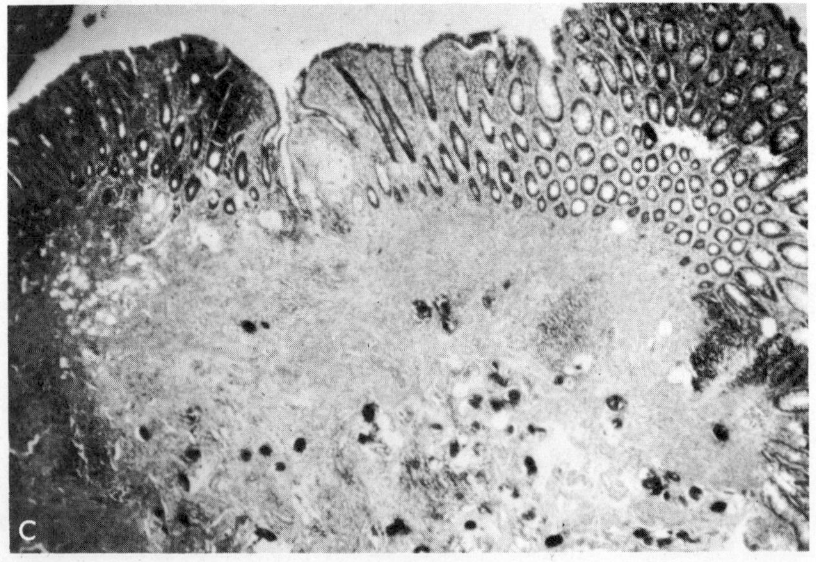
C

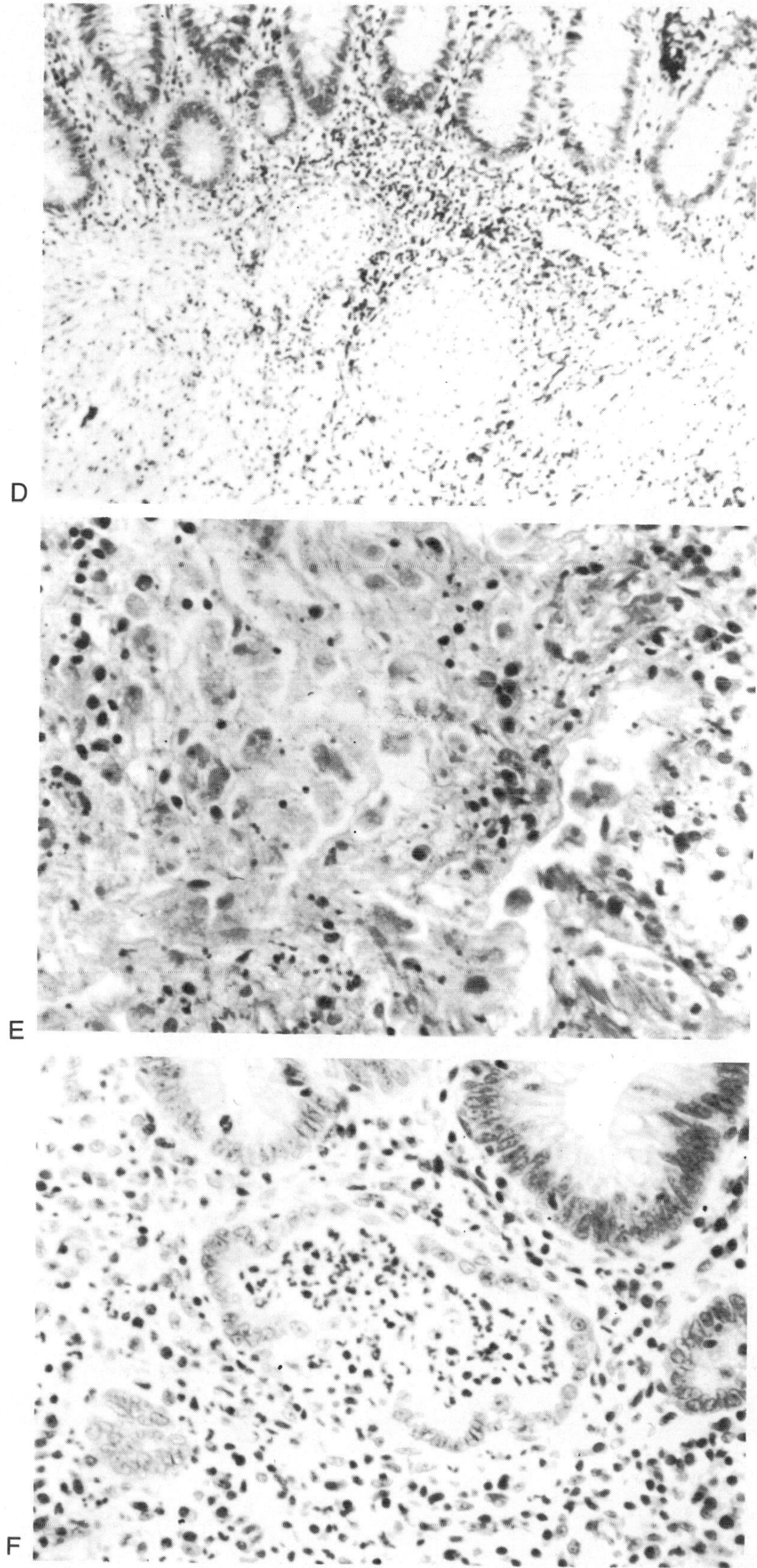
D
E
F

QUESTIONS 173–177

For each of the following, select the set of laboratory studies that best fits the clinical information.

	Basal serum gastrin (pg/ml)	Serum gastrin after secretion stimulation (pg/ml)	Basal acid output (mEq/hr)	Peak acid output (pentagastrin stimulated) (mEq/hr)
A.	350	700	35	55
B.	350	375	10	50
C.	350	300	5	15
D.	350	350	1	2
E.	75	70	10	40
F.	75	70	2	4

173. A 20-year-old female college student who has a nine-month history of epigastric pain relieved by antacids is found to have a 1-cm duodenal bulbar ulcer. In addition to the above laboratory findings, she is noted to have a two-fold increase in serum gastrin after a meal.

174. A 30-year-old male lawyer who has a six-month history of epigastric pain relieved by food or antacids; he presents with worsening abdominal pain and hematemesis.

175. A 45-year-old male accountant who has a 1-cm marginal ulcer one year after undergoing an antrectomy and Billroth II procedure for severe ulcer disease.

176. A 60-year-old male steelworker who is found to have a 1-cm antral ulcer and two duodenal ulcers by upper endoscopy; in addition, a 3-cm mass is found in the head of the pancreas by abdominal sonography.

177. A 65-year-old female postal worker who has hypothyroidism and insulin-dependent diabetes mellitus presents with hematemesis and a macrocytic anemia and is found to have a 2-cm gastric ulcer.

QUESTIONS 178–182

Match each of the following with the most appropriate lettered item.

A. Hamartomas
B. Villous adenomas
C. Inflammatory polyps
D. Adenomatous polyps

178. Greatest potential for malignancy

179. Peutz-Jeghers syndrome

180. Cronkhite-Canada syndrome

181. Familial polyposis syndrome

182. Turcot's (glioma-polyposis) syndrome

PART 4

GASTROINTESTINAL DISEASE

ANSWERS

1.(D) In the setting of acute pancreatitis, the findings of hyperglycemia, estimated fluid losses of more than 6 liters, hematocrit of less than 30, and hypoxemia have been associated with greater length of hospitalization and increased risk of mortality. Hypocalcemia with serum calcium levels of less than 8 mg/dl (not hypercalcemia) results from precipitation of calcium in areas of fat necrosis and is also a sign of severe pancreatitis. (*Cecil, Ch. 108; Sleisenger and Fordtran, Ch. 97*)

2.(D) The clinical features of the Zollinger-Ellison syndrome result from gastric acid hypersecretion secondary to chronic stimulation by gastrin. Gastrin is trophic for the gastric mucosa, and hypergastrinemia results in prominent gastric rugae. Antral gastrin-cell hyperplasia is not present in this condition. Gastric acid secretion is accompanied by excess fluid secretion and secretory diarrhea. Steatorrhea as a feature of gastrinomas is less common than diarrhea and is caused by several mechanisms due to acid hypersecretion. Pancreatic lipase is inactivated, and primary bile acids are rendered insoluble at low pH. In addition, low pH in the small intestine interferes with intrinsic factor activity and vitamin B_{12} absorption despite normal intrinsic factor secretion. (*Cecil, Ch. 100.6; Sleisenger and Fordtran, Ch. 49*)

3.(C) The historical and biochemical features of the patient's illness as well as the ultrasonographic findings are all compatible with an amebic abscess, and empiric treatment with metronidazole is the most appropriate of the choices offered. Surgical drainage via laparotomy is not appropriate or necessary for most amebic abscesses and is also generally unnecessary for most solitary pyogenic abscesses. None of the other tests offered would be expected to provide information essential to the patient's immediate management. (*Cecil, Ch. 124*)

4.(D) Since most patients with amebic abscesses respond quickly to metronidazole, the deterioration observed in this patient is reason for further evaluation. The positive serologic test may simply represent the result of an earlier amebic infection unrelated to the present illness, or the patient may have an amebic abscess that has become superinfected. Further empiric therapy is inappropriate, and aspiration is necessary to obtain material for bacteriologic studies. Laparotomy would be premature, and retrograde cholangiography, although perhaps appropriate in the future to exclude biliary tract disease as a cause of the abscess, is not the next logical step. (*Cecil, Ch. 124*)

5.(A) This patient has chronic pancreatitis demonstrated by irregularity and marked dilatation of the main pancreatic duct and secondary radicals seen on pancreatography. Although chronic alcohol abuse is the most frequent cause of chronic pancreatitis, hyperlipidemia is a major cause of both acute and chronic pancreatitis. Pancreatic calcifications are detectable in 40–60% of patients with chronic pancreatitis. Over the course of the disease, episodes of abdominal pain typically become more frequent but less severe in quality; in 30–40% of patients abdominal pain may remit completely. This patient does not have evidence of pancreatic carcinoma, in which case patient survival may be enhanced by limited field radiation therapy. Diabetes mellitus is a common complication of chronic pancreatitis. (*Cecil, Ch. 108; Sleisenger and Fordtran, Chs. 98 and 99*)

6.(D) The presence of motile trophozoites with ingested red blood cells establishes the diagnosis of invasive *Entamoeba histolytica* infection in this young, homosexual man. Indirect hemagglutination (IHA) testing and flexible sigmoidoscopic examination are not needed to establish invasive disease in this patient. Radiologic examination is often positive in amebic colitis. Air-contrast barium study may reveal a mass lesion (ameboma), ulcerations, pseudomembranes, or toxic megacolon. These lesions are nonspecific. The presence of ameboma would be a contraindication to surgery and mandates medical therapy; a rupture of the mass lesion could cause widespread dissemination and peritonitis. The proper therapy for symptomatic invasive disease is metronidazole, 750 mg three times daily for 5–10 days, plus diloxanide furoate, 500 mg three times daily for 10 days. Asymptomatic cyst passers and the sexual contacts of patients with invasive amebiasis should be treated with a 10-day course of diloxanide furoate, 500 mg three times daily. (*Cecil, Ch. 390; Bayless, pp. 268–269*)

7.(C) If the simple measures (elevation of the head of the bed, avoidance of food and fluid intake before bedtime, liquid antacids, avoidance of cigarettes and alcohol, weight loss) are not effective, then more vigorous treatment is indicated. Alginic acid-antacid, 15 ml after each meal and at bedtime, has been shown to be more effective than placebo and as effective as antacids. Parasympathomimetic agents (e.g., Bethanechol*) and H_2-receptor antagonists (e.g., Cimetidine,* Ranitidine,* Famotidine*), although not approved for therapy of heartburn, improve symptoms significantly when compared with placebo. Anticholinergic agents are contraindicated in patients with gastroesophageal reflux disease. As the disorder is associated with a hypotensive lower esophageal sphincter, the symptoms are likely to worsen with the use of anticholinergic medications. Antireflux surgery should be considered in a patient in whom an adequate trial of medical management has not brought good results in a six-month period and in whom there is good objective evidence of reflux. (*Cecil, Ch. 98; Sleisenger and Fordtran, Ch. 34*)

8.(C) A prospective comparison of several diagnostic tests of pancreatic cancer suggests that ultrasound should be performed first; if it is negative, a pancreatic function test is the next choice. A positive result from either test warrants endoscopic retrograde cholangiopancreatography (ERCP). CT scan can be substituted for ultrasonography, and angiography can be done if ERCP is unsuccessful or unavailable. Radioisotopic pancreatic scans are too insen-

**This is not listed in the manufacturer's directive.*

sitive to be useful, and visceral angiography is not appropriate as a screening test. (*Cecil, Ch. 109; DiMagno et al*)

9.(C) The delta hepatitis virus is a defective RNA virus that is dependent upon obligatory helper function of the hepatitis B virus. It has been implicated as the true cause of fulminant hepatitis in up to 30% of cases of fulminant hepatitis B worldwide. The delta virus is endemic mainly in developing countries and the Mediterranean basin, but it occurs sporadically in North America, mainly in intravenous drug addicts carrying the B hepatitis virus. Anti-delta IgG does not confer immunity to the delta virus, and its presence implies either recent resolved infection or chronic infection with this agent. (*Cecil, Ch. 121; Purcell et al*)

10.(C) There is no convincing evidence that specific diets either retard or accelerate ulcer healing. Although it was believed that small, frequent feedings might decrease gastric acid secretion by causing less gastric distention, it is now recognized that gastric acid secretion is actually greater under these circumstances than if fewer larger meals are taken. Bedtime snacks do not provide buffering capacity at night but instead increase nocturnal acid secretion and thus should be avoided. Drastic changes in diet such as low roughage or a bland diet are probably not warranted. Although milk has been used for its soothing qualities in ulcer treatment, the high protein and calcium content actually stimulates gastric acid secretion. Therefore, they should be neither encouraged nor forbidden in peptic ulcer disease. (*Cecil, Ch. 100.3; Sleisenger and Fordtran, Ch. 47*)

11.(A) In uncomplicated cirrhotic patients with noninfected ascitic fluid, the cell count is variable but usually less than 500/mm^3 with mononuclear dominance. A presumptive diagnosis of bacterial peritonitis *and* initiation of antibiotic therapy are justified when the ascitic white blood cell count exceeds 500/mm^3 with greater than 50% polymorphonuclear cells. Unfortunately, despite immediate empiric antibiotic therapy, the risk of mortality is 60–90% in these patients.

The cirrhotic patient has a greater tendency to renal failure than does a normal patient; 30% of cirrhotic patients who receive gentamicin therapy develop renal failure despite nontoxic blood levels. Moreover, there is an anticipated problem with aminoglycosides, since these agents are distributed in the free body water, which may be increased by several liters in patients with ascites. Thus, therapeutic levels may be particularly difficult to achieve, serum levels must be followed, and alternative agents should be used when feasible. Since chloramphenicol is bacteriostatic for gram-negative organisms, recurrence of infection is common. In addition, the cirrhotic patient appears more sensitive to the bone marrow suppressive side effect of this medication; it is no longer recommended as acceptable initial therapy. (*Cecil, Ch. 127; Bayless, pp. 272–273; Sleisenger and Fordtran, Ch. 26*)

12.(D) With the exception of polymorphonuclear cell concentration, the routine chemical analysis of the ascitic fluid does not usually change with the onset of spontaneous bacterial peritonitis. The absolute glucose level and total protein concentration in ascitic fluid do not change in the infected fluid compared with fluids obtained from the same patient before and/or after treatment of the infection. The rather small changes in ascitic fluid composition with spontaneous bacterial peritonitis contrast with the changes in ascites that complicate bowel perforation. In this condition the levels of lactate dehydrogenase and protein markedly increase, whereas pH and glucose decrease. (*Cecil, Ch. 127; Bayless, pp. 272–273; Sleisenger and Fordtran, Ch. 26*)

13.(B); 14.(C) The amylase:creatinine clearance ratio is derived from the general clearance formula U × V/P × T, and results in the following formula:

$$C_{am}/C_{cr}\% = \frac{\text{urine amylase}}{\text{serum amylase}} \times \frac{\text{serum creatinine}}{\text{urine creatinine}} \times 100$$

The normal range is 1 to 4%. From the data given in question 13, the C_{am}/C_{cr} ratio is 0.1%. This value is 10 times below the lower range of normal and typical of macroamylasemia, a benign chemical derangement associated with no specific disease state. In this entity, the serum amylase forms a macromolecular complex with a globulin whose size thus prevents urinary excretion. Peptic ulcer disease is a reasonable explanation for this patient's epigastric pain and deformed duodenal bulb. (*Cecil, Ch. 108; Salt and Schenker*)

15.(B) The historical and biochemical features of this case are consistent with porphyria cutanea tarda (PCT). Although probably a heterogeneous disorder, genetic or possibly acquired deficiency of uroporphyrinogen decarboxylase is believed to be important in the pathogenesis of the uroporphyrin overproduction and, hence, the skin lesions. Estrogens, iron overload, and alcohol use have all been linked with exacerbation or unmasking of the disorder. Uroporphyrin overproduction and a PCT-like symdrome have also been described in patients with hepatocellular carcinoma. Unlike the situation with acute intermittent porphyria, barbiturates do not clearly cause a worsening or unmasking of PCT. (*Cecil, Ch. 203*)

16.(C) The Norwalk group of viruses accounts for about one third of outbreaks of viral gastroenteritis in the United States and usually gives rise to vomiting and/or diarrhea that most often resolves within 48 hours. The upper small intestine is the focus of attack, and patchy mucosal lesions occur in this location with sparing of the stomach and colon. Transient malabsorption of xylose and fat have been observed during the illness, as well as reduced activity of brush border disaccharidases. Although the fecal-oral route is the primary route of transmission, some outbreaks have been traced to foods, particularly shellfish. (*Cecil, Ch. 335; Sleisenger and Fordtran, Ch. 63*)

17.(C) Diverticular disease of the large bowel is very common in Western societies and seems to increase in prevalence with age. Half the population of Europe, North America, and Australia can expect to acquire this disease. Eating a fiber-rich diet (e.g., Western vegetarians, wartime Britons) reduces the prevalence of the condition. Bleeding from complicated diverticular disease in the elderly is the most common cause of significant lower gastrointestinal blood loss. Barium enema may reveal an irregular luminal contour with a narrowed sigmoid segment, *but* barium noted outside the diverticulum establishes the diagnosis of *diverticulitis*. (*Cecil, Ch. 115; Sleisenger and Fordtran, Ch. 77*)

18.(D) The clinical picture is most compatible with cholangitis due to choledocholithiasis. Simple acute cholecystitis would not cause this much fever nor the abnormal liver function tests. Hepatic infarction and viral hepatitis are usually accompanied by more striking elevations of the SGPT and prothrombin time, and hemochromatosis typically presents in a more insidious fashion. The very high bilirubin concentration in this patient reflects markedly increased bilirubin production caused by accelerated destruction of sickled and transfused erythrocytes, as well as impaired bile flow resulting from choledocholithiasis. (*Cecil, Chs. 121, 125, and 130; Sheehy; Cameron et al*)

19. (A) Hepatic adenomas occur almost exclusively in women and are strongly associated with oral contraceptive usage. They typically present with symptoms and signs of an abdominal mass, tumor infarction, hemorrhage, or rupture. They appear as a "cold spot" on technetium-^{99}m sulfur colloid scans and may be hyper- or hypovascular on angiography. Both focal nodular hyperplasia and cavernous hemangioma are more common in women, are usually incidentally discovered, may rarely rupture, and are typically hypervascular on angiography. Focal nodular hyperplasia will often take up technetium-^{99}m sulfur colloid normally. Nodular regenerative hyperplasia produces multiple hepatic nodules and is associated with both rheumatoid arthritis and oral contraceptive use. Its most common manifestation is portal hypertension. Hepatocellular carcinoma is extremely unlikely in a young white woman. (*Cecil, Ch. 129*)

20. (D) All the disorders listed except granuloma inguinale could produce diffuse proctitis. Granuloma inguinale is a papulovesicular and ulcerating infection of the skin, perianal area, and anus and does not involve the mucosa of the rectum. Lymphogranuloma venereum, caused by *Chlamydia trachomatis,* causes a diffuse proctitis, often with accompanying inguinal lymphadenopathy, that heals with stricture formation. Gonococcal proctitis may be identified by Gram's stain and/or culture of the rectal exudate. Radiation proctitis is often nonspecific, although mucosal telangiectasia may be seen in some patients. (*Cecil, Chs. 111, 306, 307, and 308; Sleisenger and Fordtran, Ch. 65*)

21. (D) The presentation is entirely compatible with the diagnosis of Meckel's diverticulum of the ileum. The technetium scan shows uptake of the isotope by gastric mucosa, the presence of which is characteristic of many Meckel's diverticula that bleed. These remnants of the embryogenic yolk sac are usually located 50–100 cm proximal to the ileocecal valve. Bleeding is usually seen in younger patients and is treated by surgical removal of the diverticulum. (*Cecil, Ch. 102; Sleisenger and Fordtran, Ch. 54*)

22. (E) Primary sclerosing cholangitis is by far the most common cause of significant abnormalities in liver function tests and chronic liver disease in association with chronic ulcerative colitis. This condition may remain asymptomatic for many years, with a marked elevation in alkaline phosphatase being the initial clue to its presence in patients with a history of inflammatory bowel disease. Pericholangitis, although at one time thought to be a separate entity consisting of portal tract inflammation and periductular fibrosis, is now recognized as a histologic lesion mainly associated with sclerosing cholangitis. (*Cecil, Ch. 130; Zakim and Boyer, Ch. 33; Shepherd et al*)

23. (E) Endoscopic retrograde cholangiography is the single most useful approach to diagnosis in this patient, because the appearance of primary sclerosing cholangitis on cholangiography is characteristic. Technetium-^{99}m HIDA scanning and intravenous cholangiography both lack the resolution to demonstrate the diffuse biliary disease typical of sclerosing cholangitis, while oral cholecystography is useful only in delineating the gallbladder. Liver biopsy would be of value if the cholangiographic findings did not reveal sclerosing cholangitis. Sigmoidoscopy and biopsy might also be of value in identifying asymptomatic ulcerative colitis associated with sclerosing cholangitis. (*Cecil, Chs. 95 and 96; Zakim and Boyer, Ch. 33*)

24. (D) This woman has the Peutz-Jeghers syndrome, an autosomal dominant disorder characterized by congenital melanin spots on lips, buccal mucosa, palms, soles, and perianal skin and polyps of the small intestine. The polyps, which occasionally may also occur in the stomach, colon, and rectum, are benign hamartomas, not adenomas, and are not premalignant. The risk of adenocarcinoma in these patients is less than 3%, in contrast to those with Gardner's syndrome (familial polyposis), who have adenomas of the intestine and a greater than 95% risk of adenocarcinoma. Patients with the Peutz-Jeghers syndrome may be asymptomatic; however, the most common symptoms are abdominal pain, intestinal hemorrhage, and bowel obstruction. (*Cecil, Ch. 107; Sleisenger and Fordtran, Ch. 80*)

25. (C) The patient's condition is compatible with fulminant hepatic failure. Alcoholic hepatitis is almost never associated with transaminase elevations of this magnitude and is therefore the least likely cause of the illness. All the infections can cause fulminant hepatic failure, as can excess ingestion of acetaminophen. (*Cecil, Ch. 128*)

26. (C) Even if this patient's liver failure were due to acetaminophen ingestion, it is clearly too late for *N*-acetylcysteine to be of any benefit. Each of the other studies, however, would provide information potentially useful to this patient's management. (*Cecil, Ch. 128*)

27. (E) The skin rash depicted in the photographs and described in the case history is that of necrolytic migratory erythema. This lesion, along with the findings of weight loss, diarrhea, and anemia, characterizes the classic presentation of the glucagonoma syndrome. Frank diabetes occurs in 60% of patients with glucagonoma, and an additional 30% have glucose intolerance. The increased level of glucagon causes enhanced hepatic catabolism of amino acids; levels are low and hypoaminoacidemia is thought to be the etiology of the skin rash. Glucagonoma is associated with MEN 1 kindreds. At the time of presentation a majority (60–80%) of the pancreatic lesions have metastasized, most commonly to the liver and local lymph nodes. The syndrome is due to elevated levels of glucagon and *not* to vasoactive intestinal polypeptide. The so-called VIPoma produces a syndrome of watery diarrhea, hypokalemia, and hypochlorhydria (WDHA syndrome). (*Cecil, Ch. 233*)

28. (D) Patients with carcinoid tumors often have intermittent abdominal pain and diarrhea due not only to the effects of active humoral products of the tumor cells, such as serotonin, but also to kinking of bowel loops caused by tumor in the mesentery, which provokes an extensive fibrous reaction. The liver is often involved with extensive metastases. Patients may also develop endocardial fibrosis primarily involving the right heart, resulting in pulmonic stenosis and tricuspid insufficiency. (*Cecil, Ch. 107; Sleisenger and Fordtran, Ch. 82*)

29. (E) This patient has a duodenal bulbar ulcer with a large ulcer crater seen on upper gastrointestinal series. This is the initial manifestation of peptic ulcer disease in this patient. The upper GI series is of good quality and clearly shows an active ulcer. Although upper endoscopy is a highly sensitive test for diagnosing peptic ulcer disease, at this particular point in the patient's management, endoscopy would add little to the diagnosis and would not affect initial management. Unlike gastric ulcer disease, in which malignant ulcers are a common worry, duodenal ulcer disease is not associated with malignancy. Therefore, endoscopic examination and brushings for cytology are unnecessary under these circumstances.

As a group, patients with duodenal ulcer disease secrete greater amounts of gastric acid in both the basal state and when stimulated by provocative testing with histamine or pentagastrin. However, there is considerable overlap between the gastric acid secretory profiles of normal subjects and those with peptic ulcer disease. Unless one suspects a hypersecretory disorder, such as a gastrinoma, on the initial presentation of peptic ulcer disease, it is not necessary to perform acid stimulatory testing. Similarly, measurement of serum gastrin levels is not recommended in what is an otherwise normal setting for duodenal ulcer disease. If the patient has an ulcer that proves to be refractory to treatment or develops other symptoms that suggest gastric acid hypersecretion, such as diarrhea or multiple ulcers, then measurement of serum gastrin levels would be warranted. (*Cecil, Chs. 100.1 and 100.2; Sleisenger and Fordtran, Ch. 47*)

30.(A) Antacids heal peptic ulcers by neutralizing gastric acid. Studies have demonstrated that administration of liquid antacids in amounts capable of neutralizing 140 mEq of acid one and three hours after meals and before bedtime is effective therapy for the healing of duodenal ulcers. Antacid preparations vary greatly in buffering capacity, and it is important that the neutralizing properties be taken into account when these drugs are used. Antacid tablets, which have substantially less buffering capacity than liquid antacids, are generally not recommended for treatment of active ulcer disease.

The H_2-receptor antagonists, such as cimetidine and ranitidine, are potent inhibitors of gastric acid secretion and consequently are effective therapies for duodenal ulcer disease. However, the proper dosage of cimetidine is 300 mg before meals and at bedtime. Similarly, for ranitidine, the recommended dosage is 150 mg twice daily. Anticholinergic drugs decrease acid secretion and can be used in low and well-tolerated doses (such as propantheline, 15–30 mg at bedtime). However, anticholinergics by themselves are not potent enough to be considered adequate treatment for active ulcer disease. Anticholinergics are useful as adjunctive therapy and can augment the inhibitory effects of H_2-receptor antagonists. It is important to note that anticholinergics may exacerbate symptoms in patients with gastric retention or gastroesophageal reflux. (*Cecil, Ch. 100.3; Sleisenger and Fordtran, Ch. 47*)

31.(D) Bacteria play a key role in the malabsorption of tropical sprue, and bacterial overgrowth of the small intestine is an important factor in the malabsorption associated with gastrocolic fistula. Small bowel stasis commonly leads to bacterial overgrowth and subsequent malabsorption in scleroderma involving the small bowel, as well as in multiple jejunal diverticula. Although small intestinal hypomotility may result from diabetic neuropathy, bacterial overgrowth is found in only a minority of diabetic patients with diarrhea and malabsorption. In most diabetic patients with small bowel dysfunction and malabsorption, the cause is unclear and may include pancreatic insufficiency, adult celiac disease, and poorly understood factors related to autonomic dysfunction. (*Cecil, Ch. 104; Sleisenger and Fordtran, Chs. 18 and 29*)

32.(C) This patient presents the classic features of benign postoperative cholestasis, a disorder that typically follows major operations on severely ill patients who receive a number of blood transfusions. It may have a number of contributing factors, including increased bilirubin production from transfused erythrocytes and hematomas, sepsis, liver dysfunction due to intra- or postoperative hypotension, and renal failure with decreased urinary excretion of conjugated bilirubin. Jaundice of this degree resulting from halothane injury would be accompanied by marked elevations of the SGOT and prothrombin time. (*Cecil, Chs. 118 and 120; Schiff and Schiff, Ch. 38*)

33.(B); 34.(D) Patients with acute ischemic colitis are characteristically over the age of 50 and are most often affected with the abrupt onset of lower abdominal cramping pain, rectal bleeding, and—to varying degrees—vomiting and fever. Some patients give a history of similar symptoms occurring intermittently for weeks to months before. Localized or segmental ischemia is more common than extensive infarction or perforation. The areas particularly affected are those areas of bowel which lie on the "watershed" between two adjacent arterial supplies (the splenic flexure and the rectosigmoid colon). Sigmoidoscopy may reveal blue-black submucosal blebs, indicating submucosal hemorrhage. Angiography generally has *not* proved to be useful in the diagnosis of patients in this setting. Initial management consists of general supportive measures, including antibiotics.

Barium enema is not indicated at the time of the initial presentation, especially in the setting of gross blood in the patient's rectum. While the differential diagnosis certainly includes acute infections and idiopathic inflammatory bowel disease, steroids and sulfasalazine would be inappropriate in this setting. (*Cecil, Ch. 106*)

35.(D) One of the most common causes of abdominal discomfort, bloating, and postprandial vomiting following ulcer surgery is "dumping syndrome," which is also accompanied by diaphoresis, palpitations, flushing, weakness, and early satiety. This symptom complex likely results from rapid flow of fluid into the upper small intestine and release of vasoactive intestinal hormones. Other complications of peptic ulcer surgery include mechanical derangements such as gastric outlet obstruction, bezoar formation, stenosis at the anastomotic site, and partial obstruction of the afferent loop of bowel in a Billroth II anastomosis. These conditions usually cause abdominal pain, fullness, and vomiting. In addition, gastritis associated with passage of bile through the gastric remnant may cause similar symptoms. Development of cholelithiasis has been associated with vagotomy and is believed to result from vagal denervation of the gallbladder. Although chronic pancreatitis may cause postprandial abdominal pain and vomiting, it is not a complication of peptic ulcer surgery. (*Cecil, Ch. 100.4; Sleisenger and Fordtran, Ch. 53*)

36.(C) Anemia may accompany any form of ulcer surgery and usually develops over a period of many years. Often multiple deficiencies including iron, folate, and vitamin B_{12} are found. However, iron deficiency is the most common deficiency and appears to play the major role in the genesis of the anemia. Thus, most postoperative anemias are microcytic and hypochromic, and these generally occur earlier than mixed anemias or macrocytic anemias. Vitamin B_{12} deficiency with megaloblastic anemia usually requires 5–8 years to develop. The causes of these deficiencies are multiple, and all are complicated by the reduced food intake that generally accompanies ulcer surgery. Iron deficiency may result from inadequate replacement after surgery and any accompanying hemorrhage, blood loss from recurrent ulcer disease, or development of gastric carcinoma as a late complication of ulcer surgery. Malabsorption is a major cause of folate and vitamin B_{12} deficiency and results from multiple causes, including impaired digestion, bacterial overgrowth, and loss of intrinsic factor. (*Cecil, Ch. 100.4; Sleisenger and Fordtran, Ch. 53*)

37. (E) The patient has gastrointestinal bleeding, evidence of spontaneous bacterial peritonitis, and recent consumption of benzodiazepines. These as well as the other options listed could all precipitate or aggravate hepatic encephalopathy. However, hypokalemia rather than hyperkalemia (most likely secondary to spironolactone in this case), along with hypovolemia and alkalosis is the usual diuretic-induced electrolyte disorder that precipitates hepatic encephalopathy. (*Cecil, Ch. 128*)

38. (B) Duration of ulcerative colitis is the best-recognized risk factor in the development of colonic malignancy. After eight years of pancolitis there is an increase in the incidence of colon cancers when compared to age- and sex-matched groups in the general population. The age of onset seems to affect the colorectal cancer risk; patients whose ulcerative colitis began before the age of 20 have a shorter lag time before cancer develops than those whose bowel inflammation began after that age. Colitis activity is *not* related to cancer risk. In fact, it is those patients with long periods of quiescent disease who make up the majority of the colitis-cancer population. The extent of macroscopic bowel inflammation correlates directly with cancer development: Patients with disease restricted to the rectum/sigmoid colon are at very low risk, while pancolonic involvement carries the greatest risk of neoplasm. Removal of most of the colon via a subtotal colectomy does not eliminate the risk of developing cancer in the retained rectal mucosa. (*Cecil, Ch. 107; Bayless, pp. 296–301; Sleisenger and Fordtran, Chs. 78 and 81*)

39. (D) Traveler's diarrhea is usually a mild to moderately severe illness for which rapid effective therapy can be made available. Other than prudent dietary discretion, no other specific prophylactic measures should be routinely recommended. Noncarbonated bottled water cannot always be relied on; carbonated beverages are safe to recommend. Bismuth subsalicylate (Pepto-Bismol liquid or tablets) taken throughout the period of travel reduces the incidence of traveler's diarrhea by 40–60%. There is a potential for salicylate intoxication, particularly in patients who are elderly, have renal failure, or are on other medications containing salicylates. The medication would not be recommended in this 76-year-old man who takes aspirin. Trimethoprim/sulfamethoxazole is currently *not* recommended for prophylaxis. Prophylaxis against hepatitis A in the form of immune serum globulin is recommended for travelers to areas where sanitation is poor (rural Mexico). Vaccination against hepatitis B is not recommended for travelers except to protect against transmission by sexual contact in endemic areas of Africa and southeast Asia. (*Cecil, Ch. 261; Sleisenger and Fordtran, Ch. 63*)

40. (B) Carcinoid tumors arise from enterochromaffin cells that are located predominantly in the gastrointestinal mucosa. Carcinoid tumors are relatively common, but the carcinoid syndrome is rare. Carcinoid tumors are most commonly found in the appendix or rectum, but these rarely produce the carcinoid syndrome. False-positive urinary 5-HIAA determinations are common and should be suspected when the values are minimally elevated, as in this patient. Increased 5-HIAA values may follow ingestion of foods rich in serotonin (bananas, pineapples, walnuts, avocados, tomatoes, eggplant, and chocolate). A variety of medications may also yield false-positive results.

A single mediator that causes the carcinoid flush has not been identified. It is not serotonin, since inhibition of serotonin synthesis *does not* prevent flushing. Blood pressure—in contrast to the elevation in pheochromocytomas—falls during an attack. The cardiac involvement with the carcinoid syndrome is right-sided. (*Cecil, Ch. 243; Sleisenger and Fordtran, Ch. 82*)

41. (D) Hemochromatosis is distinctly unusual in a premenopausal female and is therefore the correct answer. Chronic liver disease due to alpha-methyldopa is well described, and each of the other disorders could cause the patient's illness. (*Cecil, Chs. 116 and 119*)

42. (D) There is no evidence that treating an asymptomatic patient who has chronic active hepatitis with prednisone, azathioprine, or both prolongs survival, and use of these potentially toxic agents in this patient is therefore unwarranted. The use of cholestyramine in a minimally symptomatic patient with little evidence of cholestasis, and without first trying such simple measures as emollients, is inappropriate. As long as the patient remains asymptomatic and her biochemical studies do not change, there is little reason for a repeat biopsy at arbitrary intervals. (*Cecil, Ch. 123*)

43. (B) The blood supply to the bowel wall may be severely compromised in patients with collagen vascular diseases, particularly polyarteritis nodosa and systemic lupus erythematosus, leading to perforation and peritonitis. Peritonitis without perforation resulting from subserosal arteritis is seen infrequently. Rheumatoid arthritis may be complicated by necrotizing mesenteric arteritis with ulceration, hemorrhage, perforation, and infarction of the bowel, usually in the setting of severe arthritis and high titers of rheumatoid factor. Köhlmeier-Degos disease is a rare form of systemic vasculitis involving the skin and gut. Approximately 50% of patients with this disease die of peritonitis due to bowel infarction and perforation. Familial Mediterranean fever is a disease characterized by recurrent acute polyserositis, especially peritonitis. Ulceration and perforation of the bowel do not occur. (*Cecil, Chs. 25, 104, and 209; Sleisenger and Fordtran, Chs. 101 and 102*)

44. (C) Although hematochezia usually implies colonic blood loss, brisk bleeding from an upper gastrointestinal site can also result in hematochezia. Barium enema and computerized tomography will not reveal the bleeding site in either case, and colonoscopy is difficult and usually unrevealing in an unprepared colon. Although an inferior mesenteric arteriogram might reveal a colonic site of possible blood loss, it will not identify an upper GI lesion. In addition, this patient has stopped bleeding and angiography therefore is not likely to be useful at this time. Upper GI endoscopy to look for lesions in the stomach and duodenum and the presence of blood in the upper small bowel is the best initial diagnostic step. Nasogastric tube aspiration may reveal no blood in the stomach in patients who are bleeding from the duodenum or jejunum. (*Cecil, Ch. 114*)

45. (E) Although all these lesions can result in gastrointestinal hemorrhage, villous adenomas do so rarely, and blood loss usually is not massive. Silent duodenal ulcers are a common cause of massive hemorrhage, especially in the elderly, and can present as hematochezia without hematemesis. Aortoduodenal or aortoenteric fistulas must be considered in any patient with an aortic graft. The fistulas may bleed intermittently at first and can lead to sepsis. Diagnosis is usually made by arteriography during a bleeding episode. Rarely, the source of blood loss can be seen at endoscopy if the endoscope can be passed to the area of the fistula. Therapy consists of immediate surgery, usually with bypass of the graft, followed months later by graft replacement and oversewing of the enteric fistula. Angiodysplasia of the colon can be diagnosed on selective arteriography and is a relatively common cause of hematochezia, especially in the elderly. Bleeding diverticula are another common cause of hematochezia in the elderly; they can be diagnosed by arteriography during a bleeding episode or by fortuitous identification of the bleeding site during colonoscopy. (*Cecil, Ch. 114; Sleisenger and Fordtran, Ch. 25; Meyer et al*)

46. (C) This patient has hematobilia, which results from communication of an intrahepatic vessel with the biliary tree. Blunt or penetrating trauma that fractures or lacerates hepatic parenchyma is among the most common causes of such abnormal communications, which are best diagnosed by arteriography. Other tests listed might indicate the presence but not the type of biliary disease (A and B) or would provide little useful information (D and E). (*Cecil, Ch. 130*)

47. (B) The irritable bowel syndrome is characterized by abdominal pain and altered bowel habits, usually alternating constipation and diarrhea with one of the two symptoms predominating. The syndrome is recognized as a motor disorder that is strongly influenced by emotional stress and by food intake. It is the most common gastrointestinal condition. The patient described in this question has symptoms most consistent with this diagnosis. There is nothing to suggest glucose intolerance, malabsorption, or hypergastrinemia. Symptoms of lactose intolerance may mimic in every way the symptoms of irritable bowel syndrome. In addition, lactose intolerance can aggravate the symptoms of irritable bowel syndrome. For these reasons lactose intolerance should be ruled out in patients presenting with symptoms of irritable bowel syndrome. This may be achieved by performing a lactose tolerance test (or more simply by placing the patient on a strict lactose-free diet for a trial period of two weeks). (*Cecil, Ch. 102; Bayless, pp. 342–345*)

48. (A) Wilson's disease is rarely associated with overt liver disease before 5 years of age, and Kayser-Fleischer rings can be found in patients with severe and prolonged cholestasis in the absence of liver disease. Each of the other patients exhibits clinical or biochemical features compatible with Wilson's disease. Chronic active hepatitis or fulminant hepatic failure in adolescents with Wilson's disease is frequently associated with a normal serum ceruloplasmin concentration and the absence of Kayser-Fleischer rings. Hemolysis, sunflower cataracts, and proximal tubular dysfunction are all associated with Wilson's disease. (*Cecil, Ch. 205; Zakim and Boyer, Ch. 43*)

49. (C) Fear of eating because of the predictability of onset of pain following a meal is strongly suggestive of intestinal angina. The absence of any abnormal laboratory findings or abnormal findings on the upper gastrointestinal series, endoscopy, sigmoidoscopy, and barium enema does not rule out the diagnosis of chronic intestinal ischemia. Most patients with angina are elderly and have some evidence of peripheral vascular disease. (*Cecil, Ch. 106*)

50. (E) *A. lumbricoides, F. hepatica,* and *C. sinensis* can all infest the biliary tree and cause obstruction and infection; only *Clonorchis,* which can live in its host for decades, is known to be associated with the development of cholangiocarcinoma. *S. mansoni* live as adults primarily in the rectal submucosal venous channels; they deposit eggs that find their way into the inferior mesenteric venous system, ultimately lodging in the portal venules, and are not found in the bile ducts. *S. stercoralis* may reside in the gastrointestinal tract but is not known to cause biliary disease. (*Cecil, Ch. 129; Sleisenger and Fordtran, Ch. 62*)

51. (A—True; B—True; C—False; D—False; E—False) The patient's history, presentation, and physical examination all suggest an acute gastrointestinal hemorrhage. The previous evaluations are sensitive studies and can reliably exclude large mass lesions and colonic diverticula. In contrast to the mild to moderate lower gastrointestinal blood loss, in the patient with a greater than 3-unit hematochezia episode with postural hypotension, the source of the blood loss may in fact be the upper gastrointestinal tract. This is especially true in those patients on medication known to irritate the upper gastrointestinal mucosa (e.g., salicylates, nonsteroidal agents). The most common causes of massive lower gastrointestinal bleeding are arteriovenous malformation (vascular ectasias) and diverticula in the right colon. The diagnosis of vascular ectasias is made by direct endoscopic visualization (colonoscopy) or by angiography. (*Cecil, Chs. 106 and 114; Sleisenger and Fordtran, Ch. 25*)

52. (A—True; B—False; C—False; D—True; E—True) This nuclear scan shows extravasation of the radionuclide in the area of the right colon. Since the previous scans were normal, there is an interval of 8 hours from the last scan during which bleeding into the gastrointestinal tract occurred. Although the current scan shows radionuclide only in the right colon, it is possible that blood loss from the small bowel occurred during this interval and that the blood now is passing into the right colon. This scan suggests that the bleeding is from the area of the GI tract proximal to the hepatic flexure. A small bowel lesion, particularly a distal small bowel lesion, is not excluded by this scan, given the 8-hour interval between the prior scan and this one. A repeat air-contrast barium enema examination would serve little purpose; it is unlikely that a new lesion would be demonstrated three months after a satisfactory radiographic evaluation of this area. The next step should be a pancolonoscopy following careful preparation of the colon in order to look specifically for small lesions in this area, particularly shallow ulcerations, small mass lesions, or vascular abnormalities such as vascular ectasias. These vascular ectasias are commonly encountered in elderly patients, particularly those with underlying heart disease. They are probably acquired lesions and are currently believed to be associated with nearly half of the episodes of right colonic hemorrhage. In patients with hematochezia, right-sided vascular ectasias are second only to colonic diverticular hemorrhage as a source of lower GI tract bleeding. In addition to vascular ectasias of the bowel, *E. histolytica, M. tuberculosis,* and Crohn's disease can all involve the right colon and produce significant colonic bleeding. (*Cecil, Chs. 106 and 114; Sleisenger and Fordtran, Chs. 25 and 72*)

53. (A—True; B—False; C—False; D—False; E—True) The symptom complex of sweating, weakness, tachycardia, and diarrhea following meals occurs transiently in one third or more of patients after gastric surgery. Symptoms begin soon after the patient starts a regular diet. Liquid meals, especially those containing large concentrations of carbohydrates, are most likely to evoke the symptoms of the "dumping" syndrome. Patients also note that recumbency minimizes symptoms. A low-carbohydrate, solid diet eaten in a recumbent position would minimize this patient's syndrome. (*Cecil, Ch. 102*)

54.(A—False; B—False; C—True; D—False; E—True) The age-adjusted mortality rates from carcinoma of the pancreas have increased over the past 50 years. Those factors associated with an increased risk for the development of pancreatic cancer include cigarette smoking and hereditary pancreatitis. Other forms of chronic pancreatitis, including alcoholic pancreatitis, and causes of acute pancreatitis, such as hyperlipidemia and pancreas divisum, have not been associated with pancreatic carcinoma. (*Cecil, Ch. 109; Sleisenger and Fordtran, Ch. 99*)

55.(A—True; B—True; C—False; D—True; E—True) The majority of chronic alcoholics with hyperamylasemia were found to have elevation of the salivary amylase isoenzyme component with normal pancreatic amylase levels when the amylase isoenzymes were fractionated. The exact cause of the salivary hyperamylasemia is not known, because when examined histologically, the salivary glands appeared normal without evidence of inflammation. Small amounts of amylase are produced by the lung and reproductive tract as well as the intestine and pancreas; therefore, primary lung carcinomas can produce amylase, resulting in detectable hyperamylasemia. Macroamylasemia results from amylase bound to larger serum proteins that are cleared slowly from the circulation. A distinctive laboratory feature of macroamylasemia is a low renal amylase:creatinine clearance ratio. (*Cecil, Ch. 108; Sleisenger and Fordtran, Ch. 97; Salt and Schenker*)

56.(A—False; B—True; C—False; D—True; E—False) Elevated basal gastric acid secretion can occur by stimulation of gastric parietal cells by one of three principal mechanisms: increased secretion of gastrin, increased stimulation by acetylcholine, or increased stimulation by histamine. Systemic mastocytosis is associated with increased histamine production, which acts directly on the parietal cell to stimulate acid secretion. In pernicious anemia, gastrin levels are elevated in the presence of mucosal atrophy of the body of the stomach; acid production is therefore reduced. Several known hormones normally secreted by the small intestine inhibit gastrin and gastric acid secretion; following massive small intestinal resection, these inhibitory factors are removed and gastric acid hypersecretion results. VIP inhibits gastric acid secretion, and achlorhydria is a feature of VIP-secreting tumors. Although Cushing's syndrome and adrenocorticoid therapy have been associated with peptic ulcer disease, it has not been demonstrated that this possible relationship is due to gastric acid hypersecretion. (*Cecil, Ch. 100.1; Sleisenger and Fordtran, Ch. 41*)

57.(A—False; B—False; C—False; D—True; E—True) Acute fatty liver of pregnancy, formerly believed to be almost universally fatal, is now recognized to encompass liver disease of varying severity frequently associated with a favorable outcome. Transmission of hepatitis B to the infant of the mother described might occur, but only in a minority of cases. It would be much more likely if the mother were HBeAg-positive. Unlike acute fatty liver, cholestasis of pregnancy is not known to be associated with preeclampsia. Finally, estrogen administration in humans is known to increase the cholesterol saturation of bile, and pregnancy is associated with "hypomotility" of the gallbladder, which could lead to stasis. Both these changes probably contribute to the increased prevalence of cholesterol gallstones in parous women. (*Cecil, Ch. 125*)

58.(A—True; B—False; C—True; D—True; E—False; F—True) The cause of colonic cancer is not known, but there are a number of risk factors known for the individual. The risk of colorectal carcinoma begins to increase around age 50 and roughly doubles for each succeeding decade. A number of conditions associated with increased mucosal cell turnover may lead to increased risk (e.g., inflammatory bowel disease), although inflammation limited to the rectum is apparently without increased risk of neoplasm. A history of colon cancer in a first-degree relative, "familial polyposis" syndromes, and a history of breast or female genital cancer have all been associated with increased risk. (*Cecil, Ch. 107*)

59.(All are False) Treatment of acute pancreatitis consists of analgesia, restoration and maintenance of intravascular volume, reduction of pancreatic enzyme secretion, treatment of localized complications, and elimination of causative factors. There is no evidence that any of the listed treatment modalities tested thus far affect the course of mild pancreatitis. However, several agents (anticholinergics, antibiotics, and nasogastric suction) have only been tested in cases of mild alcoholic pancreatitis; it remains to be determined if they have a role in other forms of pancreatitis. (*Cecil, Ch. 108; Sleisenger and Fordtran, Ch. 97*)

60.(A—False; B—True; C—False; D—False; E—True) This man has a pancreatic pseudocyst as a complication of acute pancreatitis. Initial treatment of uncomplicated pseudocysts is medical. Total parenteral nutrition is usually required over a six-week period as the pseudocyst either resolves or matures, making it more amenable to surgical drainage. Serial computed tomography or ultrasound examinations are helpful to follow the maturation of the pseudocyst. Antibiotics are not required for an uncomplicated resolving pseudocyst. Since most pseudocysts resolve spontaneously, needle aspiration or surgical drainage is not required in their initial management. (*Cecil, Ch. 108; Sleisenger and Fordtran, Chs. 97 and 98*)

61.(A—False; B—False; C—False; D—True; E—False) If serial CT or ultrasound examinations do not demonstrate resolution by six weeks, either surgical or percutaneous drainage of a pancreatic pseudocyst is recommended. Complications of pseudocysts that require urgent surgical intervention include bacterial infection of a pseudocyst, free pseudocyst rupture into the peritoneum, massive hemorrhage into the pseudocyst, and erosion or rupture of a pseudocyst into an adjacent organ or vessel. (*Cecil, Ch. 108; Sleisenger and Fordtran, Chs. 97 and 98*)

62.(A—True; B—False; C—True; D—False; E—True) Isoniazid hepatitis is a particularly troublesome form of drug-induced liver injury because it may not occur until many months after isoniazid has been begun, and it is usually indistinguishable from acute or chronic hepatitis on biopsy. Hepatitis occurs most frequently in the elderly and in patients who are rapid isoniazid acetylators; it bears no clear relationship to the mild transaminase elevations seen in many patients shortly after the drug is begun. (*Cecil, Ch. 122; Black et al*)

63.(A—False; B—False; C—True; D—False; E—False) The incidence of colonic adenocarcinoma increases dramatically with active pancolonic ulcerative colitis of more than 10 years' duration. The CEA is an unreliable and insensitive screening test for cancer in patients with ulcerative colitis. Not only is the serum test likely to be positive only in patients with large bulky tumors, but the CEA may be elevated in patients with active inflammatory bowel disease. The stabilized guaiac card test for occult blood should be used with patients restricting the intake of red meats and other products high in peroxidase activity. Poultry and fish will not produce a false-positive reaction with the Hemoccult cards. Dysplasia on rectal biopsy is associated with the likelihood of carcinoma of the bowel elsewhere. Although the finding of dysplasia, particularly dysplasia associated with a plaque or mass, is not an indication of and by itself for proctocolectomy, these patients must be followed carefully with frequent colonoscopy and biopsy. Repeat demonstration of severe dysplasia would be an indication for recommending colectomy. No diagnostic test can reliably exclude colonic cancer in patients with inflammatory bowel disease. Ferrous sulfate may produce a false-positive result for occult blood with the Hemoccult cards; ascorbic acid, however, is associated with false-negative tests. (*Cecil, Chs. 105.3 and 107; Sleisenger and Fordtran, Ch. 78*)

64.(A—False; B—True; C—False; D—False; E—False) Asymptomatic cholelithiasis is a relatively benign condition that is estimated to be present in about 10% of Americans. Less than 25% of patients subsequently develop severe complications, and only about one half develop any symptoms at all. The chance of death due to a future complication (less than 2%) is about offset by the chance of dying at the time of elective cholecystectomy (less than 1%). Although B is true, the risk of gallbladder cancer in a given patient with gallstones is exceedingly small and does not constitute justification for prophylactic surgery. (*Cecil, Ch. 130*)

65.(A—True; B—True; C—False; D—False; E—True) This patient has chronic alcoholic pancreatitis and pancreatic insufficiency resulting from destruction of exocrine tissue. Because of considerable exocrine reserve, steatorrhea and protein malabsorption occur in chronic pancreatitis only after 90% of the secretory capacity of the pancreas has been lost. However, symptomatic carbohydrate malabsorption is rare in chronic pancreatitis because salivary amylase remains unimpaired and pancreatic amylase is a very abundant pancreatic enzyme. The endocrine pancreas is also destroyed in chronic pancreatitis. Insulin secretion in response to an oral glucose load is impaired early in the course of the disease, and overt diabetes mellitus develops with progressive destruction of the gland. Absorption of iron and calcium is unaffected by pancreatic insufficiency. Although vitamin B_{12} malabsorption may occur from impaired proteolytic cleavage of B_{12} bound to R protein, overt vitamin B_{12} deficiency rarely develops. (*Cecil, Ch. 108; Sleisenger and Fordtran, Ch. 98*)

66.(A—True; B—False; C—False; D—True; C—True) This patient has acute alcoholic pancreatitis. Exudative pleural effusions with high levels of amylase and lipase are often seen in this disease. Although usually located in the left side, effusions may be isolated on the right or bilateral. Other pulmonary complications of acute necrotizing pancreatitis include adult respiratory distress syndrome, pulmonary edema, pneumonia, and pulmonary embolism. Narrowing of the common bile duct as it courses through the head of the pancreas may result from pancreatic edema due to active inflammation or compression from a pancreatic pseudocyst or inflammatory mass causing biliary obstruction and jaundice. If cholangitis should develop with biliary obstruction, emergency surgery should be performed. There is no correlation between the severity of acute pancreatitis (either increased mortality or length of hospitalization) and serum amylase levels. (*Cecil, Ch. 108; Sleisenger and Fordtran, Ch. 97*)

67.(A—True; B—False; C—False; D—False; E—True) Severe alpha$_1$-antitrypsin deficiency is almost entirely accounted for by the P_iZZ phenotype. About 10% of individuals with this phenotype manifest cholestasis in the first few days to weeks of life, but the majority do not have liver disease in childhood. Individuals with the P_iZZ phenotype characteristically exhibit rounded eosinophilic inclusions in the cytoplasm of periportal hepatocytes, but these also occur as an acquired defect in patients with alcoholic liver disease and are therefore not diagnostic. Cirrhotic patients with alpha$_1$-antitrypsin deficiency have an exceedingly high incidence of hepatocellular carcinoma. An increased prevalence of heterozygous MZ and SZ phenotypes is found in patients with non-B chronic active hepatitis and cryptogenic cirrhosis. (*Cecil, Ch. 125; Zakim and Boyer, Ch. 42*)

68.(A—False; B—True; C—False; D—False; E—True) The most common esophageal cancer is squamous cell carcinoma. Only 4% of the esophageal cancer is adenocarcimona. There is a distinct association between esophageal cancer and the use of alcohol and tobacco. Squamous cell carcinoma of the esophagus is also increased in incidence among patients with longstanding reflux esophagitis, achalasia, chronic strictures from caustic ingestion, and tylosis. Although the use of double-contrast barium studies of the esophagus has improved the diagnostic yield for small carcinomas of the esophagus, only direct endoscopic visalization of the esophagus with directed endoscopic biopsy and brush cytology of abnormal mucosa can adequately exclude carcinoma of the esophagus in a patient with dysphagia. Carcinoma of the esophagus is radiosensitive, with 15 to 20% five-year survival rates in patients treated with radiation therapy for carcinoma of the proximal esophagus. Middle- and distal-third esophageal squamous cell carcinoma is usually treated by esophagectomy in patients when preoperative evaluation excludes nonresectable disease. Squamous cell carcinoma of the esophagus is not responsive to single-agent chemotherapy. (*Cecil, Ch. 98; Sleisenger and Fordtran, Ch. 35*)

69.(A—False; B—True; C—True; D—False; E—True) The patient has pancreatitis that can be assumed to be severe or hemorrhagic on the basis of the physical examination and nonspecific laboratory signs of hemoconcentration, marked leukocytosis, hyperamylasemia, and elevated serum glucose. Diabetic ketoacidosis is associated with hyperamylasemia but is not itself a cause of severe clinical pancreatitis. On the other hand, hyperglycemia is frequent in severe pancreatitis of all causes. Hemorrhagic pancreatitis typically causes hypocalcemia; thus, a normal serum calcium level in this setting is a clue to previously existing hypercalcemia, such as from hyperparathyroidism. Drugs such as thiazide diuretics, azathioprine, isoniazid, corticosteroids, oral contraceptives, and methyl alcohol have been implicated as causes of pancreatitis. Thiazide diurectics can also result in hyperglycemia, hyperuricemia, and (rarely) hypercalcemia. Although "sludging" of white blood cells in small vessels occurs in acute leukemia and may be responsible for cerebral dysfunction in that disease, pancreatitis due to this mechanism has not been reported. Types I, IV, and V hyperlipoproteinemia have been associated with pancreatitis and presumably can cause pancretitis. Most hyperlipidemia-associated pancreatitis occurs in alcoholics who have been drinking heavily before the attack or who have a pre-existing hyperlipoproteinemia, especially type V. (*Cecil, Ch. 108; Sleisenger and Fordtran, Ch. 97*)

70. (A—False; B—False; C—False; D—False; E—True) There are several radiographic features of benign and malignant gastric ulcers that are helpful in their evaluation. One feature of benign gastric ulcers is that gastric folds radiate from the ulcer crater. However, the radiographic appearance of an ulcer alone is not adequate in excluding a possible malignancy, and gastroscopy with multiple biopsies of the margins of the ulcer crater should be performed. Abdominal pain or weight loss may be associated with either benign or malignant gastric ulcers. Benign gastric ulcers are more commonly found on the lesser curvature as opposed to the greater curvature of the stomach, but 25% of gastric carcinomas are also found on the lesser curvature, so this feature is not helpful in distinguishing the two diseases. Although the absence of gastric acid in the presence of a gastric ulcer suggests malignancy, 75% of patients with gastric carcinoma produce gastric acid. (*Cecil, Ch. 101; Sleisenger and Fordtran, Ch. 48*)

71. (A—True; B—True; C—False; D—False; E—True) End-to-side portacaval shunt directly decompresses the entire portal system, while distal splenorenal shunting decompresses the varices selectively, at least in the short term. Both propranolol and vasopressin reduce portal pressure, primarily by reducing splanchnic arterial blood flow, and in the case of propranolol also by reducing cardiac output. Esophageal sclerotherapy obliterates varices without affecting portal pressure. (*Cecil, Ch. 127; Cello et al*)

72. (A—False; B—True; C—False; D—True; E—True) Celiac sprue diagnosed in infancy commonly undergoes spontaneous symptomatic remission in late childhood or adolescence which is sometimes permanent, but the disease may reappear in adult life. Although only a minority of patients with celiac sprue develop dermatitis herpetiformis, almost all the patients with this skin disease, even if asymptomatic for malabsorption, will have intestinal mucosal lesions of celiac sprue that are responsive to dietary gluten exclusions. Corticosteroids usually produce marked improvement in adult celiac disease, but their use is generally reserved for patients whose disease fails to respond to a gluten-free diet. Serious complications of celiac sprue include a neurologic syndrome resembling subacute combined degeneration of the spinal cord in the absence of evidence of vitamin B_{12} deficiency and an increased incidence of intestinal and extraintestinal malignancy, including lymphomas of the bowel and squamous carcinoma of the esophagus. (*Cecil, Ch. 104; Sleisenger and Fordtran, Ch. 61*)

73. (A—True; B—False; C—False; D—True; E—False) Since 1983 the results of liver transplantation have improved dramatically, reflecting the use of cyclosporine as an immunosuppressive and improvements in patient selection, surgical technique, and aftercare. The best results (87% first-year survival) have been obtained in children with biliary atresia. Relatively few patients with fulminant hepatic failure have undergone transplantation, but the early results have been encouraging. Survival statistics for transplantation in patients with hepatobiliary malignancy have not shown much improvement since the introduction of cyclosporine. On the other hand, most patients transplanted for benign disease who survive the first three postoperative months will enjoy long-term survival. Recurrence of primary biliary cirrhosis following transplantation has been infrequently reported, and it is unclear whether this represents true recurrence or chronic rejection. (*Cecil, Ch. 128; Busuttil et al*)

74. (A—False; B—False; C—True; D—True; E—False) The barium enema shows filling of the stomach (clearly outlining gastric rugae) from the colon near the splenic flexure, a characteristic finding in gastrocolic fistula. These lesions occur most frequently following gastric or colonic surgery or in association with chronic inflammation in either the stomach or colon. Carcinomas of the stomach, pancreas, or colon may also be associated with gastrocolic fistula. The associated diarrhea is related to the constant fecal soiling of the upper gastrointestinal tract and subsequent overgrowth by colonic flora. Many of the resident colonic flora deconjugate bile salts and interfere with normal micelle formation. Thus, steatorrhea is a common feature of this disorder. Because the fistula may be relatively small, high pressures are often necessary to visualize it on barium studies. Therefore, the most reliable means of demonstrating gastrocolic fistula is by barium enema examination rather than by low-pressure upper GI series. (*Cecil, Ch. 104; Sleisenger and Fordtran, Ch. 67*)

75. (A—True; B—True; C—False; D—True; E—False) The most common findings in Whipple's disease include lymphadenopathy (40%), fever (50%), and migratory nondeforming arthritis (30–60%). Hepatosplenomegaly is uncommon in Whipple's disease, while pulmonary fibrosis is not a feature of this condition. (*Cecil, Ch. 104; Sleisenger and Fordtran, Ch. 68*)

76. (A—True; B—True; C—True; D—True; E—False) This patient has developed recurrent duodenal ulcers despite appropriate medical therapy. Episodes of pain have become more frequent and more severe and therefore may be considered refractory. Intractability is the most common cause for surgical treatment of peptic ulcer disease and may be aggravated by several factors such as ulcer penetration, pyloric obstruction and pyloric channel ulcers, postbulbar ulceration, and gastric acid hypersecretory states. Recently it has been demonstrated that salicylates and other nonsteroidal anti-inflammatory drugs are toxic to the mucosa of the stomach and duodenum and may exacerbate peptic ulcer disease. The hallmark of a gastrinoma is gastric acid hypersecretion with severe ulcer disease that is typically refractory to normal therapy for peptic ulcer disease. Since the surgical approach to patients with gastrinomas would be different from that for patients with other causes of duodenal ulcer disease, it is extremely important to identify those patients with gastrinomas before surgery is performed. Therefore, as a general rule, serum gastrin measurements should be made in patients before they undergo elective ulcer surgery.

Three common surgical approaches to the treatment of intractable peptic ulcer disease are (1) antrectomy and vagotomy, (2) vagotomy and pyloroplasty, and (3) highly selective vagotomy. Each of these operations has its own postoperative morbidity, mortality, and recurrence rate for peptic ulceration. Antrectomy and vagotomy have the lowest recurrence rate but the greatest incidence of postoperative morbidity (dumping syndrome). Vagotomy with pyloroplasty has among the highest recurrence rates and an intermediate morbidity, whereas highly selective vagotomy has the lowest incidence of morbidity but a recurrence rate approaching that of vagotomy and pyloroplasty. Before the development of potent H_2-receptor antagonists, total gastrectomy was the recommended treatment for gastrinomas. However, with a combination of medical therapy and highly selective vagotomy, total gastrectomy is usually unnecessary to control gastric acid secretion. (*Cecil, Ch. 100.4; Sleisenger and Fordtran, Chs. 47, 50, and 51*)

77. (A—False; B—True; C—False; D—True; E—True) Rectal biopsy may be diagnostic in revealing the ova of schistosomes, invasive organisms of *Balantidium coli*, and amyloid deposition in the lamina propria and walls of small blood vessels in the submucosa. Stool examination for ova will usually yield the diagnosis of ascariasis. Stool culture and microscopy for parasites, ova, and cysts will be of major value in detecting the common causes of traveler's diarrhea. (*Cecil, Ch. 103; Sleisenger and Fordtran, Chs. 29 and 62*)

78. (All are True) Each of the statements is correct. Individuals who are HBsAg-positive are at least 200 times more likely to develop hepatocellular carcinoma than those who are HBsAg-negative, making hepatitis B virus infection perhaps the strongest known risk factor for any human cancer. Although hepatocellular carcinoma associated with hepatitis B virus infection is particularly prevalent in southern Africa and southeast Asia, it also appears to be an important cause of this cancer in developed nations including the United States. Hepatitis B viral DNA has been repeatedly demonstrated in the host genome of tissue from both malignant and nonmalignant liver tissue, but the precise relationship between incorporation of the viral DNA into that of the cell and the development of cancer is unknown. (*Cecil, Ch. 129*)

79. (A—False; B—True; C—True; D—False; E—True; F—True) Pseudo-obstruction describes a syndrome that has clinical features similar to mechanical obstruction without the presence of an obstructive lesion. When it occurs as a manifestation of other disease it is termed secondary intestinal pseudo-obstruction. Diseases that involve intramural nervous tissue (either destroying it or functionally disturbing it), as well as certain endocrine, connective tissue, and neurologic disorders, may cause the problem. Certain drugs (e.g., phenothiazines, tricyclic antidepressants) may also be associated with the condition. (*Cecil, Ch. 102*)

80. (A—False; B—True; C—False; D—True; E—False) Surveillance for colonic neoplasia is currently recommended in the following circumstances: (1) to evaluate the entire colon for synchronous cancer or neoplastic polyps in a patient with a treatable cancer or neoplastic polyp; (2) as follow-up examination at 2- to 3-year intervals after resection of a colorectal cancer or neoplastic polyp and an adequate initial colonoscopy; (3) for patients with a strong positive family history of colon cancer; and (4) in patients with chronic ulcerative colitis who have pancolitis of longer than 8 years' duration, *or* who have left-sided colitis of over 15 years' duration. No surveillance is needed in patients with ulcerative colitis whose disease is limited to the rectosigmoid. Colonoscopy is generally not indicated in patients with metastatic adenocarcinoma with an unknown primary lesion in the absence of colonic symptoms. There are almost no data on which to base strong recommendations for surveillance in Crohn's disease of the colon at the present time. (*Cecil, Ch. 96; Bayless, pp. 296–301; Sleisenger and Fordtran, Ch. 80*)

81. (A—True; B—False; C—False; D—True; E—False) This patient falls into a category of patients with a symptom complex known as "nonulcer dyspepsia." This entity is characterized by epigastric fullness, discomfort, burning, or pain unrelated to bowel action and is often accompanied by belching and bloating. Two groups of patients can be identified: those with dyspepsia similar to that seen with duodenal ulcer disease, with epigastric pain occurring one to three hours after meals and relieved by antacids; and those with epigastric discomfort shortly after eating, with bloating, belching, and no relief with alkali. On endoscopic evaluation there is no mucosal evidence of peptic ulcer disease. Patients in this second group may have delayed gastric emptying and many respond to metoclopramide. Similarly in this latter group with nonulcer dyspepsia, fat intolerance is common but in itself is not a distinguishing feature from ulcer disease. Studies in which patients have been followed for the development of peptic ulcers indicate that in the absence of duodenal inflammation (duodenitis), duodenal ulcers develop in a minority of patients. Since the symptom complex is somewhat vague, it is important to exclude other disorders that may present with similar symptoms. However, in the absence of objective evidence for gallbladder disease, cholecystectomy is not indicated. (*Cecil, Ch. 100.2; Sleisenger and Fordtran, Ch. 47*)

82. (A—True; B—True; C—False; D—True; E—False) The combination of fever, weight loss, lymphadenopathy, and oral candidiasis in a homosexual male is typical for the acquired immunodeficiency syndrome (AIDS). The parasite seen in the illustrated biopsy is *Cryptosporidium*, a widespread animal parasite that is recognized as an important cause of severe, chronic diarrhea in immunocompromised hosts; it may also give rise to a benign, self-limited gastrointestinal illness in normal individuals. Cryptosporidiosis is a zoonosis, and calves and perhaps other domesticated animals are potential sources of human infection. *Cryptosporidium* attaches itself to the microvillous border of epithelial cells and does not produce ulcerative lesions. However, infestation of the biliary tract has been associated with obstructive strictures, particularly at the ampulla of Vater. The results of treatment of cryptosporidiosis with the antibiotic spiramycin in patients with AIDS have been discouraging. Symptomatic improvement has occurred in only a minority of patients, but organisms usually persist in feces with symptomatic relapse following discontinuation of therapy. (*Cecil, Ch. 103; Pitlik et al; Rodgers and Kagnoff*)

83. (A—True; B—True; C—False; D—False) Hirschsprung's disease is colonic dilatation resulting from a functional obstruction of the rectum due to congenital absence of intramural neural plexuses ("aganglionosis"). The aganglionic segment is permanently *contracted*, causing dilatation proximal to it. Congenital aganglionosis occurs in 1 of each 5000 live births, is 5 to 10 times more common in males than females, and is more common in children with congenital abnormalities, including Down's syndrome. (*Cecil, Ch. 102*)

84. (A—False; B—True; C—True; D—False; E—True) Excessive loss of serum proteins into the intestine (protein-losing enteropathy) is noted in a number of diseases affecting the gastrointestinal tract, including mucosal disease with ulceration (e.g., granulomatous enteritis) and mucosal disease without ulceration (e.g., celiac disease, Whipple's disease), and in conditions characterized by either primary or secondary lymphatic abnormalities (e.g., primary lymphangiectasia, lymphoma). In abetalipoproteinemia, failure of intestinal apolipoprotein B production results in impaired fat absorption and steatorrhea without abnormal intestinal protein loss. Cholera infection produces a toxigenic secretory diarrhea in which profound loss of water and electrolytes from the small intestine can produce circulatory collapse within hours. Loss of serum proteins is not a finding in cholera. (*Cecil, Ch. 104; Sleisenger and Fordtran, Chs. 19 and 63*)

85. (A—True; B—True; C—False; D—False; E—True) On average, 600 ml of gas is passed per rectum daily. Five gases (N_2, O_2, CO_2, H_2, and CH_4 [methane]) comprise greater than 99% of the gas passed as flatus. However, only about one third of normal individuals produce intestinal methane, whereas 80% of patients with carcinoma of the colon do so, presumably as a consequence of specialized bacterial colonization of the colon in these patients. In the majority of patients who complain of gas pains, excessive air swallowing is not responsible for either the amount of intestinal gas (which is often normal) or symptoms attributable to it; abnormal bowel motility is more likely to be responsible (irritable bowel syndrome). Bacterial metabolism appears to be the sole source of both H_2 and CH_4 production in the gastrointestinal tract, and neither germ-free rats nor newborn infants excrete these gases. (*Cecil, Ch. 94; Sleisenger and Fordtran, Ch. 17*)

86. (A—True; B—True; C—False; D—True; E—False) Bile salts are largely absorbed by the terminal ileum. Loss of terminal ileal function due to resection, disease, or bypass may cause severe diarrhea, mainly due to impairment of colonic salt and water absorption and stimulation of colonic salt and water secretion by malabsorbed bile salts. Increased hepatic synthesis of bile salts can generally compensate for bile salt losses if less than 100 cm of terminal ileum is resected, thus providing sufficient bile salts for fat absorption. In cases where more than 100 cm of terminal ileum is removed, massive bile salt loss results, and even increased hepatic synthesis will fail to provide a sufficient bile salt pool for normal dietary fat solubilization; steatorrhea will result. Hyperoxaluria with renal stone formation may result from increased oxalate absorption secondary to effects of fatty acids and bile salts on the colonic mucosa, while bile salt depletion results in lithogenic bile and about a threefold increased risk of gallstones developing. Loss of the ileocecal sphincter may allow bacterial contamination of the remaining small bowel. (*Cecil, Ch. 104; Sleisenger and Fordtran, Ch. 59*)

87. (A—True; B—False; C—False; D—True; E—False) The finding of a high-titer positive antimitochondrial antibody in a woman with cholestasis is almost always diagnostic of primary biliary cirrhosis. The diagnosis is established in this patient by the liver histology, which shows the diagnostic lesion of granulomatous nonsuppurative destructive cholangiopathy. The diagnosis of primary biliary cirrhosis is often associated with other immunologic abnormalities, including elevated serum IgM and antithyroid antibodies. Serum bile acid measurements will be predictably elevated and add nothing to the diagnostic information already available. Although several trials of D-penicillamine have been conducted in the treatment of primary biliary cirrhosis, the value of this drug in improving survival is not established. Retroperitoneal fibrosis is associated with rare cases of sclerosing cholangitis but not with primary biliary cirrhosis. (*Cecil, Ch. 126; Zakim and Boyer, Ch. 34*)

88. (A—True; B—True; C—False; D—True; E—True) The plain film shows a massively dilated transverse colon. There is also marked loss of haustral details indicative of a severe acute inflammatory process. The midtransverse colon dilatation greater than 7 cm together with the clinical course is suggestive of toxic megacolon. Toxic megacolon is commonly associated with severe acute idiopathic ulcerative colitis, and it is also seen in a variety of other acute inflammatory processes such as infections with *Shigella* and with *E. histolytica*, both of which are seen in homosexual men. Toxic megacolon can also be seen in Crohn's colitis. *Giardia lamblia* infections involve the proximal small bowel and do not produce colonic inflammatory disease. (*Cecil, Ch. 105.3; Sleisenger and Fordtran, Ch. 78*)

89. (A—False; B—True; C—False; D—True; E—True) In this patient with manifestations of acute toxicity and an acute toxic megacolon on radiography, the proctosigmoidoscopy is strongly suggestive of acute idiopathic ulcerative colitis. Nevertheless, friable mucosa can occasionally be seen in acute bowel infections. Although the absence of trophozoites on three successive stool examinations makes the likelihood of *E. histolytica* infection low, serologic testing should be done in the homosexual man to exclude amebic colitis definitely. Colonoscopy is distinctly contraindicated because of the danger of perforations of the large bowel in an acutely inflamed colon. The diagnosis in this patient would not depend on a barium enema, given the features of toxic megacolon on plain film and the appearance of acute ulcerative colitis on proctosigmoidoscopy. Moreover, barium enema has been implicated in exacerbating acute inflammatory bowel disease, although the association between barium enema and acute deterioration of ulcerative colitis has not been firmly established. Blood cultures are indicated, and broad-spectrum antibiotics should be started. Close follow-up of this patient is absolutely essential, and radiographs of the abdomen should be repeated within a short time. A deterioration of the clinical condition or a marked increase in colonic size would indicate the need for expeditious colectomy. (*Cecil, Ch. 105.3; Sleisenger and Fordtran, Ch. 78*)

90. (A—False; B—True; C—True; D—False; E—True) Prostaglandins (particularly of the E_2 variety), phenolphthalein, and chenodeoxycholic acid (a primary bile acid) are all associated with the stimulation of ion secretion and a secretory diarrhea. *Shigella* species disrupt the superficial mucosa of the colon, producing diarrhea on this basis. Villous adenomas of the left colon may produce a secretory diarrhea with associated hypokalemia. Adenocarcinoma of the rectum is not associated with a secretory diarrhea. (*Cecil, Ch. 103; Sleisenger and Fordtran, Chs. 20 and 63*)

91. (A—True; B—False; C—False; D—True; E—False) The patient has Gilbert's syndrome, a benign disorder of bilirubin production and metabolism that affects up to 7% of the population, mainly males. The diagnosis is strongly suggested by a history of mild jaundice brought on by fasting in an otherwise healthy young man with no other abnormality observed on physical examination or in liver function tests. The diagnosis requires the exclusion of overt hemolytic states, but up to 50% of patients have evidence of decreased red cell survival. Nicotinic acid administration will often exacerbate the unconjugated hyperbilirubinemia in these patients and has been used as a diagnostic test. Since the hyperbilirubinemia is unconjugated, the urine will not contain bilirubin. Liver biopsy is hardly ever required. (*Cecil, Ch. 118; Zakim and Boyer, Ch. 10*)

92. (A—False; B—False; C—True; D—False; E—True; F—False) Sequential or periodic esophagogastroduodenoscopy is currently indicated in patients with proven Barrett's esophagus; for follow-up of selected large esophageal, gastric, or stomal ulcers to demonstrate healing; and in patients with prior adenomatous gastric polyps. The procedure is of sufficiently low yield that it is generally not indicated for surveillance for malignancy in patients with gastric atrophy, pernicious anemia, treated achalasia, or prior gastric operation; surveillance for healing of benign disease, such as esophagitis or duodenal ulcer; or surveillance during repeated dilations of benign strictures. (*Cecil, Ch. 96*)

93. (A—True; B—False; C—False; D—False; E—False) Post-transfusional non-A, non-B (NANB) viral hepatitis accounts for 90% of an estimated 150,000–300,000 cases of post-transfusional hepatitis in the United States annually. In the majority of cases, the acute manifestations of infection are mild and anicteric. Chronic liver disease, however, appears more likely to develop following a mild rather than an acute, severe initial illness, and the prevalence of cirrhosis among chronically infected individuals evaluated in several studies is 10–20%. No established serologic test for NANB viral infection is available, and the diagnosis remains one of serologic exclusion. Three controlled trials of immune serum globulin in preventing transfusion-associated NANB hepatitis failed to establish the efficacy of this measure, and immune serum globulin is not recommended for prevention of transfusion-associated hepatitis. (*Cecil, Ch. 121; Dienstag*)

94. (A—True; B—False; C—False; D—True) Endoscopic retrograde cholangiopancreatography is generally not indicated in the evaluation of abdominal pain of obscure origin in the absence of objective findings or test results that suggest biliary tract or pancreatic disease. Nor is it indicated in the evaluation of suspected gallbladder disease without evidence of bile duct disease. The evaluation of a single episode of acute pancreatitis without evidence of gallstone disease should not be pursued with this testing. The examination should also not be carried out as further documentation of pancreatic malignancy that has been diagnosed by ultrasound or computed tomography scanning. (*Cecil, Ch. 96*)

95. (A—True; B—True; C—True; D—False; E—False) Liver biopsy with quantitation of hepatic iron remains the "gold standard" for diagnosis. Although the presence of stainable iron in 75% or more of hepatocytes renders the diagnosis very likely, stainable iron correlates only roughly with quantitative measurements. Particularly in alcoholic patients, in whom transferrin saturation and serum ferritin are commonly increased and minor degrees of iron overload are frequent, accurate diagnosis requires quantitative measurement of hepatic iron. Hemochromatosis is linked to certain HLA groups and therefore is probably coded for on chromosome 6. (*Cecil, Ch. 206*)

96. (All are False) Although some measures, such as vasodilator infusion, may transiently improve renal function in the hepatorenal syndrome, none of the options listed has been shown to improve survival. Hepatic transplantation may, however, be successful in some instances. (*Cecil, Chs. 127 and 128*)

97. (B) Phenytoin may give rise to acute, sometimes fatal, hepatitis characteristically accompanied by fever, lymphadenopathy, and a maculopapular rash. Hepatomegaly and jaundice are common. Histologically, the lesion resembles acute viral hepatitis. (*Cecil, Ch. 122; Zakim and Boyer, Ch. 29*)

98. (G) Oral contraceptives have been associated with hepatic vein thrombosis and the Budd-Chiari syndrome. Ascites is a cardinal feature of hepatic vein thrombosis, and hepatic enlargement is common. (*Cecil, Ch. 122; Zakim and Boyer, Ch. 29*)

99. (D) Long-term methotrexate treatment for psoriasis may lead to hepatic fibrosis and eventual cirrhosis. The evolution of this lesion may occur without symptoms or abnormalities in routine liver function tests. (*Cecil, Ch. 122; Zakim and Boyer, Ch. 29*)

100. (H) A cholestatic reaction is a well-documented complication of erythromycin estolate as well as the ethylsuccinate and lactobionate derivatives. Upper abdominal and right upper quadrant pain are often prominent and may dominate the clinical picture, leading to suspicion of acute cholecystitis. (*Cecil, Ch. 122; Zakim and Boyer, Ch. 29*)

101. (A) Figure A shows a granuloma containing acid-fast clusters of *Mycobacterium avium-intracellulare*. Atypical mycobacterial infection is commonly seen in patients with the acquired immunodeficiency syndrome. (*Cecil, Ch. 124*)

102. (F) The presence of polymorphonuclear leukocytes inside the interlobular bile ducts is characteristic of acute cholangitis. (*Wright et al, Ch. 14*)

103. (C) Figure C shows a sharply defined granuloma composed almost entirely of epithelioid cells in a patient with hepatic sarcoidosis. (*Cecil, Ch. 125*)

104. (E) This biopsy shows the characteristic early lesion of primary biliary cirrhosis, in which intact and partially degenerating interlobular bile ducts are surrounded by a mononuclear infiltrate. (*Cecil, Ch. 123*)

105. (B); 106. (D) Alcoholic cirrhosis is characteristically monolobular (micronodular) in type, whereas postnecrotic cirrhosis due to chronic hepatitis, Wilson's disease, or hemochromatosis is characteristically multilobular (macronodular), such as that shown in Figure B. (*Cecil, Chs. 123 and 126; Ishak*)

107. (C) Pancreatic ascites results from a persistent leak of pancreatic juice from a pseudocyst or disrupted pancreatic duct. It may be a late finding in acute pancreatitis or an insidious complication of chronic pancreatitis. (*Cecil, Ch. 108; Sleisenger and Fordtran, Ch. 98*)

108. (A) Fat necrosis occurs in the setting of acute pancreatitis and results from the enzymatic actions of lipase and phospholipase. Frequent areas of fat necrosis include those contiguous with the pancreas, such as peripancreatic organs, mesentery, and the retroperitoneum; however, more distant sites include fat necrosis of the bone marrow, mediastinum, pleura, and pericardium as well as periarticular fat. (*Cecil, Ch. 108; Sleisenger and Fordtran, Ch. 97*)

109. (A) Temporary obstruction of the common bile duct by passage of a gallstone is a frequent cause of acute pancreatitis. However, even multiple episodes of "gallstone pancreatitis" do not progress to chronic pancreatitis. (*Cecil, Ch. 108; Sleisenger and Fordtran, Chs. 97 and 98*)

110. (B) In achalasia there is degeneration of the ganglion cells in Auerbach's plexus, leading to increased tone and impaired relaxation of the lower esophageal sphincter; it is often associated with decreased and uncoordinated contractions in the body of the esophagus. The manometric hallmarks of the diagnosis are the high resting pressure of the lower esophageal sphincter, incomplete relaxation of the sphincter with swallowing, and simultaneous, low-amplitude contractions in the body of the esophagus. (*Cecil, Ch. 98; Bayless, pp. 37–39*)

111.(D) A normal lower esophageal sphincter tone and function in the setting of prolonged, intense contractions in the esophageal body are the hallmarks of the "nutcracker" esophagus. (*Cecil, Ch. 98; Bayless, pp. 33–37*)

112.(A) The manometric values and the description are of a *normal* esophageal motility study. (*Cecil, Ch. 98; Bayless, pp. 33–37*)

113.(E) Diffuse esophageal spasm is a combination of esophageal "colic" and dysphagia. Manometrically the condition is defined when the tracing demonstrates segmental contractions and some normal peristaltic waves interspersed with simultaneous, prolonged, high-amplitude contractions. (*Cecil, Ch. 98*)

114.(C) Systemic sclerosis (scleroderma) is a generalized disorder of connective tissue characterized by thickening and fibrosis of the skin, abnormalities of small arteries, and distinctive patterns of involvement of certain internal organs. Of the internal organ systems, the gastrointestinal tract is most often involved. Symptoms referable to the esophagus range from dysphagia to severe intractable reflux disease and stricture formation. Esophageal dysmotility is present in nearly 90% of patients with the disorder. Manometric findings reveal the absence of coordinated peristalsis, loss of amplitude of the esophageal body contractions, aperistalsis on deglutition, and a low or absent lower esophageal sphincter resting pressure. (*Cecil, Chs. 98 and 437*)

115.(C) This patient is most likely to have acute cholecystitis with cystic duct obstruction. The diagnosis can be confirmed by the absence of gallbladder visualization on a technetium-^{99}m–HIDA scan prior to surgery. Although false-negative scans (due to acute cholecystitis with a patent cystic duct) do occur, they are uncommon. (*Cecil, Ch. 130; Scharschmidt et al*)

116.(E) This patient is likely to have a retained common duct stone with biliary obstruction and infection. Endoscopic retrograde cholangiography can be both diagnostic and therapeutic in this case, as it can be combined with endoscopic sphincterotomy. Since this patient has evidence of biliary infection and cholangitis, appropriate blood cultures should be obtained and antibiotic therapy initiated prior to the procedure. Patients with more severe cholangitis or sepsis should receive antibiotic therapy and emergency surgical drainage of the biliary tree. (*Cecil, Ch. 130; Scharschmidt et al*)

117.(A) Progressive jaundice and biliary obstruction in an elderly patient with recent weight loss is likely to be due to pancreatic carcinoma. In this setting, computed tomography would be useful not only to try to localize the site of obstruction but also to identify the tumor and to allow guided percutaneous aspiration of the tumor mass and cytologic diagnosis. Although percutaneous transhepatic cholangiography could also be employed to identify the site of obstruction, and offers the additional option to drain the obstructed ducts (by placing biliary stents), it can neither identify the presumed tumor mass nor result in an histologic diagnosis. (*Cecil, Ch. 130; Scharschmidt et al*)

118.(B) The secretory diarrhea caused by VIP-secreting tumors can produce fluid losses rich in bicarbonate of up to 5 liters per day. The metabolic acidosis associated with such losses is often profound and requires vigorous intravenous replacement therapy. (*Cecil, Ch. 103; Sleisenger and Fordtran, Chs. 20 and 100; O'Dorisio and Mekhjian*)

119.(C) The most common site for both gastrinomas and VIPomas is the pancreas. Gastrinomas are also frequently located in the wall of the duodenum but may be found in other ectopic sites. VIP-secreting tumors also arise from ganglioneuromas. (*Cecil, Ch. 100.6; Sleisenger and Fordtran, Chs. 49 and 100*)

120.(A) Diarrhea in Zollinger-Ellison syndrome results directly from gastric acid and large volume fluid secretion and indirectly from the effects of gastric acid on small bowel mucosa and inactivation of bile acids and pancreatic enzymes. Therefore, diarrhea in this syndrome is improved by either inhibition of gastric acid secretion or removal of gastric acid and fluid by nasogastric suction. VIP stimulates intestinal fluid secretion; therefore, diarrhea with VIP hypersecretion is not affected by nasogastric suction. (*Cecil, Ch. 100.6; Sleisenger and Fordtran, Ch. 49*)

121.(B) A VIP-secreting tumor is believed to be the cause of the "watery diarrhea, hypokalemia, achlorhydria (WDHA) syndrome." This disease is manifest by severe secretory diarrhea and obligatory potassium loss from the colon. Because VIP inhibits gastric acid secretion, most patients have hypo- or achlorhydria. Although the definitive treatment of VIPomas is surgery, initial medical management consists of replacement of fluid losses and correction of hypokalemia. Prednisone temporarily controls the diarrhea in the majority of patients and can be used to ameliorate symptoms during the course of a patient's evaluation. (*Cecil, Ch. 103; Sleisenger and Fordtran, Chs. 20 and 100; O'Dorisio and Mekhjian*)

122.(E) Scan shows a right lower quadrant soft tissue mass compatible with a psoas abscess. The three weeks of fever, chills, and pain in a young man is suggestive of an infectious inflammatory process. The most likely etiology is a perforated appendix. (*Cecil, Chs. 107, 112, and 115*)

123.(B) Scan shows multiple soft tissue masses throughout the abdomen, particularly retroperitoneal, mesenteric, and serosal masses suggestive of diffuse abdominal metastases. (*Cecil, Chs. 107, 112, and 115*)

124.(C) Scan shows invasion of the pelvic fat by a high-density mass. This is strongly suggestive of a nonresectable rectal cancer. (*Cecil, Chs. 107, 112, and 115*)

125.(A) Scan suggests a left lower quadrant soft tissue density compatible with an abscess. The contrast-filled colon shows multiple colonic diverticula and thickening of the bowel wall, strongly suggestive of diverticulitis associated with this diverticular abscess. (The remaining CT scan of the abdomen [D] shows extensive retroperitoneal lymphadenopathy in a patient who has the acquired immunodeficiency syndrome [AIDS], there being extensive node involvement with Kaposi's sarcoma.) (*Cecil, Chs. 107, 112, and 115*)

126.(B) All antacids work by neutralizing gastric acid. Gastric acid secretion is not reduced with antacids and because for every equivalent of acid produced by the parietal cell, an equivalent of bicarbonate is also discharged into the blood, metabolic alkalosis can result. Normally this alkalosis can be compensated for by adequate renal function. (*Cecil, Ch. 100.3*)

127.(E) None of the agents listed inhibits gastrin secretion. Instead, with effective inhibition of gastric acid as seen with cimetidine, gastrin levels may increase slightly. (*Cecil, Chs. 100.1 and 100.2*)

128.(D) Prostaglandins may be beneficial in treatment of peptic ulcer by several mechanisms. In high doses, prostaglandins suppress acid secretion. Prostaglandins are cytoprotective by stimulating gastric bicarbonate secretion and increasing gastric mucus production. And finally, it has been demonstrated that prostaglandins increase mucosal blood flow. (*Cecil, Ch. 100.1*)

129.(A) The symptoms of Zollinger-Ellison syndrome result from gastric acid hypersecretion. H_2-receptor antagonists such as cimetidine are very effective in inhibiting acid secretion; most patients with hypergastrinemia can be controlled with high doses of cimetidine or ranitidine. (*Cecil, Chs. 100.3 and 100.6; Sleisenger and Fordtran, Ch. 49*)

130.(A) Patients with intestinal angina often lose substantial amounts of weight because of self-imposed reduction in food intake related to fear of the postprandial pain typical of this syndrome. (*Cecil, Ch. 106; Sleisenger and Fordtran, Ch. 101*)

131.(F) Nonocclusive intestinal infarction results from decreased splanchnic perfusion and oxygenation that may result from acute myocardial infarction, congestive heart failure, shock, or anoxia. (*Cecil, Ch. 106; Sleisenger and Fordtran, Ch. 101*)

132.(D) Mesenteric arterial embolization usually occurs in the superior mesenteric artery and is characterized by the abrupt onset of symptoms. (*Cecil, Ch. 106; Sleisenger and Fordtran, Ch. 101*)

133.(E) Patients with hypercoagulable states (e.g., antithrombin III deficiency) and portal hypertension (presumably as a complication of slowing of flow in the mesenteric veins) are at increased risk of mesenteric venous thrombosis. (*Cecil, Ch. 106; Sleisenger and Fordtran, Ch. 101*)

134.(B) Colonic ischemia generally has a good prognosis, responding to supportive care (intravenous fluids, antibiotics). Angiography is of limited value in this clinical setting. (*Cecil, Ch. 106; Sleisenger and Fordtran, Ch. 101*)

135.(C) Because Henoch-Schönlein purpura involves primarily small vessels, intestinal involvement may be characterized by patchy lesions not conforming to the anatomic distribution of the major arteries. (*Cecil, Ch. 106; Sleisenger and Fordtran, Ch. 101*)

136.(E) Both the case history and serologic findings are compatible with acute non-A, non-B hepatitis. A 4-year-old girl would be unlikely to have had previous exposure to both hepatitis A and B, making choice A unlikely, and post-transfusion hepatitis type B is currently uncommon with routine serologic screening of donor units. (*Cecil, Ch. 121*)

137.(B) Both the case history and serologic findings suggest acute hepatitis A. (*Cecil, Ch. 121*)

138.(C) A mother with chronic hepatitis B virus infection who is also positive for HBeAg is most likely to transmit the infection to her baby. (*Cecil, Ch. 121*)

139.(G) Both the case history and serologic studies are compatible with an acute delta hepatitis superimposed on chronic hepatitis B virus infection. The negative IgM anti-HBc makes simultaneously acquired delta and B virus infection unlikely. (*Cecil, Ch. 121*)

140.(A) Both the case history and serologic studies are compatible with previous hepatitis A and B virus infection from which the patient has completely recovered. Exposure to both types of infection is common in adults from developing countries. (*Cecil, Ch. 121*)

141.(C); 142.(E); 143.(H); 144.(F); 145.(D) Dermatitis herpetiformis is a pruritic skin disorder characterized by vesicles and papules; it is associated in the majority of patients with an abnormality of the jejunal mucosa identical with that of gluten enteropathy (celiac disease). The small bowel lesion returns to normal after a gluten-free diet; although the skin disorder may require additional therapy, it may also respond to gluten restriction. Erythema nodosum is seen in approximately 9% of patients with Crohn's disease, while pyoderma gangrenosum is seen in nearly 5% of patients with ulcerative colitis and is characteristic of that disease. Acanthosis nigricans, a brown-black velvety skin change localized in the axillae, nuchal folds, or groin, is associated with underlying malignancies (e.g., gastric adenocarcinoma) that tend to be aggressive and rapidly fatal. Early recognition of this cutaneous sign warrants an immediate and thorough search for underlying pathology. Nodular fat necrosis is a systemic complication of acute pancreatitis. (*Cecil, Chs. 104, 105.2, 105.3, 108, and 534*)

146.(C) The film shows a large nodular gastric mass on the greater curvature in the antrum. Cytology or endoscopic biopsy will confirm the diagnosis. Gastric cancer claims more than 14,000 lives annually and accounts for almost 3% of all newly diagnosed cancers in the United States. In Japan, however, the incidence is much greater: The mortality from gastric carcinoma in Japanese males is 66/100,000. It appears that dietary habits may affect the development of gastric cancer. This has led to recommendations to decrease ingestion of smoked, salted, or nitrate-preserved foods and to maintain a diet high in fiber and low in fat, with increased amounts of vegetables and fresh fruits. (*Cecil, Ch. 99*)

147.(A) The film shows a Billroth II anastomosis with a stomal ulceration. These ulcerations are extremely difficult to demonstrate radiographically. Often, the diagnosis of a recurrent ulcer adjacent to a gastrojejunostomy requires endoscopy. Typically, these ulcers are resistant to medical management, and an additional gastric resection or search for a nontransected vagal branch must be undertaken. (*Cecil, Ch. 100.4*)

148.(B) This film shows an asymptomatic gastric polyp. Hyperplastic polyps are the most common gastric polyp and do not progress to malignancy. Adenomatous polyps are less common, are often found in the elderly, and are often associated with achlorhydria. Adenomatous polyps smaller than 2 cm rarely show malignant changes, but the incidence of malignancy increases with larger size, and polyps 2 cm or larger should be removed. Pedunculated polyps can be safely removed by snare-cautery technique via the fiberoptic endoscope. (*Cecil, Chs. 101 and 107*)

149.(E) The film shows large, thick gastric rugae. The low basal acid output and peak acid output are strongly compatible with the diagnosis of Menetrier's disease. Definitive diagnosis usually requires full-thickness mucosal biopsy. (*Cecil, Ch. 99; Scharschmidt*)

150.(D) The film shows a benign gastric ulcer on the lesser curvature of the stomach. Chronic gastric ulcer is a recurrent disease of the stomach generally confined to a nonacidsecreting mucosa of the antrum. The average patient with gastric ulcer is older than the average patient with duodenal ulceration. The acid secretory rate in patients with gastric ulcer tends to be normal or low. (*Cecil, Chs. 100.1 and 100.2*)

151.(C) Intestinal bacterial overgrowth leads to marked increases in breath hydrogen after ingestion of lactulose, and as a result of bacterial deconjugation of bile salts, leads to increased breath $^{14}CO_2$ expiration, after administration of ^{14}C-glycine-cholate. (*Cecil, Ch. 104; Sleisenger and Fordtran, Ch. 18*)

152.(A) Expired $^{14}CO_2$ will be elevated after ^{14}C-glycine-cholate ingestion in patients with disease (e.g., Crohn's disease), resection, or bypass of the terminal ileum. (*Cecil, Ch. 104; Sleisenger and Fordtran, Ch. 18*)

153.(B) The measurement of breath hydrogen following lactose ingestion is a sensitive and specific means of establishing carbohydrate malabsorption in lactase deficiency. (*Cecil, Ch. 104; Sleisenger and Fordtran, Ch. 18*)

154.(A) Acute appendicitis should be strongly suspected in this patient. The barium enema shows a marked shift of the entire right colon to the midline, with a mass distorting the cecal mucosa suggestive of abscess in this area. The periappendiceal abscess may occur relatively soon after the perforation of the appendix. (*Cecil, Ch. 115*)

155.(B) This patient has idiopathic ulcerative colitis. The barium enema shows abnormal mucosa from the proximal transverse to the sigmoid colon. The granularity, shallow ulcerations, loss of haustral markings, and extent of the changes are entirely compatible with this disorder. (*Cecil, Ch. 105.3*)

156.(D) The patient's family history is compatible with one of the familial colonic polyposis syndromes. The barium radiograph shows scores of small, uniform, 3- to 4-mm polypoid lesions throughout the colon. These are seen in familial polyposis or in Gardner's syndrome, both of which are associated with the development of colonic malignancy early in life. The polyps are adenomatous, and in patients with Gardner's syndrome they are accompanied by benign tumors of the skin, subcutaneous tissue, and bone. (*Cecil, Ch. 107; Sleisenger and Fordtran, Ch. 80*)

157.(E) The diagnosis of intestinal tuberculosis should be strongly entertained in this patient. Tuberculosis of the gastrointestinal tract typically will involve the area of the ileocecal valve and the ascending colon. The stomach, duodenum, and other areas of the colon can also be involved in the nodular hyperplastic scarring process. This radiograph shows focal constrictions of the ascending and transverse colon with normal intervening areas. The radiographic features of intestinal tuberculosis may be difficult to distinguish from Crohn's disease, although ileal involvement alone favors the latter diagnosis. (*Cecil, Chs. 105.2 and 302*)

158.(C) The clinical features described in this patient are strongly suggestive of acute diverticulitis. The barium radiograph shows a long area of narrowing of the sigmoid colon with thickened haustra. A small amount of contrast has extended outside the lumen of the sigmoid colon and is filling the cavity of a pelvic abscess. Several diverticula are visible in the transverse and descending colon. The extent of involvement, the spasm and edema, fistulization to the pelvis, and the presence of colonic diverticula all support the diagnosis. A perforating malignancy of the sigmoid colon occasionally may present with similar clinical and radiographic features. (*Cecil, Ch. 115*)

159.(A) This patient has giardiasis with mild steatorrhea. Villous atrophy can be seen in this disorder, although it is often patchy rather than diffuse. The histologic abnormalities as well as the clinical symptoms will respond to metronidazole (250 mg three times daily for 10 days) or quinacrine hydrochloride. Current opinion probably favors the use of quinacrine initially, although both agents are effective. (*Cecil, Ch. 104; Sleisenger and Fordtran, Ch. 62*)

160.(C) This patient has tropical sprue with evidence of a megaloblastic anemia and severe malabsorption. Although iron deficiency anemia may occur, megaloblastic anemia is characteristically seen in cases with a duration longer than six months. It is usually due to folate deficiency, although vitamin B_{12} deficiency may also occur. Tetracycline and folic acid are curative, although prolonged treatment (for up to one year) may be required. In patients with megaloblastic anemia, vitamin B_{12} replacement is also given initially. (*Cecil, Ch. 104; Sleisenger and Fordtran, Ch. 66; Klipstein*)

161.(D) This patient has adult celiac sprue, which will respond to a gluten-free diet. Although pancreatic insufficiency could occur in this setting, it does not result in a decreased D-xylose absorption, villous atrophy, or severe vitamin D and calcium malabsorption with osteomalacia. Kwashiorkor (protein malnutrition) can result in villous atrophy and malabsorption but requires a severely deficient diet and is most common in young children in developing countries. (*Cecil, Ch. 104; Sleisenger and Fordtran, Ch. 61*)

162.(B) The absence of a patent portal vein in this patient precludes the use of portosystemic shunt surgery to prevent further episodes of variceal bleeding. Therefore, variceal sclerotherapy is the best available option. (*Cecil, Ch. 127*)

163.(E) The reduction in formed elements in the blood which accompanies hypersplenism secondary to portal hypertension is usually not of clinical significance and therefore is not an indication for either splenectomy or portosystemic shunting. The former, in fact, carries an appreciable risk of portal venous system thrombosis in patients with portal hypertension, while the response of hypersplenism to the latter is highly variable. (*Cecil, Ch. 127*)

164.(E) Although the risk of variceal bleeding is universal in patients with large varices, four controlled trials of prophylactic portosystemic shunting failed to show any improvement in survival in patients with esophageal varices. A benefit from prophylactic sclerotherapy in patients with large varices that have never bled has been claimed in a few studies, but this is still highly controversial and the therapy is not currently recommended. (*Cecil, Ch. 127; Burroughs et al*)

165.(B) Emergency portosystemic shunting is associated with an unacceptably high operative mortality in Child's class C patients. Sclerotherapy has at least a 75% chance of controlling acute hemorrhage and is associated with a less than 10% incidence of serious complications or death; it is therefore the preferred form of therapy in this patient. (*Cecil, Ch. 127*)

166.(C) Bleeding esophagogastric varices may arise following splenic vein thrombosis in the absence of generalized portal hypertension. Splenectomy is usually curative. (*Cecil, Ch. 127*)

167.(E) Amebic colitis commonly occurs in travelers to underdeveloped areas of the world. Its signs and symptoms mimic those of ulcerative colitis. The biopsy shows a foreign population of large ovoid cells, some with multiple nuclei, surrounded by necrotic debris. These cells are trophozoites of *Entamoeba histolytica*. Grossly, the mucosa in these patients may range from nearly normal to diffusely ulcerative. The organisms are best demonstrated by microscopy of mucus aspirated from the base of the ulcerations. (*Cecil, Ch. 105.3 and 108; Sleisenger and Fordtran, Ch. 62*)

168.(D) This patient's history is very suggestive of idiopathic inflammatory bowel disease, specifically Crohn's disease. The colonic biopsy shows diffuse mucosal and submucosal inflammation, with two submucosal granulomas in the center of the field. Although not essential for the histologic diagnosis, submucosal granulomas without caseation are strongly suggestive of Crohn's disease. Additional histologic features that may be encountered are transmural inflammation and fibrosis. Multiple affected areas of the small and large bowel may be separated by areas of uninvolved bowel ("skip" lesions). (*Cecil, Ch. 105.2*)

169.(F) Frequent short-lived episodes of abdominal cramps with mucous and bloody stools in a young or middle-aged patient suggest ulcerative colitis. The biopsy shows submucosal inflammation and one large colonic crypt filled with polymorphonuclear leukocytes. This is a classic crypt abscess of acute ulcerative colitis. Crypt abscesses are occasionally seen in other conditions such as shigellosis, ischemia, toxin exposure, and other acute inflammatory diseases of the colon. In ulcerative colitis the crypt abscesses coalesce to form larger abscesses that ulcerate. (*Cecil, Ch. 105.3*)

170.(C) Schistosomiasis commonly presents with complications of portal hypertension. Hepatocellular function is largely preserved. The rectal biopsy shows numerous submucosal, darkly stained foreign bodies strongly suggestive of the ova of *Schistosoma mansoni*. The adult females, which may live for decades, reside in the inferior mesenteric venules around the rectosigmoid. Eggs deposited by the female erode through the submucosa to the mucosa and then are deposited in the stool. Colonic mucosal appearance ranges from normal to chronically inflamed with pseudopolypoid appearance. Rectal valve biopsy is a highly accurate means of diagnosis. (*Cecil, Ch. 400*)

171.(B) Intermittent hematochezia and/or iron deficiency anemia without altered bowel habits is the common clinical presentation of an adenomatous colonic polyp. The biopsy shows a small adenomatous polyp with characteristic branching glands in the polyp head and a sizeable stalk. The vast majority of colorectal polyps are adenomatous and benign; however, with increasing size, foci of carcinoma in situ can be demonstrated. Larger polyps (>2 cm diameter) have a higher rate of malignancy and are associated with superficial mucosal ulceration and iron deficiency anemia. In general, polyps larger than 1 cm in diameter should be removed, preferably by sigmoidoscopic or colonoscopic means. (*Cecil, Ch. 107*)

172.(A) The biopsy shows submucosal inflammation and focal areas of attachment of a superficial necrotic membrane consisting of leukocytes and fibrin; it is highly suggestive of pseudomembranous colitis. Ampicillin and other antibiotics have been associated with the overgrowth of *Clostridium difficile*. This organism produces an enterotoxin that causes damage throughout the colon, particularly in the rectosigmoid region of the bowel. (*Cecil, Ch. 279; Sleisenger and Fordtran, Ch. 69*)

173–177. The pentagastrin gastric acid secretion test is performed by first collecting the basal acid output from the stomach for one hour before the subcutaneous injection of pentagastrin. The upper limit of normal for a young male is 5 mEq/hr. After injection of pentagastrin, the peak acid output is determined as the sum of the two highest consecutive 15-minute collections multiplied by 2. The upper limit of normal for peak acid output for a young male is 40 mEq/hr. Basal serum gastrin levels are normally less than 100 pg/ml. After intravenous administration of secretin (GIH, 2 U/kg), serum gastrin levels increase by 200 pg/ml or more in patients with Zollinger-Ellison syndrome. In all other individuals, gastrin levels either decrease, remain unchanged, or increase only slightly after intravenous secretin. (*Cecil, Ch. 100; Sleisenger and Fordtran, Chs. 41, 47, and 49*)

173.(B) This patient has antral G-cell hyperfunction. Although histologically gastrin cell hyperplasia cannot be demonstrated in all cases, patients have elevated basal serum gastrin levels with either a decrease or a very slight increase in gastrin levels in response to intravenous secretin. In contrast to gastrinomas, there is a marked increase in serum gastrin levels in response to a test meal. Basal and peak acid outputs are correspondingly elevated, and peptic ulcer disease is believed to be secondary to this acid hypersecretion. (*Cecil, Ch. 100.2; Sleisenger and Fordtran, Ch. 49*)

174.(E) Both basal and peak acid outputs are elevated. These findings are commonly seen in patients with duodenal ulcer disease, although there is considerable overlap with normal individuals. (*Cecil, Ch. 100.2; Sleisenger and Fordtran, Chs. 47 and 49*)

175.(C) The basal serum gastrin level is elevated but there is no increase with intravenous secretin. Both the basal and peak acid outputs increased. In the setting of previous ulcer surgery, particularly with an antrectomy, these gastrin levels are inappropriately high. The findings suggest that the antrectomy was incomplete and there is retained gastric antrum. This remaining gastric antral tissue, when removed from the body of the stomach, continues to secrete gastrin in an uninhibited manner, since it does not come in contact with intraluminal acid. (*Cecil, Ch. 100.5; Sleisenger and Fordtran, Ch. 52*)

176.(A) An increase in serum gastrin levels greater than 200 pg/ml in response to intravenous secretin is virtually diagnostic of the Zollinger-Ellison syndrome. The presence of gastric acid hypersecretion is further confirmatory evidence of the diagnosis. Since there is chronic gastrin secretion, basal acid secretion is nearly maximal. A ratio of basal acid output (BAO) to peak acid output (PAO) of greater than 0.6 is strongly suggestive of a gastrin-producing tumor. This syndrome is manifested by a severe ulcer diathesis of which multiple peptic ulcers are a common feature. The abdominal ultrasound exam localized the tumor to the pancreas, which is the most common site of sporadic gastrinomas. (*Cecil, Chs. 100.2 and 100.6; Sleisenger and Fordtran, Chs. 49 and 52*)

177.(D) This patient has atrophic gastric mucosa and a gastric ulcer. This condition is almost invariably associated with achlorhydria; as a result, serum gastrin levels are elevated. It is not uncommon for patients to have pernicious anemia and other autoimmune phenomena such as Hashimoto's thyroiditis, hyperthyroidism, hypothyroidism, and insulin-dependent diabetes mellitus. (*Cecil, Ch. 99; Sleisenger and Fordtran, Chs. 46 and 48*)

178.(B) The rate of malignancy in villous adenomas is significantly higher than in adenomatous or mixed type polyps. Therefore, regardless of size, villous adenomas should be treated by complete excision. It is also important to note that the recurrence rate is very high, approximating 25%, and patients should be closely followed by colonoscopy or barium enema examination. (*Cecil, Ch. 107; Sleisenger and Fordtran, Ch. 80*)

179.(A) Peutz-Jeghers syndrome is a familial disease of mucocutaneous pigmentation and gastrointestinal polyposis. It is inherited in an autosomal dominant manner, as are all familial polyposis diseases. As early as infancy, melanin deposits are present around the mouth, nose, and perianal area and on the lips, buccal mucosa, hands, and feet. The polyps are hamartomas, in which glandular epithelium is surrounded by smooth muscle, and are distributed in the stomach, small intestine, and colon. These polyps are not true neoplasms and the incidence of carcinoma of the colon is low, being not more than 2–3%. (*Cecil, Ch. 107; Sleisenger and Fordtran, Ch. 80*)

180.(C) The Cronkhite-Canada syndrome is an acquired, nonfamilial polyposis characterized by polyps of the stomach, small bowel, and colon and by alopecia, hyperpigmentation, nail atrophy, and protein-losing enteropathy. The polyps are histologically similar to retention polyps with inflammatory and cystic elements. Although case reports have noted that some patients have colon cancer, there is little evidence that the polyps themselves are neoplastic. (*Cecil, Ch. 107; Sleisenger and Fordtran, Ch. 80*)

181.(D) Familial polyposis syndrome is an autosomal dominant disease with a high degree of penetrance, characterized by progressive development of hundreds of adenomatous polyps of the colon. Polyps usually develop after the second decade of life and progressively increase in number. Malignant transformation is inevitable if the entire colon is not removed. (*Cecil, Ch. 107; Sleisenger and Fordtran, Ch. 80*)

182.(D) Turcot's syndrome is a familial disease involving tumors of the gastrointestinal tract and central nervous system. Patients have adenomatous polyps scattered throughout the colon, and malignant gliomas, medulloblastomas, or ependymomas of the brain. The gastrointestinal polyps have a high rate of malignant transformation. (*Cecil, Ch. 107; Sleisenger and Fordtran, Ch. 80*)

BIBLIOGRAPHY

Bartlett JG, Moon N, Chang TW, et al: Role of *Clostridium difficile* in antibiotic-associated pseudomembranous colitis. Gastroenterology 75:778, 1978.

Bayless TM (ed): Current Therapy in Gastroenterology and Liver Disease. 2nd ed. Toronto, B. C. Decker Incorporated, 1986.

Black M, Mitchell JR, Zimmerman HJ, et al: Isoniazid-associated hepatitis in 114 patients. Gastroenterology 69:289, 1975.

Burroughs AK, D'Heygere F, McIntyre N: Pitfalls in studies of prophylactic therapy for variceal bleeding in cirrhotics. Hepatology 6:1407, 1986.

Busuttil RW, Goldstein LI, Danovitch GM, et al: Liver transplantation today. Ann Intern Med 104:377, 1986.

Cameron JL, Maddrey WC, Zuidema GD: Biliary tract disease in sickle cell anemia: Surgical considerations. Ann Surg 174:702, 1971.

Cecil Textbook of Medicine. 18th ed. Wyngaarden JB, Smith LH Jr (eds): Philadelphia, W. B. Saunders Company, 1988.

Cello JP, Crass RA, Grendell JM, et al: Management of the patient with hemorrhaging esophageal varices. JAMA 256:1480, 1986.

Dienstag JL: Non-A, non-B hepatitis. I. Recognition, epidemiology, and clinical features. Gastroenterology 85:439, 1983; Dienstag JL: Non-A, non-B hepatitis. II. Experimental transmission, putative virus agents and markers, and prevention. Gastroenterology 85:743, 1983.

DiMagno EP, Malagelada J-R, Taylor WF, et al: A prospective comparison of current diagnostic tests for pancreatic cancer. N Engl J Med 297:737, 1977.

Ishak KG: Laboratory Medicine. Hagerstown, Harper and Row, 1973, pp 1–48.

Klipstein FA: Tropical sprue in travelers and expatriates living abroad. Gastroenterology 80:590, 1981.

Meyer CT, Troncale FJ, Galloway S, et al: Arteriovenous malformations of the bowel: An analysis of 22 cases and a review of the literature. Medicine 60:36, 1981.

O'Dorisio TM, Mekhjian HS: VIPoma syndrome. *In* Cohen S, Soloway RD (eds): Hormone-Producing Tumors of the Gastrointestinal Tract. New York, Churchill Livingstone, 1985, pp 101–116.

Pitlik SD, Fainstein V, Garza D, et al: Human cryptosporidiosis: Spectrum of the disease: Report of six cases and review of the literature. Arch Intern Med 143:2269, 1983.

Purcell RH, Rizzetto M, Gerin JL: Hepatitis delta virus infection of the liver. Semin Liver Dis 4:340, 1984.

Rodgers VD, Kagnoff MF: Gastrointestinal manifestations of the acquired immunodeficiency syndrome [medical progress]. West J Med 146:57, 1987.

Salt WB II, Schenker S: Amylase—its clinical significance: A review of the literature. Medicine 55:269, 1976.

Scharschmidt BF, Goldberg HI, Schmid R: Current concepts in diagnosis. Approach to the patient with cholestatic jaundice. N Engl J Med 308:1515, 1983.

Schiff L, Schiff ER (eds): Diseases of the Liver. 6th ed. Philadelphia, J. B. Lippincott Company, 1987.

Sheehy TW: Sickle cell hepatopathy. South Med J 70:533, 1977.

Shepherd HA, Selby WS, Chapman RWG, et al: Ulcerative colitis and persistent liver dysfunction. Q J Med 52:503, 1983.

Sleisenger MH, Fordtran JS (eds): Gastrointestinal Disease: Pathophysiology, Diagnosis, Management. 4th ed. Philadelphia, W. B. Saunders Company, 1988.

Wright R, Alberti KGMM, Karran S, et al (eds): Liver and Biliary Disease: Pathophysiology, Diagnosis, Management. Philadelphia, W. B. Saunders Company, 1979.

Zakim D, Boyer TD (eds): Hepatology: A Textbook of Liver Disease. Philadelphia, W. B. Saunders Company, 1982.

PART 5

HEMATOLOGY AND ONCOLOGY

CHRISTOPHER C. BENZ and CHARLES A. LINKER

DIRECTIONS: For questions 1 to 29, choose the ONE BEST answer to each question.

1. Which of the following in NOT associated with an increased incidence of breast cancer?

A. Obesity
B. Early pregnancy
C. Previous history of breast cancer
D. Family history of breast cancer

2. The presence of which one of the following abnormalities would eliminate the need for staging laparotomy in a patient with Hodgkin's disease?

A. Pleural effusion
B. Abnormal lymphangiogram
C. Reed-Sternberg cells on bone marrow biopsy
D. Splenic enlargement

3. Which of the following statements regarding immune thrombocytopenia is most correct?

A. Palpable splenomegaly is frequently present
B. Splenectomy should be reserved as a treatment of last resort, to be used only after medical therapies have failed
C. Platelet transfusions should be used only for life-threatening bleeding
D. Medications that will cause thrombocytopenia will do so within two months of their use
E. Spherocytes are usually present on the peripheral blood smear

4. Which of the following statements most correctly describes aplastic anemia?

A. When caused by medications, it is usually self-limited
B. Severity of pancytopenia is *not* prognostically useful
C. Effective treatment is often available
D. It is caused by loss of pluripotent stem cells rather than immune suppression of hematopoiesis
E. The white blood cell count falls before the platelet count

5. Which of the following statements regarding histopathologic diagnosis and classification of Hodgkin's disease is correct?

A. Older patients with systemic symptoms are likely to have lymphocyte-predominant type
B. Patients between the ages of 15 and 35 years who have predominantly mediastinal involvement are likely to have nodular sclerosis type
C. presence of Reed-Sternberg cells in an appropriate histologic setting is *not* required for the diagnosis of Hodgkin's disease
D. The histopathologic subclassifications of lymphocyte-predominant type, nodular sclerosis type, mixed cellularity type, and lymphocyte-depletion type do *not* correlate with the natural history of the disease

6. Which statement concerning hereditary spherocytosis is correct?

A. Many cases go undetected until adulthood
B. Spherocytes usually comprise 10% or more of the red blood cells on the peripheral smear
C. The spherocytes of hereditary spherocytosis can be distinguished from the spherocytes of autoimmune hemolytic anemia by the osmotic fragility test
D. Splenectomy usually eliminates spherocytes from the peripheral blood smear
E. Splenomegaly is rarely present

7. Which of the following best establishes a diagnosis of von Willebrand's disease?

A. Prolonged bleeding time and prolonged partial thromboplastin time (PTT)
B. Low level of Factor VIII coagulant activity
C. Abnormal multimeric pattern of Factor VIII antigen on agarose gel
D. Prolonged bleeding time following aspirin
E. Giant platelets on smear

8. Which statement concerning pernicious anemia is correct?

A. A normal MCV excludes the diagnosis
B. Neurologic signs may antedate significant anemia
C. Ileal absorption of the vitamin B_{12}-intrinsic factor complex is reduced
D. Non-Europeans are rarely affected
E. Gastric adenocarcinoma commonly occurs

9. Which statement best characterizes iron metabolism?

A. The majority of total body iron is stored in conjugates of ferritin
B. Absorption of iron from heme sources in food is independent of phytates and vegetable fiber

C. Absorption of iron occurs throughout the gastrointestinal tract
D. Transferrin is essential for iron absorption
E. Ferrous gluconate is more easily absorbed than ferrous sulfate

QUESTIONS 10–11

A 56-year-old Caucasian man with a prior history of alcoholism comes to you because of weight loss and right upper quadrant abdominal pain.

10. Which of the following findings consistent with tumor involving the liver would be most useful in diagnosing primary hepatocellular carcinoma?

A. Hepatomegaly with elevated carcinoembryonic antigen, anemia, and elevated alkaline phosphatase
B. Physical stigmata of cirrhosis associated with hypercholesterolemia and hepatitis B antigenemia
C. Erythrocytosis and a markedly elevated alpha-fetoprotein
D. Bloody ascites and multiple defects on technetium-^{99}m sulfur colloid liver scan

Chest roentgenogram is normal and there is no evidence of adenopathy or ascites. Radionuclide scan reveals a superficial, localized defect in the right hepatic lobe, which after percutaneous needle biopsy is described as "probable hepatocellular carcinoma."

11. Which of the following courses of action is most appropriate at this time?

A. Inform the patient and family that expected survival with this diagnosis is six months and that treatment with doxorubicin (Adriamycin) may produce tumor regression
B. Continue investigations to look for evidence of metastatic disease
C. Request angiography to further delineate the hepatic lesion
D. Request laparoscopy with directed needle biopsy to absolutely rule out a non-neoplastic hepatic lesion

12. Which statement BEST describes glucose-6-phosphate dehydrogenase (G6PD) deficiency?

A. Affected American blacks have a mild chronic hemolytic disorder that can be markedly exacerbated by exposure to certain drugs
B. One per cent of American black males are affected
C. The diagnosis is best made in the absence of hemolytic crisis
D. Heinz bodies may be present on the Wright-stained blood smear
E. Mediterranean variants of G6PD are usually clinically insignificant

13. Which of the following is most specific for the diagnosis of disseminated intravascular coagulation (DIC)?

A. Decreased fibrinogen
B. Prolonged thrombin time
C. Elevated fibrin split products
D. Prolonged euglobulin clot lysis time
E. Fragmented red blood cells on peripheral blood smear

14. Which of the following statements regarding colorectal carcinoma is correct?

A. Hematochezia may be an early clinical sign but is *not* helpful in localizing the portion of the colon involved
B. Tumors of the ileum and ascending colon tend to present earlier than left-sided colonic tumors
C. Surgery is *not* helpful in the management of patients presenting with evidence of tumor spread beyond the bowel wall
D. Radiation therapy is the most useful treatment for local recurrences, while chemotherapy is more effective for distant metastases

15. Which of the following best EXCLUDES a diagnosis of classic hemophilia A (Factor VIII_c deficiency)?

A. Absence of family history
B. Absence of bleeding episodes
C. Absence of bleeding after surgery
D. Normal partial thromboplastin time (PTT)
E. Normal prothrombin time (PT)

16. Which statement best describes autoimmune hemolytic anemia?

A. Penicillin may induce an autoantibody directed against the Rh locus
B. Erythrocytes coated with C3b are preferentially sequestered in the spleen
C. The presence of spherocytes suggests an underlying congenital hemolytic disorder
D. The finding of complement alone in the direct Coombs' test suggests an IgM-mediated disorder
E. Penicillin is the drug most commonly associated with a positive Coombs' test

17. Which of the following statements regarding the pharmacologic management of pain in a cancer patient is most appropriate?

A. When attempting to control mild to moderate pain from tumor infiltration, it is best to start with aspirin rather than acetaminophen because there may be a significant inflammatory component to the pain
B. If aspirin, 650 mg every 4 hours, is insufficient for analgesia, it is best to try adding pentazocine, 50 mg every 4–6 hours, because it has no potential for addiction
C. In the home care of a patient with advancing disease and severe pain, it is better to prescribe high doses of oral narcotics at infrequent intervals to avoid the problem of increasing drug tolerance and physical dependence
D. The addition of a phenothiazine or amitriptyline to a regularly administered narcotic dose is likely to substantially reduce the narcotic dose required

18. Which statement regarding the role of vitamin K in coagulation is correct?

A. Dietary deficiency is a common cause of vitamin K deficiency
B. Vitamin K alone cannot overcome the anticoagulant effect of warfarin
C. Postoperative antibiotic therapy is commonly implicated in causing vitamin K deficiency

D. Treatment of the vitamin K–deficient state allows new hepatic protein synthesis to occur
E. Treatment with vitamin K must be given parenterally

19. Which statement best characterizes sickle cell anemia and related syndromes?

A. Splenic sequestration crises are rare in adults with hemoglobin SS disease
B. Persons with sickle cell trait may be mildly anemic, but significant anemia should be investigated for a secondary cause
C. Persons with sickle cell trait may have mild renal insufficiency related to microinfarctions of the renal medulla
D. Patients with sickle cell anemia (hemoglobin SS) may have hemolytic crises due to folic acid deficiency or a viral infection
E. Sickled cells are rarely seen on the blood smear during asymptomatic periods

20. Which of the following is an indication for splenectomy in a patient with Felty's syndrome?

A. Thrombocytopenia
B. Worsening of arthritis
C. Recurrent bacterial infection
D. Neutrophil count less than 0.5×10^9/liter
E. Positive rheumatoid factor

21. Which statement best describes the anemia of renal failure?

A. Iron stores in the bone marrow are characteristically decreased
B. Dialysis may lead to loss of iron but not folate or vitamin B_{12}
C. Red blood cells in these patients have decreased survival when transfused to normal recipients
D. Purified erythropoietin will reliably eliminate the need for red blood cell transfusion due to renal failure
E. More frequent dialysis may correct the anemia

22. Which statement best characterizes adult hemolytic uremic syndrome (HUS)?

A. It responds to treatment with heparin
B. Renal failure is almost always reversible
C. It is associated with pregnancy and estrogen use
D. It differs hematologically from thrombotic thrombocytopenic purpura (TTP) in that the hemolytic anemia is less severe
E. The peripheral blood smear distinguishes the disorder from disseminated intravascular coagulation (DIC)

23. Which statement best characterizes chronic lymphocytic leukemia (CLL)?

A. Paraproteins secreted by the malignant cells may cause hyperviscosity
B. Patients with early-stage disease (Rai stage 0 to 1) have median survivals of 3–4 years
C. Patients with bone marrow failure due to infiltration of lymphocytes should be treated with chemotherapy
D. White blood cell counts over 200,000/mm^3 should be treated emergently with leukapheresis
E. The malignant cell is usually a T lymphocyte

QUESTIONS 24–27

A 45-year-old woman has a left breast mass, which she discovered by self-examination. She is relatively certain that the nodule was not present two months ago. She is otherwise without symptoms. On physical examination, a firm 2- by 4-cm nodule is present in the upper outer quadrant of the left breast.

24. Which of the following groups of diagnostic procedures is most appropriate in the initial preoperative evaluation?

A. Roentgenogram of the chest, serum alkaline phosphatase
B. Roentgenograms of the chest and skeleton, radionuclide bone scan
C. Roentgenogram of the chest, radionuclide bone scan, serum alkaline phosphatase
D. Roentgenogram of the chest, radionuclide bone scan, bone marrow biopsy

25. Biopsy of the lesion reveals moderately well-differentiated carcinoma, and the tumor is found to be estrogen receptor–positive. The patient undergoes mastectomy but refuses further therapy; eight months later she begins to have rib pain. Bone scan is positive in multiple areas, and biopsy of the rib lesion reveals metastatic adenocarcinoma. Which one of the following forms of therapy would you choose?

A. Chemotherapy alone
B. Surgical oophorectomy alone
C. Surgical oophorectomy and chemotherapy
D. Local radiation therapy to painful bone lesions alone

26. The patient receives appropriate therapy but continues to have pain, which is well controlled with oxycodone (Percodan). Two weeks later she develops gastrointestinal bleeding requiring multiple red cell transfusions. Which of the following statements regarding gastrointestinal bleeding in this patient is correct?

A. Breast cancer rarely metastasizes to the gastrointestinal tract
B. Since the pain is well controlled with Percodan, this medication should be continued
C. Platelet function studies will probably be normal
D. Stress ulcers are common in this type of patient

27. The gastrointestinal bleeding stops. The patient refuses further chemotherapy. Which of the following courses of action is most appropriate?

A. Advise her that an adequate trial of chemotherapy has not been completed and that you will be unable to treat her further unless she agrees to follow your instructions
B. Although an adequate trial of chemotherapy has not been completed, you should agree to continue to provide her with symptomatic care, and the possibility of subsequent chemotherapy should not be discussed further
C. You should agree to withhold chemotherapy but provide whatever supportive care seems appropriate; it is also appropriate to discuss the possibility of continuing chemotherapy on subsequent visits
D. Obtain a psychiatric consultation

28. Which of the following statements regarding estrogen receptors in breast tumors is correct?

A. Measurement of estrogen receptors in human breast tumors is principally a research tool with little clinical application as yet
B. Lack of estrogen receptors in tumors of premenopausal women means that hormone manipulation will have a less than 10% chance of being beneficial
C. The presence of estrogen receptors in tumors of premenopausal women means that hormonal manipulation has a greater than 90% chance of being beneficial
D. If a primary tumor has estrogen receptors, metastatic tumors can also be expected to have them

29. Which statement best describes the anemia of chronic disease?

A. It is usually microcytic
B. The peripheral blood smear shows red cell fragments
C. Examination of the bone marrow will differentiate it from iron deficiency anemia
D. The red blood cell survival is normal and anemia is caused by decreased production
E. The reticulocyte count distinguishes it from iron deficiency

DIRECTIONS: For questions 30 to 74, you are to decide whether EACH choice is true or false. Any combination of answers, from all true to all false, may occur. Mark the answer sheet "T" or "F" in the space provided.

30. Which of the following findings would be useful in differentiating a leukemoid reaction from chronic myelogenous leukemia (CML)?

A. Anemia
B. Splenic enlargement
C. Elevated leukocyte alkaline phosphatase
D. Bone marrow hypercellularity with an increase in granulocyte precursors
E. Elevated platelet count

31. Which of the following statements regarding transfusion reactions is/are true?

A. Anaphylaxis is usually caused by plasma proteins or drugs rather than by cellular elements
B. Severe leukoagglutinin reactions may cause pulmonary infiltrates and hemolysis
C. Hemolytic transfusion reactions can be differentiated from leukoagglutinin reactions by the absence of fever
D. Delayed hemolytic transfusion reactions can be identified by the presence of a new alloantibody at the time of hemolysis

32. Which of the following statements regarding idiopathic thrombocytopenic purpura (ITP) is/are correct?

A. Platelet survival time is decreased in patients with ITP
B. Infants born to women with ITP are frequently thrombocytopenic
C. Cultured splenic cells of patients with ITP produce antiplatelet antibodies
D. Infusion of plasma from patients with ITP produces severe thrombocytopenia in normal subjects

QUESTIONS 33–34

A 37-year-old woman with occasional postcoital spotting was found to have grade III cervical cytology on Pap smear. No other abnormality was detected after complete physical exam including bimanual pelvic exam.

33. Which of the following statements concerning the findings in this patient is/are correct?

A. Without any treatment, this lesion is likely to develop into cervical carcinoma
B. The patient's risk of developing cervical carcinoma may be increased by multiple sexual partners
C. Culdoscopy with punch biopsy is the most appropriate next step for assessment of this patient
D. It is possible that this represents cervicitis or *Trichomonas* infection and the smear should be repeated in six months

34. If this patient were later found to have invasive cervical carcinoma, which of the following statements would be true?

A. Endocervical curettage should be performed
B. Squamous cell carcinoma would be the most likely histologic type
C. Initial studies to define the extent of the neoplasm should also include a bone scan
D. Primary treatment would probably include either surgery and/or radiation therapy, but *not* chemotherapy

35. Prolongation of the template bleeding time may be caused by which of the following?

A. Uremia
B. Liver disease
C. Essential thrombocytosis
D. Platelet storage pool disease
E. Hereditary hemorrhagic telangiectasia

QUESTIONS 36–37

A 63-year-old male construction worker reports an ulcerated nodule bordering the lower lip. Biopsy reveals cancer.

36. Which of the following statements concerning skin cancers is/are correct?

A. Basal cell carcinoma is more likely than squamous cell carcinoma to arise in an area of chronic actinic damage
B. Local recurrences are of little concern if the primary lesion is completely excised and the patient avoids further solar exposure to the area
C. In areas where surgical excision is difficult or cosmetically undesirable, x-ray therapy is the treatment of choice
D. Metastatic disease following complete excision of a squamous cell carcinoma occurring in the location described above is rare

37. Which of the following statements regarding the diagnosis of a melanomatous lesion in this patient is/are correct?

A. A pigmented freckle may have been spreading superficially for years before nodularity and ulceration appeared
B. Anatomic location of the tumor, age of the patient, and type of melanoma are the primary determinants of the five-year prognosis
C. Radiation therapy should be administered subsequent to surgical resection, since the location of this lesion precludes wide local excision of the tumor
D. Further investigations to search for metastatic disease should be done at this time

38. In patients with a history suggesting a bleeding disorder, but with normal screening tests for hemostasis (prothrombin time, partial thromboplastin time, platelet count, bleeding time), which of the following disorders is/are likely?

A. Von Willebrand's disease
B. Factor X deficiency
C. Factor XIII deficiency
D. Glanzmann's thrombasthenia
E. Lupus anticoagulant

39. Which of the following statements regarding primary neoplasms of the small intestine is/are correct?

A. Premalignant conditions for some small bowel cancers include Crohn's disease and gluten-sensitive enteropathy
B. Primary adenocarcinomas are unusual; the most commonly encountered malignant tumors are metastatic

C. Small bowel tumors usually present with obstructive jaundice or flank pain
D. Unlike large bowel neoplasms, prognosis depends primarily on tumor type

40. Which of the following statements regarding neoplasms of the large intestine is/are correct?

A. The most common histopathologic type is epidermoid or squamous cell carcinoma
B. The colon is a common site of metastases from primary breast and lung carcinomas
C. History of increased dietary fat, decreased dietary fiber, ulcerative colitis, and first-degree relatives with colon cancer are each strong risk factors for the development of primary colon cancer
D. It is recommended that asymptomatic polyps be removed because of the association between colonic polyps and cancer of the colon

41. In comparing the clinical bleeding patterns caused by platelet versus coagulation defects, which of the following statements is/are correct?

A. Petechiae indicate a platelet disorder
B. Platelet bleeding tends to be more delayed
C. Hemarthroses are seen almost exclusively in congenital disorders of coagulation
D. Bleeding after tooth extractions is suggestive primarily of a platelet disorder
E. Aspirin is contraindicated only in platelet disorders

42. Which of the following statements regarding thrombotic thrombocytopenic purpura (TTP) is/are true?

A. Fever seen in patients with TTP is usually due to infection
B. The prothrombin time and partial thromboplastin time should be normal
C. Fragmentation of red blood cells on the peripheral smear suggests concomitant disseminated intravascular coagulation
D. The outcome of treatment is usually poor

43. Which of the following statements regarding aplastic anemia is/are true?

A. In most cases, a causative factor cannot be identified
B. Autoimmune hemolytic anemia may terminate in aplastic anemia
C. Aplastic anemia may be a complication during the first month of viral hepatitis
D. Antithymocyte globulin (ATG) is the treatment of choice for patients with severe aplastic anemia for whom bone marrow transplantation is not available

44. Which of the following statements regarding radiation therapy is/are correct?

A. When treating a brain tumor, it is of little clinical significance whether a kilovoltage x-ray source or a gamma radiation (cobalt-60) source is used to deliver a prescribed dose to the tumor volume
B. The formation of intracellular hydroxyl radicals and overall biologic effectiveness of radiation therapy are enhanced by hypoxic conditions
C. Because tumor cells have some ability to repair DNA breaks from radiation, it is generally better to administer a therapeutic dose in a single large fraction rather than multiple small fractions
D. The liver's poor tolerance to radiation usually prevents treatment of hepatic metastases by radiation therapy

45. Which of the following statements regarding agnogenic myeloid metaplasia is/are true?

A. Osteosclerosis commonly occurs
B. Lytic bone lesions lead to pathologic fracture
C. The Philadelphia chromosome is present in some cases
D. Abnormal red blood cell morphology (tear drops, nucleated red blood cells) suggests impending conversion to acute leukemia

46. Which of the following statements regarding "adjuvant chemotherapy" is/are correct?

A. This therapy is not curative, as it is designed to palliate patients from the symptomatic effects of disseminated malignancy
B. Adjuvant therapy has been most helpful in patients with breast cancer, sarcomas, and solid tumors of childhood
C. Beneficial effects from adjuvant therapy depend on dose intensity, and this can be associated with some life-threatening risks
D. Benefit from adjuvant chemotherapy is more likely when single rather than combination drug therapy is administered

47. Which of the following statements about antithrombin III is/are correct?

A. It inhibits activated clotting factors other than thrombin
B. Heparin is totally ineffective as an anticoagulant in its absence
C. Congenital deficiency is associated with a risk of bleeding
D. Warfarin therapy may produce falsely elevated levels

48. Which of the following statements regarding the lupus anticoagulant is/are true?

A. The partial thromboplastin time will be prolonged and will not be corrected by the addition of equal amounts of normal plasma
B. Patients with this defect have an excessive risk of both bleeding and clotting
C. The prothrombin time is usually normal or only minimally prolonged
D. Prednisone therapy of a patient with lupus will quickly eliminate this anticoagulant

49. Which of the following statements regarding histiocytic (diffuse, large-cell) lymphoma is/are true?

A. Complete response to chemotherapy with a prolonged, disease-free interval occurs in over 50% of patients
B. When it is isolated to one anatomic area, radiation therapy alone may be indicated
C. It may present with signs and symptoms of gastric carcinoma
D. It frequently progresses to a leukemic phase late in the course of disease

50. Which of the following statements about nodular non-Hodgkin's lymphoma is/are true?

A. Chemotherapy frequently produces complete remission
B. Five-year survival is greater than for diffuse non-Hodgkin's lymphoma
C. It is frequently localized to one lymph node area (stage I)
D. It frequently involves mesenteric lymph nodes

51. Which of the following statements regarding iron deficiency is/are true?

A. It is commonly caused by dietary deficiency
B. It is the most common cause of anemia among hospitalized patients in the United States
C. Oral iron repletion will correct the anemia in six months
D. Giving medicinal iron concurrent with meals nearly eliminates its usefulness

52. Which of the following statements regarding hypercalcemia of neoplastic disease is/are correct?

A. Hypercalcemia in association with neoplasms of the lung indicates metastatic disease
B. Unlike primary hyperparathyroidism, this form of hypercalcemia is usually asymptomatic
C. Serum level of immunoreactive parathyroid hormone is usually normal
D. Treatment consists of eradicating the underlying neoplasm

53. Which of the following statements regarding neutropenia is/are correct?

A. It is commonly associated with megaloblastic anemia
B. Its occurrence during chlorpromazine therapy does *not* contraindicate further use of the drug
C. Its occurrence during chloramphenicol therapy does *not* contraindicate further use of the drug
D. Some patients with severe congenital neutropenia have a benign clinical course

QUESTIONS 54–55

A 26-year-old woman has noted painless swelling in the left neck and axilla. On physical examination, enlarged, painless, discrete lymph nodes are palpable in the left cervical, supraclavicular, and axillary regions.

54. Which of the following findings would be useful in distinguishing Hodgkin's disease from non-Hodgkin's lymphoma in this patient?

A. Involvement of the oropharynx or nasopharynx
B. Spinal cord compression from extradural tumor
C. Involvement of mesenteric lymph nodes
D. Autoimmune hemolytic anemia

55. Which of the following diagnostic procedures would be useful in determining the extent of Hodgkin's disease in this patient?

A. Brain scan
B. Lymphangiogram
C. Bone marrow biopsy
D. Computed tomogram (CT scan) of the chest, abdomen, and pelvis

56. Which statement(s) regarding adult acute nonlymphocytic leukemia is/are correct?

A. An environmental cause is often evident
B. Circulating blasts are almost invariably present on the peripheral blood smear
C. A white blood count in excess of 200,000/mm^3 should be reduced slowly
D. Disseminated intravascular coagulation suggests coexistent infection
E. Treatment of young adults is now given with curative intent

57. Which of the following is/are likely to be useful in predicting relapse in patients with previously treated Hodgkin's disease?

A. Serum protein electrophoresis
B. Erythrocyte sedimentation rate
C. Leukocyte alkaline phosphatase
D. Serum copper
E. Urinary lysozyme

58. Which statement(s) is/are true of both chronic myeloid leukemia (CML) and chronic lymphoid leukemia (CLL)?

A. Many patients are asymptomatic at diagnosis when an elevated white blood count is found
B. They terminate as an aggressive lymphoid malignancy
C. Patients with favorable prognostic indicators frequently survive 10 years or longer
D. Splenic enlargement is common
E. Staging is useful in making treatment decisions

59. Which of the following drug-induced toxicities is/are clinically preventable *without* modifying dose or scheduling?

A. Vincristine alopecia
B. Methotrexate mucositis
C. Cisplatin nephropathy
D. Doxorubicin (Adriamycin) cardiotoxicity
E. 5-Fluorouracil myelosuppression

60. Which of the following statements regarding hairy cell leukemia is/are true?

A. Splenectomy may be a useful therapy when the bone marrow is completely replaced with malignant cells
B. The leukocyte alkaline phosphatase level is useful in establishing a diagnosis
C. Prolonged survival is common
D. Thrombocytopenia usually does not occur until late in the course of the disease

61. Which of the following immune abnormalities is/are associated with untreated Hodgkin's disease?

A. Impaired skin tests and mitogen-induced lymphocyte transformation
B. Lymphopenia with hypogammaglobulinemia
C. Immune hemolytic anemia or thrombocytopenia
D. Delayed risk of severe bacterial infection

62. Which of the following statements regarding the bone disease of multiple myeloma is/are true?

A. Bone scan is more sensitive than radiography in diagnosing early lesions
B. The presence of bone disease does *not* correlate with prognosis
C. Prednisone is not useful in treating hypercalcemia
D. Radiotherapy may be indicated both to palliate painful lesions and to prevent pathologic fractures

63. Which of the following statements regarding human chorionic gonadotropin (HCG) is/are correct?

A. HCG measurements are extremely important in the management of patients with trophoblastic tumors
B. Specific sensitive assays for this glycoprotein require antisera directed against the beta subunit of the molecule
C. HCG and alpha-fetoprotein always rise and fall simultaneously in the plasma of patients with trophoblastic tumors
D. HCG may be detected in patients with gastric or pancreatic cancer

64. Which of the following statements regarding primary "immunocytic" amyloid is/are correct?

A. The tongue is usually *not* involved
B. Heart disease is a more common cause of death than renal failure
C. The disease is likely to respond to colchicine
D. The ultrastructural appearance of the amyloid distinguishes this from secondary amyloid

65. Which of the following statements correctly describe(s) ways of differentiating iron deficiency from other causes of anemia?

A. Significant microcytosis occurs in iron deficiency only after significant anemia has developed
B. At comparable levels of anemia, the peripheral smear is more abnormal in iron deficiency than in thalassemia
C. A microcytic anemia with normal levels of hemoglobin A_2 and hemoglobin F is most likely iron deficiency and not thalassemia
D. Target cells and nucleated red blood cells may be seen in severe iron deficiency

66. Which of the following statements regarding subtypes of acute leukemia is/are true?

A. Terminal deoxynucleotidyl transferase (TdT) is present in nearly all cases of adult and childhood acute lymphoblastic leukemia (ALL)
B. T-cell ALL is associated with high white blood cell counts, mediastinal masses, and risk of central nervous system disease
C. Presence of Auer rods correlates with gum infiltration
D. Presence of the Philadelphia chromosome is associated with good long-term prognosis

67. Which of the following statements regarding cancer of the prostate is/are correct?

A. Every reasonable measure should be taken to eradicate a tumor that is localized to the pelvis
B. Prostatic acid phosphatase is elevated in the serum of about 90% of patients with prostate cancer
C. LHRH analogues are as effective as estrogen therapy or orchiectomy in patients with metastatic disease
D. Endocrine therapy (e.g., orchiectomy) prolongs survival in about 50% of patients with metastatic disease

68. Which of the following statements regarding thalassemia is/are true?

A. Beta-thalassemia causes more intramedullary hemolysis and subsequent bone deformity than does alpha-thalassemia
B. The longevity of patients receiving transfusion therapy is limited primarily by the development of alloantibodies that make transfusion difficult
C. Cardiac disease can be avoided if transfusion is used to avoid prolonged severe anemia
D. Hemoglobin electrophoresis is a useful way of distinguishing alpha- from beta-thalassemia

69. Which of the following immunologic complications is/are associated with chronic lymphocytic leukemia?

A. Hypogammaglobulinemia
B. Autoimmune hemolytic anemia
C. Autoimmune thrombocytopenia
D. Monoclonal immunoglobulinopathy

70. Which of the following statements regarding sarcoma is/are correct?

A. It is best treated by amputation when it occurs in a limb
B. In an adult with bone pain, it may be misdiagnosed as Paget's disease
C. When associated with other malignancies, it usually originates in a previously irradiated area
D. It is the likely diagnosis for a large intramural filling defect with normal gastroscopic exam, presenting as a painless epigastric mass

71. Which of the following statements regarding megaloblastic anemia is/are true?

A. Dietary deficiency is rarely the cause of vitamin B_{12} deficiency
B. A low serum folate level in a patient with vitamin B_{12} deficiency suggests concomitant folate deficiency
C. Hyperkalemia may occur during vitamin B_{12} deficiency
D. Macrocytic anemia without macro-ovalocytes or hypersegmented neutrophils is most likely not due to vitamin B_{12} or folic acid deficiency

72. Which of the following findings is/are useful in distinguishing acute myelogenous leukemia from acute lymphoblastic leukemia?

A. Positive staining of the leukemic cells with peroxidase and Sudan black
B. Presence of terminal deoxyribose transferase (TDT) in the leukemic cells
C. The morphologic finding of Auer rods on blood smear
D. Severe anemia and thrombocytopenia

73. Which of the following is/are associated with pure red cell aplasia?

A. Thymoma
B. Acute leukemia
C. Low serum erythropoietin levels
D. Serum antibodies directed against red cell precursors

74. Which of the following statements concerning polycythemia vera is/are true?

A. Most patients with hematocrit greater than 65% have polycythemia vera
B. An enlarged spleen should lead to the evaluation of a secondary cause of polycythemia
C. Lowering the hematocrit reduces the risk of thrombosis
D. The syndrome of erythromelalgia (painful red hands) should be treated with aspirin

DIRECTIONS: Questions 75 to 135 are matching questions. For each numbered item, choose the most likely associated lettered item from those provided. Each numbered item has ONLY ONE answer. Within each set of questions, each lettered item may be the answer to one, more than one, or none of the numbered items.

QUESTIONS 75–84

For each of the following malignancies, select the carcinogenic agent with which it is most likely to be associated.

A. Asbestos
B. Estrogens
C. Tobacco smoke
D. Schistosomiasis
E. Epstein-Barr virus
F. Ionizing radiation
G. Ultraviolet radiation
H. Mold from *Aspergillus flavus*

75. Melanoma

76. Thyroid carcinoma

77. Pancreatic carcinoma

78. Nasopharyngeal carcinoma

79. Endometrial carcinoma

80. Hepatocellular carcinoma

81. Squamous carcinoma of the bladder

82. Leukemia

83. Mesothelioma

84. Head and neck carcinoma

QUESTIONS 85–88

For each of the descriptions below, select the most appropriate disorder (A–D).

A. Essential thrombocytosis
B. Bernard-Soulier syndrome
C. Glanzmann's thrombasthenia
D. Storage pool disease

85. Normal in vitro platelet aggregation to collagen

86. Defective clot retraction

87. Associated with thromboses

88. "Aspirin-like" defect

QUESTIONS 89–96

For each of the following clinicopathologic descriptions, select the most likely associated type of non-Hodgkin's lymphoma (Rappaport classification).

A. Nodular lymphocytic, poorly differentiated type
B. Histiocytic type
C. Undifferentiated, Burkitt's type
D. Lymphoblastic type

89. Infiltrate of large, irregular, cleaved or noncleaved cells derived from lymphoid elements, usually occurring in a diffuse pattern and frequently appearing in an extranodal site

90. Diffuse pattern of aggressively disseminating T cells with round or convoluted nuclei and scanty cytoplasm, often presenting as a localized mediastinal mass

91. Infiltrates of small, cleaved, and variably sized cells of B cell origin, usually presenting in adult life as asymptomatic lymphadenopathy

92. Radiosensitive, slowly progressive lymphoma associated with prolonged survival despite early dissemination to liver, bone marrow, and peripheral blood

93. Occurring in children and young adults; when untreated, there is rapid dissemination to peripheral blood and meninges, with a median survival time of less than one year

94. Rapidly growing, diffuse infiltrate of large, uniform, and noncleaved B cells; often presenting as an abdominal mass in children

95. Occurring predominantly in later adult years; potentially curable when drug combinations that include doxorubicin are used

96. Surgery and chemotherapy with cyclophosphamide-containing drug combinations are used for effective primary treatment

QUESTIONS 97–100

For each of the following features, select the lettered item with which it is most likely to be associated.

A. Risk of bleeding
B. Risk of thrombosis
C. Risk of anaphylaxis
D. Treatment of gastric ulcers
E. Treatment of massive pulmonary embolus

97. Alpha$_2$ antiplasmin deficiency

98. Epsilon-amino caproic acid (EACA)

99. Streptokinase

100. Urokinase

QUESTIONS 101–105

Match each of the following neoplasms with the most likely associated cutaneous lesion.

A. Vitiligo
B. Ichthyosis
C. Café-au-lait spots
D. Acanthosis nigricans
E. Dermatitis herpetiformis
F. Necrolytic migratory erythema
G. Ash-leaf pattern of hypomelanosis

101. Gastric adenocarcinoma

102. Lymphoma or multiple myeloma

103. Angiofibromas and renal hamartoma

104. Glucagon-secreting pancreatic carcinoma

105. Soft tissue sarcomas or pheochromocytoma

QUESTIONS 106–109

For each of the findings below, select the condition with which it is most likely to be associated.

A. Homozygous SS disease
B. Heterozygous hemoglobin S plus alpha-thalassemia
C. Heterozygous hemoglobin S plus beta^{+}-thalassemia
D. Heterozygous hemoglobin S plus hereditary persistence of fetal hemoglobin
E. Hemoglobin SC disease

106. Hemoglobin A present

107. Hemoglobin S present, but less than 40%

108. Hyposplenism

109. Ocular complications

QUESTIONS 110–112

For each of the following diseases, select the most likely chromosomal abnormality.

A. Deletions of chromosome 5 and/or 7
B. Hyperdiploidy with more than 50 chromosomes
C. Translocation of the *abl* oncogene from chromosome 9 to chromosome 22
D. Translocation of the *myc* oncogene from chromosome 8 to the heavy chain immunoglobulin locus on chromosome 14

110. Burkitt's lymphoma

111. Acute myeloid leukemia (AML) following chemotherapy

112. Chronic myeloid leukemia (CML)

QUESTIONS 113–117

For each of the following characteristics, select the most likely type of lung cancer.

A. Oat cell carcinoma of the lung
B. Epidermoid carcinoma of the lung
C. Associated approximately equally with both of these
D. Not associated with either of these

113. Hypercalcemia

114. Carcinomatous meningitis

115. One-year history of abnormal sputum cytology without localization of primary tumor

116. Surgery most effective therapy, with overall five-year survival rate of 10–15%

117. Greater than 50% objective response rate to cytotoxic chemotherapy

QUESTIONS 118–121

For each of the following protein abnormalities, select the most likely disorder.

A. Multiple myeloma
B. Primary amyloidosis
C. Waldenström's macroglobulinemia
D. Benign monoclonal gammopathy

118. Free kappa chains in urine

119. IgM-kappa serum paraprotein

120. IgA-lambda serum paraprotein

121. Lytic bone disease

QUESTIONS 122–125

For each of the following characteristics, select the appropriate type of polycythemia.

A. Primary polycythemia
B. Secondary polycythemia
C. Both primary and secondary polycythemia

122. Increased red cell mass

123. Decreased cerebral blood flow

124. Decreased serum erythropoietin level

125. Increased leukocyte alkaline phosphatase level

QUESTIONS 126–129

Match each of the following therapies to the appropriate disorder.

A. Myelofibrosis
B. Hairy cell leukemia
C. Chronic myeloid leukemia (CML)
D. Chronic lymphocytic leukemia (CLL)

126. Interferon

127. Chlorambucil

128. Splenectomy

129. Allogeneic bone marrow transplantation

QUESTIONS 130–135

Match the following medical conditions to the drug with which they are most likely to interfere pharmacologically, leading to increased patient toxicity.

A. Cisplatin
B. Methotrexate
C. 6-Mercaptopurine
D. Cyclophosphamide
E. Doxorubicin (Adriamycin)

130. Chronic cystitis

131. Malignant effusion

132. Obstructive jaundice

133. Hyperuricemia controlled by allopurinol

134. Arthritis controlled by aspirin, 2.5 g daily

135. Systemic fungal infection being treated with amphotericin B

PART 5

HEMATOLOGY AND ONCOLOGY

ANSWERS

1.(B) Early sexual activity and early pregnancy are associated with an increased incidence of cancer of the cervix, but, in contrast, cancer of the breast is decreased in such individuals. Childless women, on the other hand, are at considerably greater risk for development of breast cancer. For reasons that are unclear, familial clustering of breast cancer is evident. Breast cancer is bilateral in 4–10% of women when first seen, and women with a history of breast cancer should be strongly encouraged to have regular examinations. Again, for unclear reasons, the incidence of breast cancer is increased in obese women. (*Cecil, Ch. 240*)

2.(C) The staging laparotomy is useful to determine the extent of the disease *if* the results of this diagnostic procedure would change the therapy plan. Stage IV disease with bone marrow involvement (as evidenced by the Reed-Sternberg cells) indicates that chemotherapy without radiation therapy is appropriate. Thus, the staging laparotomy would not change the approach to therapy of Hodgkin's disease on a patient with proven bone marrow involvement. Splenic enlargement and abnormal abdominal lymph nodes do not indicate disease that cannot be treated by radiation therapy. Pleural effusion may be the result of lymphatic obstruction without extralymphatic Hodgkin's disease. Thus, with these three abnormalities, the staging laparotomy may be useful in determining the extent of disease in order that therapy may be planned. (*Cecil, Ch. 160*)

3.(C) Although the spleen tip can occasionally be palpated in cases of immune thrombocytopenia, a significant degree of splenomegaly should make one seriously question this diagnosis. Splenectomy is one of the mainstays of treatment of this disorder and often causes less morbidity than treatment with medications. Platelet transfusions are rarely indicated in the treatment of immune thrombocytopenia. Transfused platelets have a very short survival time, just as do the patient's own platelets. Fortunately, most patients with immune thrombocytopenia have only a mild or moderate degree of clinical bleeding, and platelet transfusions are reserved for the rare cases in which life-threatening bleeding must be controlled within hours, too long to wait for a response to corticosteroid therapy. Medications must always be suspected as a cause of immune thrombocytopenia even if the patient has been taking them for a long period of time. Spherocytes are present only if immune hemolytic anemia coexists. (*Cecil, Ch. 166; McMillan*)

4.(C) Aplastic anemia is heterogeneous in nature. The defect may be either severe injury to bone marrow stem cells or immunologically mediated suppression of hematopoiesis. A number of medications may cause aplastic anemia, but, unfortunately, identifying the offending medication and stopping it does not necessarily lead to reversal of the marrow aplasia. The level of severity of pancytopenia is one of the most useful guides in establishing a patient's prognosis. Aplastic anemia may now be successfully treated in a large number of cases. For young patients with HLA-matched siblings, allogeneic bone marrow transplantation is the treatment of choice. For other patients, immunosuppressive therapy with agents such as antithymocyte globulin may be helpful. Any cell line may be the first to become subnormal. (*Cecil, Ch. 133; Camitta et al*)

5.(B) Young patients with mediastinal disease often have a nodular sclerosis variety of Hodgkin's disease. In contrast, older patients with systemic symptoms usually show the histologic variety of mixed cellularity or lymphocyte depletion. Lymphocyte-predominant Hodgkin's disease is relatively uncommon. Reed-Sternberg cells in an appropriate histopathologic setting are required to establish the diagnosis of Hodgkin's disease. Histopathologic subclassification of Hodgkin's disease is generally useful and correlates well with the natural history of the disease. (*Cecil, Ch. 160*)

6.(A) Hereditary spherocytosis is variable in severity. Although the majority of cases are detected during childhood or in early adulthood, many mild cases go undetected until late in life. Spherocytes commonly make up only a small percentage of cells on the peripheral blood smear and can easily be overlooked unless they are specifically searched for. The osmotic fragility test simply reflects the spherical shape of the cells and indicates that there is little excess membrane surface area to accommodate swelling of the cell. The Coombs' test is the best way to distinguish hereditary spherocytosis from autoimmune hemolytic anemia. Although splenectomy corrects the anemia, spherocytes still remain on the peripheral blood smear. Splenomegaly is common but is rarely massive. (*Cecil, Ch. 138*)

7.(C) An abnormal multimeric pattern of Factor VIII antigen indicates a qualitative disorder in von Willebrand's factor and is seen only in von Willebrand's disease. Although the combination of prolonged bleeding time and PTT is commonly associated with von Willebrand's disease, several combinations of disorders could also produce these abnormalities. A low Factor VIII coagulant activity is most commonly seen in classic hemophilia. Although excessive prolongation of the bleeding time following aspirin ingestion (post-aspirin bleeding time) is a good way to unmask mild von Willebrand's disease, abnormal values on this test will be seen in a variety of platelet disorders. Platelet morphology is normal. (*Cecil, Ch. 167; Zimmerman and Ruggeri*)

8.(B) Significant irreversible neurologic damage may occur owing to vitamin B_{12} deficiency with only mild anemia and mild changes on the peripheral blood smear. It is imperative to exclude vitamin B_{12} deficiency as a problem when investigating neurologic complaints consistent with that disorder. Although an elevated MCV is one of the hallmarks of pernicious anemia, many well-documented cases have been described in which the MCV was normal. In some of these cases, the patient had co-existent alpha-thalassemia trait as the explanation for the unexpectedly normal MCV. Although classically described in people of northern European descent, many young black and Hispanic women have been described with this disorder. The defect in pernicious anemia involves the secretion of intrinsic factor from the gastric mucosa. Ileal absorption of the vitamin B_{12}–intrinsic factor complex is normal. Gastric carcinoma is increased in frequency but is still very uncommon. (*Cecil, Ch. 136*)

9.(B) Heme iron is absorbed more easily than nonheme iron, and its absorption is not reduced by many substances that will reduce the absorption of medicinal or nonheme iron. The majority of total body iron is present in hemoglobin in the circulating red blood cells. Absorption of iron occurs primarily in the stomach and duodenum. Transferrin is not essential for absorption of iron from the gut. There is no difference in bioavailability of different ferrous salts. (*Cecil, Ch. 135*)

10.(C); 11.(C) In this country, although metastatic tumors to the liver from the gastrointestinal tract and elsewhere far outnumber the incidence of primary hepatocellular carcinomas, the latter may present with erythrocytosis and a markedly elevated alpha-fetoprotein, findings that virtually rule out all other malignancies. Primary liver tumors are also associated with cirrhosis, chronic hepatitis B infection, hypercholesterolemia, and elevated carcinoembryonic antigen, but these are not specific findings. In addition, metastatic liver tumors may be associated with anemia, hepatomegaly, abnormal liver function tests, and even bloody ascites. Hepatocellular carcinomas occasionally metastasize to lymph nodes in the lung but more frequently metastasize to distant parts of the liver, and these lesions will probably not be detected by radionuclide scan. Angiography will show a characteristic vascular pattern that differentiates hepatocellular carcinoma from metastatic liver tumors; in addition, this procedure is necessary for assessment of surgical resectability. Needle biopsies, whether percutaneous or directed by laparoscopy, may not be definitive of hepatocellular carcinoma, and a wedge-resected specimen may be necessary. Resection of a localized hepatocellular carcinoma remains the only chance for long-term survival and cure. Adriamycin may produce tumor regression but has shown minimal effect on the median survival time, which remains about six months. (*Cecil, Ch. 129*)

12.(C) The diagnosis of G6PD deficiency can be missed when blood is examined immediately following a hemolytic crisis. Older cells, which are most deficient in the enzyme, have already been eliminated and replaced by a cohort of younger cells, which have a higher-than-average amount of the G6PD enzyme. The disorder is best diagnosed in the steady state when the full cross-section of age distribution of red cells is present. Approximately 10% of American black males are affected. They have no evidence of chronic hemolysis and develop hematologic problems only on exposure to oxidative drugs. Heinz bodies are a useful clue to the diagnosis of oxidation-related hemolysis but are not present on the usual red blood smear. Heinz bodies can be detected only by a special procedure using a crystal violet stain. Mediterranean variants are usually more severe than that seen in American blacks. (*Cecil, Ch. 138*)

13.(A) There are few causes of decreased plasma fibrinogen level other than DIC. Congenital forms of hypofibrinogenemia are extremely uncommon, and liver disease leads to reduced synthesis of this protein only in extreme cases. Elevated fibrin split product levels, although required for diagnosis of DIC, are seen in many other disorders, and their presence may prolong the thrombin time. Although fragmented erythrocytes are occasionally a dramatic part of the DIC picture, their presence is not required to make the diagnosis, and other disorders such as TTP may cause them. (*Cecil, Ch. 166; Colman et al*)

14.(D) Most large bowel neoplasms occur in the sigmoid colon and rectum, with the least prevalent site being the transverse colon. In all cases, the most common early symptoms relate to either bleeding (e.g., anemia) or obstruction (e.g., change in bowel habits). Frank hematochezia is a clinical indication of a left-sided lesion, since blood from a lesion in the ileum or ascending colon is well mixed with stool and becomes occult. These latter tumors are often polypoid and present later than the annular lesions of the left side of the colon. Although the best hope for cure is surgical removal of a large segment of colon bearing the tumor, patients with disease extending beyond the bowel wall often require palliative surgery to relieve obstruction, compression, or bleeding. Radiation therapy and chemotherapy are being investigated as adjuvant therapy but generally are used to palliate advanced disease. Radiation therapy is most effective for localized recurrences, while chemotherapy is generally most effective for distant metastases, usually occurring in the liver. (*Cecil, Ch. 107*)

15.(C) The best screen for hemostatic competency is the performance of a patient under a challenge to the hemostatic system such as surgery. Many cases of mild hemophilia will become detected only upon such a challenge. Approximately 30% of patients with classic hemophilia A have no known family history of the disorder. Many patients with mild cases have no bleeding history if they have not undergone surgery or trauma. Since the PTT becomes prolonged only when the level of Factor VIII falls below 25%, mild cases of hemophilia may have a normal PTT. The PT is normal in hemophilia. (*Cecil, Ch. 167*)

16.(D) In cases of autoimmune hemolytic anemia, erythrocytes opsonized by IgG are preferentially sequestered in the spleen, because splenic macrophages are rich in receptors for Fc fragments. In contrast, erythrocytes opsonized by C3b are preferentially sequestered in the liver. The finding of complement only in the direct Coombs' test suggests an IgM-mediated disorder. Often the IgM adheres to the red blood cell in cooler parts of the circulation and fixes complement to the red blood cell. Upon return of the red cell to areas of core temperature, the IgM dissociates, leaving complement alone on the cell. Unlike alpha-methyldopa, which may induce autoantibody formation, penicillin acts as a hapten when bound to the red cell membrane. The antibody against the red cell pencillin has no specificity for the Rh locus. Penicillin is an uncommon cause of hemolytic anemia. Alpha-methyldopa causes a positive Coombs' test far more often. The presence of spherocytes on the peripheral blood smear is a common clue to the presence of immune hemolytic anemia and does not suggest concomitant hereditary spherocytosis. (*Cecil, Ch. 139; Frank et al*)

17.(D) When treatment of the underlying malignancy is not likely to produce complete or long-lasting relief of pain, it is important to break the cycle of pain (and the further anxiety produced by pain) and to prescribe a logical sequence of increasingly potent analgesics. Despite the practical problems of tolerance and physical dependence encountered with narcotic use, extensive concern for the addiction potential of narcotic analgesics should be avoided in treating pain in patients with advancing malignancy. For mild to moderate pain, acetaminophen is preferred over aspirin because of the latter drug's potential for gastrointestinal bleeding; there is seldom a significant inflammatory component contributing to the pain of an infiltrating tumor. Codeine is preferred over pentazocine (either alone or in combination with aspirin or acetaminophen) because of the CNS side effects and increased cost associated with the latter; pentazocine is not free of addiction liability. Pain should be treated promptly and continuously. If analgesic drug doses are spaced so far apart that pain recurs, the analgesic becomes less effective. Combinations of narcotic and non-narcotic analgesics are often more effective than either alone, and the addition of a tranquilizer or antidepressant as an adjuvant, such as phenothiazine or amitriptyline, often enhances the effect of narcotic analgesia. (*Cecil, Ch. 466; DeVita et al*)

18. (C) Since vitamin K is derived both from dietary sources and from bacteria residing in the colon, dietary deficiency alone does not cause clinical vitamin K deficiency. The most common setting is in the perioperative state, in which dietary deficiency is combined with reduction in intestinal bacteria by the use of broad-spectrum antibiotics. Vitamin K acts as a cofactor in facilitating carboxylation of clotting factors after their synthesis in the liver. The response to the treatment of vitamin K deficiency can be very rapid, because new protein synthesis need not occur. Warfarin acts as an anticoagulant by interfering with the vitamin K–dependent modification of clotting factors, and the vitamin K can completely overcome the effect of this drug. Vitamin K is effective when given by mouth. (*Cecil, Ch. 167*)

19. (A) Although splenic sequestration crises are common in young children with sickle cell anemia, adults with hemoglobin SS are hyposplenic owing to autoinfarction of the spleen and are no longer able to have excessive splenic sequestration. Persons with sickle cell trait are not anemic at all, and any anemia should be evaluated for a separate cause. Although persons with sickle cell trait may have hematuria and defects in renal tubular function, they do not have renal insufficiency. Folic acid deficiency or viral infection may cause severe anemia in patients with sickle cell disease by reducing red cell production, but they do not cause an increase in hemolysis. Sickled cells are present on smear at all times. (*Cecil, Ch. 143*)

20. (C) Splenectomy benefits approximately two thirds of patients with Felty's syndrome, but the indications for this therapy are somewhat controversial. Patients with severe neutropenia are more prone to serious infections, but it is not unusual for patients with Felty's syndrome and severe neutropenia to avoid infections for months or even years. Thus, the absolute neutrophil count cannot be used as an indication for therapy. Thrombocytopenia usually is not severe and is not predictive of benefit from splenectomy. The most clear-cut indications for therapy are recurrent bacterial infections or chronic nonhealing skin ulcers. (*Cecil, Chs. 150 and 433*)

21. (D) Clinical trials of recombinant erythropoietin have shown great success in eliminating transfusion dependence for dialysis patients. During dialysis, both iron and folic acid may become depleted. Red blood cells from these patients have normal survival in normal recipients but mildly decreased survival in the patient. Although some patients with renal failure may be iron deficient because of blood loss (either during dialysis or from a secondary cause), characteristically bone marrow iron stores are increased. Intensive dialysis does not improve anemia. (*Cecil, Ch. 134; Eschbach et al*)

22. (C) Although childhood HUS most commonly follows a diarrheal illness, the most common association in adult cases is pregnancy or use of estrogen. HUS does not differ hematologically from TTP but is distinguished primarily by the absence of neurologic abnormalities and by the presence of renal failure. Heparin is not an effective treatment; plasmapheresis is the treatment of choice. Unlike childhood HUS, which has an excellent prognosis, many cases of adult HUS are fatal or lead to permanent renal insufficiency. HUS is distinguished from DIC by the absence of coagulopathy. Fragmented red blood cells are seen in both. (*Cecil, Ch. 166*)

23. (C) The most clear-cut indication for chemotherapy treatment of CLL is bone marrow failure (Rai stage 3 to 4). Although a minority of CLL patients may have IgM paraproteins in their serum, these are never present in a great enough quantity to cause the hyperviscosity syndrome. Patients with early-stage disease have a median survival in excess of 10 years. Elevated white blood counts up to 500,000/mm^3 are usually very well tolerated, and leukapheresis is almost never indicated on an emergent basis. Almost all cases of CLL involve B lymphocytes. (*Cecil, Ch. 155*)

24. (A) The first step in planning treatment of suspected breast cancer is to define the extent of the disease. If disseminated disease is present at the outset, extensive surgical procedures are unwarranted. Roentgenogram of the chest and serum alkaline phosphatase are useful preliminary staging procedures. Radionuclide bone scans, skeletal films, and bone marrow biopsies are not useful in identifying metastatic disease, since they are abnormal in less than 10% of patients with Stage I or II breast cancer. (*Cecil, Ch. 176*)

25. (B) In a premenopausal patient with estrogen receptor–positive tumor, the likelihood of response to surgical oophorectomy is at least 50%. It is useful to know whether such a response occurs, because if it does and relapse ensues, the patient may again respond to second-line endocrine therapy. The role of chemotherapy in this disease is changing; some clinicians would treat with both chemotherapy and oophorectomy initially. The response to chemotherapy is generally at least as good as to hormonal manipulation, but skeletal metastases do not respond as well to chemotherapy. Thus, remission is more likely with oophorectomy than with chemotherapy in this patient. Chemotherapy would be indicated if she failed to respond to oophorectomy. Local radiotherapy to painful lesions is indicated if the disease is unresponsive to oophorectomy and chemotherapy. (*Cecil, Ch. 240; Legha et al*)

26. (D) Gastrointestinal bleeding is common in patients with cancer and may be due to a variety of causes. Metastases to the gastrointestinal tract should be considered. Stress ulcers are also common and may be exacerbated by gastric irritants such as aspirin, as contained in Percodan. Aspirin also produces platetet function abnormalities. Adequate pain management should be possible with other analgesics that do not contain aspirin. (*Cecil, Chs. 99, 166, and 168*)

27. (C) The care of patients with terminal diseases often presents moral dilemmas. What seems to the physician to be a rational therapeutic plan may be unacceptable to the patient. In this situation, continued supportive care should be offered. It must be remembered that patients' emotional responses to their illnesses will vary with time. A decision to stop suggested forms of therapy is not irrevocable, and at different times, under different circumstances, these decisions may change. A patient's decision to stop therapy is not an indication of psychiatric illness. (*Cecil, Ch. 168*)

28.(B) The measurement of estrogen receptors in breast tumors is of benefit in predicting response to hormonal manipulation. If tumors of premenopausal women lack estrogen receptors, hormonal manipulations will be of benefit in less than 10% of patients; in the presence of known metastatic disease, such hormonal manipulations are probably unwarranted. Unfortunately, only about 60% of premenopausal patients whose tumors are estrogen receptor–positive will respond to hormonal manipulation such as castration. Interestingly, in some patients the primary tumor will possess estrogen receptors, but metastatic tumor cells will not. Thus, it is of benefit to measure estrogen receptors in metastatic tumors as well as in the primary tumor if the primary is positive for estrogen receptors. (*Cecil, Ch. 240*)

29.(C) The anemia of chronic disease is characterized by elevated amounts of storage iron in the bone marrow, and an iron stain of the bone marrow will reliably distinguish this disorder from iron deficiency in which storage iron should be absent. In the anemia of chronic disease, red blood survival is usually mildly decreased, but there is no compensatory increase in production. Liver disease may cause anemia by itself without folic acid deficiency or other associated problems. Anemia of chronic disease is usually normocytic but may occasionally be microcytic. The red blood cell morphology is usually normal, and the reticulocyte count is not diagnostic. (*Cecil, Ch. 134*)

30.(A—False; B—True; C—True; D—False; E—False) Differentiation of CML from a secondary leukemoid reaction involves the sequential evaluation of clinical and laboratory data. Characteristically, patients with untreated CML are anemic, but diseases that cause leukemoid reactions also cause anemia. For reasons that are unclear, leukocyte alkaline phosphatase (determined by histochemical staining) is characteristically decreased or absent in CML, whereas the concentration of this enzyme is usually elevated in secondary leukemoid reactions. Splenic enlargement is characteristic of CML. Although a marked increase in cellularity and in granulocyte precursors in the bone marrow is characteristic of CML, these bone marrow findings are also seen in leukemoid reactions. Thus, morphologic examination of the blood and bone marrow does not usually aid in this differentiation. Short of bone marrow karyotype analysis, the combination of a low leukocyte alkaline phosphatase and splenomegaly makes the diagnosis of CML quite likely. High platelet counts may be seen in CML or inflammatory disorders. (*Cecil, Chs. 151 and 155*)

31.(A—True; B—False; C—False; D—True) Hemolytic transfusion reactions commonly cause fever, chills, and backache. The best way to diagnose a delayed hemolytic transfusion reaction is by identifying a new alloantibody that was not present at the time of the original cross-match. Anaphylaxis is usually due to plasma proteins or drugs. Leukoagglutinin reactions may cause severe pulmonary infiltrates but do not cause hemolysis. (*Cecil, Ch. 147; Mollison*)

32.(All are True) ITP can be classified as a thrombocytopenia of decreased platelet survival. There is strong evidence to suggest that ITP is in fact autoimmune thrombocytopenic purpura. Plasma transfusion experiments with whole plasma or with 7S gamma globulin fractions and observations concerning placental transfer of the disease strongly implicate IgG antibodies as the cause of this disorder. Tests for antiplatelet antibodies in vitro, although technically difficult, reveal such antibodies in the majority of patients with ITP. These antiplatelet antibodies also have been shown to be produced in vitro by spleen cells of patients with ITP. (*Cecil, Ch. 40; McMillan; Williams et al*)

33.(A—True; B—True; C—True; D—False); 34.(A—True; B—True; C—False; D—True) Vaginal Pap smears effectively screen for one of the most common of female neoplasms, cervical carcinoma. These smears are commonly graded I (normal), II (atypical), III (dysplasia), IV (carcinoma in situ), and V (invasive carcinoma). Premalignant changes (grades III and IV) are usually asymptomatic and may spontaneously regress, although most are believed to progress to invasive carcinoma over a subsequent period of up to 30 years. Cytologic and serologic evidence of herpes simplex Type 2 infection and exposure to multiple sexual partners are high-risk factors for the development of invasive carcinoma. While cellular atypia (grade II) commonly occurs with *Trichomonas* infection, the presence of dysplasia (grade III), especially when symptomatic, should be immediately assessed by directed biospy. Culdoscopy with punch biopsy is the most appropriate assessment of a grade III Pap smear and may be followed by cone biopsy if necessary. Endocervical curettage, chest roentgenogram, blood tests, IVP, and barium enema are important early studies to define the extent of the invasive neoplasm, which tends to involve local pelvic structures and lymph nodes before disseminating hematogenously. Bone scan is not useful in the staging of cervical carcinoma. Radiation therapy and/or surgery is the primary treatment modality for cervical cancer, and chemotherapy offers only limited, palliative value. (*Cecil, Ch. 170; DeVita et al*)

35.(A—True; B—False; C—True; D—True; E—False) Prolongation of the bleeding time may be caused either by thrombocytopenia or by a qualitative platelet dysfunction. The platelet dysfunction may be related to a defect intrinsic to the platelet or to an abnormality in a plasma factor necessary for proper functioning. In essential thrombocytosis, as in all the myeloproliferative diseases, intrinsic platelet abnormalities may occur and take a variety of forms. Storage pool disease is a congenital, qualitative platelet abnormality. Bleeding in renal failure may be related to a qualitative platelet abnormality. The exact nature of the defect remains to be determined, but recent evidence suggests that von Willebrand's factor may be implicated. Although patients with severe liver disease may have complex coagulopathies with or without indirect effect on platelets, the vast majority have normal platelet function. (*Cecil, Chs. 155 and 166*)

36.(A—True; B—False; C—False; D—False); 37.(A—True; B—False; C—False; D—True) The most common risk factor for cutaneous malignancies incuding basal cell epitheliomas, squamous cell carcinomas, and melanomas is chronic solar exposure, especially in light-complexioned individuals. Basal cell epitheliomas occur most commonly and with neglect may invade locally, but they do not metastasize. Squamous cell carcinomas are less prevalent, grow more rapidly than basal cell tumors, and occasionally metastasize, especially if located on the ear or vermilion border of the lip. Both of these tumors most often recur locally in actinic-damaged areas, even if subsequent solar exposure is avoided. X-rays enhance neoplastic change in areas of actinic damage and should be used to treat tumors only in the feeble and elderly. Melanomas have a great potential for invasion and metastasis and must be widely excised whenever possible. Treatment with radiation therapy or chemotherapy is virtually ineffective and cannot be used as an alternative to wide surgical resection. Five-year prognosis is primarily determined by evidence of metastatic spread and by the degree and depth of local skin invasion as defined by either Clark level or Breslow measurement. Other factors including age of patient, tumor location, and type of melanoma (lentigo, superficial spreading, nodular, or amelanotic) are of lesser prognostic importance. Lentigo maligna is a pigmented freckle, usually seen on the sun-exposed face of an older adult, that enlarges by lateral growth over many years before developing into a vertically invasive, nodular or ulcerating lesion. (*Cecil, Ch. 532*)

38.(A—True; B—False; C—True; D—False; E—False) Von Willebrand's disease is notoriously difficult to diagnose in mild cases, and initial screening laboratory results are frequently normal. Either repeated determinations or more sophisticated measures of von Willebrand factor function, such as ristocetin cofactor activity, may be necessary to make the diagnosis. Since the end point for the commonly performed coagulation test is formation of a fibrin clot, the activity of Factor XIII in converting the fibrin clot to a stable form is not measured. The screening test for Factor XIII deficiency is the clot solubility test performed in hyperosmolar urea. Factor X deficiency will be manifested by prolongation of the prothrombin and partial thromboplastin times. Patients with the lupus anticoagulant do not have a bleeding tendency. (*Cecil, Ch. 167; Zimmerman and Ruggeri*).

39.(A—True; B—True; C—False; D—True) The most common tumor of the small intestine is asymptomatic benign carcinoid, while the most common malignancy is a metastatic lymphoma, melanoma, or carcinoma (originating from breast, kidney, ovary, or testicle). The incidence of primary lymphoma is increased following celiac disease, whereas adenocarcinoma, a relatively rare primary tumor in the small intestine, has an increased risk in areas of the distal small bowel affected by Crohn's disease. Malignant small bowel tumors usually present with either bleeding or bowel obstruction, not jaundice or flank pain. Prognosis is poor for primary adenocarcinomas but good for primary lymphomas or leiomyosarcomas; thus, unlike neoplasms of the large bowel, prognosis with small bowel tumors depends less on tumor stage and more on tumor type. (*Cecil, Ch. 107*)

40.(A—False; B—False; C—True; D—True) Adenocarcinoma is the most common histopathologic type of large bowel neoplasm; occasionally metastases from lung and breast primaries occur, but these are uncommon. Known high-risk factors include increased dietary fat and beef protein, decreased dietary fiber, ulcerative colitis, and first-degree relatives with colon cancer. Polyps, whether associated with a familial condition (e.g., Gardner's syndrome) or not, are believed to be a premalignant condition; they are best removed when identified, even if they are asymptomatic. (*Cecil, Ch. 107*)

41.(A—True; B—False; C—True; D—False; E—False) Petechiae are an extremely important clue in the diagnosis of hemostatic disorders and are seen only in platelet disorders. Bleeding due to coagulation abnormalities characteristically occurs in a delayed fashion, and hemarthroses are almost pathognomonic of severe hemophilia. Tooth extraction is a challenge to all arms of the hemostatic system, and bleeding after extractions is characteristic of both platelet and coagulation disorders. Although aspirin in usual doses has no measurable effect on the coagulation system, but only on platelet function, aspirin is contraindicated in serious coagulation abnormalities. In disorders such as hemophilia in which thrombin generation is markedly deficient, platelet function may be more dependent on the prostaglandin pathway than in normal persons, and impairing this mode of platelet activation can have serious consequences. (*Cecil, Ch. 166*)

42.(A—False; B—True; C—False; D—False) Fever is part of the classic pentad of findings in this disorder and need not indicate an infection. Although a moderate amount of fibrin degradation products may be detectable, tests of coagulation should be normal and are critical in differentiating this syndrome from disseminated intravascular coagulation. Similarly, the finding of microangiopathic changes on the peripheral smear is of paramount importance in establishing the diagnosis and does not suggest a different disorder. Recent advances in the treatment of TTP involving the use of plasmapheresis as well as other modalities have led to complete recovery in the majority of cases. The availability of effective therapy makes it incumbent upon the clinician to rapidly and accurately diagnose TTP. (*Cecil, Ch. 166; Kacich and Linker*)

43.(A—True; B—False; C—False; D—True) Most cases of severe aplastic anemia are idiopathic. Autoimmune hemolytic anemia has not been associated with this disorder. Viral hepatitis has been associated with aplasia, but the aplasia usually occurs 2-3 months after the acute phase of the disease. ATG is a highly effective treatment with response rates of 50–60% in cases of severe aplastic anemia. It is clearly indicated when bone marrow transplantation is not an option. (*Cecil, Ch. 133; Camitta et al*)

44.(A—False; B—False; C—False; D—True) Although equal doses of radiation (rads) may be delivered to a tumor volume by either kilovolt (low-energy x-rays) or cobalt-60 (high-energy x-rays) sources, considerable differences will occur in damage to normal tissue surrounding and overlying a deeply seated tumor. Thus, low-energy x-rays will scatter more and penetrate less effectively, causing much greater injury to skin and normal brain surrounding a brain tumor. Radiotherapy causes its biologic effects by breaking DNA after formation of intracellular superoxide, or hydroxyl radicals. Hypoxic conditions reduce the formation of these reactive oxygen metabolites; in contrast, hyperbaric oxygenation may frequently enhance radiation effects. Fractionation into multiple small doses of 150–250 rads/day is generally more effective than a single large dose, probably because of differences in the ability of normal and malignant cells to repair DNA breaks. Generally, normal cells tolerate individual doses of radiation with less damage than do malignant cells. This tolerance varies considerably among normal tissues, however, and normal bone marrow and liver tissues are so sensitive that it is nearly impossible to selectively eradicate tumor cells by irradiating these organs. (*Cecil, Ch. 176*)

45.(A—True; B—False; C—False; D—False) Abnormal red blood cell morphology is one of the hallmarks of the disorder and does not suggest conversion to leukemia. The Philadelphia chromosome is present *only* in chronic myeloid leukemia and not in this disorder. Osteosclerosis is a common abnormality, but lytic bone destruction does not occur. (*Cecil, Ch. 154*)

46. (A—False; B—True; C—True; D—False) Adjuvant chemotherapy is given after surgical resection of a primary tumor, with intent to eradicate microscopic metastases and cure patients with malignancies that have a high rate of recurrence and are not curable by any therapy after recurrence. Adjuvant therapy has been shown to improve survival and probably cure selected patients with breast cancer, sarcomas, and solid tumors of childhood. Since these patients are not debilitated by metastatic disease, they tolerate chemotherapy well, but the short- and long-term life-threatening risks of aggressive (dose-intense) chemotherapy (myelosuppression and carcinogenicity) are of concern. Aggressive drug combinations rather than single agents have generally proved most effective. (*Cecil, Chs. 176 and 240*)

47. (A—True; B—True; C—False; D—True) Antithrombin III is the most important inhibitor of activated clotting factor in normal plasma. It acts by binding to the active site of all the serine proteases of coagulation, Factors XIIa, XIa, IXa, and Xa and thrombin. Heparin acts as an anticoagulant because it increases the affinity of antithrombin III for these activated factors. Congenital deficiency of antithrombin III is associated with a risk of thrombosis. Warfarin can elevate the level of antithrombin III by an unknown mechanism and can potentially mask the proper diagnosis of antithrombin III deficiency. (*Cecil, Ch. 167*)

48. (A—True; B—False; C—True; D—True) The lupus anticoagulant is usually suspected because of a prolonged partial thromboplastin time that is not corrected by the addition of normal plasma. Despite the prolonged clotting times, patients do not have an increased risk of bleeding unless there is an additional hemostatic defect. Marked prolongation of the prothrombin times suggests coexistent prothrombin deficiency, which can cause a severe bleeding diathesis. For as yet unknown reasons, the presence of lupus anticoagulant is associated with a risk of thrombosis. The lupus anticoagulant usually disappears promptly with prednisone therapy. (*Cecil, Ch. 167*)

49. (A—True; B—True; C—True; D—False) Aggressive chemotherapy is beneficial in disseminated histiocytic (diffuse, large-cell) lymphoma. Complete remission occurs in more than half the patients so treated. Patients with histiocytic lymphoma may occasionally present with disease localized to one anatomic area (stage I). It is not unusual, for instance, for histiocytic lymphoma to be localized in the gastrointestinal tract, e.g., in the stomach. For patients with carefully established stage I disease, radiation therapy alone may be curative; however, chemotherapy is often added to improve responses when primary lesions are large. Progression of histiocytic lymphoma to a leukemic phase with circulating lymphoma cells is rarely seen. (*Cecil, Ch. 158*)

50. (A—False; B—True; C—False; D—True) The classification of non-Hodgkin's lymphoma into two general groups, nodular and diffuse, has proved useful for predicting response to therapy and disease prognosis. The nodular lymphomas are usually disseminated at diagnosis and often involve lymph node areas not treated by standard radiation ports. These diseases usually respond favorably to chemotherapy, but a complete response or remission is infrequently observed. Thus, extremely aggressive chemotherapy does not seem beneficial. Despite the foregoing, patients often have a rather indolent clinical course, and the five-year survival rates for nodular lymphoma are usually greater than for patients with the diffuse varieties. (*Cecil, Chs. 157 and 158*)

51. (A—True; B—False; C—False; D—False) Although iron deficiency is the most common cause of anemia worldwide, anemia of chronic disease is more common in hospitalized patients. Dietary deficiency is the most prominent cause of iron deficiency worldwide. Medicinal iron repletion will correct the anemia in two to three months in most cases. Although absorption of medicinal iron will be reduced if it is taken with meals, it is far better to encourage this practice than to have patients reject iron because of side effects associated with taking it on an empty stomach. (*Cecil, Ch. 135*)

52. (A—False; B—False; C—True; D—False) Hypercalcemia is a relatively common metabolic abnormality in cancer patients. The earliest symptoms include polyuria, polydipsia, constipation, lethargy, and personality change. With progressive hypercalcemia, mental obtundation, coma, and death may ensue, necessitating prompt treatment with infusions of saline, diuresis with furosemide, and the occasional use of mithramycin. Solid tumors most commonly associated with hypercalcemia, including nonmetastatic lung cancer, are also refractory to primary therapy, rendering this an impractical approach to the management of hypercalcemia. There are a variety of causes for hypercalcemia in cancer patients, including ectopic production of parathyroid hormone–like materials or other tumor products such as prostaglandins and various growth factors. Most patients have normal serum values of immunoreactive parathyroid hormone, quantitated by radioimmunoassay specific for the carboxyl-region of the hormone. (*Cecil, Ch. 173; Mazzaferri et al*)

53. (A—True; B—True; C—False; D—True) Although significant neutropenia associated with the use of any medication is usually a contraindication to its continued use, chlorpromazine commonly causes a mild neutropenia that is dose-related and not necessarily a harbinger of a hematologic catastrophe. The drug can be continued, perhaps with dose adjustment, if its use is otherwise warranted. Although patients who develop severe neutropenia following a course of cytotoxic chemotherapy almost invariably get infected, this is not the case for patients with congenital neutropenia. Treatment of chronic neutropenia should be based on a history of recurrent infection rather than simply on the absolute neutrophil count. Megaloblastic anemias are a manifestation of impaired DNA synthesis that may affect all cell lines, and neutropenia of a moderate degree is commonly present. (*Cecil, Ch. 150*)

54. (A—True; B—False; C—True; D—False) Oropharyngeal or nasopharyngeal involvement occurs in approximately 20% of patients with non-Hodgkin's lymphoma. These lymph nodes are rarely involved with Hodgkin's disease. Spinal cord compression from extradural tumor occurs in patients with Hodgkin's disease as well as in those with non-Hodgkin's lymphoma. This medical emergency must be recognized early and appropriate therapy instituted in order to prevent irreversible neurologic damage in patients who otherwise might respond well to therapy. In contrast to Hodgkin's disease, which often appears to have a unicentric origin in lymph nodes above the diaphragm, other forms of malignant lymphoma frequently involve lymph tissue outside the axial skeleton lymph node areas. Mesenteric lymph node involvement is common in non-Hodgkin's lymphoma, and it frequently invades the gastrointestinal tract. Autoimmune hemolytic anemia is associated with both Hodgkin's disease and non-Hodgkin's lymphoma. Nevertheless, the most common cause of anemia in both disorders is bone marrow involvement by lymphoma. (*Cecil, Chs. 158 and 160; Williams et al, Ch. 119*)

55.(A—False; B—True; C—True; D—True) The clinical staging of Hodgkin's disease is extremely important in determining appropriate therapy. Lymphangiographic visualization of abdominal and pelvic lymph nodes to determine the extent of disease and bone marrow biopsy to ascertain whether stage IV disease of bone exists are both very important and useful diagnostic procedures. CT scans can also detect nodal enlargement and/or irregularity signifying extranodal extension, especially in chest and upper abdominal areas poorly visualized by lymphangiogram. Involvement of the brain with Hodgkin's disease is extremely rare. (*Cecil, Ch. 160*)

56.(A—False; B—False; C—False; D—False; E—True) Although the development of leukemia is occasionally associated with exposure to radiation, benzene, or prior chemotherapy, in most cases no immediate cause can be identified. In a substantial minority of cases (aleukemic leukemia), circulating leukemia cells cannot be detected even with a careful search of a peripheral smear. The diagnosis of acute leukemia is made by examination of the bone marrow. Hyperleukocytosis complicating acute myeloid leukemia is a medical emergency, and very high white blood counts should be reduced quickly. Disseminated intravascular coagulation can be a complication of leukemia itself, particularly promyelocytic and monocytic leukemias, and need not indicate a separate cause. The treatment of acute leukemia has progressed to the point that young adults should be treated with curative intent, with the expectation at the current time that approximately 20% of young adults will be cured of their disease. (*Cecil, Ch. 156*)

57.(A—False; B—True; C—True; D—True; E—True) Documentation of relapse of Hodgkin's disease in previously treated patients is often difficult. Bone or liver involvement often occurs without overt lymph node enlargement. A variety of laboratory tests have been suggested to be useful in screening patients in presumed disease remission in order to predict imminent relapse. Abnormal elevations of all the laboratory tests described here except serum protein electrophoresis have been correlated with disease activity. Although hypo- and hypergammaglobulinemia occur in Hodgkin's disease, these findings are not predictive of relapse. (*Cecil, Ch. 160*)

58.(A—False; B—True; C—False; D—True; E—False) Although many patients with CLL are diagnosed while asymptomatic, patients with CML most commonly present with symptoms of fatigue, fever, or splenic pain. CML frequently terminates in a blast crisis, which occasionally has a lymphoid phenotype. This lymphoid blast crisis is important to diagnose, because it responds reasonably well to appropriate therapy, unlike its myeloid counterpart. CLL rarely terminates in a blast crisis but may terminate as an aggressive lymphoma (Richter's syndrome). Unlike CLL, in which staging is very useful in making treatment decisions and in which patients with low stage disease have a median survival in excess of 10 years, there are no parameters that are useful in identifying long-term survivors of CML. The course of CML is much more aggressive than that of CLL, with a median survival of 3 years and only rare 10-year survivors. (*Cecil, Ch. 155*)

59.(A—True; B—False; C—True; D—False; E—False) Reducing or preventing drug-induced host toxicity improves therapeutic response rates by permitting administration of higher antitumor doses and by improving patient compliance with therapy. Hypothermic (ice) caps sufficiently decrease scalp circulation and dermal metabolism to prevent alopecia resulting from vincristine and other drugs with relatively short serum half-lives. Saline-mannitol hydration and diuresis prevent nephropathy from cisplatin; hydration and alkalinization also prevent nephropathy from high-dose methotrexate. Mucositis (including stomatitis and diarrhea) and/or myelosuppression associated with 5-fluorouracil or methotrexate therapy remain unpredictable and are prevented only by dose and schedule modifications; these occur even when leucovorin is used as a rescue agent for methotrexate. Cardiotoxicity, with clinical heart failure, occurs in an increasing fraction of patients receiving more than 500 mg/m^2 cumulative dose of doxorubicin or daunomycin. (*Cecil, Ch. 176*)

60.(A—True; B—False; C—True; D—False) Hairy cell leukemia may be an indolent disease, and prolonged survival is common with or without therapy. Pancytopenia is frequently present at diagnosis and if of moderate degree does not preclude a benign clinical course. For patients who require therapy, splenectomy is the initial treatment of choice. Splenectomy will also have a beneficial effect on the course of the disease, even when the bone marrow appears to be completely packed. The tartrate-resistant acid phosphatase (TRAP) stain is of great utility in distinguishing hairy cell leukemia from other lymphoproliferative diseases. The leukocyte alkaline phosphatase enzyme is present in neutrophils and is not affected in hairy cell leukemia. (*Cecil, Ch. 155; Quesada et al*)

61.(A—True; B—True; C—True; D—False) All patients with Hodgkin's disease have a variety of immune abnormalities that do not appear to be caused by therapy. Altered T lymphocyte function, as evidenced by loss of positivity of skin tests and impaired lymphocyte transformation to mitogens, appears to be primary. This impairment tends to become more severe with advancing disease. Recovery of immune function can occur when the disease is adequately controlled by chemotherapy, despite the immunosuppressive effects of such therapy. Most patients are lymphopenic. Altered B lymphocyte function may be manifest by autoimmune hemolytic anemia or thrombocytopenic purpura, in the presence of either hyper- or hypogammaglobulinemia. Splenectomy is performed to confirm Hodgkin's disease in the abdomen, although it induces a delayed risk of severe bacterial infections in these patients. (*Cecil, Ch. 160*)

62.(A—False; B—False; C—False; D—True) The bony lesions of myeloma are characteristically lytic with no osteoblastic reaction. Consequently, the bone scan is very insensitive in detecting these lesions. Bone disease is strongly correlated with a poor prognosis. The hypercalcemia of myeloma may often be due to a mixture of humoral factors. Prednisone is particularly useful in the treatment of hypercalcemia in myeloma. Radiotherapy plays a prominent role in the treatment of bony lesions, both in the palliation of pain and in the prevention of pathologic fractures. Symptoms of pain in weight-bearing areas should be promptly evaluated so that impending fractures can be detected and treated. (*Cecil, Ch. 163*)

63. (A—True; B—True; C—False; D—True) HCG is a hormone molecule secreted by placental trophoblastic cells. It is increased in plasma during pregnancy, but in addition it is produced by germ cell neoplasms of the ovary or testes as well as by trophoblastic tumors. Serial measurement of HCG in patients with these diseases is an effective way to measure response to therapy. HCG has alpha and beta subunits. The structure of the alpha subunit is similar to that of other hormones, and it thus may cross-react with them. Radioimmunoassays for HCG use antisera produced to the specific beta subunit. Although HCG and alpha-fetoprotein often rise and fall simultaneously in the plasma of patients with these neoplasms, discordant behavior of these two marker substances may be seen in some patients. Discordance in the level of these two substances suggests that different clones of neoplastic cells exist within the same tumor. HCG has been detected in the plasma of patients with non–germ cell tumors such as gastric or pancreatic carcinoma. (*Cecil, Ch. 172*)

64. (A—False; B—True; C—False; D—True) Primary amyloidosis may occur in the context of multiple myeloma or macroglobulinemia or without an identifiable underlying malignant plasma cell dyscrasia. The tongue and heart are prominently involved. In contrast to the secondary amyloidosis associated with familial Mediterranean fever, colchicine has not been a useful treatment. By electron microscopy, the characteristic beta pleated formation of amyloid derived from light chains is diagnostic of this disorder. (*Cecil, Ch. 163*)

65. (A—True; B—False; C—False; D—True) Moderate iron deficiency is usually normocytic, and the MCV becomes low only with significant anemia. The peripheral blood smear in thalassemia is more abnormal than that in iron deficiency, particularly with mild or moderate levels of anemia. Normal levels of hemoglobin A_2 and F exclude only beta-thalassemia and still leave the possibility of alpha-thalassemia as a cause of microcytic anemia. In severe iron deficiency, the peripheral blood smear may be markedly abnormal, with bizarre morphology, target cells, and small numbers of nucleated red blood cells. (*Cecil, Chs. 135 and 142*)

66. (A—True; B—True; C—False; D—False) The TDT is an important test in establishing the diagnosis of ALL and in differentiating this from AML. T-cell ALL is characteristically seen in adolescent males with high levels of white blood cells and mediastinal masses. Auer rods are pathognomonic of AML but are usually not seen in the monocytic variants that typically cause gum infiltration. Cases of acute leukemia in which the Philadelphia chromosome are present have a dismal prognosis. (*Cecil, Ch. 156*)

67. (A—True; B—False; C—True; D—False) After the diagnosis of prostatic cancer is established, clinical staging to determine the extent of the disease is necessary before appropriate therapy can be outlined. Clinical stage 3 or less represents disease confined to the pelvis or the prostate itself and should be treated by local measures such as surgery, radiation therapy, or both. Prostatic (tartrate-inhibitable) acid phosphatase is a useful laboratory test in such staging evaluations and is elevated in the serum of 75% of patients with palpable tumors, including those with regional or metastatic disease. Unfortunately, it is elevated in only a third of patients with occult neoplasms. When distant metastatic disease is present, hormonal manipulation by orchiectomy, exogenous LHRH analogue, or estrogen will produce objective improvement in more than one half of patients with about equal efficacy. The clinical course of metastatic prostatic cancer, however, can be quite variable, and no therapy can be shown to prolong life in such patients. (*Cecil, Chs. 172 and 236*)

68. (A—True; B—False; C—False; D—True) Severe beta-thalassemia is a much more important cause of bone deformity than is alpha-thalassemia. Hemoglobin electrophoresis usually distinguishes alpha- from beta-thalassemia because of the elevated levels of hemoglobin A_2 and F seen only in beta-thalassemia. Transfusion therapy is limited primarily by severe iron overload. Only a small minority of patients develop severe alloimmunization. (*Cecil, Ch. 142; Forget*)

69. (All are True) Chronic lymphocytic leukemia is characterized by the accumulation of immunoincompetent lymphocytes. A variety of associated immunologic complications is seen, including autoimmune disorders directed against platelet or red cells, hypogammaglobulinemia, and, in approximately 5% of patients, a monoclonal gammopathy. (*Cecil, Ch. 155*)

70. (A—False; B—False; C—False; D—True) Sarcomas of the mesodermally derived soft tissues and bone constitute approximately 10% of all malignancies and can be divided into more than a dozen different types. Of those originating in the bone, osteogenic sarcoma is the most common type, usually presenting in the second decade of life, but in older adults it is most often seen in long bones affected with Paget's disease. Radiographic evidence of cortical destruction with periosteal elevation (Codman's triangle) is a hallmark sign that should not obscure this diagnosis in pagetic patients complaining of persistent bone pain. Soft tissue sarcomas can be diverse in their clinical appearance, ranging from the raised blue or purple skin lesions of Kaposi's sarcoma to the intramural lesion of a gastric leiomyosarcoma. The latter lesion should be suspected when a palpable, painless epigastric mass shows up as a filling defect on radiography and reveals minimal mucosal defect on gastroscopy. Sarcomas are known to develop in irradiated areas; however, the doses required (≥6,000 rads) are rarely given for therapeutic purposes. The angiosarcoma known as Kaposi's sarcoma is most frequently associated with other malignancies (predominantly lymphoreticular), and this may be related to a systemic immune deficiency (AIDS especially) and/or viral infection. Most bone sarcomas are still treated with amputation; however, soft tissue sarcomas are initially treated with wide, local excision. Recent treatment protocols employing combinations of radiotherapy, chemotherapy, and limb-sparing surgery for both bone and soft tissue sarcomas are proving very successful. (*Cecil, Chs. 251 and 253; DeVita et al*)

71. (A—True; B—True; C—False; D—True) Vitamin B_{12} is so ubiquitous in the diet that only strict vegetarians (vegans) can have a dietary deficiency. Most patients with a vitamin B_{12} deficiency have normal or high folic acid levels, and a low level does suggest a second deficiency. Repletion of vitamin B_{12} is occasionally complicated by hypokalemia, which may be severe and may lead to arrhythmias. The peripheral blood picture of megaloblastic anemia is so characteristic that a macrocytic anemia without these signs is usually due to another cause, such as hematopoietic dysplasia. (*Cecil, Ch. 136*)

72. (A—True; B—True; C—True; D—False) The differentiation of acute lymphoblastic leukemia (ALL) from other forms of acute leukemia, including acute myelogenous leukemia (AML), is essential, since therapies are remarkably different. Histochemical reactions are useful in differentiating these forms of leukemia. Myeloblasts of AML usually have positive-staining reactions with peroxidase and Sudan black, whereas lymphoblasts of ALL do not stain with these reagents. In contrast, lymphoblasts usually have coarse cytoplasmic staining with periodic acid–Schiff (PAS) reagents, whereas myeloblasts do not. Esterase stains are also useful in this regard. TDT is found in high concentrations in the cells of many patients with ALL but is not present in myeloblasts. This enzyme is also found experimentally in some types of thymic lymphocytes. Its role in the pathogenesis of leukemia is unknown. Auer rods are highly refractile cytoplasmic rods that appear to derive from coalescence of azurophilic granules. They are present in only approximately one third of patients with AML, but when seen are pathognomonic for this disease. Both ALL and AML are usually detected when the patient is anemic and thrombocytopenic. (*Cecil, Ch. 156; Foon et al*)

73.(A—True; B—False; C—False; D—True) Pure red cell aplasia appears to be an autoimmune disease in which antibodies are directed against red cell precursors. It is frequently associated with thymic tumors and sometimes can be successfully treated by removal of a thymoma or by immunosuppressive agents. Bone marrow elements other than the red cells are normal, and thus, in contrast to primary myeloproliferative syndromes, transformation to acute leukemia does not occur. In response to the anemia, serum erythropoietin levels are high. (*Cecil, Ch. 133*)

74.(A—True; B—False; C—True; D—True) Although many patients with mild elevations of hematocrit do not have polycythemia vera, when the hematocrit rises above 65%, the probability of the hematologic disease is very high. Splenomegaly is characteristic of polycythemia vera rather than secondary causes. There is good evidence that reducing the hematocrit to less than 45% does reduce the risk of thrombotic complications. Erythromelalgia responds very well to treatment with aspirin. (*Cecil, Ch. 153*)

75.(G); 76.(F); 77.(C); 78.(E); 79.(B); 80.(H); 81.(D); 82.(F); 83.(A); 84.(C) Although most cancers may result from the combined effects of multiple exposures to carcinogenic agents and susceptibility states, certain agents have striking correlations with specific cancers. Tobacco smoke, principally associated with lung cancer, is also linked to carcinomas of the head and neck, pancreatic cancers, and transitional cell carcinomas of the bladder. Squamous cell carcinoma of the bladder is primarily seen in the Middle East and Africa, associated with schistosomiasis. In warm, moist areas supporting the growth of *Aspergillus flavus*, a grain-contaminating mold producing aflatoxins, there is an associated linkage with hepatocellular carcinoma. Ionizing radiation probably spares no bodily site from its carcinogenic effects, but with regard to this list of agents, it is most commonly associated with leukemia and thyroid carcinoma. Ultraviolet radiation is associated with skin cancers, including melanoma. Exogenous estrogens are associated with adenocarcinoma of the endometrium, vagina, and probably breast. Asbestos is associated with both pleural and peritoneal mesotheliomas as well as parenchymal lung carcinomas. Some viruses have been closely linked with specific malignancies, including Epstein-Barr virus, which is associated with both nasopharyngeal carcinoma and Burkitt's lymphoma. (*Cecil, Chs. 129 and 170*)

85.(B); 86.(C); 87.(A); 88.(D) Bernard-Soulier syndrome is caused by the congenital deficiency of the receptor for von Willebrand's factor. Thus, just as in von Willebrand's disease, tests of platelet aggregation are normal and the defect will not be diagnosed unless tests of platelet aggregation with ristocetin are performed. Glanzmann's thrombasthenia is caused by the congenital deficiency of the platelet receptor for fibrinogen. In the absence of fibrinogen binding, neither platelet aggregation nor clot retraction can occur. The platelet defect seen in essential thrombocytosis can paradoxically lead to both bleeding and thromboses. Storage pool disease causes an "aspirin-like" disorder because, when tested in vitro, platelets undergo a primary wave of aggregation but not a secondary wave. (*Cecil, Ch. 166*)

89.(B); 90.(D); 91.(A); 92.(A); 93.(D); 94.(C); 95.(B); 96.(C) The non-Hodgkin's lymphomas are a heterogeneous group of malignant neoplasms with distinct histopathologic subtypes, traditionally classified by morphologic features and, more recently, by immunologic techniques. Histopathologic subtyping and clinical staging are critical to establishing disease prognosis and deciding on the most effective therapy for each type of lymphoma. Doxorubicin-containing drug combinations have produced apparent cures in patients with diffuse histiocyte lymphoma. Cyclophosphamide-containing drug combinations, in conjunction with surgical reduction of localized tumor bulk, will also produce complete remissions in the majority of patients with Burkitt's lymphoma, and many of these will never relapse. (*Cecil, Chs. 157, 158, 159, and 160; DeVita et al*)

97.(A); 98.(B); 99.(C); 100.(E) Alpha$_2$ antiplasmin is the major plasma inhibitor of fibrinolysis, and congenital deficiency of this protein can lead to a bleeding diathesis. EACA is occasionally used in the treatment of subarachnoid hemorrhage and urinary tract bleeding. However, when used without concurrent heparinization in the treatment of DIC, it may lead to catastrophic thromboses. Streptokinase is a bacterial product and can occasionally cause life-threatening anaphylaxis. Although the place of fibrinolytic therapy in the treatment of thrombosis is still controversial, urokinase or tissue plasminogen activator (TPA) may be helpful in the treatment of massive pulmonary embolus. (*Cecil, Ch. 167*)

101.(D); 102.(B); 103.(G); 104.(F); 105.(C) Cutaneous lesions occasionally predate the clinical appearance of life-threatening neoplasms, and a knowledge of those associations may aid in the timely diagnosis and treatment of these malignancies. Necrolytic migratory erythema is a symmetrical, eczematous dermatitis associated with glucagon-secreting pancreatic carcinomas. When the presence of benign subcutaneous nodules and café-au-lait spots confirms the diagnosis of neurofibromatosis, there is a 5–16% chance of malignant transformation to a variety of soft tissue sarcomas, as well as the abrupt clinical appearance of hypertension signifying pheochromocytoma. Ash-leaf lesions of hypomelanosis actually predate tuberous sclerosis and the accompanying development of angiofibromas of the skin and oral cavity, gliomas of the brain, and hamartomas of the kidney. Acanthosis nigricans is usually bilateral and localized in axillae, nuchal folds, or groin and is associated with viscerally located adenocarcinomas that tend to be aggressive and rapidly fatal. The onset of ichthyosis in an adult suggests an underlying malignant process; lymphoma or multiple myeloma is found most frequently, with regression and recurrence of the tumor reflected in the activity of the dermatosis. Vitiligo may be associated with diseases of autoimmune pathogenesis, while dermatitis herpetiformis is a blistering disease associated with malabsorptive enteropathy; neither of these cutaneous disorders has an increased association with malignancy. (*Cecil, Chs. 175, 477, and 534*)

106.(C); 107.(B); 108.(A); 109.(E) When a patient is doubly heterozygous for hemoglobin S and beta$^+$-thalassemia, hemoglobin A is still produced, although in reduced amounts. The condition resulting from the combination of heterozygous hemoglobin S and alpha-thalassemia resembles sickle trait with the exception that the percentage of hemoglobin S is usually less than the 40% typically found in sickle trait patients. This lower percentage of hemoglobin S is thought to be due to more effective competition for the relatively scarce alpha chains by the normal beta globin chains. Homozygous hemoglobin S disease is usually characterized by hyposplenism in adult life. This is in contrast to the more frequent preservation of splenic function in sickle beta-thalassemia and hemoglobin SC disease. In addition to relative preservation of splenic function, hemoglobin SC disease is also notable for an increased incidence of ocular complications. The combination of hemoglobin S plus hereditary persistence of fetal hemoglobin is an asymptomatic nonanemic condition with high levels of hemoglobin F and no detectable hemoglobin A. (*Cecil, Ch. 143*)

110.(B); 111.(C); 112.(A) Several hematologic malignancies have well-described and characteristic karyotypic abnormalities. The 8,14 translocation of Burkitt's lymphoma and the 9,22 translocation of CML are the best-described entities. Treatment-related AML frequently is associated with loss of chromosomes 5 and 7. Hyperdiploidy is seen in childhood ALL and confers a favorable prognosis. (*Cecil, Chs. 152 and 156; Brodeur*)

113.(B); 114.(A); 115.(B); 116.(B); 117.(A) Hypercalcemia may occur as the result of a variety of pathophysiologic processes, including extensive bone marrow metastases and production of an ectopic hormone with parathyroid hormone–like activity. Hypercalcemia is much more commonly associated with epidermoid carcinoma of the lung and is often due to production of ectopic hormone activity. In contrast, hypercalcemia is a very unusual complication in patients with oat cell carcinoma of the lung, despite the high incidence of bone marrow metastases. Small-cell or oat cell carcinoma of the lung is usually a rapidly progressive tumor with a high propensity for metastatic disease. Without prophylactic cranial irradiation, most patients will develop symptomatic CNS metastases. Even with prophylactic cranial irradiation, some patients with small-cell carcinoma of the lung develop leptomeningeal metastases. This complication seems to occur most frequently in patients who have marrow involvement by tumor at the time of diagnosis. In contrast to small-cell carcinoma of the lung, epidermoid carcinoma of the lung sometimes appears to develop more slowly. With the more widespread use of cytologic testing, some patients have been found to shed malignant squamous epithelial cells from the lower respiratory tract, although testing, including bronchoscopy, is unable to localize a specific tumor site. Early diagnosis of epidermoid carcinoma of the lung, either by x-ray or by cytologic screening, allows a subgroup of patients to achieve a cure by surgery. In contrast, the more rapidly progressive small-cell carcinoma of the lung, with its higher metastatic potential, is seldom cured by surgery and is treated primarily with chemotherapy and radiation therapy. With combination chemotherapy, including alkylating agents and/or anthracyclines, more than half of patients with small-cell carcinoma of the lung have an objective response to chemotherapy. In patients with limited-stage small-cell cancer, chemotherapeutic response seems to increase survival. (*Cecil, Ch. 70; Haskell; Weiss*)

118.(B); 119.(C); 120.(D); 121.(A) Of the disorders listed, only multiple myeloma commonly causes lytic bone disease. Patients with benign monoclonal gammopathy may have any type of serum or urine paraprotein. Most patients with primary amyloidosis have a paraprotein in serum or urine, and Bence-Jones proteinuria is a common finding. Waldenström's macroglobulinemia is differentiated from multiple myeloma by the secretion of an IgM paraprotein. (*Cecil, Ch. 163; Kyle*)

122.(C); 123.(C); 124.(A); 125.(A) Theoretically, primary polycythemia should be easily distinguished from secondary polycythemia by the suppression of erythropoietin levels. The test is still useful, although some overlap does exist. Elevated leukocyte alkaline phosphatase may be seen in primary polycythemia. When the hematocrit rises to high levels, the rheologic properties of the blood may be unfavorable and may lead to decreased cerebral blood flow. Both primary and secondary polycythemia cause elevation of the red blood cell mass. If the red blood cell mass is normal, the patient is said to have spurious polycythemia. (*Cecil, Ch. 153*)

126.(B); 127.(D); 128.(A); 129.(C) Allogeneic bone marrow transplantation is highly successful in treating chronic phase CML. Hairy cell leukemia to date is the malignancy most responsive to interferon. Although not a routine treatment, splenectomy is a useful palliative measure in patients with myelofibrosis whose giant spleens are causing mechanical problems or high transfusion requirements. Chlorambucil is standard therapy for CLL. (*Cecil, Chs. 154 and 155; Quesada et al; Thomas et al*)

130.(D); 131.(B); 132.(E); 133.(C); 134.(B); 135.(A) Methotrexate distributes slowly into "third spaces" such as ascites or pleural effusions. The slow re-entry of drug into the systemic circulation has been associated with a prolonged half-life and unexpected toxicity. In addition, drugs such as acetylsalicylic acid (aspirin) that interfere with renal tubular secretion of methotrexate may also increase its half-life and lead to toxicity. The liver is the main site of metabolism of both doxorubicin and daunorubicin; consequently, a 75% dose reduction for bilirubin greater than 3 mg/dl is recommended. 6-Mercaptopurine is rapidly eliminated by xanthine oxidase, an enzyme inhibited by allopurinol; thus, a 75% dose reduction of 6-MP is recommended in patients requiring allopurinol. A problematic side effect of cyclophosphamide is hemorrhagic cystitis; dehydration and pre-existent cystitis can potentiate this form of toxicity. Cisplatin nephrotoxicity is associated with tubular damage similar to the nephrotoxicity that occurs in most patients receiving amphotericin B. Giving cisplatin concurrent with amphotericin B should be avoided. (*Cecil, Chs. 25, 82, and 176*)

BIBLIOGRAPHY

Brodeur GM: Molecular correlates of cytogenetic abnormalities in human cancer cells: Implications for oncogene activation. Prog Hematol 14:229, 1986.

Camitta BM, Storb R, Thomas ED: Aplastic anemia: Pathogenesis, diagnosis, treatment, and prognosis. N Engl J Med 306:645, 1982.

Cecil Textbook of Medicine. 18th ed. Wyngaarden JB, Smith LH Jr (eds). Philadelphia, W. B. Saunders Company, 1988.

Colman RW, Robboy SJ, Minna JD: Disseminated intravascular coagulation: A reappraisal. Annu Rev Med 30:359, 1979.

DeVita VT Jr, Hellman S, Rosenberg SA (eds): Cancer, Principles and Practice of Oncology. Philadelphia, J. B. Lippincott, 1985.

Eschbach JW, Egrie JC, Downing MR, et al: Correction of the anemia of end-stage renal disease with recombinant human erythropoietin: Results of a combined Phase I and II clinical trial. N Engl J Med 316:73, 1987.

Foon KA, Schroff RW, Gale RP: Surface markers on leukemia and lymphoma cells: Recent advances. Blood 60:1, 1982.

Forget BG: Molecular genetics of human hemoglobin synthesis. Ann Intern Med 91:605, 1979.

Frank MM, Schreiber AD, Atkinson JP, et al: Pathophysiology of immune hemolytic anemia. Ann Intern Med 87:210, 1977.

Haskell CM (ed): Cancer Treatment. 2nd ed. Philadelphia, W. B. Saunders Company, 1985.

Kacich R, Linker C: Thrombotic thrombocytopenic purpura. Medical Staff Conference, University of California, San Francisco. West J Med 136:513, 1982.

Kyle RA: Monoclonal gammopathy of undetermined significance. Natural history in 241 cases. Am J Med 64:814, 1978.

Legha SS, Davis HL, Muggia FM: Hormonal therapy of breast cancer: New approaches and concepts. Ann Intern Med 88:69, 1978.

Mazzaferri EL, O'Dorisio TM, LoBuglio AF: Treatment of hypercalcemia associated with malignancy. Semin Oncol 5:141, 1978.

McMillan R: Chronic idiopathic thrombocytopenic purpura. N Engl J Med 304:1135, 1981.

Mollison PL: Blood Transfusion in Clinical Medicine. 7th ed. Oxford, Blackwell Scientific Publications, 1983.

Quesada JR, Reuben J, Manning JT, et al: Alpha interferon for induction of remission in hairy-cell leukemia. N Engl J Med 310:15, 1984.

Thomas ED, Clift RA, Fefer A, et al: Marrow transplantation for the treatment of chronic myelogenous leukemia. Ann Intern Med 104:155, 1986.

Weiss RB: Small-cell carcinoma of the lung: Therapeutic management. Ann Intern Med 88:522, 1978.

Williams WJ, Beutler EL, Erslev AJ, et al (eds): Hematology. 3rd ed. New York, McGraw-Hill Book Company, 1983.

Zimmerman TS, Ruggeri ZM: Von Willebrand's disease. Prog Hemost Thromb 6:203, 1982.

PART 6

GENETIC AND METABOLIC DISEASE

RICHARD D. KLAUSNER and JURRIEN DEAN

DIRECTIONS: For questions 1 to 32, choose the ONE BEST answer to each question.

1. Each of the following statements is true about polycystic kidney disease EXCEPT

A. there is an associated hepatic fibrosis
B. the disease is inherited as an autosomal dominant trait
C. approximately 10% of affected patients have cerebral aneurysms
D. onset of clinical symptoms is usual in the fourth decade and renal dialysis and/or transplant is necessary by the fifth decade
E. it is the most common form of inherited kidney disease in the adult

2. Amniocentesis would be indicated in each of the following pregnancies EXCEPT

A. a 23-year-old woman who has a 3-year-old son with Duchenne dystrophy
B. a 23-year-old couple who have a 5-year-old son with Lesch-Nyhan syndrome
C. a 23-year-old couple who have two children affected with sickle cell anemia
D. a 25-year-old unaffected couple who have had one child with achondroplasia
E. a 39-year-old woman who is pregnant for the first time

3. Each of the following is true of cystic fibrosis EXCEPT

A. it is characterized by repeated pulmonary infections, malabsorption, and an increased risk of intestinal obstruction due to intussusception
B. diagnosis is confirmed by an elevation in the concentration of sodium and/or chloride in sweat
C. because of the recent linkage of the cystic fibrosis gene to genetic markers on the long arm of chromosome 7, prenatal diagnosis is now available for all patients at risk
D. the major morbidity and mortality are associated with pulmonary infections and the resultant cor pulmonale
E. it is the most common autosomal disease in the white population in the United States

4. What percentage of autosomal genes do a boy and his maternal aunt have in common?

A. 5%
B. 12½%
C. 25%
D. 33⅓%
E. 50%

5. The Tourette syndrome is a common neuropsychiatric disease associated with chronic tics and vocalizations. Each of the following statements is true EXCEPT

A. it is inherited as a multifactorial disease
B. no more than 30% of the patients have coprolalia
C. patients characteristically have problems with discipline and are prone to anger and violence
D. haloperidol is the therapeutic drug of choice
E. onset is most commonly in the first decade of life

6. Which of the following corresponds to the karyotype 47,XX, +21?

A. Down's syndrome
B. Noonan's syndrome
C. Klinefelter's syndrome
D. Bloom's syndrome
E. Turner's syndrome

7. Different alleles of *N*-acetyltransferase result in two different human phenotypes that differ in their ability to acetylate and metabolize certain drugs, including each of the following EXCEPT

A. isoniazid
B. hydralazine
C. salicyl-azo-sulfapyridine
D. dapsone
E. phenytoin

8. A newborn infant of unaffected 26-year-old parents died recently in a hyperammonemic coma and was diagnosed as having ornithine carbamyl transferase deficiency (OCT). The mother is again pregnant and comes to you for counseling. Which of the following is correct?

A. The best available option at this time is prenatal diagnosis and elective abortion
B. The mother should be treated with sodium benzoate and restriction of dietary protein during pregnancy
C. Fifty per cent of her sons but none of her daughters will be at risk of having OCT
D. The neonate should be treated with sodium benzoate and restriction of dietary protein
E. Metabolic acidosis is characteristically seen after treatment of neonatal hyperammonemia

9. Each of the following statements concerning the thalassemic syndromes is true EXCEPT

A. deletion of the gene occurs more commonly in beta-thalassemia than in alpha-thalassemia
B. beta-thalassemia can be caused by a point mutation leading to premature termination of globin transcription
C. beta-thalassemia can be caused by a point mutation, leading to defective splicing of precursor globin mRNA
D. unbalanced chain synthesis results in ineffective erythropoiesis
E. patients with beta-thalassemia trait are asymptomatic

10. The pedigree illustrated is most consistent with which one of the following patterns of inheritance?

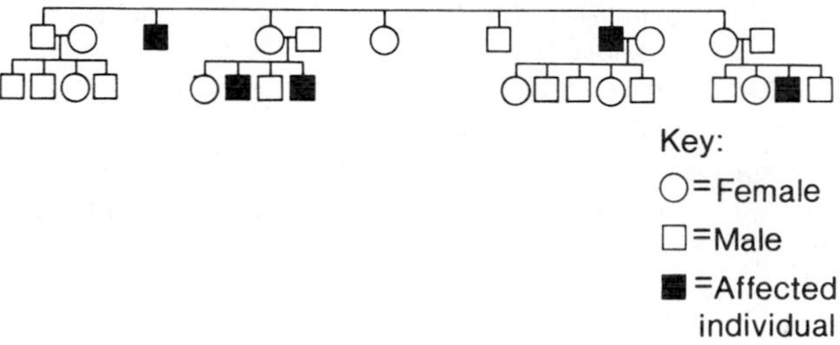

Key:
○=Female
□=Male
■=Affected individual

A. Autosomal recessive
B. Autosomal dominant
C. X-linked recessive
D. X-linked dominant
E. Polygenic

11. Each of the following statements is true of von Gierke's disease EXCEPT

A. it results from a deficiency of glucose-6-phosphatase
B. it is associated with hypoglycemia
C. it is inherited as an X-linked recessive
D. it is associated with hyperlipidemia
E. it is associated with hyperuricemia

12. You are asked to see a 9-year-old girl with short stature, a webbed neck, and a systolic murmur. You should consider each of the following diagnoses EXCEPT

A. trisomy 13
B. trisomy 21
C. Turner's syndrome
D. Noonan's syndrome
E. fetal hydantoin syndrome

13. Each of the following is true of Menke's syndrome EXCEPT

A. it is inherited as an X-linked recessive trait
B. treatment with parenteral copper reverses the clinical course of the disease
C. abnormal copper transport results in low levels of serum copper and ceruloplasmin
D. abnormal copper transport results in abnormal copper accumulation in the duodenum and jejunum
E. prenatal diagnosis is possible by observing abnormal copper metabolism in cultured amniotic cells

14. An asymptomatic 20-year-old woman has one brother with cystic fibrosis. Neither of her parents is affected. The chance that she is a carrier is

A. 25%
B. 33⅓%
C. 50%
D. 66⅔%
E. 75%

15. Each of the following syndromes is associated with photosensitivity EXCEPT

A. Bloom syndrome
B. Cockayne syndrome
C. erythropoietic protoporphyria
D. congenital erythropoietic porphyria
E. hereditary hemorrhagic telangiectasia

16. Which of the following statements about gout is FALSE?

A. Monosodium urate crystals in leukocytes are generally found in synovial fluid during acute arthritis
B. The majority of patients have normal excretion of uric acid in the urine
C. The prevalence of arthritis, but not nephrolithiasis, is correlated with the serum urate level
D. Nephropathy is probably *not* caused by associated nephrolithiasis alone
E. Urine acidity predisposes toward nephrolithiasis

17. Which of the following statements concerning severe combined immunodeficiency disorders (SCID) is correct?

A. They are clinically associated with eczema and megakaryocytic thrombocytopenic purpura
B. They are inherited as autosomal dominant genetic diseases
C. Patients receiving monthly injections of gamma globulin have normal immunologic functions
D. Thirty per cent of patients have an associated adenosine deaminase deficiency with SCID
E. Thirty per cent of patients with adenosine deaminase deficiency have SCID

18. Which of the following statements about Wilson's disease is FALSE?

A. Penicillamine is the treatment of choice
B. It is inherited as an autosomal recessive trait
C. Although liver disease is common, the onset is rarely acute
D. The most common neurologic symptoms include loss of coordination and movement disorders
E. Liver accumulation of copper results from the failure of biliary excretion of the metal

19. Each of the following enzymatic defects is known to produce hyperuricemia EXCEPT

A. hypoxanthine-guanine phosphoribosyl transferase (HPRT) deficiency
B. muscle phosphorylase deficiency
C. glucose-6-phosphatase deficiency (G6PD)
D. phosphoribosyl pyrophosphate synthetase abnormalities
E. partial HPRT deficiency

20. Which of the following statements about acute intermittent porphyria (AIP) is FALSE?

A. It is an autosomal dominant trait
B. The biochemical defect results in a deficiency of porphobilinogen deaminase

C. Abdominal pain is usually the first clinical symptom
D. Because of the enzyme deficiency, patients have excess excretion of porphobilinogen
E. Clinical expression usually first occurs after puberty

21. Which of the following clinical manifestations of the Lesch-Nyhan syndrome is NOT seen in patients with partial deficiency of HPRT?

A. Renal calculi
B. Gouty arthritis
C. Mental retardation
D. Self-mutilation
E. Tophi

22. Which of the following statements concerning xeroderma pigmentosum is FALSE?

A. The patients have a high incidence of sunlight-induced cutaneous malignancies
B. Heterozygotes are asymptomatic
C. One genetically distinct group of patients develops neurologic disorders
D. The disease is due to hypersensitivity of DNA to initial UV-induced damage
E. Photophobia is common early in the disease

23. Ocular manifestations are observed in each of the following EXCEPT

A. Fabry's disease
B. Marfan's syndrome
C. HPRT deficiency
D. Wilson's disease
E. Xeroderma pigmentosum

24. Which of the following statements concerning familial hypercholesterolemia is FALSE?

A. Heterozygotes are rarely clinically affected
B. Serum LDL cholesterol is elevated from birth
C. Tendon xanthomas are present
D. The disorder is the result of defective receptors for LDL
E. Migratory polyarthritis may be present

25. Each of the following is true about homozygous α_1-antitrypsin deficiency EXCEPT

A. it is due to the failure of the protein to be excreted from the liver
B. the majority of patients will develop panacinar emphysema
C. it can cause neonatal hepatitis
D. some severely affected patients have normal levels of the serum protein
E. it is inherited via two co-dominant autosomal alleles

26. Phytanic acid storage (Refsum's) disease is characterized by each of the following EXCEPT

A. enhanced synthesis of phytanic acid
B. peripheral neuropathy
C. failure to oxidize phytanic acid
D. accumulation of exogenous phytanic acid
E. retinitis pigmentosa

27. Each of the following defects has been found for the LDL receptor in familial hypercholesterolemia EXCEPT

A. failure to synthesize the receptor
B. failure to correctly transport the receptor to the cell surface
C. failure to degrade the receptor after internalization
D. failure to internalize the receptor
E. abnormal binding of ligand

28. In patients with severe neurologic or neuromuscular dysfunction, it may be necessary to treat an attack of acute intermittent porphyria with intravenous hematin. Which of the following mechanisms is thought to be responsible for the rapid response observed following hematin infusion?

A. Reversal of the neurotoxic effects of porphobilinogen
B. Stimulation of uroporphyrinogen synthetase activity
C. Suppression of delta-aminolevulinic acid (ALA) synthetase activity
D. Increase in urinary porphyrin excretion
E. Increased peripheral metabolism of porphyrins

29. Restriction fragment length polymorphisms (RFLP's) can help with the diagnosis of each of the following EXCEPT

A. Huntington's disease
B. Duchenne muscular dystrophy
C. beta-thalassemia
D. Wilson's disease
E. phenylketonuria

30. Which of the following statements about hereditary hemochromatosis is FALSE?

A. The heterozygote frequency is between 8 and 13%
B. Hypogonadism is frequently due to failure to secrete gonadotropins
C. Diabetes mellitus is caused by iron overload
D. In untreated patients with liver involvement, the risk of developing hepatocarcinoma is significant
E. The responsible gene is linked to the HLA locus on chromosome 6

31. Each of the following is true about phenylketonuria (PKU) EXCEPT

A. heterozygote frequency is about 1 in 50 Caucasians
B. the only known defect is in the gene for hepatic phenylalanine hydroxylase
C. a single molecular defect in the responsible gene is found in all patients
D. mental retardation is the major clinical manifestation

32. Each of the following statements about the genetic basis of Duchenne's muscular dystrophy is correct EXCEPT

A. it is the most common X-linked fatal genetic disease
B. diagnostic restriction fragment length polymorphisms provide the basis for both carrier detection and prenatal diagnosis
C. Becker's muscular dystrophy, in contrast to Duchenne's, is not localized to Xp21
D. some patients have large chromosomal deletions associated with abnormalities such as glycerol kinase deficiency

DIRECTIONS: For questions 33 to 60, you are to decide whether EACH choice is true or false. Any combination of answers, from all true to all false, may occur. Mark the answer sheet "T" or "F" in the space provided.

33. Type I diabetes mellitus (insulin-dependent diabetes mellitus) is seen in patients with a genetically susceptible background. Which of the following statements is/are true?

A. More than 90% of affected Caucasian patients have the DR3 and/or DR4 haplotype at the HLA locus
B. There is a higher incidence of disease in children of affected fathers than in children of affected mothers
C. Hyperosmolar coma occurs more commonly in affected patients than does ketoacidosis
D. The concordance of the disease among identical twins is greater than 90%

34. A couple has a 5-year-old mentally retarded daughter with galactosemia. The parents are unaffected and they wish to have another child. Which of the following would be included in appropriate counseling?

A. Reassurance that their child is a new "mutation" and that the recurrence risk is that of the general population
B. Advising each parent to have a karyotype to look for a deletion in 11p
C. Advising that amniocentesis should be performed during pregnancy to detect galactose-1-phosphate uridyl transferase
D. Advising that the mother should be placed on a low galactose diet during pregnancy

35. Which of the following is/are true about Huntington's disease?

A. It is inherited in an autosomal recessive manner
B. Using restriction length fragment polymorphisms (RFLP's), the defective gene has been mapped to chromosome 4
C. The recombination frequency between the RFLP and the Huntington's disease gene precludes the use of linkage analysis for genetic counseling
D. Affected patients appear normal at birth but feed poorly and have marked neurologic and developmental impairment by age five

36. The human genome is composed of approximately 3×10^9 base pairs of DNA on 46 chromosomes. Which of the following statements is/are true?

A. Genetic recombination takes place during the prophase of the second meiotic division
B. More than 90% of the genome is thought to code for structural proteins and enzymes
C. Mutations resulting in abnormal receptors are usually inherited as mendelian recessive diseases
D. More than 2000 autosomal loci have been mapped on the human gene map

37. Which of the following is/are true about prenatal hazards and congenital malformation?

A. Methylmercury causes abnormalities in brain development during the first trimester of gestation
B. Pregnant women treated with hydantoins for control of a seizure disorder are at greater risk of having children with congenital heart disease, cleft lip, and nail and digital hypoplasia
C. Prenatal exposure to cytomegalovirus can lead to deafness and mental retardation
D. Patients with artificial heart valves who are receiving vitamin K antagonists should take effective measures to avoid pregnancy

38. A 27-year-old Caucasian woman gave birth to a boy with a unilateral cleft lip and cleft palate. The baby died at 2 months of age from aspiration pneumonia. Your genetic counseling of the parents should include

A. a karyotype of father and mother
B. a determination of prenatal exposure to hydantoins
C. information that both parents are morphologically normal, there being a recurrence risk of 4%

39. Which of the following is/are true of epidermolysis bullosa?

A. The dominant form has been linked to a restriction fragment polymorphism on chromosome 9 and can now be detected prenatally
B. The major clinical manifestation is blister formation after minimal trauma
C. Only the X-linked variant leads to permanent scarring
D. Even with linkage analysis, genetic counseling of patients at risk is complicated by the late onset of clinical manifestations

40. Which of the following statements concerning Klinefelter's syndrome is/are true?

A. More than 95% of patients have gynecomastia
B. Most patients have hypospadias and hypoplasia of external genitalia
C. Diagnosis can be made at birth on the basis of characteristic dysmorphology
D. Most patients have severe mental retardation

41. A 28-year-old woman with a family history of Huntington's disease is married to her 30-year-old second cousin. She is now pregnant and consults you for prenatal diagnosis of Huntington's disease. Which of the following situations would present an ethical dilemma?

A. The fetus is affected and each parent wants to know his/her risk of also being affected
B. The fetus is affected and the parents want other relatives at risk to be notified
C. The fetus is affected and one parent but not the other wants to know if they have the abnormal gene
D. The fetus is affected but the parents do not want other members of their families to know

42. Homocystinuria is inherited as an autosomal recessive disease. Which of the following statements is/are true?

A. Homocystinuria is caused by a deficiency of cystathionine β-synthase
B. Homocystinuria is caused by a deficiency of 5,10-methylenetetrahydrofolate reductase
C. Thromboembolic events are a major cause of death
D. Osteoporosis and scoliosis are frequent complications of homocystinuria

43. Which of the following inherited syndromes is/are associated with deafness?

A. Treacher Collins syndrome
B. Waardenburg's syndrome
C. Alport's syndrome
D. Usher's syndrome

44. Orotic aciduria occurs in which of the following conditions?

A. Deficiencies of orotate phosphoribosyltransferase and orotidine 5'-phosphate decarboxylase
B. Therapy with allopurinol
C. Ornithine transcarbamylase deficiency
D. Carbamyl phosphate synthetase deficiency

45. Which of the following statements is/are true of sickle cell anemia?

A. It is inherited as an autosomal recessive disease, and heterozygotes do not have clinical manifestations of the disease
B. Prenatal diagnosis is based on a restriction enzyme site in fetal DNA created by the sickle mutation in the B-globin gene
C. Newborns rarely have clinical manifestations because of their relatively higher levels of hemoglobin A_2
D. Balanced polymorphism is thought to explain the preservation of the deleterious sickle gene in black populations
E. Hemoglobin SF disease is the second most common form of sickling disorder and has qualitatively similar clinical manifestations

46. Laurence-Moon-Biedl syndrome is associated with which of the following findings?

A. Obesity
B. Retinitis pigmentosa
C. Hypogonadism
D. Polydactyly

47. Which of the following is/are true of familial cancer syndromes, in contrast to nonfamilial cancers?

A. Tumors have an earlier age of onset
B. Tumors are more commonly multifocal (bilateral, if applicable)
C. An affected individual is more likely to have a second cancer
D. The concordance of cancer in identical twins is greater than 90%
E. In almost all pedigrees that have been reported, the incidence of cancer appears to follow the inheritance pattern of autosomal recessive

48. Which of the following statements about cystinosis is/are true?

A. All patients develop nephropathy
B. It is inherited as an autosomal recessive trait
C. It is the result of accumulation of cystine in cellular lysosomes
D. Cystine accumulates in the cell due to enhanced synthesis of this amino acid
E. The early manifestations of cystinotic nephropathy are renal tubular defects

49. Which of the following clinical states is/are associated with gout?

A. Hypertension
B. Rheumatoid arthritis
C. Obesity
D. Diabetes mellitus

50. Hematologic abnormalities occur in which of the following disorders?

A. Pyruvate kinase deficiency
B. Hereditary hemochromatosis
C. Familial hypercholesterolemia
D. Dihydrofolate reductase deficiency

51. Which of the following is/are true of joint involvement in gout?

A. Untreated attacks will often last for weeks
B. Podagra is experienced by the vast majority of patients
C. Polyarticular arthritis is rarely, if ever, seen
D. The majority of untreated patients will experience a recurrence after the first attack

52. Which of the following genetic diseases is/are linked to the HLA locus?

A. Wilson's disease
B. Adenosine deaminase deficiency
C. Hereditary hemochromatosis
D. 21-hydroxylase deficiency
E. α_1-Antitrypsin deficiency

53. Which of the following statements regarding glucose-6-phosphate dehydrogenase (G6PD) deficiency is/are true?

A. Inheritance is X-linked
B. Administration of sulfa drugs induces hemolysis
C. It is associated with neurologic deterioration
D. Enzyme deficiency is most easily documented immediately following an episode of hemolysis

54. Which of the following is/are true about purine metabolism in humans?

A. Xanthine oxidase is found in high concentrations in all organs of the body
B. Uric acid is produced by the oxidation of xanthine
C. Inosine monophosphate can be converted to both adenosine and guanosine monophosphate
D. Salvage pathways result in the synthesis of ribonucleotides from free purines

55. Which of the following statements is/are true about AMP deaminase deficiency?

A. It is inherited as an autosomal recessive trait
B. It is clinically characterized by a peripheral neuropathy
C. Enzyme deficiency results in the failure to convert AMP into CMP
D. Patients complain of muscle fatigue and postexercise cramps
E. Patients demonstrate excessive rises in blood NH_3 upon exercise

56. Uric acid calculi are associated with which of the following abnormalities?

A. Increased uric acid excretion
B. Persistently alkaline urine

C. Highly concentrated urine
D. Renal tubular acidosis

57. Which of the following statements is/are true about hereditary spherocytosis?

A. It is inherited as a sex-linked recessive trait
B. Patients do *not* respond to splenectomy
C. 80% of patients have transfusion-dependent anemia
D. Patients can experience aplastic crises
E. Patients rarely develop clinically apparent gallbladder disease

58. Which of the following drugs is/are CONTRAINDICATED in patients with acute intermittent porphyria, variegate porphyria, and hereditary coproporphyria?

A. Phenothiazines
B. Barbiturates
C. Sulfonamides
D. Intravenous glucose

59. Which of the following statements about tyrosinase-negative oculocutaneous albinism is/are true?

A. Visual acuity is normal
B. Hair color will darken with age
C. Nystagmus and photophobia are present
D. Serum tyrosine levels are elevated

60. Which of the following statements regarding familial Mediterranean fever is/are correct?

A. It is inherited in an autosomal dominant manner
B. It is more common in people of Mediterranean or Middle Eastern origin than in the general population living in the United States
C. It is a self-limited, acute, febrile illness accompanied by peritonitis, arthritis, or pleuritis
D. Among patients living in the United States, amyloidosis is a rare complication of this disorder

DIRECTIONS: Questions 61 to 94 are matching questions. For each numbered item, choose the most likely associated lettered item from those provided. Each numbered item has ONLY ONE answer. Within each set of questions, each lettered item may be the answer to one, more than one, or none of the numbered items.

QUESTIONS 61–64

For each of the following clinical descriptions, select the appropriate tumor.

A. Multiple endocrine adenomatosis, type 1
B. Retinoblastoma
C. Wilms' tumor
D. Neuroblastoma

61. A subset of affected patients has associated aniridia and a deletion in the p13 band on chromosome 11

62. The most common tumor of childhood, which generally occurs sporadically but is also inherited as an autosomal dominant disease

63. Inherited as an autosomal dominant disease with a subset having a deletion on chromosome 13 at band q14

64. Increased susceptibility to developing osteosarcoma as a second tumor

QUESTIONS 65–68

A number of genetic diseases are associated with abnormalities of the gastrointestinal tract. For each of the following clinical situations, select the appropriate genetic syndrome.

A. Gardner's syndrome
B. Neurofibromatosis
C. Peutz-Jeghers syndrome
D. Turcot's syndrome

65. Benign tumors, most commonly in the stomach and jejunum, which rarely protrude into the lumen

66. Colorectal polyps associated with osteomas and exostoses of the skull, mandible, and long bones as well as soft tissue tumors of the skin

67. Mucocutaneous pigmentation associated with intestinal polyps, most commonly in the jejunum and ileum, which are rarely premalignant

68. An autosomal dominant disease associated with a high risk of colorectal cancer

QUESTIONS 69–71

Pharmacogenetic studies have demonstrated the existence of phenotypes that differ in their ability to metabolize drugs. Match each of the following clinical situations with the appropriate syndromes.

A. Glucose-6-phosphate dehydrogenase deficiency
B. Chlorpropamide-alcohol flushing
C. Malignant hyperthermia
D. Pseudocholinesterase deficiency

69. A 35-year-old woman anesthetized with halothane for elective surgery who dies suddenly on the operating table prior to the first incision

70. A 35-year-old man being treated with primaquine for malaria who develops anemia

71. Prior to anesthesia, a 35-year-old woman who is treated with succinylcholine chloride and develops prolonged apnea

QUESTIONS 72–74

The phakomatoses syndromes often have characteristic changes in pigmentation. Match each of the following clinical descriptions with the appropriate syndrome.

A. Sturge-Weber syndrome
B. Tuberous sclerosis
C. Neurofibromatosis
D. von Hippel-Lindau disease

72. Lesch nodules in the iris of the eye

73. Hypomelanotic macules (ash leaf spots)

74. Facial nevus flammeus (purple flat angiomas)

QUESTIONS 75–78

For each of the patients with genetic disease described below, select the most appropriate therapy.

A. Phlebotomy
B. Penicillamine
C. Androgens
D. Castration
E. Hematin
F. Progesterone

75. A 9-year-old girl who has short stature and a webbed neck; karyotype reveals a 40,XO/46,XY mosaicism

76. A 20-year-old woman who has episodic abdominal pain, often associated with generalized nonpitting edema

77. A 20-year-old woman who has abdominal pain and acute psychosis 36 hours after starting use of oral contraceptives; serum sodium is 120 mEq/L

78. A 40-year-old man who has impotence, hypogonadism, mildly elevated SGOT, and symmetric arthritis affecting the second and third metacarpophalangeal joints

QUESTIONS 79–82

For each of the patients described below, select the most likely associated malformation.

A. Aortic stenosis
B. Coarctation of the aorta
C. Atrioventricular canal
D. Pulmonic stenosis
E. Patent ductus arteriosus

79. An infant with hypotonia, brachydactyly, and trisomy for a small acrocentric autosome

80. A 10-year-old boy who has hypertelorism, downward eye slant, mild mental retardation, pectus excavatum, and a webbed neck

81. A 15-year-old girl who has a webbed neck, cubitus valgus, gonadal dysgenesis, short stature, normal intelligence, and 45 chromosomes; as a newborn, she was noted to have pedal edema

82. A 20-year-old man who has a coarse voice, thickened lips, stellate iris, and mental retardation; he has a history of neonatal hypercalcemia

QUESTIONS 83–85

Match each mode of inheritance with the appropriate disease.

A. Autosomal dominant
B. X-linked
C. Autosomal recessive

83. Cystic fibrosis

84. HPRT deficiency

85. Porphyria cutanea tarda

QUESTIONS 86–88

Match each disorder of the complement system with the appropriate clinical syndrome.

A. C3 deficiency
B. C1 inhibitor deficiency
C. C8 deficiency

86. Observed in patients with recurrent or persistent infections with *Neisseria*

87. Recurrent attacks of transient, acute-onset edema are localized to different areas of the skin

88. Patients have recurrent episodes of severe infections with both gram-negative and gram-positive organisms

QUESTIONS 89–91

Match each description with the appropriate syndrome of abnormal bilirubin metabolism.

A. Criggler Najjar syndrome type I
B. Gilbert's syndrome
C. Dubin-Johnson syndrome

89. Elevated levels of unconjugated bilirubin presenting with kernicterus

90. Mild conjugated hyperbilirubinemia and jaundice which increase with illness

91. Mild benign unconjugated hyperbilirubinemia

QUESTIONS 92–94

Match each of the following clinical descriptions with the appropriate lysosomal enzyme deficiency.

A. Arylsulfatase A deficiency
B. Glucocerebrosidase deficiency
C. α-Galactosidase-A deficiency

92. A 12-year-old boy who has episodes of pain and paresthesias in the trunk and extremities. On physical examination the patient is noted to have vascular skin lesions in a bathing suit distribution

93. A 21-year-old man who presents with a clinical picture of progressive loss of neural function over an 18-month period, characterized by loss of memory, disorganized thinking, and personality changes. His general motor ability has slowed

94. A 30-year-old man who has splenomegaly, anemia, leukopenia, and thrombocytopenia. He has mild hepatomegaly with slight elevations of serum levels of liver enzymes. He has noted back and leg pains for several years; roentgenograms show evidence of aseptic necrosis of the head of the femur

PART 6

GENETIC AND METABOLIC DISEASE

ANSWERS

1.(A) Adult polycystic kidney disease is inherited as an autosomal dominant trait. Unlike childhood polycystic disease, it is not associated with hepatic fibrosis, although liver cysts are not uncommon. Approximately 10% of affected patients have cerebral artery aneurysms, and a small percentage die from subarachnoid bleeding. Typically, symptoms (flank pain, renal mass, hematuria, etc.) appear in the fourth decade and overt renal failure in the fifth decade. *(Cecil, Ch. 91; Heptinstall, pp. 83–140)*

2.(D) Amniocentesis is useful for the prenatal diagnosis of genetic diseases with known biochemical abnormalities. The biochemical defect causing achondroplasia is unknown. The disease is inherited as an autosomal dominant. If the parents are unaffected, the child must represent a new spontaneous mutation. Subsequent children should not be at greater risk of having achondroplasia than the general population. Amniocentesis is indicated for women over the age of 35 because of the increased risk of having children with chromosomal abnormalities. It has also been used for selective abortion of male fetuses of women who are obligatory carriers of Duchenne dystrophy. It is of particular use in diagnosing specific biochemical defects such as sickle cell anemia. *(Cecil, Ch. 36; Smith, pp. 248–251)*

3.(C) Cystic fibrosis is the most common autosomal recessive disease among whites in the United States. It is associated with obstructive pulmonary disease, pancreatic insufficiency, intestinal obstruction, cirrhosis of the liver, and infertility. The clinical diagnosis is confirmed by elevated levels of sodium or chloride or both in sweat. Recently, the cystic fibrosis gene has been linked (within 1% recombination) to two genetic markers on chromosome 7. However, these markers will be 96% accurate only for prenatal diagnosis in fully informant pedigrees and not in all patients at risk. *(Cecil, Ch. 66; Stanbury et al, pp. 1889–1917; Beaudet et al)*

4.(C) The percentage of autosomal genes shared by any two relatives is a direct function of their degree of relation, i.e., as given by the equation

$$C = 0.5^n$$

where n is the degree of relation and C is the percentage of genes in common. Thus, first-degree relatives (e.g., sibling–sibling, parent–offspring) share 50% of their genes, and second-degree relatives (e.g., nephew–aunt) share 25% of their autosomal genes. Calculations of this sort are important in determining the increased risk for a deleterious recessive disorder among the offspring of a consanguineous mating. *(Vogel and Motulsky, pp. 414–416)*

5.(A) The Tourette syndrome is inherited as an autosomal dominant disease with as much as 1% of the population being carriers of the gene. The age of onset is usually between 3 and 12. It is characterized by chronic tics and vocalizations, although no more than 30% of the patients have coprolalia. Patients often have problems with discipline and are prone to anger, violence, exhibitionism, and obsessive-compulsive behavior. Haloperidol has been particularly useful in treating this syndrome, and incremental doses are used to reach a goal of 70–90% suppression of tics. *(Cecil, Ch. 472; Comings and Comings)*

6.(A) By conventional nomenclature, this shorthand notation describes a female XX with 47 chromosomes, including an extra chromosome 21. The clinical diagnosis is Down's syndrome. *(Cecil, Ch. 36)*

7.(E) Different rates of acetylation were first described in the metabolism of isoniazid in patients with tuberculosis. Subsequently, the consequences of "fast" and "slow" acetylation on the metabolism and biologic effectiveness of a variety of drugs, including hydralazine, salicyl-azo-sulfapyridine and dapsone, were described. Phenytoin is metabolized by the para-oxidation of a phenyl ring and not by acetylation. *(Emery and Rimoin, pp. 1389–1400)*

8.(D) The most common urea cycle disorder is due to a deficiency of ornithine carbamyl transferase (OCT), which is characterized by hyperammonemia and severe orotic aciduria. The absence of a metabolic acidosis helps to exclude organic acidemias, which can have a similar presentation. OCT deficiency is inherited as an X-linked dominant trait. Prenatal diagnosis is not available for this condition. Recently, neonatal treatment with sodium benzoate and restriction of dietary protein has markedly improved the prognosis for patients with OCT. The mother is an obligatory carrier and will transmit the disease to 50% of her sons; 50% of her daughters will be carriers, and, depending on the pattern of mosaicism, the clinical manifestations in these daughters will range from normal to severely affected. *(Cecil, Chs. 192 and 197; Batshaw et al; Stanbury et al, pp. 402–438)*

9.(A) Thalassemias are inherited anemias that are caused by decreased synthesis of globin chains. Deletion of the genes coding for the a-globin chains is the most common cause of alpha-thalassemia. A variety of point mutations can cause beta-thalassemia and result in a decrease in B-globin transcription. These include point mutations that cause premature termination or incomplete splicing of precursor B-globin mRNA's. The resultant imbalance in a/B globin chain synthesis results in ineffective erythropoiesis and subsequent anemia. Most patients with the beta-thalassemia trait are clinically asymptomatic, although they may exhibit a slight anemia. *(Cecil, Ch. 142; Emery and Rimoin, pp. 1032–1043)*

10.(C) This is most likely an X-linked recessive trait, since only males are affected. Transmission is through females who are normal, and there is no evidence of father-to-son transmission. *(Cecil, Ch. 33)*

11.(C) Von Gierke's disease is the most common glycogen storage disease and results from a deficiency in glucose-6-phosphatase. It is inherited as an autosomal recessive trait. Patients have prominent abdomens and massive hepatomegaly. Commonly, patients exhibit profound fasting hypoglycemia as well as associated hyperlipidemia and hyperuricemia. *(Cecil, Ch. 179; Stanbury et al, pp. 141–166)*

12. (A) Trisomy 13 is characterized by bilateral cleft lip and palate, microphthalmia, hexadactyly, and early death. Few patients live beyond the first year of life. Growth in patients with trisomy 21 is usually slow for the first decade of life; their necks often appear short and there can be associated cardiac anomalies. Noonan's syndrome has a phenotype similar to that of Turner's syndrome but has a normal karyotype and is transmitted as an autosomal dominant trait. The fetal hydantoin syndrome has been associated with webbed neck and both aortic and pulmonic stenosis. A detailed history and a karyotype should help to confirm the diagnosis. *(Cecil, Chs. 36 and 211; de Grouchy and Turleau, pp. 224–231, 336–349; Smith, pp. 414–417)*

13. (B) Menkes' syndrome is associated with abnormal hair, progressive cerebral degeneration, hypopigmentation, bone changes, and an increased risk of arterial rupture and/or thrombosis. It is inherited as an X-linked recessive disease and is associated with abnormal copper metabolism. There appears to be an inability to adequately absorb copper from the gastrointestinal tract, which results in the accumulation of copper in the mucosal cells of the upper GI tract and low levels of circulating copper and ceruloplasmin. Parenteral administration of copper does not reverse the clinical progression of the disease; most patients die in early childhood. *(Stanbury et al, pp. 1251–1268; Emery and Rimoin, pp. 1323–1325)*

14. (D) Assuming that both the woman's parents are carriers for the autosomal recessive cystic fibrosis gene, the expected phenotypic ratios among their offspring would be 1:2:1 (homozygous normal:carrier [asymptomatic]:affected). Since any asymptomatic offspring is known not to be affected, it follows that an unaffected offspring has a one-third chance of being homozygous normal and a two-thirds chance of being a carrier. *(Cecil, Ch. 33)*

15. (E) Congenital erythropoietic porphyria (autosomal recessive) is associated with severe photosensitivity and hemolysis. Erythropoietic protoporphyria (autosomal dominant) has mild to moderate photosensitivity and no hemolysis but is usually associated with significant hepatic damage. Bloom syndrome (autosomal recessive) is associated with short stature, malar hypoplasia, and telangiectatic erythema in the face which is exacerbated by sunlight. Cockayne syndrome (autosomal recessive) is associated with progressive mental deterioration, progressive hearing loss, retinal pigmentation, and dermal photosensitivity. Hereditary hemorrhagic telangiectasia (autosomal dominant with varying penetrance) is associated with multiple telangiectasias on the tongue, lips, face, conjunctiva, nasal mucosal surfaces, and fingertips. There is no associated photosensitivity. *(Cecil, Ch. 203; Stanbury et al, pp. 1301–1384; Smith, pp. 88–89, 116–117, 389)*

16. (C) The prevalence and incidence of both arthritis and nephrolithiasis correlate with the serum level of uric acid. *(Cecil, Ch. 195; Stanbury et al, Ch. 58)*

17. (D) Severe combined immunodeficiency (SCID) is in all likelihood a group of disorders. From 30 to 35% of them are inherited in an X-linked manner, and the rest as autosomal recessive traits. SCID patients have a severe impairment of both humoral and cellular immunity. Unless specific measures are taken, the children usually die within the first few years of life. Thirty per cent of SCID patients have an associated adenosine deaminase (ADA) deficiency, and 85 to 90% of patients with ADA deficiency have SCID. No effective therapy is available at present. The Wiskott-Aldrich syndrome is another immunodeficiency state associated with eczema and megakaryocytic thrombocytopenic purpura, which is inherited as an X-linked trait. A third immunodeficiency state, X-linked agammaglobulinemia, has been successfully treated with monthly gamma globulin injection. *(Cecil, Ch. 419; Stanbury et al, pp. 1157–1183)*

18. (C) Liver disease is common in Wilson's disease, especially when the disease presents in the pediatric age group. Acute hepatitis is a frequent presentation. *(Cecil, Ch. 205; Stanbury et al, pp. 1251–1261)*

19. (B) HPRT deficiency, both complete and partial, leads to hyperuricemia due to excessive production of uric acid. Patients with increased catalytic activity of phosphoribosyl pyrophosphate synthetase produce increased amounts of uric acid due to raised levels of phosphoribosyl-1-pyrophosphate, a substrate in the initial step in purine biosynthesis. Glucose-6-phosphatase deficiency (von Gierke's disease) increases uric acid production; the mechanisms are unknown. Muscle phosphorylase deficiency is not associated with hyperuricemia. *(Cecil, Ch. 195; Stanbury et al, pp. 1043–1143)*

20. (D) The majority (~90%) of patients with porphobilinogen deaminase deficiency never develop clinical symptoms of AIP. In patients with latent disease there is no increase in urinary porphobilinogen. In ill patients the urinary excretion of both α-levulinic acid (ALA) and porphobilinogen rises dramatically. Clinical symptoms usually begin with abdominal pain and include behavioral changes and neurologic impairments. *(Cecil, Ch. 203; Stanbury et al, pp. 1337–1351)*

21. (D) Patients with partial deficiency of the enzyme do not manifest self-mutilation. Many such patients have no neurologic abnormalities, but up to 20% exhibit mental retardation, seizures, and ataxia. Gouty arthritis with tophi is seen. *(Cecil, Ch. 196; Stanbury et al, pp. 1115–1138)*

22. (D) Xeroderma pigmentosum is an autosomal recessive disorder characterized by a high incidence of sunlight-induced malignancies. Other skin manifestations include freckles, telangiectasia, dermal sclerosis, and hypopigmentation. Heterozygotes are unaffected. Early in the disease photophobia is common and can lead to keratitis and opacities. Two clinical forms exist. One form is characterized by neurologic manifestations including progressive mental retardation, movement disorders, and sensorimotor defects. The basis of the disease is a failure to repair damaged DNA. The rate of initial UV-induced DNA damage is identical to that seen in unaffected individuals. *(Cecil, Ch. 534; Stanbury et al, Ch. 57)*

23. (C) In Fabry's disease (α-galactosidase-A deficiency) multiple ocular abnormalities are seen, including lenticular opacities (present in heterozygote female patients as well) and retinal and conjunctival vascular lesions. Virtually all patients with Marfan's syndrome have ectopia lentis, which is usually bilateral. Kayser-Fleischer rings—yellow-brown deposits at the corneal linkers—are characteristic physical findings in Wilson's disease. It is present in virtually all patients with neurologic symptoms and in the majority of patients with only liver disease. Patients with xeroderma pigmentosum frequently have conjunctivitis and photophobia. No ocular problems are associated with HPRT deficiency. *(Cecil, Ch. 196)*

24. (A) About one in 500 Americans is a heterozygote for familial hypercholesterolemia. These patients have elevated levels of LDL cholesterol from birth and show an increased risk of developing atherosclerotic coronary artery disease. Patients frequently have characteristic xanthomas over tendons, especially the Achilles and extensor tendons of the hands. Recurrent attacks of polyarthritis with inflammation of the wrists, ankles, knees, and interphalangeal joints are seen. The molecular defect responsible for the disease involves abnormalities of the cell surface receptor for LDL, resulting in lowered cellular clearance of LDL particles. *(Cecil, Ch. 183; Stanbury et al, pp. 672–711)*

25. (D) Roughly 95% of the people in the United States are homozygous for the M form of α_1-antitrypsin. The most common cause of deficiency in the United States is homozygosity for the Pi^z form of α_1-antitrypsin. The Z protein, compared to the normal M protein, has a single amino acid substitution which impairs the ability of the protein to be secreted by the liver. All patients have 80–90% reductions in the levels of circulating α_1-antitrypsin. More than 80% of patients will develop panacinar emphysema. Liver disease is common, and up to one fifth of affected infants will have neonatal hepatitis. *(Cecil, Ch. 125; Stanbury et al, Ch. 64)*

26. (A) Refsum's disease is an autosomal recessive disorder that causes accumulation of phytanic acid. This is a result of the failure to oxidize dietary phytanic acid. Dietary restriction results in symptomatic and biochemical improvement. Patients develop peripheral neuropathies and central neurologic manifestations. Retinitis pigmentosa, first manifest as night blindness, is common. *(Stanbury et al, pp. 731–747)*

27. (C) Multiple genetic defects have been defined as the basis for familial hypercholesterolemia. All involve the structural gene for the low-density lipoprotein receptor, and all result in the failure of the receptor to adequately clear LDL from the circulation. This process requires a normal number of cell-surface receptors that bind the LDL and internalize it via the process of receptor-mediated endocytosis. Often homozygotes have inherited two distinct genetic defects. Multiple abnormalities in the gene encoding the LDL receptor have been observed. These result in a variety of phenotypes including failure to synthesize receptor and abnormal receptors that fail to be correctly processed and transported to the plasma membrane or fail to bind LDL once on the cell surface. A small set of patients expresses normal amounts of receptors that bind LDL but fails to internalize. Degradation of the LDL receptor after internalization is not part of the endocytic pathway of this receptor. *(Cecil, Ch. 183; Stanbury et al, Ch. 33)*

28. (C) The increased activity of ALA synthetase in patients with acute intermittent porphyria is thought to be secondary to decreased feedback inhibition and/or derepression due to the primary block in heme synthesis. i.e., uroporphyrinogen synthetase deficiency. Following the administration of hematin, there is immediate feedback inhibition and later repression of ALA synthetase, with subsequent decrease in ALA and porphobilinogen synthesis. No direct effect on urinary excretion, metabolism, or toxicity of porphyrins occurs. *(Cecil, Ch. 203; Dhar et al)*

29. (D) Restriction fragment length polymorphisms (RFLP's) represent genetic diversity of the population of DNA sequences that define sites for recognition and digestion by restriction endonucleases around specific regions of genomic DNA. To analyze RFLP's, high molecular weight DNA from individuals' cells is digested to completion with one or several restriction endonucleases. Enzymes used are generally those that recognize specific sequences of six or more nucleotides. The digested DNA is separated by electrophoresis through agarose gels on the basis of fragment size (or length). After the separated DNA is transferred to a filter, specific DNA segments are detected by the use of a radioactively labeled segment of DNA corresponding to a particular gene or defined genomic fragment. This "probe" will hybridize to the corresponding restriction fragment that contains the gene in question, resulting in a pattern of hybridization specific for the restriction enzyme used. Probes derived from known genes or of defined chromosomal regions have been used to correlate the inheritance of abnormal genes for each of the entities cited, except Wilson's disease. *(Thompson and Thompson)*

30. (C) Hereditary hemochromatosis is an autosomal recessive disease causing increased intestinal absorption of iron. The heterozygote frequency is between 8 and 13% in several recent series. Many of the patients have hypogonadism; this is most often due to failure to secrete gonadotropins. Patients who develop cirrhosis are reported to have an incidence of hepatocarcinoma approaching 30%. Patients do not show renal involvement. Type II diabetes seen in these patients is due to the occurrence of two common diseases in the same family. The gene for the disease, while not molecularly defined, can be localized to the HLA locus on chromosome 6p21. *(Cecil, Ch. 206; Stanbury et al, pp. 1269–1298)*

31. (C) Phenylketonuria (PKU) is an autosomal recessive disorder with a frequency in the United States of about 1 in 10,000 births. The cause is defective hepatic phenylalanine hydroxylase, resulting in impaired oxidative metabolism of phenylalanine with consequent hyperphenylalaninemia. The major clinical manifestation is mental retardation. Patients may also demonstrate seizures and abnormal behavior. The genetic defect varies in different kindred. One point mutation has recently been reported in a Danish population. This point mutation leads to incorrect splicing of the gene, with translation of a truncated protein. *(Cecil, Ch. 188; Stanbury et al, Ch. 12)*

32. (C) Duchenne's muscular dystrophy affects 1 in 3000 to 3500 live-born males. Using X-chromosome–specific genomic DNA probes, a very reliable restriction fragment length polymorphism test has emerged for the detection of carriers and for prenatal diagnosis in up to 90% of families at risk. Both Duchenne's and the clinically milder Becker form map to the p21 band of the X-chromosome. In some patients DMD is seen in conjunction with other disorders, including glycerol kinase deficiency, adrenal hypoplasia, chronic granulomatosis, and retinitis pigmentosa. These patients have large deletions around Xp21. *(Cecil, Ch. 513)*

33. (A—True; B—True; C—False; D—False) Type I diabetes mellitus is strongly associated with the DR3 and DR4 haplotype, which suggests that a gene or group of genes near the HLA locus is important for establishing a permissive genetic background. Children of affected fathers have a higher incidence of disease than children of affected mothers; this appears to be a reflection of a preferential transmission of the paternal HLA DR4 haplotype. The concordance in monozygotic twins of type I diabetes mellitus is on average less than 50% but varies from 40% (DR3/DR4-negative) to 70% (DR3/DR4-positive). In contrast, concordance among identical twins with type II diabetes mellitus is almost 100%. Patients with type I diabetes mellitus are more prone to ketoacidosis than to hyperosmolar coma. The reverse is true of type II diabetes. *(Cecil, Ch. 231; Stanbury et al, pp. 99–117; Eisenbarth; Vadheim et al)*

34.(A—False; B—False; C—True; D—True) Galactosemia is most often caused by a deficiency in galactose-1-phosphate uridyl transferase but can also be caused by a deficiency in galactokinase. Both deficiencies are inherited as autosomal recessive traits. In most cases the parents of an affected child are both heterozygous for the enzyme deficiency, and this can be substantiated by finding an intermediate enzymatic activity in their peripheral blood. During subsequent pregnancies the heterozygous mother should be placed on a low galactose diet to forestall galactose toxicity in an affected child. Amniocentesis can be used to detect an affected fetus by measuring the transferase activity in amniotic cells. *(Cecil, Ch. 178; Stanbury et al, pp. 167–191)*

35.(A—False; B—True; C—False; D—False) Huntington's chorea is inherited as an autosomal dominant disease which has a mean age of onset around 35 to 42 years (although roughly 3% have onset before the age of 15). Often psychiatric symptoms precede overt neurologic manifestation. Using well-documented pedigrees, the defective gene has been closely linked to a restriction fragment length polymorphism (RFLP) on chromosome 4. However, because of recombination, this linkage is no greater than 95% accurate, which (along with the variable age of onset) complicates genetic counseling of clinically normal but potentially affected members of a pedigree. *(Cecil, Ch. 470; Conneally; Martin and Gusella)*

36.(A—False; B—False; C—False; D—True) Genetic recombination takes place during the prophase of the *first* meiotic division. No more than 10% of the human genome is thought to code for structural proteins and enzymes. Most often, mutations in receptors are inherited as autosomal dominant diseases. Almost 3000 autosomal loci have been mapped to the human genome. *(Cecil, Chs. 33 and 36)*

37.(A—False; B—True; C—True; D—True) Methylmercury poisoning is, perhaps, the best-documented example of an environmental agent adversely affecting human development. However, the disruption of brain development by methylmercury is seen if exposure occurs during the later months of gestation rather than in the first trimester. The fetal hydantoin syndrome is seen in newborns exposed to hydantoins in the first trimester of pregnancy and is associated with heart disease, clefting, abnormal midfacial development, and digital abnormalities. The severe deafness and mental retardation associated with cytomegalovirus infection is seen in 0.05 to 0.1 per 1000 live births, or approximately 5–10% of infected newborns. Vitamin K antagonists administered during pregnancy can cause coumarin embryopathy (nasal hypoplasia, epiphyseal stippling, and eye abnormalities) or fetal hemorrhage in a substantial number of fetuses. It does not appear that the substitution of low-dose heparin in the first trimester will facilitate a safer pregnancy. *(Cecil, Chs. 217, 341, and 493; Kalter and Warkany; Iturbe-Allessio et al)*

38.(All are True) Cleft lip and palate occur not only by themselves but also as a manifestation of other genetic diseases, including trisomy 13 and the fetal hydantoin syndrome. A previously undetected balanced translocation in one of the parents could cause trisomy 13. If both parents are unaffected, the recurrence risk of subsequent children having cleft lip and cleft palate is 4%. *(Cecil, Ch. 38; Smith, pp. 174–175)*

39.(A—False; B—True; C—False; D—False) Epidermolysis bullosa is a collection of genetic skin diseases that can be inherited as autosomal dominant, autosomal recessive, and X-linked diseases. Spontaneous blistering or blistering after minor trauma is the major clinical manifestation of the disease and is apparent early in life. In some variants, permanent scarring of the skin can result in contractures and scarring of mucosal surfaces, which can interfere with feeding and nutrition. The nature of the inherited defect remains to be elucidated and has not yet been located on a chromosome. *(Cecil, Ch. 534; Stanbury et al, pp. 1441–1442; Der Kaloustian and Kurban, pp. 80–87)*

40.(A—False; B—True; C—False; D—False) Klinefelter's syndrome is a chromosomal abnormality with a karyotype of 47,XXY. The genital abnormalities that can be seen at birth are nonspecific, and the diagnosis usually is not made until puberty. Fewer than one third of patients have gynecomastia, and most have normal intelligence. *(Cecil, Ch. 235; de Grouchy and Turleau, pp. 392–395)*

41.(A—False; B—True; C—True; D—True) Huntington's disease is inherited as an autosomal dominant trait, and symptoms do not usually become apparent until the fourth decade. Symptoms include choreic movements, progressive dementia, and emotional problems, and patients at risk usually have experienced this devastating disease firsthand in their parents. Prenatal diagnosis rests on the ability to link certain markers on chromosome 4 with symptomatic disease. The diagnosis requires the analysis of DNA from multiple members and generations of a pedigree. There is considerable controversy among geneticists and among patients as to whether or not affected, but not as yet symptomatic, patients should be tested and told of their diagnosis. Not only does the possibility of false-positive and false-negative results exist in the linkage analysis currently available for diagnosis, but the confrontation of the disease by affected patients can lead to severe emotional upheaval. There are no clear-cut answers to these questions, and each case must be handled separately. *(Shapiro et al)*

42.(All are True) Homocystinuria is inherited as an autosomal recessive trait and can be caused by a deficiency in cystathionine β-synthase as well as by a deficiency of 5,10-methylenetetrahydrofolate reductase. Treatment with pyridoxine (vitamin B_6) has been effective in many patients with cystathionine β-synthase deficiency. In the untreated state, the major manifestations of homocystinuria include dislocation of the optic lens, osteoporosis, scoliosis, mental retardation, and thromboembolism, which can often be life-threatening. *(Cecil, Ch. 194; Stanbury et al, pp. 552–559)*

43.(All are True) Treacher Collins syndrome is inherited as an autosomal dominant trait and is associated with micrognathia, malar hypoplasia, downward sloping eyes, microtia with deformed pinnae, and variable conductive deafness. The Waardenburg syndrome is inherited as an autosomal dominant trait and is associated with a white forelock, heterochromia, hypertelorism, and variable perceptive deafness in 20% of affected patients. Alport's syndrome is thought to be inherited as an autosomal dominant trait with chronic nephritis; 50% of patients have progressive perceptive deafness. Usher's syndrome is inherited as an autosomal recessive trait and is associated with bilateral and severe perceptive deafness present at birth as well as progressive retinitis pigmentosa. *(Cecil, Ch. 89; Emery and Rimoin, pp. 562–575)*

44. (A—True; B—True; C—True; D—False) Deficiencies of orotate phosphoribosyltransferase and orotidine 5′-phosphate decarboxylase lead to hereditary orotic aciduria—a disorder characterized by megaloblastic anemia, leukopenia, and growth retardation. Ornithine transcarbamylase deficiency, a urea cycle defect, produces orotic aciduria owing to overflow of carbamyl phosphate from the urea cycle into the pyrimidine pathway. Carbamyl phosphate synthetase deficiency, another urea cycle defect, leads to decreased carbamyl phosphate synthesis and does not result in orotic aciduria. Allopurinol therapy produces orotic aciduria by inhibiting orotidine 5′-phosphate decarboxylase activity. *(Cecil, Ch. 197; Stanbury et al, pp. 1166–1221)*

45. (A—True; B—True; C—False; D—True; E—False) Sickle cell anemia is a homoglobinopathy that results from a point mutation in the B-globin gene, causing the replacement of a normal glutamic acid with a valine residue. The disease is inherited as an autosomal recessive trait, and roughly 8-10% of American blacks are carriers. In Africa, the gene frequently is almost 45%, and the persistence of this clearly deleterious gene has been ascribed to a balanced polymorphism (a resistance to *Plasmodium falciparum* malaria). Heterozygotes have no clinical manifestations of the disease, and the presence of relatively high levels of hemoglobin F, both in certain populations (e.g., sickle cell anemia in Saudi Arabia) and in newborns, considerably lessens the severity of the disease. Prenatal diagnosis can be made on fetal DNA after digestion with Mst II, a restriction enzyme that will cut at the point mutation of the S- but not the B-globin gene. SC disease, not SF disease, has qualitatively similar clinical manifestations but is much less severe than SS disease. *(Cecil, Ch. 143; Stanbury et al, pp. 1695–1710)*

46. (All are True) This autosomal recessive disorder is also associated with mental retardation. The condition must be distinguished from Fröhlich's syndrome, in which there are clear-cut abnormalities in the hypothalamic-pituitary axis. *(Cecil, Ch. 211)*

47. (A—True; B—True; C—True; D—False; E—False) In keeping with Knudson's two-hit hypothesis, familial cancer syndromes are most commonly inherited as autosomal dominant traits with 60% penetrance. The occurrence of cancer is earlier in affected pedigrees, and the cancers that develop are more likely to be multifocal or bilateral. Affected patients are also more likely to have a second cancer. Concordance among identical twins is less than 15%. *(Cecil, Ch. 170; Emery and Rimoin, pp. 1401–1426)*

48. (A—False; B—True; C—True; D—False; E—True) Cystinosis is an autosomal recessive disease that results from the accumulation of cystine within lysosomes. The biochemical defect is most likely the failure to transport cystine out of lysosomes after protein degradation has occurred within these organelles. There are three clinical forms of the disease. In infantile nephropathic cystinosis, infants develop renal disease first manifest as Fanconi-like tubular defects. There are a late-onset form and a benign form in which no renal disease is seen. *(Cecil, Ch. 187; Stanbury et al, pp. 1844–1866)*

49. (A—True; B—False; C—True; D—True) Rheumatoid arthritis is rarely seen in patients with gouty arthritis. All the other disorders show a higher-than-expected incidence in patients with gout. *(Cecil, Ch. 195; Stanbury et al, pp. 1043–1113)*

50. (A—True; B—False; C—False; D—True) No hematologic abnormalities are seen in patients with hereditary hemochromatosis or familial hypercholesterolemia. Patients with pyruvate kinase deficiency have a chronic hemolytic anemia. Dihydrofolate reductase deficiency is a rare disorder generally fatal in utero. Infants who survive have severe megaloblastic anemia. *(Cecil, Ch. 131; Stanbury et al, pp. 513–514, 1606–1628)*

51. (A—False; B—True; C—False; D—True) Attacks of acute gouty arthritis are characteristically self-limited; they resolve without therapy in a few days to (rarely) several weeks. Ninety per cent of patients experience podagra at some time during the course of the disease. Polyarticular arthritis is not the rule but is seen in 10 to 20% of patients. Eighty per cent of patients experience a recurrence within two years of the first attack. *(Cecil, Ch. 195; Stanbury et al, pp. 1043–1059)*

52. (A—False; B—False; C—True; D—True; E—False) Hereditary hemochromatosis is closely linked to the HLA-A locus. The most common associated haplotype is A3. Steroid 21-hydroxylase deficiency is linked to the B region of the HLA locus. Bw 47 is the most commonly associated haplotype. *(Stanbury et al, pp. 90–91)*

53. (A—True; B—True; C—False; D—False) The gene coding for human G6PD is X-linked. There are more than 80 defined variants of this enzyme. The two most clinically significant forms of G6PD deficiency are those associated with either the African variant (which affects 10% of black American males) or the Mediterranean variant (frequency among white males, approximately one in 1000). Hemolysis following exposure to any of a variety of oxidizing drugs (including sulfas) is characteristic of these disorders. Hemolysis in the Mediterranean form is much more severe and is elicited by a larger number of drugs. The disorder common among blacks is due primarily to enzyme instability, and since the hemolysis affects only older red cells, it is functionally self-limited. Younger erythrocytes possess sufficient enzyme activity to avoid drug-induced hemolysis, and patients frequently have increased G6PD activity (per red cell) after a hemolytic episode. Neurologic deterioration is not a feature of this disorder. *(Cecil, Ch. 138; Vogel and Motulsky, pp. 201–204, 257)*

54. (A—False; B—True; C—True; D—True) Xanthine oxidase, which can convert xanthine to uric acid, is found in large amounts only in the liver. Inosine monophosphate can be converted to both AMP and GMP by two-step enzymatic processes. Purine bases can be reacted with pyrophosphoribose phosphate to produce ribonucleotides. *(Cecil, Ch. 196; Stanbury et al, pp. 1064–1068)*

55. (A—True; B—False; C—False; D—True; E—False) Deficiency of muscle AMP deaminase, which catalyzes the conversion of AMP to IMP, is a rare autosomal recessive trait characterized by muscle fatigue and postexercise cramps and myalgias. In contrast to normal subjects, exercise does not lead to a rise in muscle production of NH_3 and IMP. *(Cecil, Ch. 196; Stanbury et al, Ch. 54)*

56. (A—True; B—False; C—True; D—False) Uric acid stones are most likely to occur in patients with excessive purine biosynthesis and increased uric acid excretion; in individuals with persistently acid urine; and in patients who excrete highly concentrated urine. There is no association between renal tubular acidosis and uric acid calculi. *(Cecil, Ch. 195; Stanbury et al, pp. 268, 283)*

57.(A—False; B—False; C—False; D—True; E—False) Hereditary spherocytosis is an autosomal dominant trait characterized by mild to moderate hemolytic anemia with splenomegaly. Patients rarely have severe transfusion-requiring anemia and virtually always respond to splenectomy with clinical improvement. Gallbladder disease is a common problem. Aplastic crises, while seen in the minority of patients, represent one of the most devastating and unexplained concomitants of this disorder. *(Cecil, Ch. 138; Stanbury et al, Ch. 72)*

58.(A—False; B—True; C—True; D—False) These types of hepatic porphyria may be exacerbated following administration of barbiturates or sulfonamides, as well as many other types of drugs. Intravenous glucose may abort an attack, and phenothiazines are the preferred treatment for pain. *(Cecil, Ch. 203; Stanbury et al, pp. 1166–1221)*

59.(A—False; B—False; C—True; D—False) Oculocutaneous albinism represents at least 10 clinically distinct disorders. All have decreased pigmentation of the skin, eyes, and hair. Involvement of eyes includes decreased visual acuity, nystagmus, and photophobia. In tyrosinase-negative albinism there is no visual pigment, and this does not change with time. Visual problems including strabismus, nystagmus, photophobia, and poor visual acuity are generally severe. Serum tyrosine levels are normal. The syndrome is inherited as an autosomal recessive trait. *(Cecil, Ch. 534; Stanbury et al, Ch. 15)*

60.(A—False; B—True; C—True; D—True) Familial Mediterranean fever is an autosomal recessive disorder of unknown etiology. The acute onset of fever is most often accompanied by painful peritonitis, pleuritis, and/or arthritis. For unexplained reasons, amyloidosis is rarely seen in patients with familial Mediterranean fever living in the United States, although these individuals develop the characteristic acute inflammatory episodes. Patients from the same ethnic background exhibit a high incidence of amyloidosis in Israel and the Middle East. *(Cecil, Ch. 209)*

61.(C); 62.(C) Wilms' tumor is the most common tumor of childhood; although it is usually sporadic, it is also inherited as an autosomal dominant disease. Approximately 1% of affected patients have associated aniridia and a deletion in the p13 band on chromosome 11. *(Cecil, Ch. 93; Emery and Rimoin, pp. 1401–1426)*

63.(B); 64.(B) Approximately 30% of the time retinoblastoma is inherited as an autosomal dominant disease; the rest of the time it appears to be sporadic. In a relatively small subset of patients, the disease is associated with a deletion in band q14 on chromosome 13. Affected patients have an increased incidence of secondary tumors, including osteosarcoma, fibrosarcoma, Ewing's sarcoma, and Wilms' tumor. *(Cecil, Chs. 36 and 171; Emery and Rimoin, pp. 1401–1425; Orkin)*

65.(B) Neurofibromatosis is inherited as an autosomal dominant disease and is characterized by café-au-lait spots, multiple fibromas, and neurofibromas, as well as frequent skeletal abnormalities. In about 25% of affected patients, neurofibromas are found in the stomach or jejunum. Although they are usually subserosal, ulceration can lead to bleeding, and these lesions have been associated with obstruction due to intussusception as well as bowel perforation. *(Cecil, Ch. 534; Berk et al, Ch. 138; Ricardi)*

66.(A) Gardner's syndrome is inherited as an autosomal dominant disease and is characterized by polyps found primarily in the large colon and rectum. The syndrome is also associated with extracolonic features including skeletal abnormalities, soft tissue tumors, and dental anomalies, which include odontomas and supernumerary as well as unerupted teeth. Because of the very high risk (approaching 100%) of developing cancer, colorectal resection is a common mode of therapy. *(Cecil, Ch. 107; Berk et al, Ch. 138)*

67.(C) Peutz-Jeghers syndrome is an autosomal dominant disorder that is characterized by dark brown or blue-black pigmented patches on the lips, oral mucosa, hands, and feet associated with gastrointestinal polyps most commonly found in the jejunum and ileum. The risk of malignant transformation appears to be small, and these patients should be followed symptomatically. *(Cecil, Ch. 107; Berk et al, Ch. 138)*

68.(A) Turcot's syndrome has a high incidence of colorectal cancer but is thought to be inherited as an autosomal recessive disease. Peutz-Jeghers syndrome is rarely associated with colorectal cancer. *(Cecil, Ch. 107; Berk et al, Ch. 138)*

69.(C) Malignant hyperthermia is inherited as an autosomal dominant trait and is usually manifest after anesthesia with halothane and/or succinylcholine chloride. Affected patients develop muscle spasms, hyperthermia, acidosis, and sudden death. *(Emery and Rimoin, pp. 1389–1400)*

70.(A) Glucose-6-phosphate dehydrogenase deficiency is inherited as an X-linked recessive trait and is associated with hemolysis, hematuria, and anemia in affected males after the ingestion of a variety of drugs, including primaquine, sulfa drugs, and some analgesics. *(Cecil, Ch. 138; Stanbury et al, pp. 1629–1653)*

71.(D) Pseudocholinesterase deficiency is inherited as an autosomal recessive trait that results in a decreased ability to metabolize suxamethonium or succinylcholine chloride and can lead to prolonged apnea. *(Emery and Rimoin, pp. 1389–1400)*

72.(C) Neurofibromatosis (autosomal dominant) is associated with café-au-lait spots, axillary freckling, multiple cutaneous neurofibromas, and characteristic Lesch nodules in the iris. Affected patients have an increased incidence of gliomas and intracranial meningiomas. *(Cecil, Ch. 477; Emery and Rimoin, pp. 313–320)*

73.(B) Tuberous sclerosis (autosomal dominant) is associated with facial adenoma sebaceum, epilepsy, and mental retardation. Characteristically these patients also have ash leaf spots that can best be detected under ultraviolet light. *(Cecil, Ch. 477; Emery and Rimoin, pp. 313–320)*

74.(A) Sturge-Weber syndrome is not known to be inherited. It is characterized by cutaneous capillary hemangiomas, most often in the distribution of the trigeminal nerve. The syndrome is also associated with angiomas of the underlying meninges and generalized seizures. *(Cecil, Ch. 477; Emery and Rimoin, pp. 313–320)*

75–78. It is important to recognize that many genetic disorders (including those that mimic other, more common diseases) are amenable to therapeutic intervention, often with dramatically beneficial results.

75.(D) The characteristic karyotype of Turner's syndrome is 45,XO; however, it should be noted that the Turner's phenotype is associated specifically with deletion of the short arm of the X chromosome, whereas gonadal dysgenesis per se is due to deletion of the long arm of the X chromosome. Frequently, patients with Turner's syndrome have a mosaic karyotype, the most common of which is 45,XO/46,XX. Patients with mosaic karyotypes that include a cell line possessing the Y chromosome are at extreme risk of a neoplastic transformation in a dysgenetic gonad. Thus, the gonads should be removed as soon as this diagnosis is made. *(Cecil, Chs. 36 and 237)*

76. (C) This patient has hereditary angioedema due to C1 inhibitor deficiency. Androgens have been found not only to prevent attacks of edema and abdominal pain but to cause a reversal of the biochemical defect. There is a rapid reappearance of the functional form of the serum C1 esterase inhibitor. *(Cecil, Ch. 420; Stanbury et al, pp. 1745–1749)*

77. (E) This patient has acute intermittent porphyria. Exacerbations of this syndrome sometimes correlate with the menstrual cycle, and in many patients an attack may be precipitated by the use of oral contraceptives. The neurologic consequences of an acute exacerbation of acute intermittent porphyria include abnormalities of the neurohypophysis, such as the syndrome of inappropriate ADH secretion. *(Cecil, Ch. 203; Stanbury et al, pp. 1166–1209)*

78. (A) Deposition of iron in hemochromatosis can result in hypofunction of the anterior pituitary with consequent hypogonadotropic hypogonadism, which is often apparent long before clinically overt signs of hepatic or pancreatic dysfunction appear. Thus, organic impotence and/or hypogonadism in a middle-aged man should raise the suspicion of hemochromatosis. One of the few clinical consequences of hemochromatosis which does not respond to phlebotomy is the arthritis that characteristically affects the second and third metacarpophalangeal joints and is often associated with positive rheumatoid factor. *(Cecil, Ch. 206; Stanbury et al, pp. 1127–1159)*

79–82 Dysmorphic syndromes are often associated with abnormalities of major organ systems, and the pattern of involvement can be specific for a particular syndrome. Adequate medical care requires awareness and anticipation of the affiliated organ abnormalities and the potential medical complication characteristic of the disorder.

79. (C) The major cause of early death in trisomy 21 is cardiovascular malformation; nearly half of those with cardiac abnormalities die in infancy. *(Cecil, Chs. 36 and 49; Smith, pp. 10–13)*

80. (D) Often called "male Turner's syndrome," Noonan's syndrome is actually an autosomal dominant trait and occurs in both sexes with equal frequency. Mild mental retardation is characteristic. *(Cecil, Ch. 211; Smith, pp. 102–103)*

81. (B) Turner's syndrome is usually associated with normal intelligence. Neonatal lymphedema (responsible for webbing of the neck and other phenotypic traits) is characteristic. *(Cecil, Chs. 36 and 237; Smith, pp. 72–75)*

82. (A) Supravalvular aortic stenosis is often seen in William's syndrome (idiopathic hypercalcemia of pregnancy), which is not hereditary. *(Smith, pp. 100–101)*

83. (C); 84. (B); 85. (A)

86. (C) Deficiency has been described in a small number of kindreds. Patients have recurrent *Neisseria* infections, presumably due to impaired opsonization of the bacteria.

87. (B) C1 inhibitor deficiency causes an autosomal dominant disease, hereditary angioedema, characterized by recurrent episodes of edema of the skin, GI tract, and respiratory tract. The most severe problem is acute respiratory obstruction.

88. (A) C3 deficiency is a rare disorder resulting in severe compromise of the ability to fight bacterial infections. Patients suffer both gram-positive and gram-negative infections.

89. (A); 90. (C); 91. (B)

92. (C) This patient has Fabry's disease, an X-linked deficiency of α-galactosidase activity. Galactose-terminal glycosphingolipid accumulates in lysosomes of a variety of cell types. This is particularly marked in vascular endothelial cells. Vascular skin lesions called angiokeratomas are common. Patients generally succumb to renal or, less commonly, cardiac or cerebrovascular disease. *(Cecil, Ch. 184; Stanbury et al, Ch. 45)*

93. (A) Arylsulfatase A deficiency is the most common biochemical cause of metachromatic leukodystrophy. In rare patients the onset of the disease is delayed beyond the second decade of life. Mental deterioration is the most marked characteristic of the adult-onset form. Gait disturbances are common. *(Cecil, Ch. 492; Stanbury et al, Ch. 44)*

94. (B) Glucocerebrosidase, which catalyzes the cleavage of glucose from glucosylceramide, is deficient in patients with Gaucher's disease. Resulting accumulation of glucocerebroside in reticuloendothelial cells leads to the finding of the Gaucher cells. There are three clinical forms of the disease, each inherited as an autosomal dominant trait. This patient has type I, or adult non-neuropathic, form. Splenomegaly with hypersplenism is common, as is mild to moderate liver dysfunction. Bony complications and symptoms are common. Severity and progression of the disease are quite variable in this form. *(Cecil, Ch. 185; Stanbury et al, Ch. 42)*

BIBLIOGRAPHY

Beaudet A, Bowcock A, Buchwald M, et al: Linkage of cystic fibrosis to two tightly linked DNA markers: Joint report from a collaborative study. Am J Hum Genet 39:681, 1986.

Berk JE, Haubrich WS, Kalser MH, et al: Bockus Gastroenterology. 4th ed. Philadelphia, W.B. Saunders Company, 1985.

Cecil Textbook of Medicine. 18th ed. Wyngaarden JB, Smith LH Jr (eds). Philadelphia, W.B. Saunders Company, 1988.

Comings DE, Comings BG: Tourette syndrome: Clinical and psychological aspects of 250 cases. Am J Hum Genet 37:435, 1985.

Conneally PM: Huntington disease: Genetics and epidemiology. Am J Hum Gen 36:506, 1984.

de Grouchy J, Turleau C: Clinical Atlas of Human Chromosomes. New York, John Wiley & Sons, 1984.
Der Kaloustian VM, Kurban AK: Genetic Disease of the Skin. Berlin, Springer-Verlag, 1979.
Eisenbarth GS: Type I diabetes mellitus. N Engl J Med 714:1360, 1986.
Emery AEH, Rimoin DL: Principles and Practices of Medical Genetics. Edinburgh, Churchill Livingstone, 1983.
Heptinstall RH: Pathology of the Kidney. Boston, Little, Brown and Company, 1983.
Iturbe-Alessio I, Fonseca MC, Mutchinkik O, et al: Risk of anticoagulation therapy in pregnant women with artificial heart valves. N Engl J Med 315:1390, 1986.
Kalter H, Warkany J: Congenital malformations. N Engl J Med 308:424, 308:491, 1983.
Martin JB, Gusella JF: Huntington's disease. N Engl J Med 315:1267, 1986.
Mudd SH, Skovby F, Levy HL, et al: The natural history of homocystinuria due to cystathionine B-synthase deficiency. Am J Hum Genet 37:1, 1985.
Orkin SH: Reverse genetics and human disease. Cell 47:845, 1986.
Ricardi VM: Von Recklinghausen neurofibromatosis. N Engl J Med 305:1617, 1981.
Shapiro LT, Comings DE, Jones OW, et al: New frontiers in genetic medicine. Ann Intern Med 104:527, 1986.
Smith DW: Recognizable Patterns of Human Malformation. 3rd ed. Philadelphia, W.B. Saunders Company, 1982.
Stanbury JB, Wyngaarden JB, Fredrickson DS, et al: The Metabolic Basis of Inherited Disease. New York, McGraw-Hill Book Company, 1983.
Thompson JS, Thompson MW: Genetics in Medicine. 3rd ed. Philadelphia, W.B. Saunders Company, 1980.
Vadheim CM, Rotter JI, Maclaren NK, et al: Preferential transmission of diabetic alleles within the HLA complex. N Engl J Med 315:1314, 1986.
Vogel R, Motulsky AG: Human Genetics: Problems and Approaches. New York, Springer-Verlag, 1979.

PART 7

ENDOCRINOLOGY AND DIABETES MELLITUS

KENNETH R. FEINGOLD and ROBERT KLEIN

DIRECTIONS: For questions 1 to 62, choose the ONE BEST answer to each question.

1. In a 24-year-old man, both symptoms and physical examination are suggestive of acromegaly; the patient is referred to you for evaluation. A random growth hormone level is 16 ng/ml (normal = 0–10). Which of the following is the next step?

A. Referral to a neurosurgeon
B. Referral for radiation therapy
C. Glucose suppression test
D. Treatment with bromoergocryptine
E. Treatment with somatostatin infusion

2. A 45-year-old, obese woman is given a routine skull roentgenogram following a car accident; an enlarged sella turcica is noted. Endocrine testing shows no abnormalities and computed tomography (CT scan) reveals an empty sella. Which of the following is appropriate management of this patient?

A. Transsphenoidal surgery
B. Radiation therapy
C. Bromoergocryptine therapy
D. Hormone replacement
E. Reassurance

3. A 12-year-old boy is referred to you for evaluation of diabetes insipidus. Physical examination reveals exophthalmos; skull roentgenograms show punched-out lesions. The most likely diagnosis is

A. meningioma
B. sarcoidosis
C. hemochromatosis
D. histiocytosis X
E. pituitary apoplexy

4. A 24-year-old, insulin-dependent diabetic man is treated with 45 units NPH insulin every morning and evening. Although laboratory data show a hemoglobin A_1 level of 7.6% (normal = 4–8%), he reports that his home measurement of plasma glucose levels—measured three times daily, at 7:00 AM, 11:00 AM, and 5:00 PM—are consistently greater than 180 mg/dl. The most likely explanation for these findings is

A. renal glycosuria
B. hyporeninemic hypoaldosteronism
C. nocturnal hypoglycemia
D. diabetic gastroparesis
E. insulin resistance

5. You are called in consultation to see a 17-year-old boy with persistent 2% glycosuria; plasma glucose values are consistently less than 120 mg/dl. Which of the following is the most likely explanation of this patient's condition?

A. Werner's syndrome
B. Insulin resistance
C. Renal glycosuria
D. Maturity-onset diabetes of the young
E. None of the above

6. A 36-year-old man with an 18-year history of insulin-dependent diabetes has been admitted to the hospital for severe hypoglycemia four times in the past six months. In the hospital, insulin-induced hypoglycemia shows failure to recover (nadir plasma glucose is 32 mg/dl; 20 minutes later, plasma glucose is 34 mg/dl). The most likely explanation for the failure to raise blood glucose levels in response to hypoglycemia is

A. glucocorticoid deficiency alone
B. epinephrine deficiency alone
C. glucagon deficiency and glucocorticoid deficiency
D. epinephrine deficiency and glucocorticoid deficiency
E. epinephrine deficiency and glucagon deficiency

7. You are asked to evaluate a 38-year-old woman who has classic symptoms of hypoglycemia with documented low plasma glucose levels. During a supervised fast in the hospital she is noted to develop hypoglycemia after four hours. Plasma insulin and C-peptide levels drawn at the time of symptoms are both markedly elevated. Which of the following is the most appropriate diagnostic test?

A. Glucose tolerance test
B. Glucagon stimulation test
C. Tolbutamide stimulation test
D. Superior mesenteric angiography
E. Measurement of insulin-like growth factors

8. A 58-year-old woman with non–insulin-dependent diabetes is currently being treated with insulin, 240 units daily. She is 61 inches tall and weighs 260 pounds. Hemoglobin A_1 levels are 15% and fasting glucose levels are 280–325 mg/dl. Which of the following is the most likely cause of the insulin resistance?

A. Insulin antibodies
B. Cushing's syndrome

C. High caloric intake
D. Destruction of insulin at the injection site
E. Antibodies to the insulin receptor

9. You are asked to see a 23-year-old man who has insulin-dependent diabetes of 10 years' duration; he has swelling over the abdomen, at the site where he injects insulin. Physical examination shows lipohypertrophy. The patient's current insulin regimen consists of human insulin, given twice per day. Which of the following is the most appropriate therapy?

A. Switch to purified pork insulin
B. Mix hydrocortisone in the insulin injections
C. Achieve desensitization with low doses of human insulin intradermally
D. Rotate insulin injection sites
E. Give reassurance

10. A 43-year-old man who has elevated plasma glucose levels, glossitis, weight loss, and anemia is noted to have a rash (see figure below). This rash first occurred two years ago; it appears sporadically, and has been noted on the face, abdomen, and buttocks. The most likely diagnosis is

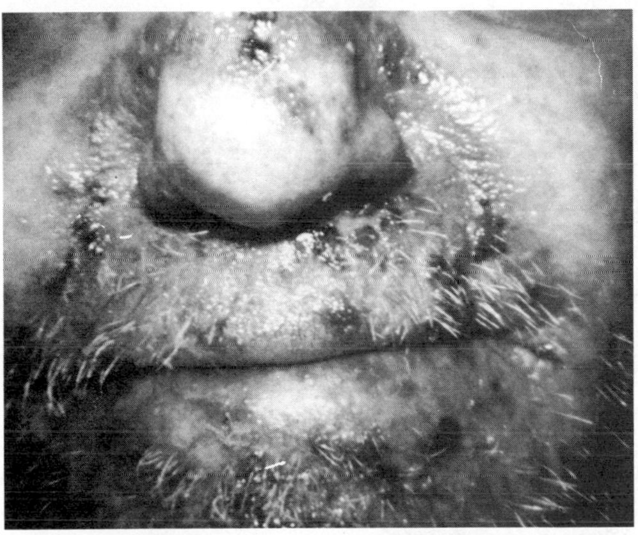

A. glucagonoma
B. pheochromocytoma
C. Cushing's syndrome
D. carcinoid syndrome
E. necrobiosis lipoidica diabeticorum

11. A 60-year-old diabetic woman is admitted to the hospital with a large ulcer overlying the third metatarsal joint of the right foot. Examination shows purulent drainage and surrounding cellulitis. Which of the following is the most appropriate antibiotic therapy?

A. Sulfamethoxazole-trimethoprim
B. Penicillin G
C. Cloxacillin
D. Gentamicin
E. Cefoxitin

12. A 24-year-old woman with insulin-dependent diabetes has a skin lesion (see figure above right) that is located over the pretibial regions bilaterally. The most likely diagnosis is

A. eruptive xanthoma
B. pretibial myxedema

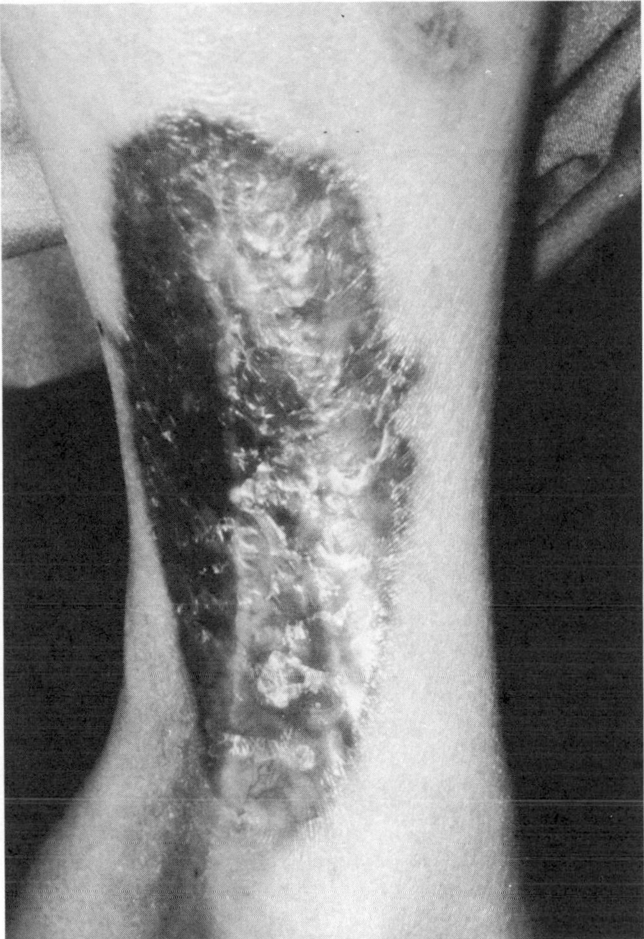

C. diabetic dermopathy
D. bullosis diabeticorum
E. necrobiosis lipoidica diabeticorum

13. A 26-year-old woman with insulin-dependent diabetes is admitted to the hospital in a coma; laboratory studies indicate diabetic ketoacidosis. Physical examination shows periorbital swelling, bloody nasal discharge, and black necrotic nasal mucosa. Antibiotic therapy with which one of the following would be appropriate?

A. Isoniazid
B. Gentamicin
C. Penicillin G
D. Amphotericin B
E. Chloramphenicol

14. You see a 30-year-old man for evaluation of impotence. There is a strong family history of diabetes and peripheral vascular disease. The patient also reports he has frequent headaches. Nocturnal penile tumescence shows the presence of nocturnal erections. Which of the following is the most likely etiology of the impotence?

A. Hypogonadism
B. Diabetes mellitus
C. Vascular insufficiency
D. Panhypopituitarism secondary to a pituitary tumor
E. None of the above

15. A 23-year-old man is referred to you for evaluation of hypogonadism. Physical examination shows a eunuchoidal male with anosmia. Serum testosterone and LH levels are low. Which of the following is the most likely diagnosis?

A. Prolactinoma
B. Myotonic dystrophy
C. Kallman's syndrome
D. Klinefelter's syndrome
E. None of the above

16. A 34-year-old man is referred to you for evaluation of infertility. Physical examination shows a tall, obese man with bilateral gynecomastia and small, firm testes. Which one of the following diagnostic studies is most appropriate?

A. Semen analysis
B. Testicular biopsy
C. Leukocyte karyotyping
D. Response to HCG administration
E. Response to GNRH administration

17. A 46-year-old man is referred to you for evaluation of infertility. Laboratory studies reveal azoospermia and normal levels of plasma testosterone, LH, and FSH. Which of the following is the most likely diagnosis?

A. Varicocele
B. Myotonic muscular dystrophy
C. Kartagener's syndrome
D. Obstruction of the vas deferens
E. None of the above

18. A 33-year-old woman who has acute myelogenous leukemia, with a white blood cell count of 76,000/mm^3, is noted to have fasting plasma glucose of 24 mg/dl. She reports no symptoms compatible with hypoglycemia. Which of the following is the most appropriate diagnostic test?

A. Glucose tolerance test
B. 72-hour supervised fast
C. Intravenous tolbutamide test
D. Intravenous glucagon test
E. None of the above

19. A 27-year-old man is referred to you for evaluation of infertility. History and physical examination do not suggest a likely etiology. Which of the following is the next most appropriate diagnostic test?

A. Semen analysis
B. Serum prolactin
C. Serum testosterone
D. Roentgenograms of the sella turcica
E. None of the above

20. A 56-year-old woman is referred to you for evaluation of polydipsia. During a water deprivation test, maximum serum osmolality was 298 mOsm/kg and maximum urine osmolality was 400 mOsm/kg. One hour after administration of aqueous pitressin, 5 units subcutaneously, urine osmolality was 500 mOsm/kg. The most likely diagnosis is

A. primary polydipsia
B. partial ADH deficiency
C. complete ADH deficiency
D. nephrogenic diabetes insipidus
E. none of the above

21. A 30-year-old woman with lymphoma is admitted to the hospital with confusion and lethargy. Laboratory studies show serum sodium of 117 mEq/L and urine osmolality of 630 mOsm/kg. Which of the following is the most appropriate initial therapy?

A. Demeclocycline, orally
B. Lithium carbonate, orally
C. Isotonic saline, intravenously
D. Hypertonic saline, intravenously
E. Water restriction

22. A 23-year-old man is admitted to the hospital for evaluation of polyuria. During a dehydration test the patient developed maximum urine osmolality of 200 mOsm/kg, with serum osmolality of 301 mOsm/kg. One hour after administration of aqueous pitressin, 5 units subcutaneously, urine osmolality is 205 mOsm/kg. Which of the following is appropriate therapy?

A. DDAVP
B. Clofibrate
C. Chlorpropamide
D. Thiazide diuretics
E. Vasopressin in oil

23. A 38-year-old man with active pulmonary tuberculosis is evaluated for treatment. Routine laboratory studies show serum sodium of 124 mEq/L; further data show urine osmolality of 560 mOsm/kg. Which of the following is the most appropriate first step in treatment?

A. Water restriction
B. Administration of lithium carbonate
C. Administration of demeclocycline
D. Administration of hypertonic saline, intravenously
E. Administration of hypertonic saline and furosemide (Lasix), intravenously

24. A 13-year-old boy is referred to you for evaluation of gynecomastia. History and physical examination do not indicate a likely etiology. Which of the following is the best next step?

A. Leukocyte karyotyping
B. Measure serum HCG
C. Measure serum prolactin
D. Measure serum testosterone
E. None of the above

25. A 36-year-old man who underwent successful renal transplantation six months ago is referred to you for evaluation of persistent hypercalcemia (serum calcium levels 11.5–12 mg/dl on multiple occasions). Serum PTH levels are markedly elevated. Roentgenograms of the hand show subperiosteal resorption. Which of the following is the most appropriate therapy?

A. Administration of calcitriol
B. Administration of oral calcium supplements
C. Administration of phosphate-binding antacids
D. Parathyroidectomy
E. None of the above

26. A 73-year-old man has a two-year history of pain and stiffness in the right hip. Recently he has developed hearing loss. He has noted an increase in hat size. Blood tests show calcium 9.6 mg/dl, phosphorus 4.1 mg/dl, and alkaline phosphatase 470 IU/L (normal = 0–120). Which of the following tests would be most helpful in establishing the diagnosis?

A. Fasting serum growth hormone level
B. Radionuclide bone scan
C. Computed tomography (CT scan) of the pituitary
D. Ultrasound examination of the abdomen
E. Roentgenograms of the skull and pelvis

27. Which of the following is the most characteristic and diagnostically useful roentgenographic feature of osteomalacia?

A. Generalized bone demineralization
B. Subperiosteal bone resorption
C. Vertebral compression fractures
D. "Pseudofractures" (Milkman's lines or Looser's zones)
E. None of the above

28. A 40-year-old woman is referred to you for the evaluation of lethargy, cold intolerance, constipation, dry skin, and 10-pound weight gain. Physical examination shows slow reflexes, enlarged tongue, and slight goiter. Which of the following is the best test to confirm the clinical impression of primary hypothyroidism?

A. Measurement of serum T_4
B. Measurement of serum T_3
C. Measurement of serum TSH
D. Measurement of serum thyroglobulin
E. Test for antithyroidal antibodies

29. A 35-year-old woman has a swelling in the neck. She reports no obstructive symptoms (hoarseness, dyspnea, or dysphagia). Physical examination shows a thyroid gland two times normal size. Thyroid function tests are normal and ^{123}I scan reveals an enlarged thyroid gland with inhomogeneous uptake of tracer. Which is the most appropriate step at this time?

A. Iodine administration
B. Propylthiouracil administration
C. Ablative therapy with ^{131}I
D. Thyroxine replacement therapy
E. Total thyroidectomy

30. The best treatment for recurrent kidney stones secondary to renal hypercalciuria is

A. sodium phosphate
B. hydrochlorothiazide
C. penicillamine
D. sodium bicarbonate
E. potassium citrate

31. A 38-year-old man is brought to the emergency room by his wife because of lassitude and drowsiness. His wife says that he has been on a heavy drinking binge since losing his job one month ago. The patient reports frequent episodes of numbness and tingling around the mouth, but describes no other symptoms. Physical examination is notable for hepatomegaly, generalized hyperreflexia, and positive Chvostek sign. Laboratory studies include normal electrolytes, calcium 6.7 mg/dl, phosphorus 2.5 mg/dl, albumin 3.7 mg/dl, and SGOT 150 U/ml. The most likely cause of the hypocalcemia is

A. hypomagnesemia
B. renal hypercalciuria
C. malabsorption of calcium
D. decreased dietary calcium intake
E. primary hypoparathyroidism

32. A 45-year-old woman is incidentally noted to have a right adrenal mass measuring 10 cm in diameter after computed tomography (CT scan) of the abdomen. Urine metanephrines and low-dose dexamethasone suppression tests are normal. Which of the following is the next most appropriate step?

A. High-dose dexamethasone test
B. Percutaneous adrenal vein sampling
C. Chemotherapy
D. Right adrenalectomy
E. No further action at this time; schedule patient's return in six months for check-up

33. A 60-year-old woman has sudden onset of hoarseness and massive, painless neck swelling. The patient has a 20-year history of hypothyroidism secondary to Hashimoto's thyroiditis; she has received chronic thyroid replacement therapy with L-thyroxine, 150 μg daily. At present she reports no symptoms of thyroid dysfunction. The most likely diagnosis is

A. acute viral infection
B. multinodular goiter
C. factitious thyrotoxicosis
D. acute suppurative thyroiditis
E. lymphoma of the thyroid

34. A 17-year-old woman is seen for the evaluation of hirsutism. Plasma 17-hydroxyprogesterone level is 5 μg/dl (normal <0.2 μg/dl). Computed tomography (CT scan) of the abdomen reveals a 2-cm left adrenal mass. Which of the following is proper management of this patient?

A. Administration of mitotane
B. Administration of oral contraceptive
C. Administration of cyproterone acetate
D. Trial of dexamethasone suppression
E. Left adrenalectomy

35. A 47-year-old man is admitted to the hospital for evaluation of hypertension and hypokalemia. After the patient has been restricted to a 120 mEq/day sodium diet for one week, plasma aldosterone levels are twice normal. Which of the following is the next most appropriate step?

A. Fludrocortisone suppression test
B. Cortrosyn (ACTH) stimulation test
C. Measurement of plasma renin activity
D. Computed tomography (CT scan) of the adrenal glands
E. Treatment with spironolactone

36. A 56-year-old woman is admitted to the hospital because of confusion and lethargy. Laboratory studies on admission show serum calcium, 15.6 mg/dl; serum phosphate, 4.4 mg/dl; creatinine, 2.8 mg/dl; and blood urea nitrogen, 74 mg/dl. Administration of which of the following is the most appropriate initial therapy?

A. Glucocorticoids
B. Calcitonin
C. Mithramycin
D. Normal saline, intravenously
E. Lasix (furosemide)

37. A 27-year-old white woman with Graves' disease is treated with radioiodine for hyperthyroidism. One year later she becomes hypothyroid and is subsequently maintained on L-thyroxine, 150 μg daily. Three months ago she began to experience eye irritation, particularly on awakening in the morning. She is now clinically euthyroid with serum thyroxine and thyroid-stimulating hormone (TSH) values within the normal range. Visual acuity is normal and there is no diplopia. Conjunctival injection and chemosis are present, as well as mild exophthalmos (front of cornea 22 mm anterior to the lateral orbital ridge). All the following may be of therapeutic value for this patient EXCEPT

A. 6-inch elevation of the head of the bed
B. methylcellulose eyedrops

C. a thiazide diuretic at bedtime
D. reduction of the L-thyroxine to 50 μg daily
E. taping the eyelids closed during sleep

38. A 70-year-old boardinghouse tenant is found stuporous in his room by fellow lodgers. The label on an empty bottle in his room indicates that it once contained thyroxine. On examination in the hospital the patient is comatose; pulse rate is 52 per minute; rectal temperature is 30°C. There is a midline, transverse scar in the lower neck. Rales are heard at the base of the left lung. Emergency management of this patient should include all the following EXCEPT

A. L-thyroxine, 2 μg/kg intravenously
B. raising body temperature rapidly with a heating blanket
C. evaluation and treatment of infection
D. measurement of arterial blood PO_2 and PCO_2
E. monitoring serum sodium levels

39. A 47-year-old man is seen because of wasting, weakness, and persistent hypokalemia. A late-afternoon plasma cortisol measurement is 58 μg/dl (normal = 5–15). The most likely etiology of the hypercortisolism is

A. Cushing's disease
B. adrenocortical carcinoma
C. adrenocortical adenoma
D. glucocorticoid therapy
E. ectopic ACTH syndrome

40. A 49-year-old woman has weakness and hypertension. Serum calcium is 12.8 mg/dl (normal = 8.9–10.1); serum phosphate, 1.9 mg/dl (normal = 2.5–4.5); serum chloride, 111 mEq/L (normal = 98–108); serum parathyroid hormone concentration, 478 pg/ml (normal = 10–150). On physical examination a 2-cm nodule can be felt in the left lobe of the thyroid gland. This nodule most likely represents which one of the following?

A. A palpable parathyroid adenoma
B. Metastatic cancer of the lung
C. A parathyroid carcinoma
D. A thyroid adenoma
E. A lymphoma arising from the thyroid gland

41. A 43-year-old woman is referred to you for evaluation of a nodule, 2.5 cm in diameter, in the left lobe of the thyroid gland. She was treated for enlarged tonsils with radiotherapy when 8 years old. Thyroid function tests are normal; a thyroid scan reveals that the nodule is cold. Which of the following is the most appropriate management of this patient?

A. TRH stimulation test
B. Ultrasound examination
C. Needle biopsy of the nodule
D. Thyroid surgery
E. L-Thyroxine administration with close observation

42. A 32-year-old man with insulin-dependent diabetes mellitus is admitted to the hospital for the evaluation of marked renal insufficiency. Blood urea nitrogen (BUN) is 123 mg/dl and creatinine is 9.8 mg/dl. Two years before admission, he was noted to have proteinuria and mild renal insufficiency (BUN 25 mg/dl, creatinine 1.6 mg/dl). Six months before admission, BUN was 30 mg/dl and creatinine was 1.8 mg/dl. Which of the following is the LEAST likely cause of renal failure in this patient?

A. Bladder atony
B. Urinary tract infection
C. Uncontrolled hypertension
D. Rapidly progressive glomerulonephritis
E. Natural progression of diabetic glomerulopathy

43. An elderly diabetic man with mild renal insufficiency was brought to the emergency room because of confusion. Blood glucose was 27 mg/dl. He was treated with glucose intravenously for 24 hours, discharged, and instructed not to take any medication. Six hours after discharge he is brought back to the emergency room in a coma. Blood glucose is now 18 mg/dl. Which of the following oral hypoglycemic agents is the patient most likely to be using?

A. Tolbutamide
B. Chlorpropamide
C. Tolazamide
D. Acetohexamide
E. Glipizide

44. A 17-year-old girl consults you because of amenorrhea. Menarche was spontaneous at age 12, and she has had cyclic menses until two months ago when menses ceased. She describes no other symptoms and reports no recent sexual exposure. Physical examination is unrevealing. Which one of the following would you do next?

A. Measure chorionic gonadotropin in urine or blood
B. Assess pituitary function including skull radiographs
C. Measure serum estrogen and gonadotropins
D. Assess vaginal cytology and cervical mucus for estrogen effects
E. Administer progesterone in oil, 100 mg intramuscularly, and observe for menses

45. You are asked to see a 37-year-old man for the evaluation of polyuria (approximately 20 liters/24 hours). Plasma osmolality is 270 mOsm/kg and spot urine osmolality is 140 mOsm/kg. Which of the following is the most likely diagnosis?

A. Central diabetes insipidus
B. Nephrogenic diabetes insipidus
C. Primary polydipsia
D. Diabetes mellitus
E. None of the above

46. An asymptomatic 72-year-old man is noted on routine chest roentgenographic examination to have a sclerotic rib abnormality consistent with Paget's disease. Further studies show normal calcium and phosphate levels and serum alkaline phosphatase of 210 U/L (normal <120 U/L). Which of the following is the most appropriate step?

A. Administration of mithramycin
B. Administration of prednisone
C. Administration of diphosphonates
D. Administration of calcitonin
E. No therapy indicated

47. A 34-year-old man is referred to you because of infertility. Libido and potency are normal. There is no history of drug or radiation therapy. Routine physical examination is unremarkable. Serum testosterone is 0.57 μg/dl (normal = 0.3–1.2); serum luteinizing hormone (LH), 9 mIU/ml (normal = 4–19); and follicle-stimulating hormone (FSH), 75 mIU/ml (normal = 4–27). Which of the following is correct?

A. Complete pituitary evaluation is indicated
B. Gonadotropin-releasing hormone (Gn/RH) will improve fertility

C. Prolonged testosterone enanthate therapy will improve fertility
D. The infertility is almost certainly irreversible
E. Testicular biopsy should be performed to establish the diagnosis

48. You are asked to see a 15-year-old girl because of failure to begin menses and insufficient sexual development, which has caused her to withdraw from social contacts. In contrast to her peers she has had no breast enlargement, and she is acutely embarrassed by her "abnormality." Physical examination shows a few fine strands of pubic hair, which she had not noticed, and small islands of breast tissue below the areolae. The remainder of the examination reveals no abnormalities. Which one of the following would you order next?

A. Karyotyping
B. Full pituitary evaluation
C. Pelvic ultrasound to detect the presence of ovaries
D. Serum gonadotropin and estrogen measurements
E. None of the above

49. A 46-year-old woman notes the recent appearance of increased body hair. Physical examination shows increased facial and body hair, male-pattern baldness, clitoral hypertrophy, a deep voice, and a palpable abdominal mass located in the left upper quadrant. The most likely diagnosis is

A. polycystic ovary disease
B. congenital adrenal hyperplasia
C. Cushing's disease
D. adrenal carcinoma
E. idiopathic hirsutism

50. A 43-year-old chronic alcoholic man was admitted to the hospital for evaluation of Cushing's syndrome. Findings on physical examination included hypertension, a buffalo hump, abdominal striae, easy bruising, and cushingoid facies. Morning and evening cortisol levels on admission were 37 μg/dl and 29 μg/dl, respectively, and after an overnight 1-mg dexamethasone suppression test, the 8 AM cortisol level was 24 μg/dl. The next diagnostic test should be

A. a high-dose dexamethasone suppression test
B. computed tomography (CT scan) of the adrenal glands
C. metyrapone test
D. repetition of 1-mg overnight dexamethasone test in one week
E. measurement of ACTH levels

51. A 56-year-old woman has had polyuria and polydipsia for three months. Height is 63 inches; weight is 195 pounds. Physical examination shows no evidence of either micro- or macrovascular disease. Fasting glucose is 236 mg/dl and urinalysis shows 1% glycosuria without other abnormalities. Which of the following is the most appropriate initial therapy?

A. Tolbutamide, 500 mg orally three times per day
B. 25 units NPH insulin every morning
C. 25 units NPH insulin every morning and 10 units NPH every evening
D. Calorie-restricted diet
E. None of the above

52. A 41-year-old woman has pain localized over the thyroid gland that radiates to the left ear. She has also had fever, chills, and malaise for one week. Physical examination shows an enlarged and painful thyroid gland. Thyroid hormone levels are normal and radioactive iodine uptake is low. Which of the following is the most likely diagnosis?

A. Graves' disease
B. Hashimoto's thyroiditis
C. Lymphocytic thyroiditis
D. Subacute thyroiditis
E. None of the above

53. A previously undiagnosed patient is found to have ketoacidosis after five weeks of polyuria. Plasma glucose is 485 mg/dl; blood urea nitrogen is 29 mg/dl; serum electrolytes show sodium 142, potassium 3.9, chloride 98, and bicarbonate 12 mEq/L. After therapy with saline, intermittent intramuscular insulin, and bicarbonate, the patient develops generalized weakness, hypoventilation, and cardiac irritability. What is the most likely cause of this complication?

A. Hypoglycemia
B. Hyponatremia
C. Magnesium depletion
D. Hypokalemia
E. Hypophosphatemia

54. A 55-year-old man noted a mass in his neck while shaving. Physical examination is normal except for a firm, 5-cm oval nodule in the left lobe of the thyroid gland. The right lobe cannot be felt. Serum thyroxine is 8.4 μg/dl (normal = 5–11); resin T_3 uptake, 1.04 (normal = 0.85–1.15); free thyroxine index, 8.7 (normal = 4.7–10.5); and thyroid-stimulating hormone (TSH), 1.9 μU/ml (normal = 0–6). Radioisotope thyroidal scan is shown in the accompanying illustration. Which of the following actions is most appropriate?

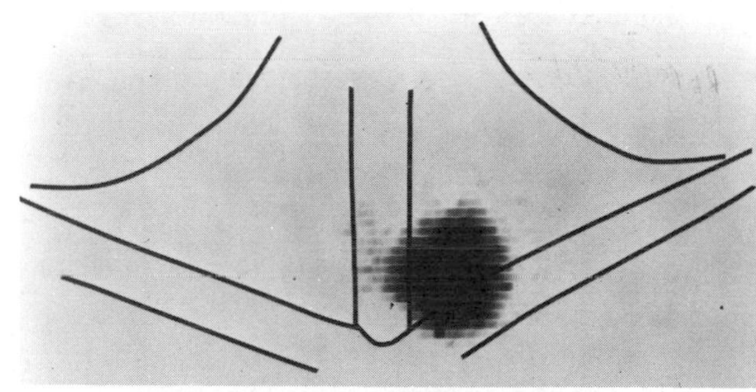

A. Measurement of antithyroid antibodies
B. Measurement of serum T_3
C. Aspiration biopsy of nodule
D. Radioiodine ablation of nodule
E. Surgical excision of nodule after propylthiouracil treatment

55. A 57-year-old woman is referred to you because of hypercalcemia (calcium, 11.5 mg/dl). The patient's history includes carcinoma of the breast that was treated by mastectomy two years ago. Three months ago she was noted to have a recurrence of cancer in the axillary lymph nodes and was successfully treated with radiotherapy. Extensive studies revealed no other evidence of malignancy at that time; specifically, there was no evidence of bone metastases. Current laboratory studies show serum calcium, 11.5 mg/dl; serum phosphate, 2.0 mg/dl; and PTH, 107 μl Eq/ml (normal = 0–40) Which of the following is the most appropriate next step?

A. Measurement of 25-OH vitamin D levels
B. Measurement of the tubular resorption of phosphate
C. Neck exploration
D. Chemotherapy
E. Mithramycin administration

56. A 27-year-old asymptomatic man is referred to you for evaluation of persistent hypercalcemia (calcium, 11.0–12.0 mg/dl) following parathyroid surgery. Serum PTH levels have all been consistently between 30 and 45 μl Eq/ml (normal = 0–40). Urine calcium excretion is 38 mg/24 hours. Which of the following is the most appropriate course of action?

A. Glucocorticoid suppression test
B. Measurement of phosphate clearance
C. Arteriography and venous catheterization of thyroid and mediastinal veins
D. Neck exploration
E. Family studies

57. A 24-year-old woman is brought to the emergency room hypotensive and in coma. Plasma glucose is 60 mg/dl, serum sodium 120 mEq/L, and serum potassium 4.4 mEq/L. Two years ago the patient developed galactorrhea and amenorrhea, and underwent pituitary irradiation for a prolactinoma. Although galactorrhea ceased, amenorrhea has persisted. Three days ago she began taking L-thyroxine, 0.3 mg daily, which her gynecologist had prescribed for symptoms typical of hypothyroidism. Which of the following is the most appropriate emergency therapy for this patient?

A. Methimazole, 100 mg by nasogastric tube, followed by saturated solution of potassium iodide, ten drops every eight hours
B. Hydrocortisone, 100 mg intravenously every six hours, with normal saline sufficient to replace 10 to 20% of the extracellular volume
C. 50% Dextrose in water, 50-ml bolus intravenously
D. L-Thyroxine, 300 μg intravenously
E. 3% Saline solution, 2 liters intravenously over two hours

58. A 55-year-old woman with diabetes mellitus of 20 years' duration suddenly develops diplopia. Examination of extraocular movements reveals paresis of external rotation of her left eye, as illustrated below. You also discover a symmetric, stocking-type of anesthesia in the lower extremities. You find no other abnormalities on neurologic examination. Which one of the following should you do?

A. Advise the patient that the double vision will probably resolve spontaneously in several weeks
B. Obtain computed tomography (CT scan) of the brain to rule out a mass lesion
C. Consider this a potential neurosurgical emergency and arrange for immediate hospitalization
D. Obtain a neurology consultation to rule out a systemic demyelinating disease
E. Advise the patient that she has had a small stroke and that her double vision is probably permanent

59. A 68-year-old diabetic man is admitted to the hospital in a coma. Glucose is 540 mg/dl, sodium 120 mEq/L, potassium 4.4 mEq/L, chloride 85 mEq/L, and bicarbonate 20 mEq/L. Blood urea nitrogen is 60 mg/dl. The LEAST likely cause of the coma is

A. liver failure
B. opiate overdose
C. subdural hematoma
D. brain stem infarction
E. hyperosmolar diabetic coma

60. A 31-year-old woman, a medical researcher, is admitted to the hospital because of hypoglycemia. Blood glucose on admission was 28 mg/dl, plasma insulin was 220 μU/ml, and plasma C-peptide levels were undetectable. Which of the following is the most appropriate next step?

A. Exploratory surgery
B. Computed tomography (CT scan) of the pancreas
C. Tolbutamide tolerance test
D. Diazoxide therapy
E. None of the above

61. A 47-year-old diabetic man is found to have a serum potassium that ranges between 5.3 and 5.9 mEq/L. Other serum electrolytes are sodium 141 mEq/L, chloride 113 mEq/L, and bicarbonate 15 mEq/L. Renal function is moderately impaired (creatinine clearance, 37 ml/min). The most likely etiology of the hyperkalemia in this patient is

A. renal insufficiency
B. Addison's disease
C. 18-hydroxylation defect
D. hyporeninism
E. spironolactone therapy

62. Which of the following is the most common presentation of primary hyperparathyroidism?

A. Muscular weakness
B. Renal stone formation
C. Central nervous system impairment
D. Bone pain
E. No symptoms

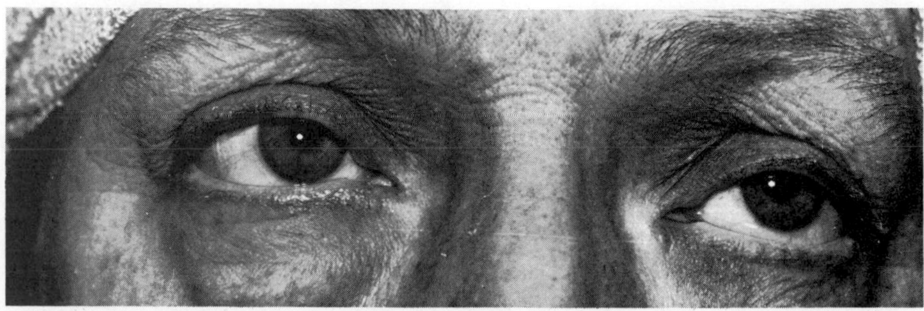

DIRECTIONS: For questions 63 to 103, you are to decide whether EACH choice is true or false. Any combination of answers, from all true to all false, may occur. Mark the answer sheet "T" or "F" in the space provided.

63. Elevated prolactin levels can cause

A. impotence
B. gynecomastia
C. osteopenia
D. amenorrhea
E. acanthosis nigricans

64. Which of the following is/are likely to be responsible for elevated serum prolactin levels in a 36-year-old woman?

A. Phenothiazines
B. Heroin addiction
C. Renal failure
D. Ovarian failure
E. Hyperthyroidism

65. Craniopharyngiomas are characterized by

A. calcification
B. visual defects
C. hyperthyroidism
D. suprasellar location
E. usual onset after age 60

66. Acromegaly is associated with

A. anosmia
B. joint pain
C. hypotension
D. increased body odor
E. carpal tunnel syndrome

67. A 62-year-old man has decreased libido and impotence. Past medical history shows that three years ago he had a nasopharyngeal carcinoma that was treated with radiotherapy. Laboratory data include serum testosterone of 0.15 μg/dl (normal = 0.3–1.2) and serum luteinizing hormone of 5 mIU/ml (normal = 4–19). Appropriate initial work-up should include which of the following?

A. Serum T_4 measurement
B. HCG stimulation test
C. TRH stimulation test
D. GNRH stimulation test
E. Insulin-induced hypoglycemia

68. A 36-year-old man who has an 18-year history of diabetes with autonomic neuropathy complains of severe sweating following meals. Which of the following is/are among appropriate treatment possibilities?

A. Clonidine
B. Antihistamines
C. Beta blockers
D. Anticholinergics
E. Systemic steroids

69. Which of the following drugs is/are known to cause hypoglycemia?

A. Ethanol
B. Aspirin
C. Streptomycin
D. Clofibrate
E. Pentamidine

70. Which of the following medications is/are likely to impair metabolic control in diabetic patients?

A. Phenytoin
B. Gentamicin
C. Dexamethasone
D. Hydrochlorothiazide
E. Estrogenic oral contraceptives

71. Which of the following is/are characteristic of proliferative diabetic retinopathy?

A. Microaneurysms
B. Flame hemorrhages
C. Neovascularization
D. Hard waxy exudates
E. Cotton wool exudates

72. In patients with hypoglycemia secondary to extrapancreatic tumors, which of the following malignancies is/are frequently observed?

A. Sarcomas
B. Hepatomas
C. Breast cancer
D. Hodgkin's disease
E. Transitional carcinoma of the bladder

73. Difficulties caused by diabetic autonomic neuropathy include

A. constipation
B. Charcot joints
C. diabetic amyotrophy
D. retrograde ejaculation
E. cardiorespiratory arrest

74. Which of the following is/are associated with insulin-dependent diabetes?

A. Obesity
B. Antibodies against islet cells
C. Increased frequency of HLA D3 and D4
D. Peak age of onset in the fourth decade
E. Greater than 90% concordance in identical twins

75. A 58-year-old man with poorly controlled diabetes is admitted to the hospital because of severe epigastric pain radiating through the back. Initial laboratory studies show plasma glucose of 460 mg/dl and grossly lipemic plasma. Which of the following is/are also likely to be found?

A. Hyponatremia
B. Lipemia retinalis
C. Eruptive xanthoma
D. Tendinous xanthoma
E. Necrobiosis lipoidica diabeticorum

76. Gynecomastia is observed in association with which of the following?

A. Tolbutamide
B. Heroin addiction
C. Hypothyroidism
D. Testicular tumors
E. Lung cancer

77. Low serum testosterone levels are observed in patients with

A. cryptorchidism
B. hemochromatosis

C. hyperprolactinemia
D. germinal cell aplasia
E. isolated FSH deficiency

78. Androgen therapy in male patients is associated with which of the following adverse effects?

A. Gynecomastia
B. Peliosis hepatis
C. Angioneurotic edema
D. Atrophy of the prostate
E. Congestive heart failure

79. Which of the following is/are seen frequently in patients with Nelson's syndrome?

A. Gynecomastia
B. Hyperpigmentation
C. Visual field defects
D. Kartagener's syndrome
E. Excessive perspiration

80. A 40-year-old woman is referred to you for evaluation of severe watery diarrhea (>4 liters/day). Laboratory studies show serum potassium of 2.4 mEq/L and markedly elevated serum vasoactive intestinal peptide. Which of the following abnormalities is/are likely to be seen?

A. Asthma
B. Achlorhydria
C. Hypoglycemia
D. Hypercalcemia
E. Necrolytic migratory erythema

81. Frequent manifestations of hypopituitarism include

A. erythema
B. oily hair
C. hyperpigmentation
D. decreased sexual hair
E. fine wrinkling around the eyes

82. Which of the following suggest(s) the presence of vitamin D deficiency?

A. Hypocalcemia
B. Hyperphosphatemia
C. Elevated levels of PTH
D. Reduced alkaline phosphatase levels
E. Low serum concentrations of 25-hydroxyvitamin D

83. Hypoparathyroidism is associated with which of the following?

A. Hypomagnesemia
B. Immunodeficiency
C. Addison's disease
D. Vitamin D deficiency
E. Mucocutaneous candidiasis

84. Which of the following is/are included among risk factors for osteoporosis?

A. Obesity
B. Cigarette smoking
C. High protein intake
D. High alcohol consumption
E. Decreased physical activity

85. Which of the following is/are among indications for institution of calcitonin therapy in Paget's disease?

A. Alkaline phosphatase level greater than three times normal
B. Deafness
C. Bone pain
D. Osteolytic bone lesions
E. High-output cardiac failure

86. Reduced levels of corticosteroid-binding globulin (CBG, or transcortin) are likely to result from

A. pregnancy
B. cirrhosis
C. hyperthyroidism
D. nephrotic syndrome
E. oral contraceptive use

87. Which of the following is/are true of cortisol-secreting adenomas?

A. They secrete a wide variety of steroids
B. They are usually large at the time of diagnosis
C. They are usually composed of zona fasciculata–like cells
D. They are suppressed by high doses of dexamethasone
E. Their histologic appearance easily distinguishes them from adrenal carcinomas that secrete cortisol

88. In a patient with a solitary thyroid nodule, which of the following is/are associated with increased likelihood of malignancy?

A. Male gender
B. History of childhood neck irradiation
C. Fixation of nodule to surrounding tissues
D. Development of recurrent laryngeal nerve paresis
E. Lack of radioisotope uptake in nodule ("cold nodule")

89. Which of the following is/are frequently observed in elderly patients with hyperthyroidism?

A. Thick tongue
B. Absent goiter
C. Marked weight loss
D. Apathetic behavior
E. Heart rate less than 100 bpm

90. A 35-year-old woman has diffuse thyroid gland enlargement. Serum free T_4 level is reduced and serum TSH is elevated. Antimicrosomal and antithyroglobulin antibodies are elevated. This patient is at an increased risk for developing which of the following?

A. Pernicious anemia
B. Cushing's syndrome
C. Sjögren's syndrome
D. Systemic lupus erythematosus
E. Idiopathic thrombocytopenic purpura

91. Appropriate management of a patient with medullary carcinoma of the thyroid includes

A. evaluation for pheochromocytoma
B. subtotal thyroidectomy to remove all palpable tumor
C. follow-up thyroglobulin measurements
D. follow-up with provocative testing of serum calcitonin levels
E. provocative testing and measurement of immunoreactive calcitonin levels in all primary relatives of the patient

92. You see a 47-year-old man with a blood pressure of 270/120 mm Hg in preparation for the surgical removal of a pheochromocytoma. Which of the following would be appropriate to include in treatment of this patient?

A. Diuretics
B. Methyldopa
C. Propranolol
D. Phenoxybenzamine
E. Salt restriction

93. A 54-year-old man with an artificial heart valve who is receiving chronic anticoagulation therapy is referred to you because of the acute development of fever, abdominal pain, nausea and vomiting, and hypovolemia. Laboratory data show serum potassium of 6.1 mEq/L and white blood cell count of 16,000/mm^3 with 8% eosinophilia. Management of this patient should include which of the following?

A. Hydrocortisone, 100 mg intravenously
B. Fludrocortisone, 0.1 mg orally
C. Rapid ACTH stimulation test
D. Volume repletion with intravenous saline
E. Esophagogastroscopy

94. A 32-year-old alcoholic woman is hospitalized for pneumonia; past medical history is notable for endogenous depression and a seizure disorder for which she receives phenytoin. Physical examination shows hypertension, plethoric facies, and centripetal obesity. Fasting AM cortisol after oral dexamethasone, 1 mg at midnight, is 12 μg/dl (normal <5). Which of the following is/are among the possible reasons for the abnormal response to dexamethasone?

A. Alcoholism
B. Depression
C. Acute illness
D. Cushing's syndrome
E. Anticonvulsant therapy

95. A 28-year-old man undergoes neck exploration for asymptomatic hypercalcemia and hyperparathyroidism; at surgery, all four parathyroid glands are found to be abnormal and three and one-half glands are removed. This patient is at risk for developing which of the following endocrine abnormalities?

A. Headache and tunnel vision
B. Headaches and bizarre behavior relieved by food
C. Paroxysmal tachycardia and hypertension
D. Azoospermia and gynecomastia
E. Calcified thyroidal mass

96. An 18-year-old woman, deaf from birth, is referred to you for the evaluation of a slowly enlarging goiter. Thyroid tests reveal low normal serum T_4 level and an elevated serum TSH level. Which of the following is/are likely?

A. Low TBG levels
B. Increased iodide uptake
C. Abnormal circulating iodoproteins
D. Positive perchlorate discharge test
E. Impaired iodide uptake by the thyroid

97. A 56-year-old man is admitted to the hospital for evaluation of hypoglycemia. After six hours of fasting, he develops symptoms of hypoglycemia and has blood glucose of 27 mg/dl. A simultaneously obtained plasma insulin measurement shows no detectable level. Which of the following is/are possibly causing the hypoglycemia?

A. Uremia
B. Insulinoma
C. Alimentary hypoglycemia
D. Addison's disease
E. Extrapancreatic malignancy

98. A 55-year-old man is brought to the emergency room after an automobile accident. Skull roentgenograms show an enlarged sella turcica. Which of the following diagnostic studies is/are appropriate?

A. Serum FSH
B. Serum T_4 and free T_4
C. Serum prolactin
D. Serum testosterone
E. Computed tomography (CT scan) of the pituitary

99. A hypertensive 27-year-old man is seen for evaluation of a thyroid nodule. His grandmother, father, and one brother are reported to have had thyroid cancer. A sister and aunt died for unexplained reasons after minor surgical procedures. This patient is likely to have which of the following abnormalities?

A. Hypocalcemia
B. Hypoglycemia
C. Elevated serum T_3 levels
D. Elevated serum prolactin levels
E. Elevated urinary metanephrines

100. After careful endocrine testing, a 41-year-old man is shown to have panhypopituitarism. The appropriate treatment of this patient includes

A. L-thyroxine, 150 μg orally once per day
B. hydrocortisone, 50 mg orally at 9 AM, and 50 mg orally at 9 PM
C. fludrocortisone, 0.1 mg orally once per day
D. testosterone enanthate, 150 mg intramuscularly every two weeks
E. use of a medical-alert bracelet

101. A 36-year-old man is referred to you because of infertility. Seminal fluid analysis reveals a sperm count of less than 1 million/ml (normal >20). Serum FSH is 49 mIU/ml (normal = 4–27) and serum testosterone is within the normal range. Which of the following disorders is/are consistent with the laboratory results?

A. Kartagener's syndrome
B. Klinefelter's syndrome
C. Sertoli-cell–only syndrome
D. Testicular irradiation
E. Mumps orchitis

102. An adolescent girl has muscular weakness. She is short and obese, and has a round face and ocular strabismus. Roentgenogram of the hands is shown below. Serum calcium is 7.5 mg/dl (normal = 8.9–10.1), and serum phosphate is 5.5 mg/dl (normal = 2.5–4.5). Which of the following is/are likely to be found in this patient?

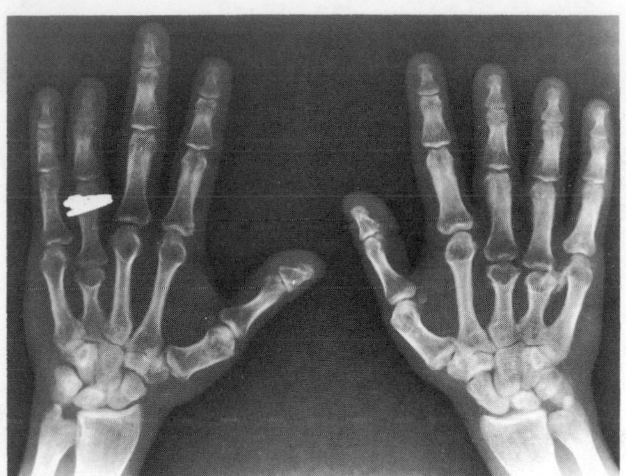

A. Increased serum parathyroid hormone (PTH) concentration
B. Basal ganglia calcification on skull film
C. A normal urinary cyclic AMP response to PTH
D. Subnormal intelligence
E. Family members of the same phenotype

103. A 56-year-old woman is admitted to the hospital because of lethargy and confusion. Initial laboratory studies show serum sodium of 114 mEq/L. Further studies show serum osmolality of 248 mOsm/kg and urine osmolality of 745 mOsm/kg. Which of the following disorders is/are associated with these findings?

A. Hepatitis
B. Meningitis
C. Hypothyroidism
D. Addison's disease
E. Carcinoma of the lung

DIRECTIONS: Questions 104 to 137 are matching questions. For each numbered item, choose the most likely associated lettered item from those provided. Each numbered item has ONLY ONE answer. Within each set of questions, each lettered item may be the answer to one, more than one, or none of the numbered items, unless otherwise specified.

Questions 104–107

For each of the following sets of laboratory values, select the most appropriate condition (A–C).

A. Normal
B. Diabetes mellitus
C. Impaired glucose tolerance

	Fasting Plasma Glucose (mg/dl)	After 75-gram Glucose Tolerance Test (mg/dl) 30 min	60 min	90 min	120 min
104.	125	175	197	220	210
105.	125	175	220	180	160
106.	125	175	220	210	205
107.	125	175	180	160	120

QUESTIONS 108–112

For each of the following clinical circumstances, choose the most likely set of laboratory values. *(Note: Use each lettered item only once.)*

	Serum Calcium (mg/dl) (normal = 8.5–10.5)	Serum Phosphorus (mg/dl) (normal = 2.5–4.5)	Immunoreactive PTH (pg/ml) (normal = 10–40)
A.	8.8	5.8	750
B.	7.5	2.0	120
C.	6.5	6.5	120
D.	10.9	2.5	120
E.	14.4	2.8	40

108. A 25-year-old obese woman who has round facies, mental retardation, and short fourth and fifth metacarpal bones

109. A 35-year-old woman with chronic renal failure who receives hemodialysis treatments three times weekly

110. A 45-year-old man who has pancreatic insufficiency and intestinal malabsorption

111. A 50-year-old woman who has a history of gastrinoma and pituitary tumor

112. A 65-year-old man with squamous cell carcinoma of the lung who is admitted to the hospital for weakness, lethargy, and constipation

QUESTIONS 113–117

For each of the following clinical descriptions, match the most appropriate set of laboratory values. *(Note: Use each lettered item only once.)*

	Potassium	ACTH	Cortisol	Plasma Renin Activity	Aldosterone
A.	↓	nl	nl	↑	↑
B.	↓	nl	nl	↓	↑
C.	↑	↑	↓	↑	↓
D.	↑	nl	nl	↓	↓
E.	↑	nl	nl	↑	↑

↑ = Increased; ↓ = decreased; nl = normal

113. A 5-year-old boy who accidentally ingests 15–20 potassium chloride tablets

114. A 30-year-old man who has polyuria, lassitude, muscle weakness, and hypertension

115. A 35-year-old man with insulin-dependent diabetes mellitus and hypothyroidism who develops weight loss, fatigue, and increasing pigmentation of the skin and buccal mucosa

116. A 54-year-old woman who has essential hypertension controlled with hydrochlorothiazide

117. A 60-year-old woman who has diabetes mellitus and moderate renal insufficiency

QUESTIONS 118–122

For each of the following clinical conditions, choose the most likely set of laboratory values. *(Note: Use each lettered item only once.)*

	LH (mIU/ml (normal = 4–19)	FSH (mIU/ml) (normal = 4–27)	Estradiol (pg/ml) (normal ≤ 40)	Prolactin (ng/ml) (normal = 5–25)
A.	6	5	12	150
B.	15	20	35	10
C.	35	25	120	12
D.	100	80	10	10
E.	6	5	10	22

118. Amenorrhea, anorexia nervosa

119. Amenorrhea, galactorrhea, headaches

120. Amenorrhea, hirsutism, acne, enlarged ovaries without virilism

121. Amenorrhea, hypothyroidism, Addison's disease

122. Amenorrhea following cesarean section

QUESTIONS 123–127

For each of the following clinical situations, choose the most likely set of laboratory values. *(Note: Use each lettered item only once.)*

	T_4 (μg/dl) (normal = 5–11)	T_3 (ng/dl) (normal = 100–200)	TSH (μU/ml) (normal = 0.8–5.0)
A.	10.5	365	0.2
B.	15.7	290	25.0
C.	10.1	70	4.0
D.	12.5	225	3.5
E.	3.2	50	1.2

123. A 25-year-old woman with a hydatidiform mole, who has nervousness, weight loss, and decreased heat tolerance

124. A 27-year-old asymptomatic woman who is eight months pregnant

125. A 35-year-old man who has a six-month history of fatigue, nervousness, fine tremor, and weight loss

126. A 47-year-old woman who has hypertension being treated with high doses of propranolol

127. A 55-year-old man who has a two-year history of fatigue, cold intolerance, severe headache, and worsening tunnel vision

QUESTIONS 128–131

A 23-year-old man who has a nine-year history of insulin-dependent diabetes mellitus is currently taking 35 units of NPH insulin every morning. He routinely measures his blood glucose at home before breakfast, lunch, and dinner and at bedtime. For each of the following typical blood glucose profiles, select the most appropriate alteration in insulin therapy.

A. Add 5 units of regular insulin to morning NPH
B. Decrease morning NPH to 30 units
C. Switch to twice-daily NPH—25 units in morning, 15 units in evening
D. No change
E. Switch to twice-daily NPH—35 units in morning, 25 units in evening

	Blood Glucose (mg/dl)			
	7 AM	11 AM	5 PM	9 PM
128.	350	175	160	270
129.	130	300	210	150
130.	130	160	150	110
131.	40	290	170	80

	Plasma Cortisol 8:00 AM	Plasma Cortisol 5:00 PM	Plasma ACTH 8:00 AM	Urinary 17-OH Corticoids	Urinary 17-keto-steroids	*Urinary 17-OH Corticoids After Dexamethasone*	
						0.5 mg every 6 hr	*2.0 mg every 6 hr*
(Normal)	*(8–25 μg/dl)*	*(5–10 μg/dl)*	*(<80 pg/ml)*	*(3–7 mg/gcr*)*	*(<20 mg/day)*	*(<2 mg/gcr*)*	*(<2 mg/gcr*)*
A.	27	25	65	19	27	15	6
B.	15	21	20	14	10	15	16
C.	12	8	92	15	25	<2	<2
D.	25	23	20	18	343	16	23
E.	55	42	250	45	114	47	48
F.	35	30	75	6	12	<2	<2

*gcr = gram of creatinine.

QUESTIONS 132–137

For each of the following patients who are being evaluated for the possibility of Cushing's syndrome, select from the table above (A–F) the most likely associated set of laboratory values. *(Note: Use each lettered item only once.)*

132. A 5-year-boy with phallic enlargement, accelerated growth, and high blood pressure

133. A 24-year-old woman with sleep disturbance, easy fatigability, central obesity, abdominal striae, and an adrenal mass on computed tomography (CT scan)

134. An overweight 26-year-old woman receiving oral contraceptives

135. A 41-year-old woman with amenorrhea, acne, beard growth, deep voice, and a palpable mass in the left flank

136. A 52-year-old woman with a basophilic pituitary adenoma

137. A 55-year-old man with cough, weakness, hypokalemia, and a lung mass on roentgenogram of the chest

PART 7

ENDOCRINOLOGY AND DIABETES MELLITUS

ANSWERS

1.(C) Since random elevated growth hormone levels may at times be observed in healthy patients, more definitive diagnostic procedures are required before the diagnosis of acromegaly can be confirmed. The failure to suppress growth hormone levels to less than 5 ng/ml after glucose ingestion would confirm the diagnosis of acromegaly. Plasma somatomedin C levels would also be helpful in definitively diagnosing acromegaly. *(Cecil, Ch. 226; Melmed et al)*

2.(E) The majority of patients with the empty sella syndrome have no abnormalities of pituitary function. The major clinical significance of the empty sella syndrome is to avoid misdiagnosing a pituitary tumor. No treatment other than reassurance is required in most patients with the syndrome. *(Cecil, Ch. 226)*

3.(D) Histiocytosis X is a non-neoplastic histiocytic reaction to unknown stimuli. The classic triad in this disorder is punched-out skull lesions, exophthalmos from histiocytic invasion of the retro-orbital space, and diabetes insipidus. The disease is usually responsive to radiation therapy and treatment with prednisone or vinblastine. *(Cecil, Ch. 227)*

4.(C) The hemoglobin A_1 level depends on the plasma glucose concentration for the six to ten weeks preceding measurement. Normal hemoglobin A_1 level in a patient who is known to be hyperglycemic during the day suggests nocturnal hypoglycemia. Low nocturnal plasma glucose concentrations and elevated daytime levels result in average plasma glucose being within the normal range, hence, a normal hemoglobin A_1 level. A lack of accuracy in the home plasma glucose measurement could also account for these findings. *(Cecil, Ch. 231; Health and Public Policy Committee)*

5.(C) This patient does not have diabetes mellitus. The glycosuria is due to a defect in the transport of glucose in the proximal renal tubule which leads to glucose in the urine. This disorder is inherited as an autosomal recessive, and the incidence is approximately 1 in 500. This condition is benign and should not be confused with diabetes mellitus. *(Cecil, Chs. 84 and 231)*

6.(E) Glucagon is the hormone chiefly responsible for the glucose recovery from acute hypoglycemia. In glucagon-deficient individuals, epinephrine can compensate for the absence of glucagon, and glucose recovery is almost normal. The deficiency of epinephrine, glucocorticoids, or growth hormone alone does not significantly affect glucose recovery from hypoglycemia in patients with an adequate glucagon response. In patients deficient in both epinephrine and glucagon, recovery from hypoglycemia is profoundly impaired. This is clinically important because many patients with longstanding diabetes and autonomic insufficiency have impaired secretion of both glucagon and epinephrine in response to hypoglycemia; they are therefore susceptible to serious hypoglycemic reactions. *(Cecil, Ch. 231; Cryer and Gerich)*

7.(D) The data provided indicate that this patient has an insulinoma. Stimulatory diagnostic tests using either glucagon or tolbutamide are occasionally useful in this diagnosis when fasting is equivocal, but they are unlikely to provide further useful information in this case and are potentially harmful. Glucose tolerance tests and measurement of insulin-like growth factors are not indicated in the evaluation of a patient with an insulinoma. In this patient, the diagnostic efforts should be directed toward localizing the tumor using such techniques as ultrasound, computed tomography (CT scan), arteriography, and selective pancreatic venous catheterization. *(Cecil, Ch. 232; Nelson)*

8.(C) All the conditions listed can cause insulin resistance; however, high caloric intake and associated obesity are by far the most common cause of insulin resistance. If this patient followed a weight reduction diet, it is very likely that the insulin requirements would decrease greatly. It is even possible that with dietary therapy the diabetes might be acceptably controlled without insulin treatment. *(Cecil, Ch. 231; Grunfeld)*

9.(D) Lipohypertrophy occurs secondary to the direct metabolic effects of insulin which lead to increased fat synthesis. It is thus observed regardless of the insulin preparation used and is most commonly observed when the site of insulin injection is not varied. There is frequently local hypesthesia over the hypertrophied site, and the patient usually chooses to inject this area to lessen discomfort. It should be noted that insulin absorption from a hypertrophied site may differ from that from unaffected locations. The treatment of choice is to rotate sites and avoid injection into the hypertrophied area. *(Cecil, Ch. 231; Huntley)*

10.(A) Glucagonomas cause a clinical syndrome called necrolytic migratory erythema. It is characterized by distinctive cutaneous lesions appearing on the face, abdomen, buttocks, or extremities, with multiple crusts, scaling macules and papules, bullae, and generalized erythema. These lesions tend to remit and recur over time. It is important to recognize this skin lesion so that appropriate evaluation for a glucagonoma can begin. *(Cecil, Ch. 233; Bolt et al)*

11.(E) Infected diabetic foot ulcers frequently contain multiple microorganisms, including aerobic gram-positive and gram-negative bacteria and anaerobic bacteria. Many of these anaerobic and gram-negative organisms are not sensitive to penicillin G or cloxacillin, so these antibiotics are not ideal choices. Similarly, gentamicin and sulfamethoxazole-trimethoprim do not offer effective coverage against the wide spectrum of organisms that are commonly observed in diabetic foot ulcers. Cefoxitin, however, offers relatively broad coverage, including anaerobes; in mild to moderate infections it is a suitable therapeutic choice. *(Cecil, Ch. 231; Gleckman and Roth)*

12.(E) NLD is a plaque-like lesion with a central yellow area surrounded by a brownish border. It is usually located in the pretibial regions but may occur at any site. The lesion occurs most commonly in young females and may ulcerate with minor trauma. Steroid therapy, either topically or intralesionally, can be helpful. Evidence that platelet inhibitors are useful has not been demonstrated in control trials. *(Cecil, Ch. 231; Huntley)*

13.(D) Rhinocerebral mucormycosis is a rare fungal infection that is usually seen during or following an episode of diabetic ketoacidosis. The organisms responsible for this disorder are from the genera *Mucor, Rhizopus,* and *Absidia.* The therapy of choice is amphotericin B coupled with aggressive debridement. *(Cecil, Ch. 231; Lehrer et al)*

14.(E) Although A–D are all causes of impotence, the presence of nocturnal erections strongly suggests psychogenic impotence. In evaluating patients with impotence it is very useful to determine if they are having normal erections at any time; this indicates an intact system and suggests that the cause of the impotence is not physiological. *(Cecil, Ch. 235; Morley)*

15.(C) Kallman's syndrome is characterized by hypogonadism with low levels of plasma testosterone, FSH, and LH. Both the FSH and LH increase in response to GNRH, and the syndrome is thought to be due to a failure of the hypothalamus to produce GNRH. Anosmia and hyposmia are commonly observed and point toward the diagnosis. Because anosmia is often not recognized by patients, the sense of smell must be tested in all patients with delayed puberty or eunuchoidal features. *(Cecil, Ch. 235)*

16.(C) The patient is most likely to have Klinefelter's syndrome, a disorder characterized by tall stature, small firm testes, azoospermia, gynecomastia, elevated gonadotropin levels, and decreased serum testosterone levels. Obesity, varicose veins, mild mental deficiency, social maladjustment, diabetes mellitus, and pulmonary disease occur more frequently than in the general population. The syndrome is secondary to the presence of two or more X chromosomes, and the most common karyotype is 47 XXY, but mosaic forms and other abnormalities are observed. Leukocyte karyotyping is the diagnostic test of choice. *(Cecil, Ch. 235).*

17.(D) Azoospermia with normal laboratory studies strongly suggests obstruction of sperm transport; urologic consultation is indicated. In Kartagener's syndrome (sinusitis, bronchiectasis, and situs inversus) the sperm are nonmotile because of a defect in microtubule structure which also causes immobility of the cilia in the bronchi. Varicoceles may result in oligospermia and abnormalities of sperm morphology, but azoospermia is not seen. In myotonic muscular dystrophy, abnormalities in hormone levels are observed. *(Cecil, Ch. 235; Swerdloff et al)*

18.(E) The most likely diagnosis in this patient is artifactual hypoglycemia secondary to excessive glycolysis by leukocytes. The most appropriate diagnostic test is a repeat measurement of plasma glucose with prompt separation of the plasma from the cells and rapid measurement of the glucose level. *(Cecil, Ch. 232)*

19.(A) Evaluation of sperm concentration, motility, and morphology is of critical importance in the evaluation of infertility in males. Hormonal tests, such as serum prolactin and testosterone levels, are indicated only if the semen analysis is abnormal. Roentgenograms of the sella are indicated only if hormonal studies point toward a pituitary abnormality. *(Cecil, Ch. 235; Swerdloff et al)*

20.(B) Dehydration in this patient results in a serum osmolality slightly greater than the normal range and a modest increase in urine osmolality but not to the degree usually expected with dehydration (urine osmolality >700–800 mOsm/kg). That the urine osmolality is greater than the serum osmolality indicates some ADH effect. After injection of vasopressin, urine osmolality increased by 25%, thus demonstrating that the renal tubules are responsive to ADH. Together these data indicate that the secretion of endogenous ADH is suboptimal, suggesting the diagnosis of partial ADH deficiency. *(Cecil, Ch. 227; Moses and Notman)*

21.(D) Patients with inappropriate ADH, severe hyponatremia, and *symptoms* should be treated vigorously. Intravenous administration of 3% saline to raise serum sodium levels by approximately 2 mEq per hour is indicated. If congestive heart failure is likely or develops, furosemide (Lasix) should be administered simultaneously. Once the initial hyponatremia improves and the symptoms abate, water restriction should be instituted. If intravenous fluids are required, isotonic saline rather than hypotonic fluids should be used. Demeclocycline and lithium carbonate may be useful agents in the management of the inappropriate ADH syndrome in those patients who do not respond well to fluid restriction. *(Cecil, Ch. 227; Narins)*

22.(D) Failure to respond to pitressin administration indicates that this patient has nephrogenic diabetes insipidus. Nephrogenic diabetes insipidus can be treated with thiazides or other diuretics that produce sodium depletion and cause a fall in GFR. This decrease in GFR results in an enhanced proximal tubular sodium reabsorption and decreased delivery of sodium to the ascending loop of Henle, which consequently reduces the capacity to dilute the urine. In conjunction with diuretics, a decreased sodium intake is essential to obtain satisfactory results. The other therapies are effective only in the treatment of central diabetes insipidus. *(Cecil, Ch. 227; Moses and Notman)*

23.(A) The patient has inappropriate ADH production secondary to pulmonary tuberculosis. All the therapies described are useful in treating patients with inappropriate ADH, but in this patient who has no symptoms and only a modest decrease in serum sodium, the restriction of water is the most appropriate initial therapy. Choices D and E are useful in rapidly raising serum sodium levels in patients who either are symptomatic or have very low serum sodium levels. Choices B and C are drugs that inhibit the effect of vasopressin on the kidney and have been useful in the treatment of chronic symptomatic inappropriate ADH secretion. These agents should not be used in patients in whom the syndrome of inappropriate ADH is mild, asymptomatic, or probably of short duration. Since both these drugs have serious potential complications, water restriction, when possible, is the treatment of choice. *(Cecil, Ch. 227; Narins)*

24.(E) It should be recognized that transient gynecomastia is a frequent occurrence during normal puberty. In an otherwise asymptomatic adolescent boy, extensive diagnostic studies are not indicated. *(Cecil, Ch. 235; Wilson et al)*

25.(D) The patient has severe secondary hyperparathyroidism, as manifested by subperiosteal bone resorption and increased serum levels of immunoreactive PTH. For renal transplant patients with this disorder, parathyroidectomy is the treatment of choice. It is widely believed that hypercalcemia will decrease transplant survival and it is therefore essential to treat the elevated calcium levels. *(Cecil, Ch. 249)*

26. (E) This patient has several characteristic clinical features of Paget's disease, including musculoskeletal pain, increase in hat size, hearing loss, and elevated serum alkaline phosphatase activity. Roentgenograms of clinically involved areas (skull and pelvis) will be most helpful in establishing the diagnosis. Although the bone scan is the most sensitive means to detect active lesions of Paget's disease, it is not a specific diagnostic test. *(Cecil, Ch. 251; Strewler)*

27. (D) Pseudofractures are a pathognomonic radiologic feature of osteomalacia. These radiolucent lines are most often found along the inner aspects of the femoral neck, the pubic rami, the ribs, and the outer edge of the scapula. Pseudofractures probably result from demineralization of bone along the distribution of blood vessels or from unhealed microfractures at points of stress. In severe cases pseudofractures can progress to complete fractures, thereby resulting in substantial deformity and disability. Reduced bone density is not a reliable indication of osteomalacia, since some patients (especially those with chronic renal failure) will have increased rather than decreased radiologic bone density. *(Cecil, Ch. 246; Frame and Parfitt)*

28. (C) The most sensitive test for diagnosing primary hypothyroidism is an elevated TSH level. TSH-induced hypersecretion of T_3 relative to T_4 can result in serum T_3 levels within the normal range. On rare occasions, serum T_4 is also in the low-normal range. Tests for antithyroid antibodies are helpful in determining the etiology but not the diagnosis of hypothyroidism. Serum thyroglobulin may be elevated in any patient with an enlarged thyroid or following acute trauma to the thyroid. *(Cecil, Ch. 229)*

29. (D) This patient has a diffuse, nontoxic (multinodular) goiter. Young (<40 years old) euthyroid patients with diffuse thyroid enlargement should be started on thyroxine replacement therapy to suppress TSH. In some patients, this treatment may block further thyroid enlargement as well as cause regression of goiter. In older patients, TSH suppression only occasionally results in an improvement in physical symptoms; furthermore, autonomously functioning hyperplastic nodules are more common in the elderly, and attempts to suppress TSH can result in iatrogenic hyperthyroidism. Hyperthyroid patients with multinodular goiter are best treated with radioactive iodine. However, if a low RAI uptake limits the efficacy of ^{131}I treatment, then surgery should be performed after appropriate preparation with antithyroid drugs (iodine, PTU). Iodine administration can induce thyrotoxicosis in patients with nontoxic goiter and thus should be avoided. *(Cecil, Ch. 229; Rojeski and Gharib)*

30. (B) Recognition and treatment of hypercalciuria in a patient with recurrent nephrolithiasis is important, since hypercalciuria directly contributes to stone formation by raising urine saturation. Thiazides are unique among diuretics in their ability to augment renal tubular calcium resorption; they thereby can correct the renal leak of calcium responsible for renal hypercalciuria. Thiazides are very effective in preventing the formation of new kidney stones. *(Cecil, Ch. 90; Coe)*

31. (A) Decreases in body magnesium stores result in decreased secretion of parathyroid hormone and are the most likely cause of hypocalcemia in an alcoholic patient. Reduced dietary intake of calcium and malabsorption of calcium due to intestinal disease do not cause hypocalcemia in patients with normal parathyroid function. In renal hypercalciuria, secondary hyperparathyroidism is evoked by urinary losses of calcium. Elevated levels of PTH increase renal production of 1,25-dihydroxy vitamin D, producing increased intestinal absorption of calcium. *(Cecil, Ch. 247; Agus et al)*

32. (D) Management of incidental adrenal masses depends on the size of the lesion. When the adrenal mass is small (<6 cm) and not biochemically active, the lesion can be observed, if solid, or aspirated, if cystic. However, a larger mass (>6 cm) should be removed surgically because of the greater potential for malignancy. Preoperative evaluation for a functioning adrenal adenoma or pheochromocytoma is important in planning perioperative management of the patient (i.e., antihypertensive therapy, steroid taper, etc.). *(Cecil, Ch. 230; Copeland)*

33. (E) An uncommon but important consideration in the differential diagnosis of goiter is lymphoma of the thyroid. History of Hashimoto's thyroiditis in an older patient (> 50 years) with rapid enlargement of the thyroid suggests lymphoma of the thyroid. Thyroid fine-needle aspirate should establish the diagnosis. Although lymphoma can cause painful enlargement of the thyroid, it frequently is painless. On the other hand, neck pain is the most common presenting symptom of subacute thyroiditis and acute suppurative thyroiditis. Factitious thyrotoxicosis is not associated with thyroid enlargement. In a patient receiving thyroid replacement therapy, massive growth of the thyroid secondary to multinodular goiter is unlikely. *(Cecil, Ch. 229; Hamburger et al)*

34. (D) Congenital adrenal hyperplasia resulting from 21-hydroxylase deficiency results in marked elevations of 17-hydroxyprogesterone. However, this steroid precursor can also be secreted in large amounts by certain ovarian and adrenal neoplasms. Proper management of the patient at this time would be to administer dexamethasone, 0.5 mg four times daily, for three days. Suppression of the elevated 17-hydroxyprogesterone by this maneuver confirms the diagnosis of 21-hydroxylase deficiency. Surgical exploration of an adrenal mass should be undertaken only after the diagnosis of congenital adrenal hyperplasia has been excluded. Antiandrogens such as cyproterone acetate and oral contraceptives have had limited success in the treatment of idiopathic hirsutism. Mitotane is a chemotherapeutic agent used to treat metastatic adrenal carcinoma. It should be noted that congenital adrenal hyperplasia can lead to asymmetric enlargement of adrenal glands; the enlargement of a single gland should not be confused with tumor. *(Cecil, Ch. 237; Rittmaster and Loriaux)*

35. (C) This patient shows elevated plasma aldosterone levels and a history compatible with the syndrome of primary aldosteronism. However, before a diagnosis is made, it is crucial to measure the plasma renin activity. In primary aldosteronism plasma renin activity is low, whereas in secondary aldosteronism plasma renin activity is increased. Such disorders as renal artery stenosis or renin-secreting tumors can present with hypertension, hypokalemia, and increased plasma aldosterone levels due to increased renin secretion; primary aldosteronism must be differentiated from these disorders. *(Cecil, Ch. 230; Ferriss et al)*

36. (D) All choices (A–E) have been used in the treatment of patients with hypercalcemia, but the initial and most important therapeutic approach is hydration with isotonic sodium chloride. Rehydration will result in an increase in renal calcium excretion and sometimes lower serum calcium concentrations to an acceptable range. Other therapeutic options can be added to hydration if the serum calcium response is inadequate. *(Cecil, Ch. 247; Lee et al)*

37.(D) The patient has mild ophthalmopathy associated with Graves' disease. The disease is not severe enough to warrant therapy with glucocorticoids or surgical decompression of the orbit, but elevation of the head of the bed and the use of methylcellulose eyedrops may be of value. Since the symptoms are worse in the morning, it is possible that the palpebral fissures are not completely closed during sleep, and taping the eyelids closed at bedtime may help. Bed elevation and administration of diuretics may reduce conjunctival edema. Although the natural course of the disease is not influenced by these measures, it is generally the impression that hyperthyroidism or hypothyroidism, particularly the latter, may exacerbate ophthalmopathy. Reduction of exogenous thyroxine replacement to induce hypothyroidism is therefore contraindicated. *(Cecil, Ch. 229)*

38.(B) In myxedema coma, hypothermia should be treated by covering the patient with a blanket to induce gradual, passive warming. Active warming with a heating blanket may lead to shock and death. The best method for administration of thyroid hormone in this condition is unclear. The present consensus, however, is for the rapid intravenous injection of a large dose of L-thyroxine. Infection is often an important factor in precipitating myxedema coma, and should be carefully looked for and vigorously treated. Respiratory depression is also commonly seen in this condition, and when myxedema coma is suspected the measurement of arterial blood gas tensions is mandatory. Ventilatory assistance may be necessary. Because of diminished free-water clearance in hypothyroidism, and because of the reduced insensitive loss of water during severe hypothyroidism, these patients are at risk of developing hyponatremia and water intoxication. *(Cecil, Ch. 229; Werner and Ingbar)*

39.(E) In most cases of ectopic ACTH syndrome, the typical features of Cushing's syndrome are absent. The clinical picture is dominated by wasting, weakness, and other manifestations of malignancy. Peristent hypokalemia and very high plasma cortisol levels are also commonly observed. Oat cell carcinoma of the lung is the most common cause of the syndrome, but numerous other tumors have also been associated with it. *(Cecil, Ch. 230)*

40.(D) The patient clearly has hyperparathyroidism. Even in patients who eventually prove to have large parathyroid adenomas, however, the tumor is rarely palpable in the neck. Such palpable masses usually prove to be coexisting and unrelated thyroid nodules. *(Cecil, Ch. 247)*

41.(D) The incidence of thyroid cancer is 50- to 300-fold increased in patients with previous radiotherapy to the thyroid gland. Because of this marked increase in the frequency of malignancy, surgical exploration should be performed in all patients with a well-demarcated thyroid nodule. Needle biopsies are of limited use in patients with a history of radiotherapy; it has been observed that the palpable nodule can be benign, but surrounding thyroid tissue may harbor a malignancy. *(Cecil, Ch. 229)*

42.(E) The progression of renal insufficiency secondary to diabetic glomerulopathy in a particular diabetic patient follows a predictable pattern. A sudden worsening in renal function should prompt an extensive search for other factors that could account for the clinical course. In this patient, it is unlikely that diabetic glomerulopathy accounts for the sudden and accelerated decrease in renal function. *(Cecil, Ch. 231)*

43.(B) Profound and prolonged hypoglycemia is most likely to occur in patients taking chlorpropamide, especially if renal function is compromised. The duration of the hypoglycemic action of chlorpropamide is much greater (60 hours) than that of the other hypoglycemic agents, and it is excreted primarily by the kidneys. Because of these characteristics, the use of chlorpropamide should be avoided in elderly patients, in patients with renal insufficiency, or in any individuals who are at increased risk of hypoglycemia. *(Cecil, Ch. 232; Boyden and Bressler)*

44.(A) Despite the patient's denial of sexual activity, pregnancy cannot be discounted. It remains the chief cause of "secondary amenorrhea" and should *always* be excluded before other expensive and possibly contraindicated procedures are undertaken. *(Cecil, Ch. 237)*

45.(C) The most likely cause of the polyuria is primary polydipsia because the plasma osmolality is less than normal. In the other disorders (A, B, and D), the plasma osmolality is either normal or increased. Also, when diabetes mellitus induces polyuria, the urine osmolality is very high owing to the presence of glucose. *(Cecil, Ch. 227; Moses and Notman; Robertson et al)*

46.(E) Paget's disease is a relatively common bone disease in patients over the age of 70. Approximately 20% of patients are asymptomatic during the course of the disease. All the drugs listed (A–D) are used to treat Paget's disease, but in this asymptomatic patient with only a mild increase in alkaline phosphatase, treatment is not indicated. *(Cecil, Ch. 251; Wallach)*

47.(D) This patient has elevated FSH despite normal testis size, normal testosterone, and normal LH. These findings are compatible with germinal cell aplasia (Sertoli-cell–only syndrome). Biopsy is unnecessary. This condition is occasionally seen after cytotoxic drugs or radiation therapy; when it occurs spontaneously, it is irreversible and the patients are infertile. The diagnosis may be confirmed by finding azoospermia in the ejaculate. There is no evidence to indicate pituitary dysfunction or that any form of treatment will improve fertility. *(Cecil, Ch. 235)*

48.(E) This girl is beyond the usual age of menarche (12.6 years), but early signs of beginning sexual maturation (early pubic hair and breast development) are present. It is reasonable to assume that menarche will occur spontaneously, and careful observation is an appropriate decision. Only if no further progression occurs or if other signs of pituitary dysfunction appear (such as growth cessation) would pituitary or gonadal investigations be appropriate. Induction of menses with gonadal steroids may be appropriate because of the patient's psychological burden of difference from her peers. In that case, more careful laboratory definition of pituitary and gonadal function might be contemplated. *(Cecil, Ch. 237)*

49.(D) Virilism in adult females is commonly due to either adrenocortical or ovarian tumors. The presence of a palpable left upper quadrant abdominal mass strongly suggests that the virilization is due to an adrenocortical carcinoma. Polycystic ovary syndrome, idiopathic hirsutism, and Cushing's disease do not cause true virilization. Congenital adrenal hyperplasia is not associated with a large abdominal mass, and the onset of androgen excess usually begins earlier in life. *(Cecil, Ch. 238; Givens)*

50. (D) Chronic alcoholic patients may develop physical stigmata resembling Cushing's syndrome (pseudo-Cushing's syndrome). They may present with all the physical stigmata of Cushing's syndrome, and biochemical studies may reveal hypercortisolemia, elevated ACTH levels, impaired diurnal cortisol variation, and inadequate cortisol suppression after dexamethasone administration. The abnormal biochemical findings rapidly return toward normal with abstinence but reappear upon resumption of alcohol ingestion. It is essential to avoid misdiagnosis, and therefore the evaluation of alcoholic patients with suspected Cushing's syndrome should be carried out only after they have undergone a period of abstinence. The overnight dexamethasone test should be repeated. *(Cecil, Ch. 230; Wright; Cook et al)*

51. (D) The major focus of therapy in obese patients with newly diagnosed non-insulin-dependent diabetes mellitus (NIDDM) is caloric restriction and weight loss. This group of patients may note a marked improvement in hyperglycemia with diet alone; therefore, it is important to determine the effectiveness of caloric restriction before initiating treatment with either insulin or oral agents. *(Cecil, Ch. 231)*

52. (D) The history, physical examination, and laboratory results are typical of subacute thyroiditis. This illness often follows a viral infection by several weeks. Occasionally, patients are hyperthyroid secondary to the release of hormone during the destruction of the gland. The hyperthyroidism is usually of short duration (<2 months) and can be followed by hypothyroidism, which sometimes persists. Aspirin is useful in the treatment of subacute thyroiditis, but in a significant number of patients prednisone therapy is required. *(Cecil, Ch. 229)*

53. (D) Although all these problems may develop in ketoacidosis, a normal serum potassium at the time of presentation with moderately severe acidosis should alert one to the severe total body potassium depletion seen in a chronically untreated patient. This may be aggravated by treatment. *(Cecil, Ch. 231)*

54. (B) Solitary thyroid nodules raise the question of malignancy. This potential is so markedly reduced in hyperfunctioning nodules ("hot nodules") that no biopsy is needed. If the patient is euthyroid, no therapy is needed; if he is hyperthyroid, surgical removal or radioiodine ablation is appropriate. Since the free thyroxine index in this patient is normal, we now need to assess serum T_3. If it is normal, only observation is indicated; if elevated, we may presume early and (as yet) mild "T_3 thyrotoxicosis," and the nodule should be removed or destroyed. *(Cecil, Ch. 229)*

55. (C) It is important to remember that primary hyperparathyroidism is a common disorder. Tumors can induce hypercalcemia by various mechanisms, but in some patients with malignant disease the hypercalcemia is due to coexistent primary hyperparathyroidism. In this patient, the hypercalcemia is very likely due to primary hyperparathyroidism because of (1) the lack of evidence of metastatic disease, which is almost always observed in the hypercalcemia associated with breast cancer but not necessarily with other tumors; and (2) the marked increase in serum PTH levels. PTH levels in patients with the hypercalcemia of malignancy have been reported to be undetectable, normal, or slightly elevated. An increase in PTH to the level observed in this patient strongly suggests the presence of hyperparathyroidism. Previous calcium levels would be very helpful in the evaluation of this patient, because an increased calcium dating for many months or years would strongly point to primary hyperparathyroidism. The treatment of choice for primary hyperparathyroidism is surgery. *(Cecil, Ch. 247; Agus et al)*

56. (E) The most likely diagnosis of this patient is familial hypocalciuric hypercalcemia. This disorder is inherited as an autosomal dominant trait and is characterized by asymptomatic hypercalcemia, hypocalciuria, and normal or slightly elevated PTH levels. The documentation of hypercalcemia and hypocalciuria in immediate relatives would confirm the diagnosis and avoid further invasive procedures. The clinical course is benign. *(Cecil, Ch. 247; Marx et al)*

57. (B) Vigorous thyroid replacement therapy in a patient with panhypopituitarism can precipitate an adrenal crisis. Before replacing thyroid hormone in such a patient, secondary adrenal insufficiency should always be ruled out, and the replacement dosage of thyroxine should be initially small and increased gradually. If treatment is begun before cortisol secretory status is known, prophylactic glucocorticoids should be given while results are pending. *(Cecil, Ch. 226)*

58. (A) Diabetes affects the nervous system in many ways, the most common being the peripheral neuropathy demonstrated in this patient's feet. In addition, the marked predilection of the diabetic to atherosclerosis predisposes to single peripheral nerve infarction with sudden loss of motor and sensory function. This frequently involves one of the oculomotor nerves, as in this patient, producing acute ophthalmoplegia. Fortunately, collateral circulation usually corrects most or all of the deficit in weeks or months. *(Cecil, Ch. 231)*

59. (E) The osmolality of the patient, in spite of the elevated glucose, is not increased; therefore, hyperosmolar coma is not a likely cause of coma in this patient. In order for hyperglycemia to account for coma, the osmolality must be at least 350 mOsm/kg. *(Cecil Ch. 231; Foster)*

60. (E) The patient described has factitious hypoglycemia secondary to surreptitious administration of insulin. This condition is most common in young women with a medical background, and the patients may have no obvious psychological problems. The characteristic findings are hypoglycemia with very high insulin levels and suppressed C-peptide levels. Insulin antibodies are frequently present if insulin administration has been occurring for a sufficient period. However, it must be recognized that the presence of insulin antibodies is not pathognomonic for factitious insulin administration; several patients have been described with spontaneous hypoglycemia associated with insulin antibodies arising spontaneously on an autoimmune basis (insulin autoimmune hypoglycemia). *(Cecil, Ch. 232; Fajans and Floyd)*

61. (D) All the conditions listed can cause hyperkalemia, but in a diabetic with metabolic acidosis and moderately impaired renal function, the most likely etiology is hyporeninemic hypoaldosteronism. Plasma renin levels are low and do not increase normally in response to sodium restriction. This absence of renin, and hence angiotensin II, results in the failure of the zona glomerulosa to secrete aldosterone in response to sodium restriction and postural changes. This hyporeninism can occur in other kidney diseases in addition to diabetes. The basis for the impaired renin response is unknown. Diabetic patients rarely have a defect in the adrenal synthesis of aldosterone. *(Cecil, Ch. 231; Schambelan and Sebastian)*

62. (E) Hyperparathyroidism results in all the symptoms listed. Nevertheless, most patients with this condition are asymptomatic and are detected because hypercalcemia is found on biochemical screening tests. *(Cecil, Ch. 247)*

63. (A—True; B—False; C—True; D—True; E—False) In women, hyperprolactinemia can cause galactorrhea, oligomenorrhea or amenorrhea, and infertility. The cause of the amenorrhea is related to an interference by prolactin with the normal positive feedback effect of estradiol on GNRH secretion. In men, hyperprolactinemia results in impotence and decreased libido. Gynecomastia does not occur secondary to hyperprolactinemia. Longstanding hyperprolactinemia has been associated with decreased bone density in both men and women. *(Cecil, Ch. 226; Martin et al; Greenspan et al)*

64. (A—True; B—True; C—True; D—False; E—False) Elevated serum prolactin levels can occur secondary to a wide variety of factors. In addition to prolactin-secreting pituitary tumors, numerous drugs such as alpha-methyldopa, reserpine, phenothiazines, oral contraceptives, and opiates can induce hyperprolactinemia. Such medical conditions as hypothyroidism, renal failure, cirrhosis, thoracic spine lesions, and chest wall trauma or surgery have also been associated with elevated prolactin levels. Lastly, CNS disorders such as sarcoidosis, epileptic seizures, histiocytosis, trauma that results in stalk sections, and large pituitary or parasellar tumors that interfere with the hypothalamic pituitary portal blood flow can lead to hyperprolactinemia. It is important, therefore, not to assume that an elevation in plasma prolactin levels necessarily indicates the presence of a prolactin-secreting pituitary tumor. *(Cecil, Ch. 226; Martin et al)*

65. (A—True; B—True; C—False; D—True; E—False) Craniopharyngiomas usually occur in a suprasellar location but may extend into the sella turcica. The peak incidence is in the second decade, but they can occur at any age. Increased intracranial pressure is commonly observed in children, whereas in adults, visual defects are common. Approximately half of adult patients have endocrine deficiencies of anterior pituitary hormones. Diabetes insipidus and such hypothalamic syndromes as obesity, anorexia, etc., occasionally occur. The tumor is frequently calcified on routine roentgenogram, which is helpful in suggesting the diagnosis. *(Cecil, Ch. 226)*

66. (A—False; B—True; C—False; D—True; E—True) Acromegaly is characterized by acral enlargement, increased soft tissue growth leading to coarsening of the facial features and enlargement of the hands and feet, bony enlargement, increased sweating and sebaceous gland activity leading to increased body odor, joint pain secondary to osteoarthritis, and nerve entrapments including carpal tunnel syndrome. Hypertension is observed in approximately 25% of acromegalic patients. *(Cecil, Ch. 226; Melmed et al)*

67. (A—True; B—False; C—False; D—False; E—True) The patient is most likely to have hypopituitarism secondary to radiation therapy. This is supported by the levels of serum testosterone and LH, which indicate secondary hypogonadism. In such a case it is important to clarify whether there are other hormonal deficiencies. To determine thyroid function, T_4 measurement is the most desirable test. In evaluating ACTH secretion, it is important to identify patients with partial adrenal insufficiency in whom an inadequate cortisol response to stress may occur: The best stimulus is insulin-induced hypoglycemia with measurement of the cortisol response. If there are contraindications to insulin-induced hypoglycemia such as cerebral vascular disease, a cosyntropin or metyrapone stimulation test can provide useful information. Further evaluation of the pituitary gonadal axis is not indicated in the initial evaluation. *(Cecil, Ch. 226; Abboud)*

68. (A—True; B—False; C—False; D—True; E—False) Gustatory sweating is occasionally observed in diabetics with severe autonomic neuropathy; it can be generalized or occur in localized areas. This disorder can be very uncomfortable and distressing to the patient and will often respond to treatment with either anticholinergic drugs or clonidine. *(Cecil, Ch. 231; Janka et al)*

69. (A—True; B—True; C—False; D—False; E—True) The drugs that most commonly cause hypoglycemia are insulin and sulfonylureas. However, it should be recognized that other commonly used drugs can also occasionally lead to hypoglycemia. Alcohol can inhibit hepatic gluconeogenesis and thereby lead to fasting hypoglycemia. Aspirin, in large doses, can increase peripheral glucose utilization and cause hypoglycemia. Pentamidine destroys the pancreatic beta cells, leading to a transient hyperinsulinemia and hypoglycemia. Long-term pentamidine therapy can destroy sufficient pancreatic beta cells to lead to permanent diabetes mellitus. *(Cecil, Ch. 232; Nelson)*

70. (A—True; B—False; C—True; D—True; E—True) Numerous drugs can affect metabolic control in patients with diabetes mellitus. Insulin release is impaired by phenytoin and diuretics; in the latter case the disorder is related to hypokalemia. Insulin resistance is induced by dexamethasone (and other glucocorticoids) and oral contraceptives. *(Cecil, Ch. 231; Grunfeld and Chappell)*

71. (A—False; B—False; C—True; D—False; E—False) The hallmark of proliferative diabetic retinopathy is new vessel formation, i.e., neovascularization. Microaneurysms, hard waxy exudates, cotton wool exudates, hemorrhages, and edema may be observed in patients with proliferative retinopathy, but these lesions are also observed in patients with background (nonproliferative) retinopathy. *(Cecil, Ch. 231; Herman et al)*

72. (A—True; B—True; C—False; D—False; E—False) The most common extrapancreatic tumors that cause hypoglycemia are fibromas, sarcomas, hepatomas, carcinomas of the gastrointestinal tract, and adrenal carcinomas. Although the mechanism of hypoglycemia is not clear, it may, in some cases, be related to the production of insulin-like growth factors. *(Cecil, Ch. 232; Nelson)*

73. (A—True; B—False; C—False; D—True; E—True) Autonomic neuropathy may affect a variety of organs and cause a multitude of disorders. The entire gastrointestinal tract may be affected, leading to esophageal dysfunction, delayed gastric emptying, altered small bowel motility, diarrhea, and constipation. Additionally, bladder dysfunction, impotence, retrograde ejaculation, orthostatic hypotension, syncope, and, rarely, cardiorespiratory arrest also are observed. Diabetic amyotrophy is a form of neuropathy that leads to atrophy and weakness of the large muscles of the upper leg and pelvic girdle; it resembles a primary muscle disease. Charcot joints develop secondary to the loss of sensation; they typically occur in the feet and ankles of diabetics with longstanding severe peripheral neuropathy. *(Cecil, Ch. 231)*

74.(A—False; B—True; C—True; D—False; E—False) The peak age of onset of insulin-dependent diabetes is approximately age 12, and most insulin-dependent diabetics are of normal weight. At the onset of diabetes, 80% of insulin-dependent diabetics have antibodies against islet cells in the serum. With increasing duration of diabetes, the prevalence of islet cell antibodies decreases. In comparison to nondiabetic controls, the frequency of HLA D3 and D4 is increased in Caucasians with insulin-dependent diabetes. In identical twins, the concordance rate for insulin-dependent diabetics is approximately 40–50%, while in non–insulin-dependent diabetics the concordance rate is greater than 90%. *(Cecil, Ch. 231; Eisenbarth)*

75.(A—True; B—True; C—True; D—False; E—False) This patient has the chylomicronemia syndrome, clinically characterized by severe abdominal pain, frequently secondary to pancreatitis. The marked elevation in chylomicrons leads to lipemic plasma; lipemia retinalis, a whitish appearance of the retinal vessels; and eruptive xanthoma. Hyponatremia may occur due to elevations in both plasma glucose levels and triglyceride concentrations. This disorder is seen in poorly controlled diabetics because the enzyme lipoprotein lipase, crucial for the metabolism of circulating triglyceride-rich lipoproteins, is not present in sufficient quantities in the insulinopenic state. With improvements in glycemic control, there is a marked decrease in plasma triglyceride levels, but frequently the patient has an underlying abnormality in lipid metabolism such that complete normalization of plasma triglycerides is not observed. *(Cecil, Ch. 231; Chait et al)*

76.(A—False; B—True; C—False; D—True; E—True) Gynecomastia can occur secondary to deficient production of testosterone or increased production of estrogen. In lung cancer and testicular tumors, increased testicular estrogen secretion results from elevations in plasma HCG produced by the tumor. Use of heroin and marijuana can cause gynecomastia by decreasing serum testosterone levels and increasing estrogen levels. Such drugs as digitalis, cimetidine, spironolactone, alkylating agents, isoniazid, methyldopa, tricyclic antidepressants, and diazepam have also been reported to cause gynecomastia. Hyperthyroidism increases androgen production, resulting in the increased peripheral formation of estrogens and, thus, gynecomastia. *(Cecil, Ch. 235; Wilson et al)*

77.(A—False; B—True; C—True; D—False; E—False) Hyperprolactinemia has been associated with low serum testosterone levels, most likely due to the inhibition of LH secretion by prolactin. Hemochromatosis lowers serum testosterone most commonly by affecting pituitary secretion of gonadotropins, but direct effects on the testes can also occur. Germinal cell aplasia and unilateral cryptorchidism are associated with infertility and increased FSH levels, but serum testosterone levels are usually within the normal range. Isolated FSH deficiency is associated with infertility, but serum testosterone levels are normal. *(Cecil, Ch. 235; Lipsett)*

78.(A—True; B—True; C—False; D—False; E—True) Orally administered androgens can lead to elevations in liver enzymes; jaundice may occasionally be observed. Rarely, oral androgen therapy leads to the development of peliosis hepatis (blood-filled cysts in the liver). Sodium retention is a consequence of androgen therapy, and in patients with underlying heart disease, congestive heart failure can occur. Gynecomastia is common in children given androgens and is occasionally seen in adults, probably because androgens are converted to estrogens. Androgens lead to prostate growth and on occasion can lead to the development of benign prostatic hypertrophy. Hereditary angioneurotic edema is treated with androgens; these increase the levels of the inhibitor of the first component of complement. *(Cecil, Ch. 235; Wilson and Griffin)*

79.(A—False; B—True; C—True; D—False; E—False) Nelson's syndrome develops in patients with Cushing's disease who have been treated with bilateral adrenalectomy. Because of the lack of feedback inhibition, an aggressive ACTH-secreting tumor develops in the pituitary. The tumor is locally invasive and frequently leads to visual field defects. Marked elevations in plasma ACTH levels are seen, and the patients can develop profound hyperpigmentation from ACTH or β-lipotropin hypersecretion. *(Cecil, Ch. 226; Cook)*

80.(A—False; B—True; C—False; D—True; E—False) The patient described has a tumor that is producing vasoactive intestinal peptide (VIPoma), which is characterized by watery diarrhea, hypokalemia, and achlorhydria. In addition, approximately two thirds of such patients have hypercalcemia and many are hyperglycemic. The clinical picture is due to elevations in circulating vasoactive intestinal peptide levels. With successful removal of the pancreatic islet cell tumor, the vasoactive intestinal peptide levels decrease, the symptoms disappear, and the abnormal laboratory values revert to normal. *(Cecil, Ch. 233)*

81.(A—False; B—False; C—False; D—True; E—True) Hypopituitarism is a composite of several hormonal deficiencies. Lack of ACTH results in decreased pigmentation and in symptoms of adrenal insufficiency. Decreased gonadotropin production and deficiency in adrenal function result in a decrease in sexual hair. Hypothyroidism, stemming from thyrotropin deficiency, leads to dry, sometimes coarse, hair. The combination of hypothyroidism and hypogonadism results in fine wrinkling of the skin, noticeable particularly around the eyes. In hypopituitarism the skin is frequently pale, chiefly because of hypothyroidism. *(Cecil, Ch. 226)*

82.(A—True; B—False; C—True; D—False; E—True) Vitamin D deficiency results in decreased intestinal absorption of calcium and phosphate. In conjunction with the resulting secondary hyperparathyroidism, it leads to an increase in bone resorption, urinary phosphate excretion, and renal tubular reabsorption of calcium. The net result tends to be low serum calcium and phosphate levels and elevations in the serum concentrations of PTH and alkaline phosphatase. Finding a low 25-hydroxyvitamin D level in combination with these biochemical abnormalities confirms the diagnosis of vitamin D deficiency. *(Cecil, Ch. 245)*

83.(A—True; B—True; C—True; D—False; E—True) Hypoparathyroidism is associated wtih Addison's disease and mucocutaneous candidiasis as part of the polyendocrine autoimmune deficiency syndrome. Hypoparathyroidism can also occur in association with thymic hypoplasia and immunodeficiency (DiGeorge syndrome), a condition resulting from dysmorphogenesis of the third and fourth pharyngeal pouches, leading to hypoplasia or aplasia of the thymic and parathyroid glands. More commonly, hypoparathyroidism can occur in patients with severe and prolonged hypomagnesemia because magnesium is required for the release of parathyroid hormone from the parathyroid glands. Magnesium replacement can restore parathyroid function. *(Cecil, Chs. 241 and 247; Trence et al)*

84. (A—False; B—True; C—True; D—True; E—True) Various environmental risk factors for bone loss have been identified. These include high protein intake, high alcohol consumption, cigarette smoking, and decreased physical activity. Obesity is protective, possibly because of the increased local stress to the spine and, in postmenopausal women, because of the increased conversion in fat tissue of adrenal androgens to estrogens. *(Cecil, Ch. 250; Riggs and Melton)*

85. (A—False; B—True; C—True; D—True; E—True) Relief of bone pain, healing of osteolytic bone lesions, reduction of increased cardiac output, and stabilization of auditory acuity have all been convincingly documented during long-term calcitonin treatment of Paget's disease. Elevations in alkaline phosphatase levels in asymptomatic patients with Paget's disease do not require therapeutic intervention. *(Cecil, Ch. 251; Strewler)*

86. (A—False; B—True; C—False; D—True; E—False) CBG concentrations in plasma are regulated by hormones and other factors. However, there appears to be no obligatory need for this transport protein, as physiologic stimuli that regulate cortisol levels respond to the free level of hormone. When CBG levels are primarily elevated or depressed there are parallel changes in the total cortisol levels in plasma, but the free cortisol concentration remains unchanged. This is important to remember when evaluating states of glucocorticoid excess or deficiency. CBG is increased in pregnancy and hyperthyroidism and by estrogens and oral contraceptives. CBG levels are reduced in liver disease, multiple myeloma, obesity, and the nephrotic syndrome. *(Cecil, Ch. 242; Aron et al)*

87. (A—False; B—False; C—True; D—False; E—False) Cortisol-secreting adenomas can frequently be distinguished from adrenal carcinomas on clinical grounds: They are usually small (<6 cm in diameter) and typically secrete cortisol alone. Adrenal carcinomas that secrete cortisol are usually large at the time of diagnosis and may first be noticed as a palpable abdominal mass. Although adenomas are usually composed of zona fasciculata–like cells, they may exhibit considerable pleomorphism; thus, the histologic appearance does not predict benign or malignant behavior. The diagnosis of adrenal carcinoma is dependent on the demonstration of local tumor invasion or metastatic spread. Neither adrenal cortical carcinomas nor adenomas suppress during the high-dose dexamethasone suppression test. *(Cecil, Ch. 242; Carpenter)*

88. (All are True) Youth, male gender, history of neck irradiation, and a functionless ("cold") nodule are all associated with increased likelihood that a solitary nodule is malignant. Additionally, history of rapid growth, evidence of recurrent nerve paresis, obvious involvement of lymph nodes, or fixation of the nodule to surrounding tissues should also lead to careful evaluation for malignancy. *(Cecil, Ch. 229)*

89. (A—False; B—True; C—True; D—True; E—True) Clinical manifestions of hyperthyroidism in elderly patients are substantially different from those observed in younger patients. The term "apathetic thyrotoxicosis" has been coined for this syndrome. Symptoms of weight loss, myopathy, and congestive heart failure are common components of this syndrome. Although atrial fibrillation is common in the elderly thyrotoxic patient, the heart rate, in contrast to that of younger patients, is typically less than 100 bpm. *(Cecil, Ch. 229; Tibaldi et al)*

90. (A—True; B—False; C—True; D—True; E—True) The patient described has the typical clinical presentation of hypothyroidism secondary to Hashimoto's thyroiditis. This disease is believed to result from autoimmune phenomena because of the increased prevalence of disorders such as Sjögren's syndrome, SLE, ITP, and pernicious anemia in patients with Hashimoto's thyroiditis. Involvement of other endocrine glands can result in diabetes mellitus, Addison's disease, etc. *(Cecil, Ch. 229; Kidd et al)*

91. (A—True; B—False; C—False; D—True; E—True) Although medullary carcinoma of the thyroid occurs sporadically, it may also be inherited as an autosomal dominant trait as part of the multiple endocrine neoplasia syndrome types 2 and 3. These syndromes include medullary carcinoma of the thyroid and pheochromocytomas; therefore, the presence of pheochromocytoma should be considered in all patients with a medullary carcinoma. To rule out familial medullary carcinoma, calcitonin levels should be measured during a provocative test in all primary relatives of patients regardless of family history. Medullary carcinoma is usually polycentric and frequently bilateral, necessitating a total thyroidectomy for definitive therapy. Follow-up with provocative testing of calcitonin levels is required in all patients. *(Cecil, Ch. 248; Wells et al)*

92. (A—False; B—False; C—True; D—True; E—False) Patients are usually prepared for surgery by administration of an alpha-adrenergic antagonist such as phenoxybenzamine in doses sufficient to produce a normal blood pressure. If arrhythmias are a problem, a beta-adrenergic antagonist such as propranolol can be added to the preoperative regimen. Administration of diuretics or salt restriction is contraindicated in patients with pheochromocytomas, since the normal physiologic response to excessive adrenergic stimulation is diuresis, and most patients with pheochromocytomas are already severely fluid-depleted.

In addition, a number of drugs should be avoided in patients with known or suspected pheochromocytomas. Certain drugs such as opiates, ACTH, glucagon, saralasin, and histamine can directly stimulate release of catecholamines from the tumor. Such sympathomimetic amines as methyldopa can induce the release of catecholamines from neuronal stores, and drugs that inhibit neuronal uptake of catecholamines, such as tricyclic antidepressants and guanethidine, can enhance the effects of circulating catecholamines. *(Cecil, Ch. 242; Bravo and Gifford)*

93. (A—True; B—False; C—True; D—True; E—False) This patient has acute adrenal cortical insufficiency resulting from adrenal hemorrhage. If adrenal cortical insufficiency is suspected, a rapid ACTH stimulation test should be performed to confirm the diagnosis. Volume depletion and electrolyte abnormalities should be corrected immediately and general supportive measures instituted. Precipitating factors should be assessed and corrected. After completion of the stimulation test, which takes approximately 30 minutes, hydrocortisone should be given intravenously. Mineralocorticoid replacement is unnecessary, both because high doses of cortisol have sufficient mineralocorticoid effects and because fluid and electrolytes are being replaced intravenously. *(Cecil, Ch. 230)*

94.(All are True) The overnight 1-mg dexamethasone suppression test is an excellent screening procedure for detecting the presence of Cushing's syndrome. However, false-positive responses can occur with acute illness, depression, alcoholism, and anticonvulsant therapy. Anticonvulsants, especially phenytoin and phenobarbital, accelerate hepatic metabolism of dexamethasone. Concurrent illness, depression, or alcoholism can mimic all the biochemical characteristics of Cushing's syndrome. Thus, to avoid misdiagnosis, the dexamethasone suppression test should be repeated when the patient's condition is stable, without fever or other aggravating factors. *(Cecil, Ch. 230; Aron et al)*

95.(A—True; B—True; C—True; D—False; E—True) The surgical finding of diffuse parathyroid gland hyperplasia is frequently observed as part of the multiple endocrine neoplasia (MEN) syndromes. Almost all patients with MEN type 1 have parathyroid gland abnormalities and can also have associated islet cell tumors of the pancreas and/or pituitary tumors. The symptom complex of "headaches and bizarre behavior relieved by food" is classic for an insulinoma, and large pituitary tumors are sometimes seen with mass lesion–type symptoms of headaches and tunnel vision. Parathyroid gland abnormalities also occur as part of the MEN type 2 syndrome, in which medullary carcinoma of the thyroid ("calcified thyroid mass") is a universal finding. Pheochromocytomas ("paroxysmal tachycardia and hypertension") also occur as part of the MEN type 2 syndrome. Azoospermia and gynecomastia are not components of either MEN syndrome. *(Cecil, Chs. 241 and 247; Lamers and Froeling)*

96.(A—False; B—True; C—False; D—True; E—False) This patient has a genetic defect in thyroid hormone synthesis known as Pendred's syndrome, characterized by the inability of the thyroid to carry out organic iodinations. The goiter results in the increased uptake of iodide which can be discharged almost completely by perchlorate administration. The deafness, which may be present at birth or develop during childhood, is not due to hypothyroidism per se. In fact, most patients with this syndrome are euthyroid. The cause of the association between deafness and abnormalities in the thyroid gland is unknown. *(Cecil, Ch. 229)*

97.(A—True; B—False; C—False; D—True; E—True) Hypoglycemia secondary to extrapancreatic malignancy, endocrine deficiency states, hepatic disease, renal disease, and malnutrition is associated with an appropriate reduction in plasma insulin levels. In contrast, hypoglycemia secondary to insulinoma is associated wtih elevated plasma insulin concentrations. Alimentary hypoglycemia is occasionally observed in patients who have undergone gastric surgery, and typically occurs 1½ to 3 hours after eating. Excessive insulin secretion in response to early hyperglycemia is the mechanism for this disorder. *(Cecil, Ch. 232)*

98.(A—False; B—True; C—True; D—True; E—True) In a patient with an enlarged sella discovered incidentally, it is most important to determine (1) if there is hypersecretion of any pituitary hormones, (2) if there is impaired pituitary function, and (3) the anatomy of the lesion. Unstimulated measurement of most pituitary hormones (ACTH, FSH, LH, TSH, and GH) is not adequte for demonstrating impairment of pituitary function, because low plasma concentrations overlap with the normal range. Impaired secretion of these pituitary hormones is best documented by determining end-organ function of the thyroid, adrenal glands, and gonads. If abnormalities in end-organ function are noted, further stimulatory tests are indicated. The possibility of hypersecretion of growth hormone, prolactin, and ACTH should be evaluated, but hypersecretion of the other pituitary hormones (FSH, LH, TSH) is very rare and should not be routinely investigated. *(Cecil, Ch. 226; Cook)*

99.(A—False; B—False; C—False; D—False; E—True) The patient is most likely to have multiple endocrine neoplasia (MEN) type 2 syndrome, characterized by medullary carcinoma of the thyroid, pheochromocytomas (frequently bilateral), and hyperparathyroidism secondary to hyperplasia. Since the syndrome is inherited as an autosomal dominant trait, it is important to screen periodically the families of patients with this disorder for early diagnosis in other family members. Urinary metanephrines or VMA measurements, serum calcium levels, and calcitonin concentrations after either pentagastrin or calcium infusion should be determined in all relatives at risk for this syndrome. *(Cecil, Ch. 241; Pont)*

100.(A—True; B—False; C—False; D—True; E—True) Patients with pituitary insufficiency do not require treatment with mineralocorticoids (fludrocortisone). ACTH is not the major factor that regulates the secretion of aldosterone by the adrenal gland, and thus mineralocorticoid replacement is unnecessary. The appropriate dose of hydrocortisone varies from patient to patient, but is usually in the range of 20 mg in the morning and 10 mg at night. Male patients with panhypopituitarism require thyroid and testosterone replacement. A Medical Alert bracelet can be life-saving in patients with panhypopituitarism, by alerting emergency room personnel to the need for glucocorticoids during stress. *(Cecil, Ch. 226)*

101.(A—False; B—True; C—True; D—True; E—True) Kartagener's syndrome is characterized by situs inversus, chronic sinusitis, bronchiectasis, and nonmotile sperm. This syndrome is due to a structural abnormality in both the tail of the sperm and the cilia of the respiratory tract. Testicular irradiation, Sertoli-cell–only syndrome, and mumps orchitis are characterized by normal Leydig cell function and impaired spermatogenesis. This results in the laboratory findings of normal serum testosterone levels and increased serum FSH concentrations. In Klinefelter's syndrome the testosterone levels are usually low, but a substantial number of patients show testosterone levels within the normal range and have essentially normal secondary sex characteristics. *(Cecil, Ch. 235; Lipsett)*

102.(A—True; B—True; C—False; D—True; E—True) The hand film shows a short fourth metacarpal on the left, and short third and fourth metacarpals on the right. This, together with the other features described, is diagnostic of pseudohypoparathyroidism. The underlying renal abnormality in this condition is tubular resistance to the action of PTH. One manifestation of this resistance is a subnormal excretory response of cyclic AMP in the urine following an injection of PTH. As is generally seen in conditions with end-organ resistance, the serum concentration of the hormone to which resistance is present, in this case PTH, is elevated. Basal ganglia calcification is a manifestation of longstanding hypoparathyroidism and pseudohypoparathyroidism. Subjects with pseudohypoparathyroidism are frequently of subnormal intelligence. The disease is familial, but the genetics of the inheritance are unclear. *(Cecil, Ch. 247)*

103. (A—False; B—True; C—True; D—True; E—True) This patient shows the biochemical abnormalities of the syndrome of inappropriate ADH. It has numerous causes, which can be divided into several broad categories: (1) tumors (e.g., lung, pancreas, prostate); (2) pulmonary disease (e.g., pneumonia, tuberculosis, fungal infections); (3) CNS disease (e.g., meningitis, head injuries, brain abscess); (4) endocrine abnormalities (hypothyroidism and hypoadrenalism); and (5) drug toxicity (e.g., vincristine, carbamazepine, clofibrate, phenothiazines, cyclophosphamide, chlorpropamide, nicotine). It is important that reversible and treatable etiologies be sought in patients with the syndrome of inappropriate ADH. *(Cecil, Ch. 227; Moses and Notman; Robertson et al)*

104. (B); 105. (C); 106. (B); 107. (A) The National Diabetes Data Group has recommended the following criteria for establishing the diagnosis of diabetes mellitus:

1. Fasting venous plasma glucose concentration greater than 140 mg/dl on at least two occasions, OR
2. Presence of the classic symptoms of diabetes together with a gross and unequivocal elevation of plasma glucose, OR
3. On two occasions, following the oral ingestion of 75 grams of glucose, both the two-hour venous plasma glucose concentration and one other sample being greater than 200 mg/dl

An impaired glucose tolerance exists if on two occasions the fasting plasma glucose is less than 140 mg/dl and if the 30-, 60-, or 90-minute plasma glucose level exceeds 200 mg/dl, along with a two-hour plasma glucose level between 140 and 200 mg/dl. *(Cecil, Ch. 231; National Diabetes Data Group)*

108. (C); 109. (A); 110. (B); 111. (D); 112. (E) 108. This patient has the classic manifestations of pseudohypoparathyroidism, which is characterized by resistance to the effects of PTH. This results in hypocalcemia, hyperphosphatemia, and elevated iPTH levels. **109.** Secondary hyperparathyroidism occurs in patients with chronic renal failure. Renal disease results in a reduction in the filtered load of phosphate which, if dietary intake of phosphate is maintained, produces an increase in plasma phosphorus levels. The elevated plasma phosphorus concentration leads to a reciprocal fall in plasma-ionized calcium concentration and a corresponding increase in PTH secretion. In addition, immunoreactive PTH levels in uremia are often very high because of the decreased renal clearance of biologically inactive carboxyl-terminal fragments of PTH. **110.** Disease states in which intestinal calcium absorption is reduced result in hypocalcemia and compensatory secondary hyperparathyroidism. Hypophosphatemia is frequent in this setting because of poor nutritional intake and inhibition by PTH of renal proximal tubular reabsorption of phosphate. **111.** The history of a pancreatic islet cell tumor and a pituitary tumor suggests the diagnosis of multiple endocrine neoplasia (MEN) syndrome, type 1. As the incidence of parathyroid gland abnormalities in patients with MEN 1 approaches 100%, such a patient should be examined closely for evidence of abnormal parathyroid gland function. This patient has hypercalcemia, hypophosphatemia, and increased PTH levels, which indicate mild hyperparathyroidism. **112.** The hypercalcemia of malignancy is occasionally associated with detectable levels of iPTH in the normal to high-normal range despite marked elevations of serum calcium. Hypercalcemia of malignancy seems to be most frequently caused by secretion of a protein that is not PTH but which has considerable structural homology to it. *(Cecil, Chs. 241, 245, 247, and 249; Agus et al)*

113. (E); 114. (B); 115. (C); 116. (A); 117. (D) 113. A physiologic increase in renin and aldosterone production occurs during excessive potassium intake as part of the body's defense against hyperkalemia. **114.** Hypertension with symptomatic hypokalemia (lassitude, muscle weakness, polyuria) is the hallmark of primary aldosteronism. Autonomous production of aldosterone leads to reduced renin levels and hypokalemia. Cortisol production and ACTH levels are normal in primary aldosteronism. **115.** Addison's disease is a component of the polyglandular failure syndrome. The decreased production of adrenal steroids results in secondary increases in ACTH and renin levels. Aldosterone deficiency results in hyperkalemia. **116.** Administration of diuretics can produce a state of secondary hyperaldosteronism by reducing renal artery perfusion pressure and/or renal tubular sodium chloride concentration, either of which stimulates renin release. **117.** The syndrome of hyporeninemic hypoaldosteronism is often seen in diabetic patients with moderate renal failure. The decreased production of renin and aldosterone results in hyperkalemia. ACTH and cortisol levels are normal. *(Cecil, Ch. 230; Batlle and Kurtzman)*

118. (E); 119. (A); 120. (C); 121. (D); 122. (B) 118. Amenorrhea often occurs in women with anorexia nervosa and in women who participate in regular, strenuous exercise (ballet dancing, long-distance running). The etiology of amenorrhea in these women is poorly understood, but at present is supposed to be hypothalamic in origin. Estradiol and gonadotropin levels are usually low-normal in these conditions. Prolactin levels are normal. **119.** These are typical symptoms of a prolactinoma. Elevated prolactin levels can lead to secondary suppression of LH and FSH secretion, with resultant reduction in estradiol levels. **120.** These are manifestions of the Stein-Leventhal (polycystic ovary) syndrome. Hormonal findings typically show increased serum LH (greater than FSH) concentration and normal prolactin. The diseased ovaries secrete high concentrations of androstenedione, which is converted peripherally to estrogen. **121.** The clinical picture is of primary ovarian failure, a frequent component of the autoimmune polyendocrine failure syndrome. Serum gonadotropins, freed of feedback inhibition, are very high. **122.** This is amenorrhea traumatica, which can occur after any insult to the uterus that results in outflow tract obstruction. All hormonal functions are normal. *(Cecil, Ch. 237; Neinstein; Schriock)*

123. (B); 124. (D); 125. (A); 126. (C); 127. (E) 123. In patients with a hydatidiform mole or choriocarcinoma, high levels of TSH can be secreted by the tumor, resulting in thyrotoxicosis. Surgical removal of the tumor will relieve the hyperthyroidism. **124.** Total serum levels of thyroid hormone (T_4 and T_3) are determined by both the quantity and affinity of circulating thyroid hormone–binding proteins (thyroxine-binding globulin [TBG], thyroxine-binding prealbumin [TBPA], and albumin), and the quantity of hormone secreted by the gland. Levels of TBG are increased during pregnancy; consequently, total T_4 and T_3 levels are increased. However, serum *free* T_4 and T_3 levels remain unchanged, as reflected by the normal serum TSH level. **125.** Thyrotoxicosis in which serum T_4 levels are normal and serum T_3 levels are increased is termed T_3 toxicosis. Some patients with hyperthyroidism (Graves' disease, multinodular goiter, or hyperfunctioning adenoma) can have T_3 toxicosis that precedes the emergence of increases in T_4. It should be noted that the TSH level is very low, reflecting feedback on the pituitary. **126.** A number of pharmacologic agents can reduce the peripheral conversion of T_4 to T_3, including propylthiouracil, iodinated contrast agents used for oral cholecystography, amiodarone, propranolol, and high doses of glucocorticoids. This blockage of conversion results in high-normal T_4 levels, decreased T_3 levels, and normal TSH levels. **127.** In a patient with the symptoms of hypothyroidism and a pituitary tumor, the diagnosis of secondary hypothyroidism should be made. It is important in such cases to identify any other deficiencies of pituitary hormone secretion before instituting therapy. Thyroid hormone replacement can exacerbate mild ACTH insufficiency and provoke a full-blown Addisonian crisis. *(Cecil, Ch. 229)*

128.(C); 129.(A); 130.(D); 131.(B) 128. Blood glucose levels are unacceptably high before bedtime and breakfast. This indicates that the duration of action of NPH insulin is not sufficient in this patient to result in acceptable blood glucose control for the entire day. The most appropriate therapeutic change is to administer NPH insulin twice daily. It is important when making this change to remember to lower the morning insulin dosage so that the total daily insulin dosage is not greatly increased at one time. Approximately two thirds of the insulin should be given in the morning and one third in the evening, but there is great individual variation. **129.** Blood glucose levels are unacceptably high at 11 AM. This indicates that the morning NPH is not acting early in the day; therefore, the most appropriate therapeutic measure is to add a small dose of regular insulin to the morning NPH insulin. **130.** Blood glucose values are in an acceptable range at all times; a change in insulin dosage is not indicated. **131.** Blood glucose concentrations before breakfast are too low; a reduction in insulin dosage is indicated. Note that the elevated 11 AM blood glucose may be secondary to hypoglycemia (Somogyi phenomenon), and, most important, that this hyperglycemia may improve with a reduction in insulin dose. *(Cecil, Ch. 231)*

132.(C) This patient has isosexual precocious pseudopuberty caused by congenital adrenal hyperplasia. The hypertension points to an adrenal 11-hydroxylase deficiency that leads to serum and urinary accumulation of 11-deoxycortisol and 11-deoxycorticosterone. Measurement of these compounds would aid diagnosis, as does the easy suppressibility of urinary 17-OH and ketosteroids. Basal 17-ketosteroids are elevated because of increased adrenal androgen synthesis; the 17-OH steroids are increased because 11-deoxycortisol, although inert metabolically, is excreted as a 17-OH corticoid. Plasma cortisol (measured by specific means) is in the low-normal range because sufficient adrenal function is present for excessive stimulation to produce cortisol (albeit at the price of causing the adrenogenital syndrome). *(Cecil, Ch. 230)*

133.(B) This patient has typical Cushing's syndrome. The adrenal mass (usually not palpable, but detectable by computed tomography or arteriography) points to an adrenal origin of the cortisol excess. Plasma cortisol shows no diurnal variation and ACTH is low. Basal 17-OH corticoid excretion is high and does not suppress with either low- or high-dose dexamethasone. These data confirm the diagnosis. The low urinary 17-ketosteroids make a carcinoma unlikely. The patient probably has an adrenal adenoma, and unilateral adrenalectomy will cure the condition. *(Cecil, Ch. 230)*

134.(F) Oral contraceptives raise plasma transcortin levels. As a result, plasma cortisol levels are high but other measures of adrenal function (ACTH, urine excretion, suppressibility) are normal. *(Cecil, Ch. 230)*

135.(D) Adrenocortical carcinoma is a likely diagnosis in this patient with signs of virilism and a palpable flank mass. These tumors can produce excess cortisol but generally are inefficient synthesizers of steroids. As a result, large amounts of 17-ketosteroids are excreted and are the hallmark of this condition. *(Cecil, Chs. 230 and 238)*

136.(A) Failure of urinary 17-OH corticoids to suppress when the patient is given low-dose dexamethasone establishes the diagnosis of Cushing's syndrome. The decrease in 17-OH corticoids (>50% fall from baseline) after high-dose dexamethasone makes Cushing's disease highly likely. Plasma cortisol levels are elevated, and diurnal variation is absent; urinary steroid excretion is high, consistent with this diagnosis. Plasma ACTH is measurable but not elevated in many cases of Cushing's disease, although it does increase markedly after adrenalectomy. *(Cecil, Ch. 230)*

137.(E) This patient has ectopic ACTH syndrome owing to a lung cancer. Many tumors, especially oat cell carcinoma of the lung, have been shown to secrete ACTH. Typical body habitus of Cushing's syndrome may be lacking, but marked elevation of plasma and urinary 17-OH and ketosteroids is the rule. Plasma ACTH may be very high (in contrast to pituitary Cushing's disease). Dexamethasone does not suppress cortisol secretion. *(Cecil, Ch. 230)*

BIBLIOGRAPHY

Abboud CF: Laboratory diagnosis of hypopituitarism. Mayo Clin Proc 61:35, 1986.

Agus ZS, Wasserstein A, Goldfarb S: Disorders of calcium and magnesium homeostasis. Am J Med 72:473, 1982.

Aron DC, Tyrrell JB, Fitzgerald PA, et al: Cushing's syndrome: Problems in diagnosis. Medicine 60:25, 1981.

Batlle DC, Kurtzman NA: Clinical disorders of aldosterone metabolism. DM 30:1, 1984.

Bolt RJ, Tesluk H, Esquivel C, et al: Glucagonoma—an underdiagnosed syndrome? West J Med 144:746, 1986.

Boyden T, Bressler R: Oral hypoglycemia agents. Adv Intern Med 24:53, 1979.

Bravo EL, Gifford RW Jr: Pheochromocytoma: Diagnosis, localization and management. N Engl J Med 311:1298, 1984.

Carpenter PC: Cushing's syndrome: Update of diagnosis and management. Mayo Clin Proc 61:49, 1986.

Cecil Textbook of Medicine. 18th ed. Wyngaarden JB, Smith LH Jr (eds). Philadelphia, W.B. Saunders Company, 1988.

Chait A, Robertson HT, Brunzell JD: Chylomicronemia syndrome in diabetes mellitus. Diabetes Care 4:343, 1981.

Coe F: Treatment of hypercalciuria. N Engl J Med 311:116, 1984.

Cook DM: Pituitary tumors—current concepts of diagnosis and therapy. West J Med 133:189, 1980.
Cook DM, Kendall JW, Jordan R: Cushing syndrome: Current concepts of diagnosis and therapy (Medical Progress). West J Med 132:111, 1980.
Copeland DM: The incidentally discovered adrenal mass. Ann Intern Med 98:940, 1983.
Cryer PE, Gerich JE: Glucose counterregulation, hypoglycemia, and intensive insulin therapy in diabetes mellitus. N Engl J Med 313:232, 1985.
Eisenbarth GS: Type I diabetes mellitus: A chronic autoimmune disease. N Engl J Med 314:1360, 1986.
Fajans SS, Floyd JC Jr: Diagnosis and medical management of insulinomas. Annu Rev Med 30:313, 1979.
Ferriss JB, Brown JJ, Fraser R, et al: Primary hyperaldosteronism. Clin Endocrinol Metab 10:419, 1981.
Foster DW: Insulin deficiency and hyperosmolar coma. Adv Intern Med 19:159, 1974.
Frame B, Parfitt AM: Osteomalacia: Current concepts. Ann Intern Med 89:966, 1978.
Givens JR: Hirsutism and hyperandrogenism. Adv Intern Med 21:221, 1976.
Gleckman RA, Roth RM: Diabetic foot infections—prevention and treatment (Topics in Primary Care Medicine). West J Med 142:263, 1985.
Greenspan SL, Neer RM, Ridgway EC, et al: Osteoporosis in men with hyperprolactinemic hypogonadism. Ann Intern Med 104:777, 1986.
Grunfeld C: Insulin resistance: Pathophysiology, diagnosis and therapeutic implications. Spec Top Endocrinol Metab 6:193, 1984.
Grunfeld C, Chappell DA: Hypokalemia and diabetes mellitus. Am J Med 75:553, 1983.
Hamburger JI, Miller JM, Kini SR: Lymphoma of the thyroid. Ann Intern Med 99:685, 1983.
Health and Public Policy Committee, American College of Physicians: Glycosylated hemoglobin assays in the management and diagnosis of diabetes mellitus. Ann Intern Med 101:710, 1984.
Herman WH, Teutsch SM, Sepe SJ, et al: An approach to the prevention of blindness in diabetes. Diabetes Care 6:608, 1983.
Huntley AC: The cutaneous manifestations of diabetes mellitus. J Am Acad Dermatol 7:427, 1982.
Ingbar SH, Braverman LE (eds): Werner's The Thyroid: A Fundamental and Clinical Text. 5th ed. Philadelphia, J.B. Lippincott Company, 1986.
Janka HU, Standl E, Mehnert H: Clonidine effect on diabetic gustatory sweating. Ann Intern Med 91:130, 1979.
Kidd A, Okita N, Row VV, et al: Immunologic aspects of Graves' and Hashimoto's diseases. Metabolism 29:80, 1980.
Lamers CBHW, Froeling PGAM: Clinical significance of hyperparathyroidism in familial multiple endocrine adenomatosis type I (MEA I). Am J Med 66:422, 1979.
Lee DBN, Zawada ET, Kleeman CR: The pathophysiology and clinical aspects of hypercalcemic disorders (Medical Progress). West J Med 129:278, 1978.
Lehrer RI, Howard DH, Sypherd PS, et al: Mucormycosis. Ann Intern Med 93:93, 1980.
Lipsett MB: Physiology and pathology of the Leydig cell. N Engl J Med 303:682, 1980.
Martin MC, Schriock ED, Jaffe RB: Prolactin-secreting pituitary adenomas (Medical Progress). West J Med 139:663, 1983.
Marx SJ, Spiegel AM, Levine MA, et al: Familial hypocalciuric hypercalcemia: The relation to primary parathyroid hyperplasia. N Engl J Med 307:416, 1982.
Melmed S, Braunstein GD, Chang RJ, et al: Pituitary tumors secreting growth hormone and prolactin. Ann Intern Med 105:238, 1986.
Morley JE: Impotence. Am J Med 80:897, 1986.
Moses AM, Notman DD: Diabetes insipidus and syndrome of inappropriate antidiuretic hormone secretion (SIADH). Adv Intern Med 27:73, 1982.
Narins RG: Therapy of hyponatremia: Does haste make waste? N Engl J Med 314:1573, 1986.
National Diabetes Data Group: Classification and diagnosis of diabetes mellitus and other categories of glucose intolerance. Diabetes 28:1039, 1979.
Neinstein LS: Menstrual dysfunction in pathophysiologic states (Clinical Review). West J Med 143:476, 1985.
Nelson RL: Hypoglycemia: Fact or fiction? Mayo Clin Proc 60:844, 1985.
Pont A: Multiple endocrine neoplasia syndromes (Medical Progress). West J Med 132:301, 1980.
Riggs BL, Melton LJ III: Involutional osteoporosis. N Engl J Med 314:1676, 1986.
Rittmaster RS, Loriaux DL: Hirsutism. Ann Intern Med 106:95, 1987.
Robertson GL, Aycinena P, Zerbe RL: Neurogenic disorders of osmoregulation. Am J Med 72:339, 1982.
Rojeski MT, Gharib H: Nodular thyroid disease: Evaluation and management. N Engl J Med 313:428, 1985.
Schambelan M, Sebastian A: Hyporeninemic hypoaldosteronism. Adv Intern Med 24:385, 1979.
Schriock E, Martin MC, Jaffe RB: Polycystic ovarian disease (Medical Progress). West J Med 142:519, 1985.
Strewler GJ: Paget's disease of bone. Medical Staff Conference, University of California, San Francisco. West J Med 140:763, 1984.
Swerdloff RS, Overstreet JW, Sokol RZ, et al: Infertility in the male. Ann Intern Med 103:906, 1985.
Tibaldi JM, Barzel US, Albin J, et al: Thyrotoxicosis in the very old. Am J Med 81:619, 1986.
Trence DL, Morley JE, Handwerger BS: Polyglandular autoimmune syndromes. Am J Med 77:107, 1984.
Wallach S: Treatment of Paget's disease. Adv Intern Med 27:1, 1982.
Wells SA Jr, Dilley WG, Farndon JA, et al: Early diagnosis and treatment of medullary thyroid carcinoma. Arch Intern Med 145:1248, 1985.
Werner SC, Ingbar SH (eds): The Thyroid. 4th ed. New York, Harper and Row, 1978.
Wilson JD, Aiman J, MacDonald PC: The pathogenesis of gynecomastia. Adv Intern Med 25:1, 1980.
Wilson JD, Griffin JE: The use and misuse of androgens. Metabolism 29:1278, 1980.
Wright J: Endocrine effects of alcohol. Clin Endocrinol Metab 7:351, 1978.

PART 8

INFECTIOUS DISEASE

HENRY MASUR

DIRECTIONS: For questions 1 to 50, choose the ONE BEST answer to each question.

1. A 30-year-old male prostitute comes to your office because of fever, chills, and headache of several days' duration. He has had no sexual contact for five weeks, and has noted no ulcers and no other symptoms except for burning on urination. Physical examination reveals only tender, matted inguinal nodes bilaterally which are draining purulent material from several discrete sites. Gram's stain of the purulent material shows many polymorphonuclear leukocytes but no organisms. Which of the following tests would be helpful to establish the most likely etiology?

   A. Serum VDRL
   B. Culture of the pus for herpesviruses
   C. Culture of the pus for anaerobic bacteria
   D. Culture of the pus for routine aerobic bacteria
   E. Complement fixation test for lymphogranuloma venereum (LGV)

2. An 84-year-old woman is brought to the emergency room from a nursing home where she was found one evening in her bed confused and hypotensive. In the emergency room the rectal temperature is 37.7°C, blood pressure is 70/20 mm Hg, pulse is 160 per minute. She is unresponsive but has no other physical findings. Which of the following would suggest sepsis as the cause for this patient's hypotension and confusion, in contrast to other causes of hypotension?

   A. A low systemic vascular resistance and a high cardiac output
   B. A high systemic vascular resistance and a low cardiac output
   C. A pulmonary capillary wedge pressure prior to administration of fluids of 26 mm Hg
   D. An arterial blood pH of 7.1
   E. A serum lactate level of 22 mmol/L

3. A 28-year-old man with acute myelogenous leukemia is admitted to the hospital two weeks after receiving chemotherapy; temperature is 40.0°C and blood pressure is 150/90 mm Hg. He has been neutropenic (granulocyte count less than $100/mm^3$) for seven days, but has been feeling relatively well at home. He is now fatigued with no localizing symptoms or signs after thorough evaluation. Which of the following would definitely NOT be an acceptable empiric antimicrobial regimen?

   A. Imipenem
   B. Cefotaxime
   C. Ceftazidime
   D. Piperacillin and tobromycin
   E. Clindamycin and ticarcillin and gentamicin

4. A 42-year-old healthy man plans a four-week trip to rural Colombia to buy gems. Which of the following suggestions would not affect the likelihood of his developing diarrhea?

   A. Avoiding raw shellfish
   B. Avoiding raw or poorly cooked meat
   C. Avoiding unboiled water for drinking or tooth-brushing
   D. Avoiding consumption of raw ground vegetables like lettuce and tomatoes
   E. Taking bismuth subsalicylate, 60 cc four times daily

5. A 29-year-old previously healthy man who takes no medications has had mild fatigue, night sweats, and temperature spikes to 38.0°C for four weeks but has been able to continue working as a salesman. On physical examination he has generalized lymphadenopathy with firm, nontender nodes. Which of the following is correct?

   A. A Sabin-Feldman dye test titer of 1:64 would confirm that toxoplasmosis is the cause of the lymphadenopathy
   B. A positive ELISA for HIV performed on one occasion would confirm that HIV is the cause of the lymphadenopathy
   C. A lymph node biopsy and blood culture that grew *Mycobacterium avium-intracellulare* would strongly suggest that this patient has AIDS
   D. A Western blot test following repeated positive ELISA tests would confirm that this patient has AIDS
   E. An OKT4/OKT8 ratio determination on peripheral lymphocytes would help narrow the differential diagnosis

6. To establish a diagnosis of *Pneumocystis* pneumonia in a patient with diffuse pulmonary infiltrates, which of the following techniques is likely to provide a specific and unequivocally diagnostic result?

   A. Sputum examination using Giemsa stain
   B. Serology
   C. Sputum culture
   D. Gallium scan
   E. Pulmonary function tests including diffusing capacity

7. A 50-year-old woman is convalescing in the hospital from a cholecystectomy. Because she has no bowel sounds, an intravenous cannula has been in place for five days so that she can receive fluids. The patient's temperature rises to 39.5°C on the fifth postoperative day. No source is

apparent, so therapy with clindamycin and gentamicin is begun. The next day two blood cultures drawn separately are reported to be growing gram-positive cocci in clusters. What is the best management of the antimicrobial regimen for this patient?

A. Continue the clindamycin and gentamicin until the organism is identified and susceptibilities are determined
B. Add ampicillin to the current regimen
C. Add vancomycin to the current regimen
D. Add nafcillin to the current regimen
E. Switch the antibiotic regimen from clindamycin and gentamicin to the fixed combination ticarcillin–clavulanic acid.

8. Vancomycin has good activity and would be acceptable therapy for infections due to each of the following EXCEPT

A. *Staphylococcus aureus*
B. *Staphylococcus epidermidis*
C. *Streptococcus faecalis*
D. *Bacteroides fragilis*
E. *Clostridium difficile*

9. Which of the following statements about gentamicin, tobramycin, and amikacin is NOT correct for this group of three drugs?

A. All can cause renal damage
B. All can cause cochlear damage
C. All can cause granulocytopenia
D. All can cause vestibular damage
E. All must be dose-adjusted for patients in renal failure

10. Nosocomial infections occur in approximately what percentage of hospitalized patients nationally?

A. 0.01–0.1%
B. 1–2%
C. 5–10%
D. 25–50%
E. Greater than 50%

11. Which statement about infections due to *Clostridium diphtheriae* is NOT correct?

A. They can no longer be acquired in the United States
B. Transmission is by respiratory droplets or skin exudate
C. Myocarditis and neuritis are caused by a toxin elaborated by the organism rather than by direct microbial invasion
D. Diagnosis must usually be based on clinical grounds, so that treatment can be started promptly
E. Therapy of choice is diphtheria antitoxin and penicillin

12. Which of the following is true about typhoid fever?

A. The disease is extremely unlikely to occur in someone who has been immunized against *Salmonella typhi* in the past three years
B. The diagnosis is unlikely if the patient does not have diarrhea or a history of diarrhea in the recent past
C. The reservoir for *S. typhi* is man or animals
D. Chloramphenicol, ampicillin, and trimethoprim-sulfamethoxazole would all be acceptable therapeutic alternatives
E. Chronic carriers cannot be successfully treated medically; cholecystectomy must be performed

13. A 30-year-old woman came to the emergency room yesterday with nausea, vomiting, chills, and a fever of 38.3°C. She was sent home with an antiemetic but no specific therapy. The laboratory reports that the stool is growing a non-typhi *Salmonella*. Which of the following is true about the disease and management?

A. The source of the *Salmonella* was almost certainly another human
B. The positive blood culture indicates an intravascular focus of infection
C. Blood cultures are almost never positive except in immunosuppressed or debilitated patients
D. The patient should be brought into the hospital for immediate intravenous antibiotic therapy
E. If antibiotic therapy were necessary, trimethoprim-sulfamethoxazole would likely be useful

14. A 19-year-old man has fever and crampy abdominal pain that migrates from the mid-epigastrium to the right lower quadrant. At surgery the appendix is normal. Several days postoperatively the patient reports arthralgias and develops erythema nodosum. Which of the following is NOT true about the most likely diagnosis?

A. The etiologic agent can be cultured from blood, stool, or the surgical specimen
B. Special culture techniques are needed in the microbiology laboratory to grow the organism
C. Antibiotic therapy is not clearly effective
D. The likely reservoir is another human
E. Outbreaks of disease due to the etiologic agent have been reported in the United States

15. Which of the following is true about plague?

A. The organism has been eradicated from the United States but not from Asia, Africa, or South America
B. The causative agent is a gram-positive rod
C. Its most common mode of transmission is flea bite
D. Pneumonic plague has not occurred in this century
E. Ampicillin is the therapy of choice

16. A 29-year-old Mexican man has a grand mal seizure for the first time in his life. He recovers uneventfully by the next day, but a CAT scan shows several space-occupying lesions. Physical examination reveals several subcutaneous nodules that are calcified on roentgenogram. This patient most likely acquired this lesion by eating what type of poorly cooked food?

A. Pork
B. Beef
C. Chicken
D. Lamb
E. Snails

17. Intravenous acyclovir is effective therapy for each of the following EXCEPT

A. herpes simplex encephalitis
B. herpes simplex proctitis
C. herpetic whitlow (herpes simplex paronychia)
D. disseminated cytomegalovirus disease
E. localized herpes zoster of recent onset (24 hours) in a patient with Hodgkin's disease

18. Homosexual males (without HIV infection) who are sexually active have documented predisposition to all of the following infectious diseases EXCEPT

A. Herpes simplex
B. *Chlamydia trachomatis* infection
C. Hepatitis B
D. Cytomegalovirus infection
E. Epstein-Barr virus infection

19. An 80-year-old man, bedridden in a nursing home, is admitted to a general medical ward with fever and confusion, and blood cultures grow *Streptococcus faecalis*. A likely source of the bacteremia would be which one of the following?

A. A decubitus ulcer over his heel
B. A dental abscess
C. Chronic sinusitis
D. Empyema of the gallbladder
E. A tender paronychia

20. All the following types of diarrhea are likely to respond to antimicrobial therapy EXCEPT

A. Whipple's disease
B. eosinophilic enteritis
C. celiac disease
D. tropical sprue
E. bacterial overgrowth of the small bowel

21. To establish the etiologic agent for retinochoroiditis in a 24-year-old man who is otherwise healthy, which of the following tests would be most helpful?

A. Sabin-Feldman dye test
B. Blood cultures for bacteria
C. Serum cryptococcal antigen
D. Conjunctival scraping
E. Aqueous humor aspiration for culture

22. Adenine arabinoside (ara-A) is clearly the drug of choice for which of the following infections?

A. Herpes simplex encephalitis
B. Cytomegalovirus retinochoroiditis
C. Disseminated herpes zoster
D. Epstein-Barr virus pneumonia
E. None of the above

23. A diagnosis of Rocky Mountain spotted fever could best be confirmed rapidly at most hospitals, prior to initiation of therapy, by which of the following tests?

A. Blood culture
B. Routine histology
C. Culture from a skin biopsy
D. Serology
E. None of the above

24. Coccidioidomycosis occurs most frequently in what region of the United States?

A. Northeast
B. Southeast
C. Gulf states
D. Northwest
E. Southwest

25. What is the most common clinical presentation of sporotrichosis?

A. Solitary pulmonary nodule
B. Diffuse pneumonia
C. Calcified hepatic granulomas
D. Lymphocutaneous
E. Chronic meningitis

26. Which of the following would be the most likely underlying disease in an apparently healthy 33-year-old man receiving no drugs, who has oral candidiasis on routine physical examination?

A. Lymphoma
B. DiGeorge's syndrome
C. Alcoholism
D. Chronic renal failure
E. HIV infection

27. The appropriate therapy for cutaneous scabies would be which of the following?

A. Lindane
B. Nystatin
C. Topical tetracycline
D. Pyrvinium pamoate
E. Topical idoxuridine

28. Bone marrow suppression and/or cytopenias are well-recognized complications of all of the following drugs EXCEPT

A. chloramphenicol
B. pentamidine
C. flucytosine
D. clindamycin
E. pyrimethamine

29. Each of the following is a well-recognized complication of infectious mononucleosis EXCEPT

A. meningoencephalitis
B. transverse myelitis
C. hepatitis
D. agranulocytosis
E. acalculous cholecystitis

30. A 22-year-old man consults you because of a painful lesion on the penis. The lesion is not indurated and has a necrotic, dirty-appearing base. There is tender left inguinal lymphadenopathy. Gram's stain of material from the base of the lesion reveals parallel arrays of small, gram-negative coccobacilli. Which of the following is the most appropriate treatment?

A. Cephalexin
B. Benzathine penicillin
C. Procaine penicillin plus probenecid
D. Sulfisoxazole
E. Chloramphenicol

31. A 16-year-old boy is brought to your office 12 hours after he was bitten on the hand by a cat while playing at a friend's house. The hand is markedly swollen. The wound is purulent and draining and surrounded by fiery-red cellulitis. There is axillary adenopathy. Gram's stain of the exudate would most likely reveal

A. gram-positive cocci in chains
B. gram-positive cocci in clusters
C. gram-negative rods
D. a mixture of gram-positive cocci in pairs, chains, clusters; long, slender, gram-negative rods; and gram-positive rods
E. large, gram-positive rods with terminal spores

32. Each of the following uses of prophylactic antibiotics is appropriate EXCEPT

A. cefazolin, 1.0 g intravenously every six hours starting one hour before planned total hip arthroplasty and continuing for 48 hours thereafter
B. cefazolin, 1.0 g intravenously every six hours starting one hour before planned vaginal hysterectomy and continuing for 48 hours thereafter
C. cefazolin, 1.0 g intravenously every six hours starting four hours before planned cardiac catheterization and continuing for 48 hours thereafter
D. oral nonabsorbable antibiotics starting several days before a planned colectomy
E. *no* prophylactic antibiotics given to a patient prior to elective craniotomy for removal of a meningioma

33. A 23-year-old woman in the first trimester of pregnancy attends a suburban lunch party during which she picks up and comforts a fractious child who is later found to have rubella. A hemagglutination inhibition (HI) titer is performed at once on the woman's blood, and proves negative. You should now

A. offer an abortion, if the mother so wishes
B. administer cytosine arabinoside (ara-A)
C. administer rubella vaccine and gamma globulin
D. administer human immune serum globulin
E. wait two to three weeks and repeat the HI titer

34. Which of the following is most appropriate to assess the response to therapy of a patient with neurosyphilis?

A. CSF cell count and VDRL titer
B. CSF cell count, protein, and VDRL titer
C. CSF cell count, glucose, and protein
D. CSF fluorescent treponemal antibody-absorbed (FTA-ABS) titer
E. Serum FTA-ABS titer and CSF VDRL titer

35. A 26-year-old female anthropologist who is 14 weeks' pregnant will be leaving in four weeks for a two-year assignment in the Amazon basin near the Brazil-Peru border. Which of the following is among the measures that should be recommended to her?

A. Yellow fever vaccine
B. Chloroquine for malaria prophylaxis
C. Sulfadoxine-pyrimethamine (Fansidar) for malaria prophylaxis
D. Cholera immunization
E. Paratyphoid immunization

36. A 36-year-old previously healthy male business executive returns from a trip to Thailand, Vietnam, and Indonesia with rigors and temperature spikes of 40.5°C. Peripheral smear shows plasmodia. About 10% of erythrocytes are parasitized, many with multiple organisms and appliqué forms. Which one of the following regimens would be best?

A. Chloroquine orally daily until the fever is reduced for at least 48 hours, followed by a two-week course of primaquine
B. Chloroquine orally, 2.5 g over 48 hours, followed by a two-week course of primaquine
C. Quinine intravenously for seven to ten days, followed by a two-week course of primaquine
D. Quinine intravenously for seven to ten days, in conjunction with three to five days of both sulfadiazine and pyrimethamine
E. Quinine intravenously, alone, for seven to ten days

37. *Staphylococcus epidermidis* is commonly the etiologic agent of which one of the following?

A. Furunculosis
B. Prosthetic valve endocarditis (PVE)
C. Endocarditis in drug-addicted individuals
D. Cellulitis in immunologically normal individuals
E. Urinary tract infections in patients with ileostomies

38. Examination of a peripheral blood smear can usually establish the diagnosis of which one of the following?

A. Babesiosis and tularemia
B. Babesiosis and leptospirosis
C. Borreliosis and toxoplasmosis
D. Borreliosis, babesiosis, and malaria
E. Lyme disease

39. Which of the following is true about the management of bacterial endocarditis?

A. Most vegetations visible at autopsy could have been seen on echocardiogram
B. Blood cultures often require three to six weeks' incubation before many streptococci or staphylococci are recognizable
C. Blood cultures should become negative within 24 hours of institution of appropriate antimicrobial therapy
D. The microbiologic cure rate of endocarditis due to sensitive viridans streptococci should be over 95% if adequate amounts of penicillin are used for four to six weeks
E. Vegetations visible by echocardiography are an absolute indication to replace the valve immediately in order to avoid embolization

40. In bacterial meningitis due to an unidentified, non-lactose-fermenting gram-negative bacillus, which initial regimen would be best?

A. Gentamicin and cephalothin intravenously
B. Tobramycin and carbenicillin intravenously, plus carbenicillin intrathecally
C. Tobramycin and ticarcillin intravenously, plus tobramycin intrathecally
D. Trimethoprim-sulfamethoxazole and piperacillin intravenously
E. Vancomycin and chloramphenicol intravenously

41. You are asked to see a 38-year-old, insulin-dependent, diabetic woman who was brought to the emergency room having ketoacidosis with a warm, crepitant soft tissue process extending from the perirectal area down the buttock to the thigh. Within the first few hours of hospitalization to treat her infection, which one of the following would you recommend?

A. Place the patient in a hyperbaric chamber and administer high-dose penicillin
B. Aspirate the soft tissue for a culture specimen; institute therapy with penicillin and aminoglycoside
C. Order surgical wide debridement and treat with clindamycin, ampicillin, and an aminoglycoside
D. Order surgical wide debridement and treat with nafcillin
E. Obtain cultures, then treat the patient with penicillin, clindamycin, and an aminoglycoside; order a surgical drainage procedure when the infection organizes into discrete abscesses

42. An 18-year-old male college student has severe headache and fever. Cerebrospinal fluid (CSF) shows 3750 cells/mm^3 with 90% neutrophils. Examination of centrifuged CSF shows diplococci in almost every high-power microscopic field. Which of the following is true?

A. The likelihood of developing infection due to some serotypes of this organism could be decreased by immunization
B. All individuals who have been at lectures with this patient during the past several days should receive prophylaxis with rifampin
C. Most secondary or co-primary cases occur within two weeks of the index case
D. Minocycline is as safe and effective as rifampin for prophylaxis
E. Sulfa drugs no longer have any role in the prophylaxis or treatment of this infection

43. Which of the following is true about *Candida* esophagitis?

A. Barium swallow can establish this diagnosis specifically
B. More than 25% of patients have no identifiable risk factors
C. It is rare in the absence of clinically apparent oral candidiasis
D. Therapy with at least 1 g of intravenous amphotericin B is indicated
E. Esophageal rupture and substantial hemorrhage are recognized complications

44. Which one of the following groups should receive isoniazid prophylaxis?

A. Individuals over 35 years of age with a positive PPD (5TU)
B. Individuals with a positive PPD and diabetes mellitus
C. Individuals with granulomas on chest x-ray but a negative PPD (5TU) tested on two occasions six months apart
D. Individuals with fever of unknown origin and granulomas in the liver and bone marrow on recent biopsies
E. Individuals with a cavitary lung lesion and positive sputum smear for acid-fast bacilli but *no* pulmonary or systemic symptoms

45. Amphotericin B would be the initial drug of choice, with or without a second drug, for each of the following EXCEPT

A. *Candida* sepsis
B. cryptococcal meningitis
C. rhinocerebral mucormycosis
D. lymphocutaneous sporotrichosis
E. pulmonary blastomycosis

46. In which one of the following has flucytosine been shown most convincingly to be clinically useful?

A. Mucocutaneous candidiasis
B. Cryptococcal meningitis
C. Pulmonary aspergillosis
D. Rhinocerebral mucormycosis
E. *Candida* meningitis

47. Which one of the following could NOT establish a diagnosis of trichinosis?

A. Skin test
B. Bentonite flocculation test
C. Thick and thin blood smears
D. Hematoxylin and eosin staining of a muscle biopsy
E. Squash preparation of fresh muscle from a biopsy

48. Each of the following viruses is frequently associated with the common cold EXCEPT

A. picornaviruses
B. rotaviruses
C. myxoviruses
D. reoviruses
E. adenoviruses

49. A hospital employee receives a deep needle stick from a needle just used to draw blood from a patient who is HBsAg positive for hepatitis B. Which one of the following should the employee be given after the wound is cleaned to provide optimal protection against hepatitis B?

A. Hepatitis B immunization alone
B. Hyperimmune globulin (HBIG) given in one dose if the employee becomes HBsAg positive
C. HBIG given in one dose simultaneously with hepatitis B immunization at the time of HBsAg seroconversion
D. HBIG given in two doses at the time of the initial injury and again 20 to 30 days later
E. HBIG in four consecutive monthly doses starting at the time of injury

50. A nurse in the intensive care unit has had painful swelling of the left index finger adjacent to the nail for ten days without improvement, despite surgical drainage and six days of therapy with oral cephalexin (Keflex). There are multiple small pustules on the tip of the finger; Gram's stain shows no organisms. The most likely etiology is

A. varicella zoster
B. herpes simplex
C. *Pseudomonas aeruginosa*
D. *Legionella*
E. *Mycoplasma*

DIRECTIONS: For questions 51 to 93, you are to decide whether EACH choice is true or false. Any combination of answers, from all true to all false, may occur. Mark the answer sheet "T" or "F" in the space provided.

51. Which of the following is/are true about infectious mononucleosis?

A. Antibody-positive individuals are permanent carriers of Epstein-Barr virus (EBV)
B. The source of infection is contaminated body fluids, usually oropharyngeal secretions
C. Seropositive individuals can develop symptomatic disease after re-exposure to EBV
D. Asymptomatic infection occurs less frequently than symptomatic disease
E. EBV infection occurs more commonly in developed than in developing countries

52. Which of the following is/are true about azidothymidine (zidovudine, formerly known as AZT)?

A. Anemia is a frequent adverse reaction
B. Hepatitis is a frequent adverse reaction
C. It is effective against herpes viruses as well as HIV
D. *Pneumocystis* pneumonia rarely, if ever, occurs in HIV-infected patients who have received at least six weeks of therapy at a dose of 200 mg orally five times daily
E. It decreases the number of clinically recognized serious opportunistic infections in patients who have had *Pneumocystis* pneumonia when compared to patients receiving placebo

53. Which of the following is/are true about the epidemiology and transmission of leprosy?

A. The disease has the highest prevalence in Asia and Africa
B. The disease is endemic in Hawaii
C. The disease is endemic in Texas, Louisiana, and Florida
D. The risk of transmission is no greater for a household family member of a patient with leprosy than for anyone else in the same community
E. An animal reservoir for *Mycobacterium leprae* appears to exist among armadillos

54. Which of the following is/are true about primary tuberculosis?

A. Most primary infections are asymptomatic
B. Most primary infections cannot be detected radiographically
C. Primary disease can manifest as pleurisy with effusions
D. Cavity formation is not a manifestation of primary disease
E. The severity of primary infection is related to age

55. Which of the following is/are true about isoniazid therapy?

A. The drug is bactericidal against *Mycobacterium tuberculosis*
B. Peripheral neuropathy is more commonly seen in fast acetylators
C. Neuropathy can be prevented by administration of pyridoxine
D. Primary drug resistance is especially high among Oriental and Hispanic immigrants to the United States
E. Asymptomatic transaminase elevations are an indication to stop the drug

56. Which of the following is/are true about the diagnosis and treatment of brucellosis?

A. *Brucella* species can be grown in standard media in over 50% of untreated patients
B. Blood culture isolation of *Brucella* species is not safe to attempt unless special biosafety facilities are available
C. *Brucella* agglutination test is a reliable method for establishing the diagnosis
D. The drug of choice for therapy is ampicillin
E. The optimal duration of therapy for uncomplicated brucellosis is two to three weeks

57. Which of the following is/are true about nocardiosis?

A. The etiologic agent is spread by inhalation of airborne organisms
B. Disease occurs only in immunocompromised patients
C. Pulmonary disease is the most common clinical manifestation
D. The organism will grow only on selective media specific for *Nocardia*
E. The treatment of choice is tetracycline

58. Which of the following is/are true about actinomycosis?

A. Serology is a useful and available technique for establishing the diagnosis
B. Isolation of the organism from any clinical specimen is an indication that treatment is required
C. The organism cannot be seen by Gram's stain
D. The "sulfur granules" discharged from *Actinomyces* abscesses consist of a mucinous secretion but not intact organisms
E. Therapy of choice is an aminoglycoside

59. Which of the following is/are true about anthrax?

A. Cases of infection acquired in the United States are rare over the past 10 years
B. The organism is a common environmental contaminant in dust, dirt, and vegetation in many parts of the world
C. Microscopic examination of lesion exudate reveals gram-positive rods
D. Therapy of choice is tetracycline
E. The disease is rarely fatal even if untreated

60. Which of the following is/are true about Q fever?

A. The etiologic agent, *Coxiella burnetii*, is a rickettsia
B. The disease is usually transmitted to humans by ticks
C. The disease can often present in humans as pneumonia

D. The etiologic agent can be readily cultured by most clinical microbiology laboratories
E. Tetracyclines and chloramphenicol are effective therapy

61. Which of the following would be typical and characteristic for a diagnosis of spinal epidural abscess in a 60-year-old woman with diabetes mellitus?

A. A history of back pain preceding the development of muscle weakness
B. Motor and sensory impairment
C. Normal cerebrospinal fluid cell count, protein, and glucose below the level of the presumed block
D. A normal myelogram but abnormal CT scan
E. Isolation of *Staphylococcus aureus* from blood cultures

62. A 74-year-old woman with diabetes mellitus has severe left ear pain and a left seventh nerve palsy following meningismus. She looks "toxic." Which of the following is/are true?

A. *Pseudomonas aeruginosa* is a likely cause of her syndrome
B. The infection may have originated in the external auditory canal
C. Necrotizing osteitis of the temporal bone is a feature of this illness
D. Mortality associated with this syndrome is considerable
E. There is no role for surgical debridement

63. Which of the following is/are true about *Legionella* infections?

A. The etiologic agent is a bacterium that can be grown on artificial medium
B. The organisms are usually transmitted from person to person
C. *Legionella pneumophila* is the only *Legionella* species that is pathogenic for humans
D. The organisms probably did not cause human disease until the 1970's
E. *Legionella* infects only the lungs

64. Which of the following is/are true about aspiration pneumonia?

A. If the sputum is not foul and purulent, the patient probably does not have aspiration pneumonia
B. Sputum culture for aerobic and anaerobic bacteria is useful for identifying the etiologic agent
C. Abscess formation is a well-recognized sequela of severe aspiration pneumonia
D. The role of corticosteroids in improving prognosis has been clearly shown
E. Large pleural effusions are unusual in association with aspiration pneumonia

65. Which of the following is/are true about mucormycosis?

A. Mucormycosis is almost never seen in patients other than granulocytopenic patients
B. The diagnosis can often be made by blood culture if a selective fungal medium is used
C. Amphotericin B is the only drug with proven efficacy when used as a single agent
D. Mortality is substantial with any form of invasive mucormycosis

66. Which of the following is/are true about poliomyelitis?

A. The disease no longer can be acquired in North America
B. Humans are the only known natural hosts of poliovirus
C. Nonparalytic, asymptomatic infection is more common than paralytic disease
D. Oral polio vaccine produces humoral and intestinal immunity
E. The killed vaccine is advantageous compared to oral vaccine, in that vaccine-related cases of polio do not occur as a result of immunization

67. Which of the following is/are true about herpes zoster?

A. The etiologic virus is identical to the causative agent of varicella
B. Zoster can develop after exposure to varicella
C. Varicella can develop after exposure to zoster
D. Typically, lesions crust over 5–10 days after initial appearance
E. Dissemination occurs more often in neutropenic patients than in those with defective cell-mediated immunity

68. Which of the following is/are true about Lyme disease?

A. The disease is geographically confined to the eastern United States
B. Erythema chronicum migrans is the characteristic skin lesion associated with Lyme disease, but it does not invariably occur
C. The disease is transmitted by ticks
D. The disease is caused by a gram-negative rod that has yet to be grown
E. The therapy of choice is oral tetracycline

69. Which of the following is/are true about trachoma?

A. It is caused by *Chlamydia*
B. It is transmitted by fingers and fomites
C. It occurs in hundreds of millions of people worldwide
D. Bacterial superinfection contributes to corneal damage
E. Topical or oral tetracycline can be effective therapy

70. Which of the following is/are true about infections due to *Mycoplasma pneumoniae*?

A. The pulmonary disease is characterized by a disabling, paroxysmal cough
B. The chest roentgenogram is usually more abnormal than the chest physical examination
C. Large pleural effusions are characteristically present
D. Patients who are neutropenic are predisposed to severe, life-threatening disseminated disease
E. Diagnosis can be confirmed by blood culture in 25–40% of cases

71. Which of the following is/are true about dengue?

A. The disease is increasing in frequency in the United States
B. Person-to-person spread is the most common route of transmission
C. Hemorrhagic fever occurs only in association with second or subsequent episodes

D. Therapy is largely supportive
E. Mortality for cases in the United States is greater than 40%

72. Which of the following is/are true about tetanus?

A. The life-threatening manifestations occur as a direct result of invasion by the *Clostridium tetani* organism
B. Patients with suspected disease should be treated with penicillin or erythromycin
C. Patients with suspected disease should be treated with human tetanus immunoglobulin
D. Active immunization should be administered to patients who recover from tetanus
E. Surgical wound debridement, if necessary, should be carried out after administration of human tetanus immunoglobulin

73. Which of the following is/are true about botulism?

A. Home-canned foods, meat, and preserved fish are all commonly responsible for cases of botulism
B. Incubation period can be as long as 10 weeks
C. Individuals with the shortest incubation period usually have the most severe disease
D. Bulbar musculature is affected before peripheral musculature
E. Nausea, vomiting, and abdominal pain occur commonly

74. Which of the following is/are true about *Clostridium difficile*–induced disease?

A. The presence of *C. difficile* organisms in the stool is almost always associated with disease
B. Clinical manifestations range from mild diarrhea to severe, life-threatening bloody diarrhea with fever and abdominal pain
C. The preferred diagnostic test is a tissue culture assay of stool to demonstrate a cytopathic toxin
D. The *C. difficile*–induced diarrhea or colitis is rarely associated with antibiotics other than clindamycin
E. Metronidazole and bacitracin are acceptable alternative therapies to vancomycin

75. Which of the following is/are true about *Cryptosporidium* and cryptosporidiosis?

A. The causative organism is a protozoon
B. The causative organism produces primarily gastrointestinal disease
C. The organism is found only among AIDS patients
D. Cattle are a natural reservoir for cryptosporidia
E. There is no effective therapy for cryptosporidiosis

76. Which of the following is/are true about osteomyelitis?

A. Hematogenously caused osteomyelitic disease occurs with increased frequency at the extremes of age
B. *Staphylococcus aureus* is the most common pathogen
C. Anaerobic bacteria rarely if ever cause osteomyelitis
D. *Mycobacterium tuberculosis* is still a major cause of spinal osteomyelitis

77. Which of the following is/are recognized toxicities of acyclovir?

A. Hepatitis
B. Renal tubular obstruction
C. Interference with calcium metabolism
D. Anemia
E. Abdominal cramps

78. Which of the following is/are true about rabies?

A. In the United States, dogs near the Mexican border are the only significant reservoir of infection
B. The incubation period is almost always less than 30 days
C. Recovery of humans with proven rabies is rare
D. Health care personnel should take precautions against contact with body fluids of potentially infected patients
E. Duck embryo virus vaccine should be given to veterinarians and others with occupational exposure to potentially infected animals

79. Which of the following is/are true about viral meningitis and meningoencephalitis?

A. Mumps is the single most common recognized cause of viral meningitis and meningoencephalitis
B. Coxsackie and echoviruses are spread primarily by hand-to-mouth contact resulting in family clusters of illness
C. Viral meningitis is never associated with more than 1000 cells/mm³ in the cerebrospinal fluid, nor are there ever more than 50% neutrophils
D. The incidence of meningitis or meningoencephalitis associated with hospitalized patients with mumps parotitis is approximately 50%

80. Which of the following drugs is/are likely to be useful in the prevention of traveler's diarrhea?

A. Iodochlorhydroxyquin (Entero-Vioform)
B. Doxycycline
C. Trimethoprim-sulfamethoxazole
D. Subsalicylate bismuth (Pepto-Bismol)
E. Amoxicillin

81. Which of the following drugs would be acceptable treatment for pneumonia resulting from a witnessed aspiration during intubation of a chronically hospitalized patient?

A. Clindamycin and tobramycin
B. Metronidazole, cephalothin, and gentamicin
C. Vancomycin and amikacin
D. Cefoxitin and gentamicin
E. Piperacillin

82. Which of the following is/are more characteristic of prosthetic valve endocarditis than native valve endocarditis?

A. Abscesses in the perivalvular ring
B. *Staphylococcus epidermidis* and diphtheroids as common etiologic agents
C. Arrhythmias due to invasion of the conducting system by the causative organism
D. Inability to cure the endocarditis with antimicrobial therapy alone
E. Frequency of culture-negative endocarditis

83. Which of the following is/are true concerning cat-scratch disease?

A. Lymphadenopathy is not associated with fever, malaise, or headache
B. A gram-negative bacillus has been recognized in

lymph node specimens and appears to be the etiologic agent
C. Disease usually develops about two weeks after contact with a young cat
D. Characteristically, pus aspirated from affected nodes acutely is sterile
E. Antimicrobial therapy is not known to be effective

84. Which of the following is/are true concerning *Haemophilus influenzae*?

A. Nonencapsulated organisms can cause localized disease
B. Encapsulated organisms cause invasive disease, but almost all pathogens are type B
C. Successful treatment of *H. influenzae* meningitis almost always results in elimination of the organism from the upper respiratory tract
D. *H. influenzae* type B does *not* cause community outbreaks, but does produce secondary cases among susceptible individuals in day-care centers or in families
E. *H. influenzae* is the only *Haemophilus* species that has been shown conclusively to cause human disease

85. Which of the following is/are true about tuberculous lymphadenitis?

A. Patients may lack any systemic symptoms
B. Diagnosis should be established by aspiration of a node
C. Etiologies may include typical or atypical mycobacteria
D. Control of bovine tuberculosis has substantially decreased the frequency of cervical tuberculous lymphadenitis

86. Which of the following is/are true about gonorrhea?

A. A man having sexual contact with an infected woman has a much lower likelihood of developing gonorrhea than a woman who has intercourse with an infected man
B. Untreated gonococcal infection will persist for the patient's lifetime
C. Among infected men with urethral infection, about 10% are asymptomatic
D. Among women with endocervical or urethral infection, about 10% are asymptomatic

87. Which of the following is/are true about psittacosis?

A. It is usually acquired by inhalation
B. The incubation period is 45 to 90 days
C. Treatment with sulfadiazine or pyrimethamine is effective
D. Isolation of the organism is dangerous and requires special facilities
E. It is caused by an organism that can grow only in tissue culture, not in artificial media

88. Which of the following is/are true about HIV infection?

A. Transmission among homosexual males correlates directly with the number of male sexual contacts
B. Transmission among homosexual males correlates directly with the practice of receptive anal intercourse
C. Transmission among homosexual males correlates directly with the use of such recreational drugs as amyl nitrate
D. Transmission from males to females can occur but not from females to males unless rectal intercourse is practiced
E. Transmission via infected blood products will no longer occur if blood products are screened by current serologic techniques

89. Which of the following statements regarding syphilitic aortitis is/are true?

A. It causes characteristic calcification in the arch of the aorta
B. It is one cause of dissecting aortic aneurysm
C. It occurs as a result of congenital syphilis
D. It is associated with neurosyphilis in about 75% of cases
E. It can cause aortic stenosis

90. *Aspergillus fumigatus* is recovered repeatedly from small specimens of mucoid sputum obtained from a patient who complains of intermittent wheezing and dyspnea. Which of the following is/are likely to be true?

A. Precipitins to *Aspergillus* are present in the serum
B. Counterimmunoelectrophoresis (CIE) will show *Aspergillus* antigen in the blood and sputum
C. Eosinophilia is present in the peripheral blood
D. The patient should receive a course of amphotericin B intravenously

91. Antiviral agents effective in prophylaxis or therapy of viral infections include

A. amantadine
B. thiosemicarbazone
C. adenine arabinoside (ara-A)
D. idoxuridine

92. A patient recovering from untreated secondary syphilis has approximately a

A. 7% chance of developing neurosyphilis
B. 10% chance of developing cardiovascular syphilis
C. 25% chance of relapsing, with recurrent manifestations of secondary syphilis
D. 30% chance of developing tertiary syphilis

93. Acute gastroenteritis due to rotaviruses

A. usually occurs during winter months
B. is unusual in patients over four years of age
C. usually causes leukocytes to appear in stools
D. has an incubation period of one to four days

DIRECTIONS: Questions 94 to 170 are matching questions. For each numbered item, choose the most likely associated item from those provided. Each numbered item has ONLY ONE answer. Within each set of questions, each lettered item may be the answer to one, more than one, or none of the numbered items.

QUESTIONS 94–98

For each of the following diagnostic techniques, select the organism or disease that would be most readily and accurately identified.

A. Cutaneous leishmaniasis
B. *Diphyllobothrium latum*
C. Amebic liver abscess
D. Babeosis
E. Enterobiasis

94. Serology

95. Biopsy

96. Blood smear

97. Stool examination

98. Cellophane tape test

QUESTIONS 99–103

For each of the drug regimens listed below, select the form of endocarditis that would be treated most effectively.

A. *Streptococcus viridans* endocarditis (native valve)
B. *Streptococcus faecalis* endocarditis (native valve)
C. *Staphylococcus aureus* endocarditis (native valve)
D. *Candida* endocarditis (native valve)
E. Native valve endocarditis of unknown cause

99. Nafcillin, 2 g every 4 hours for four to six weeks

100. Nafcillin, 2 g every 4 hours, plus ampicillin, 2 g every 4 hours, plus gentamicin, 1 mg/kg every 8 hours, for four to six weeks

101. Penicillin G, 2 million units every 6 hours, plus streptomycin, 10 mg/kg every 12 hours, for two weeks

102. Ampicillin, 2 g every 4 hours, plus gentamicin, 1 mg/kg every 6 hours, for four to six weeks

103. Surgical valve replacement plus antimicrobial therapy

QUESTIONS 104–108

For each of the following antimicrobial regimens, select the clinical syndrome that would be optimally treated.

A. Urinary sepsis in an 80-year-old penicillin-allergic nursing home resident
B. Fever and hypotension in a neutropenic cancer patient
C. Diffuse pulmonary infiltrates and hypoxemia in a healthy college student
D. Acute meningitis of unknown cause in a healthy college student
E. Oral candidiasis in an AIDS patient

104. Piperacillin and tobramycin

105. Erythromycin

106. Ampicillin and chloramphenicol

107. Ketoconazole

108. Vancomycin and gentamicin

QUESTIONS 109–114

For each of the following microorganisms, select the organ systems that are most severely involved.

A. Skin, lymph nodes
B. Lungs
C. Soft tissue, cornea
D. Liver, spleen, bone marrow
E. Liver, gastrointestinal tract
F. Gastrointestinal tract

109. *Clostridium difficile*

110. *Pneumocystis*

111. *Sporothrix schenckii*

112. *Leishmania donovani*

113. *Onchocerca volvulus*

114. Yellow fever virus

QUESTIONS 115–120

For each of the following diseases, select the most appropriate therapeutic drug.

A. Penicillin
B. Tetracycline plus streptomycin
C. Aminoglycosides
D. Ceftazidime
E. Dapsone, rifampin, clofazimine
F. Sulfa and pyrimethamine
G. Tetracycline

115. Brucellosis

116. Leptospirosis

117. Tularemia

118. Listeriosis

119. Diphtheria

120. Leprosy

QUESTIONS 121–125

For each of the following diseases, select the vector that can transmit the etiologic agent.

A. Hard ticks (Ixodidae)
B. Soft ticks (Argasidae)
C. Centipedes
D. Lice

121. Rocky Mountain spotted fever

122. Tularemia

123. Babesiosis

124. Lyme disease

125. Relapsing fever

QUESTIONS 126–131

For each of the following immunizations, select the patient population that would be most likely to benefit.

A. Any traveler to the developing world
B. Everyone who is immunocompetent and not vaccinated for many years
C. Only laboratory workers doing research on the agent
D. Travelers to certain areas of equatorial Africa and South America
E. Travelers planning to swim in fresh water lakes in the developing world
F. Abattoir workers

126. Smallpox vaccination

127. Gamma globulin

128. Diphtheria vaccine

129. Polio vaccine

130. Tetanus immunization

131. Yellow fever vaccine

QUESTIONS 132–137

Match the clinical syndrome associated with HIV infection with the description that is most appropriate. (*Note:* Use each lettered item only once.)

A. Toxoplasmosis
B. Cytomegalovirus
C. Kaposi's sarcoma
D. Oral leukoplakia
E. Aseptic meningitis
F. Disseminated *Mycobacterium avium-intracellulare*

132. It is probably caused by Epstein-Barr virus

133. It most often presents clinically as retinitis

134. It most often presents with focal neurologic deficits

135. It occurs within 3–14 days of initial acquisition of HIV disease

136. It can be diagnosed by cultivation of blood using lysis-centrifugation or radiometric techniques

137. Among HIV-infected patients, it is often recognized among homosexual males, but rarely among females, intravenous drug abusers, or transfusion recipients.

QUESTIONS 138–143

For each of the following respiratory diseases, select the clinical description that most closely applies.

A. Pharyngitis
B. Croup
C. Bronchitis
D. Epiglottitis

138. Occurs exclusively in children

139. Most commonly caused by parainfluenza types 1, 3, 2 and only very rarely influenza A and B or respiratory syncytial virus

140. Most common, caused by many viruses, including rhinoviruses, influenza, coronavirus, and adenovirus

141. Antibiotics are invariably indicated

142. Airway obstruction is a potential complication for adult patients

143. *Streptococcus pyogenes* is a common bacterial cause; *Neisseria gonorrhoeae* and *Corynebacterium diphtheriae* are less common causes

QUESTIONS 144–148

For each of the following statements, select the lettered item to which it applies.

A. Rheumatic fever
B. Poststreptococcal glomerulonephritis
C. Both of the above
D. Neither of the above

144. Known to follow streptococcal impetigo

145. Known to follow streptococcal pharyngitis

146. Prevented by penicillin therapy

147. Probably immunologic in origin

148. Prophylactic therapy is required to prevent recurrences

QUESTIONS 149–153

For each of the infections listed below, select the cerebrospinal fluid data with which it is most likely to be associated. *Note:* Use each set of CSF findings only once.

Leukocytes	Protein	Glucose	Culture
A. Few to 1000's; lymphocytes predominate (PMN's seen early in disease)	Elevated	Usually normal	Usually negative
B. Several to 1000's; PMN's predominate	Elevated	Usually decreased (<⅔ of serum value)	Usually diagnostic
C. Few to 100's; lymphocytes predominate	Elevated	Markedly decreased (usually <40 mg/dl)	Diagnostic in ~50% of cases
D. None to several hundred; lymphocytes predominate	Elevated	Decreased in ≈ 50% of cases	Usually negative
E. Few to several hundred; usually mixed PMN's and lymphocytes	Elevated	Usually normal	Usually negative

149. Fungal meningitis (*Cryptococcus, Coccidioides*)

150. Bacterial meningitis

151. Viral meningitis

152. Brain abscess

153. Tuberculous meningitis

QUESTIONS 154–159

Below are six descriptions of ulcers occurring on the genitals. For each, select the most appropriate diagnosis.

A. Syphilis
B. Herpes simplex virus type 2
C. Behçet's syndrome
D. Chancroid
E. Lymphogranuloma venereum
F. Granuloma inguinale

154. A vesicle forms on the penis, breaks down to form a small ulcer, and heals in a week; the patient then develops enlarged, matted, painful inguinal nodes, which later discharge pus through two sinus tracts

155. A single painless, clean-based, indurated ulcer with raised, firm borders at the anal margin in a male homosexual; there is no inguinal adenopathy

156. Five shallow, very painful ulcers on the shaft of the penis, 3 mm across and 2 mm apart, healing and then recurring three times in seven months

157. Two painful, exudative, nonindurated ulcers at the border of the glans penis, with regional lymphadenopathy; material from the ulcer is negative on dark-field examination; aspirate from a suppurating inguinal lymph node grows a species of *Haemophilus*

158. A single circular, painless ulcer with a sharply demarcated margin on the shaft of the penis; material from the ulcer is negative on dark-field examination, but pleomorphic coccobacilli can be found within monocytes

159. Four painless, punched-out ulcers on the scrotum in a patient with concomitant oral ulcers and superficial thrombophlebitis

QUESTIONS 160–166

For each of the following infections, select the isolation technique recommended by the Centers for Disease Control.

A. Strict isolation
B. Respiratory isolation only
C. Enteric precautions only
D. Contact isolation
E. Blood and body fluid precautions only

160. Methicillin-resistant *Staphylococcus aureus* infection of mediastinal wound

161. Pulmonary tuberculosis

162. Hepatitis A

163. Meningococcal disease

164. Disseminated herpes zoster

165. Measles

166. Hepatitis B

QUESTIONS 167–170

For each of the following diseases, select the appropriate incubation period.

A. 1–2 days
B. 2–6 days
C. 3–20 days
D. 10–90 days
E. 38–140 days
F. 60–120 days

167. Lymphogranuloma venereum (LGV)

168. Primary syphilis

169. Secondary syphilis

170. Genitorectal gonorrhea

PART 8
INFECTIOUS DISEASE

ANSWERS

1.(E) Lymphogranuloma venereum (LGV) is a sexually transmitted infection that characteristically presents with an ulcerative genital lesion a few days to several weeks after sexual exposure. Frequently, however, the ulcer or papule is not noticed, and the manifestation that brings the patient to medical attention is the development of inguinal adenopathy 2–6 weeks after sexual contact. Draining fistulas are characteristic of LGV. The etiologic agent, *Chlamydia trachomatis*, can be grown in tissue culture, but this test is not generally available. The complement fixation serology is generally available. A titer of 1:16 is highly suggestive. Paired samples that demonstrate a four-fold titer rise to 1:64 or greater are diagnostic. (*Cecil, Ch. 307*)

2.(A) Hemodynamic shock can be caused by a variety of processes, including hypovolemia, sepsis, anaphylaxis, and cardiac disorders (valvular, myocardial, or pericardial). When tissues are not adequately perfused, all patients in severe shock develop a metabolic acidosis with elevated lactate levels. Septic shock characteristically produces a high cardiac output, low systemic vascular resistance, and low pulmonary capillary wedge pressure. A high pulmonary capillary wedge pressure suggests a cardiac etiology rather than hypovolemia or sepsis. Swan-Ganz catheters are used with increasing frequency to assess patients with hypotension, both because they provide helpful diagnostic information and because they provide objective parameters for assessing the adequacy of therapy. (*Cecil, Chs. 44 and 259*)

3.(B) Neutropenic patients are susceptible to a wide variety of gram-positive and gram-negative organisms. Thus, when they are febrile they must receive a broad-spectrum empiric regimen. This regimen can be modified when the etiologic agent is identified to assure optimal activity against the etiologic agent, although it must remain broad-spectrum with good anti-*Pseudomonas* activity until the neutrophil count returns to a level above 1000/mm^3. Imipenem and ceftazidime are broad-spectrum agents with anti-*Pseudomonas* activity which are acceptable regimens for neutropenic, febrile patients, despite the lack of extensive data to show that they are as good as combination regimens that include an aminoglycoside (gentamicin, tobramycin, or amikacin) plus a penicillin with anti-*Pseudomonas* activity (ticarcillin, carbenicillin, piperacillin, azlocillin, mezlocillin). Cefotaxime is a broad-spectrum third-generation cephalosporin, but it lacks much activity against *Pseudomonas aeruginosa* and therefore is *not* an acceptable regimen as a single agent. (*Cecil, Ch. 258; Mandell et al, pp. 1680–1687*)

4.(B) In developing countries, major causes of diarrhea are (1) fecal contamination of food grown in fields where human feces are deposited indiscriminantly or for fertilizer, and (2) fecal contamination of rivers, streams, and harbors where drinking water or shellfish are obtained. Human feces in these areas often contain *Salmonella, Shigella, Campylobacter*, and a variety of viruses including those that cause hepatitis A. Thus, avoiding raw vegetables, unboiled drinking water, and raw shellfish can greatly decrease the likelihood of diarrheal illnesses. Bismuth subsalicylate is an effective but somewhat impractical prophylaxis, considering the amount needed for long trips. Undercooked meat can transmit trichinosis, toxoplasmosis, and taenia, but it is usually not associated with diarrheal illnesses when freshly prepared. (*Cecil, Ch. 261; Mandell et al, pp. 1698–1705*)

5.(C) The appropriate evaluation of generalized lymphadenopathy in a symptomatic individual includes lymph node biopsy and serologies for diseases such as mononucleosis, toxoplasmosis, cytomegalovirus, syphilis, and AIDS. The ELISA test for HIV (HTLV-III/LAV) is very sensitive but not very specific. To confirm the presence of HIV infection, a Western blot (or similarly specific technique) should be performed to assure that the result is specific for this virus. The presence of HIV (HTLV-III/LAV) infection in the patient does not guarantee that this virus is the cause of the lymphadenopathy, nor does a positive serology indicate that the patient has AIDS. AIDS is a clinical syndrome, and many virus-infected patients do not have the clinical syndrome of AIDS. Especially in a symptomatic patient, a biopsy of a lymph node should be performed. Since *Mycobacterium avium-intracellulare* occurs so rarely in nonpulmonary tissue in association with any disease other than AIDS, its isolation from a lymph node in a previously healthy individual would strongly suggest the diagnosis of AIDS. A Sabin-Feldman dye test titer of 1:64 is characteristic of chronic infection of longstanding duration (years) rather than acute infection; lymphadenopathy occurs only in association with acute infection except in extraordinarily rare situations. An OKT4/OKT8 ratio determination on peripheral lymphocytes has little diagnostic use in any situation, since so many diseases and drugs can alter either the number of T4-positive lymphocytes or the number of T8-positive lymphocytes. (*Cecil, Chs. 157, 346, 385*)

6.(A) *Pneumocystis carinii* derived from human specimens cannot be grown in vitro, nor is there a reliable serology. To establish the diagnosis, the organism must be visualized in pulmonary secretions or tissue. Recently it has been shown that careful examination of sputum can reveal *Pneumocystis* in at least 50% of AIDS patients ultimately shown to have *Pneumocystis* pneumonia. The presence of *Pneumocystis* in pulmonary secretions or tissues should always be assumed to indicate that *Pneumocystis* is etiologically associated with pulmonary dysfunction. Gallium scanning can indicate the presence of pulmonary inflammation due to any cause; it is thus nonspecific. Lung diffusing capacity is decreased in patients with *Pneumocystis* pneumonia as well as in patients with many other lung diseases. Pulmonary function abnormalities are thus not specific for *Pneumocystis* pneumonia. (*Cecil, Ch. 386*)

7.(C) When gram-positive cocci in clusters are grown from the blood, consideration must be given to *Staphylococcus aureus* or *S. epidermidis*, especially in patients who have intravenous lines that have been in place for more than three days. Intravenous catheter sepsis can occur even when the catheter site appears to be unremarkable and uninflamed. Clindamycin does not provide activity against *S. epidermidis* and is not an optimal agent for *S. aureus*. Nafcillin is an excellent agent for *S. aureus* and for some *S. epidermidis*. Vancomycin would be a preferable agent, since the likelihood of a vancomycin-resistant *S. aureus* or *S. epidermidis* is extraordinarily low. The clindamycin and gentamicin could be stopped in another day or two when the gram-positive organism is unequivocally identified and it is clear that the patient does not have polymicrobial sepsis. Clavulanic acid binds to beta-lactamases, providing the fixed combination of clavulanic acid–ticarcillin with activity against most *S. aureus* but not against many *S. epidermidis* isolates. (*Cecil, Chs. 260 and 271; Mandell et al, pp. 1612–1620*)

8.(D) Vancomycin has excellent activity against aerobic gram-positive cocci including *Staphylococcus epidermidis, S. aureus*, and *Streptococcus faecalis*. It has good activity against many clostridia and is the therapy of choice for *Clostridium difficile* colitis. It has poor activity against many anaerobes, however, and is not considered adequate therapy for most anaerobic infections. (*Cecil, Chs. 28, 279, and 282; Pratt and Fekety, pp. 142–144*)

9.(C) Aminoglycosides as a group are toxic for both vestibular and cochlear function. They also cause renal damage and occasionally cause curare-like effects. Since they are excreted in the urine, the dose must be adjusted for patients in renal failure. Toxicity can be reduced by carefully monitoring serum peak and trough levels. Granulocytopenia can probably occur in association with aminoglycoside therapy but is not a common occurrence. (*Cecil, Ch. 28; Pratt and Fekety, pp. 153–183*)

10.(C) Nosocomial infections, defined as infections that were not present or incubating upon hospital admission, occur in 5–10% of the 40 million people who are hospitalized in the United States. In acute care hospitals, urinary tract infections are responsible for 35–40%, postoperative wound infections 20%, pulmonary infections 15%, blood stream infections 5–10%, and other infections 15–20%. (*Cecil, Ch. 260; Bennett and Brachman*)

11.(A) Diphtheria is caused by a gram-positive bacillus that is spread by respiratory droplets or close contact with respiratory secretions or skin exudate. The organism causes a local diphtheritic lesion in the pharynx or skin. An elaborated toxin causes the myocarditis and neuritis. Therapy with antitoxin and penicillin or erythromycin should be initiated as soon as the diagnosis is suspected, since the infection can be rapidly fatal. The disease can still be acquired in the United States from indigenous or immigrant populations. (*Cecil, Ch. 277; Centers for Disease Control, 1985b*)

12.(D) Typhoid fever is caused by *Salmonella typhi*, which is spread by flies, fomites, food, feces, and fingers. Humans are the only reservoir; there is no animal reservoir. Diarrhea is not an invariable finding. Chloramphenicol is the standard therapy, although trimethoprim-sulfamethoxazole and ampicillin may be used. Ampicillin-resistant strains are relatively common, however, so ampicillin is a less desirable therapy until drug susceptibilities are known. Immunization is only 70% effective and is associated with considerable inflammation at the injection site. About two thirds of chronic carriers, defined as those excreting *S. typhi* for at least one year, can be successfully treated with a six-week course of ampicillin. (*Cecil, Ch. 283; Bryan et al*)

13.(E) Non-typhoidal *Salmonella* infections are common causes of upper or lower gastrointestinal disorders in the United States. Meat-producing animals and poultry are common sources. Gastroenteritis with abrupt onset of nausea and vomiting is a common presentation. Bacteremia occurs occasionally in healthy individuals, although its presence should stimulate a search for a source, especially if the *Salmonella* is *S. cholerasuis*. Therapy for *Salmonella* gastroenteritis should emphasize fluid replacement. Antibiotic therapy may be used for patients with prolonged symptoms or those who are debilitated or immunosuppressed. A short course of oral ampicillin or amoxicillin or trimethoprim-sulfamethoxazole can be useful, although there is a growing frequency of ampicillin-resistant *Salmonella*. (*Cecil, Ch. 284*)

14.(D) *Yersinia enterocolitica* typically presents as fever associated with diarrhea or abdominal pain. A terminal ileitis or mesenteric adenitis or both can develop and present very much like appendicitis. Findings at surgery are nonspecific, but stool, blood, and the surgical specimen are likely to grow the organism if the sample is incubated at low temperatures (4°C for stool). Since most cases are self-limiting and are diagnosed retrospectively, it is difficult to ascertain if therapy is useful. The reservoirs for this organism are domestic and farm animals. Food- and water-borne epidemics of *Y. enterocolitica* infection occur. (*Cecil, Ch. 291*)

15.(C) Plague is an endemic zoonosis of the Americas, Africa, and Asia. *Yersinia pestis* is an aerobic gram-negative rod. Sylvatic rodents in the Southwest United States are an important reservoir. Infection occurs by the bite of infected fleas or, less commonly, when infected animals are ingested. Primary inhalational plague is rare but it does occur. When bacteremic patients cough they can aerosolize the organism and produce the pneumonic form of plague, which is fatal if therapy is delayed more than 20 hours. Streptomycin is the therapy of choice. (*Cecil, Ch. 291*)

16.(A) Cysticercosis is a common cause of grand mal seizures in young adults in many parts of the world. Ingestion of poorly cooked pork is the usual vehicle for infection with *Taenia solium*. Ingestion of the cysticerca leads to intestinal infection with one adult worm which releases gravid proglottids into the intestinal contents; thus the human is the intermediate host. Humans become a definitive host when they ingest eggs and the eggs produce larva in the small bowel which migrate in the bloodstream to distant sites including brain and soft tissues. Humans consume eggs by ingesting fecally contaminated food, by autoinoculation from rectum to mouth, or perhaps by reverse peristalsis of eggs. (*Cecil, Ch. 395; Mandell et al, p. 1581*)

17.(D) Acyclovir has excellent activity against herpes simplex virus at serum levels that can be achieved by administering 15 mg/kg/day in three divided doses. The drug has been successfully used to treat a wide variety of herpes simplex infections. Herpes zoster is not as sensitive to acyclovir as herpes simplex. Higher doses are needed, usually 30 mg/kg/day in three divided doses. Acyclovir does not have enough activity against cytomegalovirus to be clinically effective. (*Cecil, Chs. 29, 340, and 343; Pratt and Fekety, pp. 474–478*)

18.(E) Herpes simplex virus and *Chlamydia trachomatis* are both frequent causes of proctitis among homosexual males. Hepatitis B and cytomegalovirus infections are also recognized to occur with much higher frequency among sexually active homosexuals compared to sexually active heterosexuals. There is no evidence that Epstein-Barr virus infects or causes disease among homosexual males who are HIV-seronegative any more frequently than among heterosexual males. Among HIV-seropositive homosexual males, however, EBV infection may have a role in producing hairy leukoplakia, lymphadenopathy, or Kaposi's sarcoma. (*Cecil, Chs. 305 and 346; Mandell et al, pp. 1667–1674*)

19.(D) *Streptococcus faecalis* is part of normal bowel flora. Its role in causing purulent abdominal infections is controversial. Bacteremias due to *S. faecalis* often arise from the biliary or urinary tracts, however, which must be examined in anyone with unexplained *S. faecalis* bacteremia. Endocarditis is also a major concern to be investigated. *S. faecalis* rarely causes disease of the skin, oral cavity, or upper airway. (*Cecil, Ch. 268; Mandell et al, pp. 1152–1155*)

20.(B) Eosinophilic gastroenteritis, characterized by malabsorption, gastrointestinal bleeding, protein-losing enteropathy, and infiltration of the small bowel mucosa by eosinophils, is probably an allergic response, since it occurs more often in individuals with other allergies. For the other diseases listed, antimicrobial therapy is often helpful. (*Cecil, Chs. 103 and 104*)

21.(A) The most common recognized cause of retinochoroiditis in young adults is toxoplasmosis. Patients typically have a Sabin-Feldman dye test of 1:64–1:512, which indicates a chronic infection that was acquired many years previously. Most often the infection was acquired congenitally, but the clinical disease does not manifest until the third or fourth decade of life. Other infectious agents that need to be considered include syphilis, tuberculosis, cytomegalovirus, and histoplasmosis. Aqueous humor aspirates or vitreous humor aspirates rarely yield the etiologic agent in any situation, although the ratio of antibody in the aqueous humor to antibody in the serum might be of some diagnostic help. (*Cecil, Ch. 385; Mandell et al, pp. 1540–1548*)

22.(E) Adenine arabinoside (ara-A) has good in vitro activity against herpes simplex. It effectively reduces mortality due to herpes simplex encephalitis from 70% to 30–40%. It has some activity clinically against herpes zoster, but little or none against cytomegalovirus and Epstein-Barr virus. The drug is relatively insoluble, must be given in large amounts of fluid, can suppress the bone marrow, and can cause neurologic disturbances. Acyclovir is equally effective for herpes simplex and herpes zoster infections. Because acyclovir is safer and easier to administer, it has replaced adenine arabinoside as the drug of choice for herpes simplex and herpes zoster infections. There is no clear role for adenine arabinoside at this time. (*Cecil, Chs. 29, 340, and 343; Mandell et al, pp. 270–285*)

23.(E) Rocky Mountain spotted fever is caused by *Rickettsia rickettsii*. The syndrome can be rapidly fatal; thus, when a patient presents with a compatible syndrome, therapy with a tetracycline antibiotic should be initiated immediately. Few medical centers have the facilities to grow *Rickettsia* safely in cell cultures. The organism cannot be seen in routine histologic sections, although fluorescent antibody techniques for detecting the organism are becoming more widely available. Serologies are useful only in retrospect, since titers do not rise until the end of the first week of clinical illness. (*Cecil, Chs. 320 and 322*)

24.(E) Coccidioidomycosis, the second most common endemic mycosis in the United States, occurs in the Southwestern United States, Mexico, and parts of Central and South America. About 80–95% of the population in parts of California and Arizona are skin test positive. (*Cecil, Ch. 370*)

25.(D) Sporotrichosis is a noncontagious mycosis of the skin and regional lymphatics that results from percutaneous inoculation of *Sporothrix schenckii*. In about 75% of cases a single lesion presents on an exposed skin surface, usually following trauma. A pimple, wart, pustule, ulcer, or abscess fails to heal and spreads up the extremity, manifesting as subcutaneous nodules over thickened lymphatics. Pulmonary sporotrichosis can occur, but it is unusual. (*Cecil, Ch. 374*)

26.(E) Oral candidiasis, diagnosed on the basis of white plaques in the mouth which have yeast on methylene blue or Gram's stained smears, can occur secondary to corticosteroid therapy, diabetes mellitus, or antibiotic therapy. Oral candidiasis is often the initial manifestation of HIV-induced immune dysfunction: About 60% of HIV-seropositive patients with oral candidiasis will develop AIDS within six months. It would be unusual for oral candidiasis to be the initial manifestation of lymphoma. DiGeorge's syndrome is unusual and is obvious early in childhood. (*Cecil, Chs. 346, 375, and 419*)

27.(A) Scabies is a dermatologic infestation caused by the mite *Sarcoptes scabiei*, which burrows into the skin and can reproduce there. Intense pruritus begins two to six weeks after initial exposure. Treatment includes antipruritic drugs and an acaricide preparation such as lindane. (*Cecil, Ch. 414*)

28.(D) Clindamycin is not associated with bone marrow suppression commonly, although occasional cases of cytopenia have been reported. Chloramphenicol, pyrimethamine, and flucytosine all suppress bone marrow function in a dose-related, predictable fashion. Pentamidine is being reported more and more often with leukopenia. (*Cecil, Ch. 28*)

29.(E) Neurologic and hematologic complications of infectious mononucleosis are quite often recognized. Neurologic complications include meningoencephalitis, transverse myelitis, Guillain-Barré syndrome, and Bell's palsy. Hematologic complications include thrombocytopenia, hemolytic anemia, agranulocytosis, and aplastic anemia. Hepatitis, often with jaundice, is a characteristic feature of mononucleosis, but biliary disease is not recognized to be an association. (*Cecil, Ch. 342*)

30.(D) This is a classic presentation of a patient with chancroid (soft chancre). The disease is caused by *Haemophilus ducreyi*, a gram-negative pleomorphic bacillus. Classically, patients present with a painful genital lesion that has a necrotic base and nonindurated edges. Lymphadenopathy occurs in about 50% of patients, usually unilaterally (two thirds of those with adenopathy). The therapy of choice is sulfisoxazole, 1 g four times daily for 10 to 14 days. Alternatively, tetracycline, 500 mg four times daily, can be used. (*Cecil, Ch. 309; Mandell et al, pp. 1281–1282*)

31.(C) The most likely etiologic agent in this setting is *Pasteurella multocida*, an aerobic, gram-negative bacillus that is part of the oral flora of many cats and dogs. Infections with this organism occur more commonly after cat bites than after dog bites. The interval between the injury and the onset of symptoms is short (less than 24 hours). The infection progresses rapidly, and by the time the patient seeks medical attention the wound is usually purulent, with a surrounding cellulitis; local adenopathy is commonly present, and there may be associated systemic symptoms such as fever and malaise. The most rapid way of making a diagnosis is by demonstration of gram-negative rods of Gram's stain of the wound, although definitive diagnosis depends upon culturing the organism. *Staphylococcus aureus* and streptococci cause most infections that become clinically evident more than 24 hours after a bite injury, and Gram's stain in that setting will show gram-positive cocci in pairs, chains, and clusters. *(Mandell et al, pp. 1294–1295)*

32.(C) Several studies have shown that prophylactic antibiotics, in order to be effective, should be started immediately before surgery. The exception to this is oral, nonabsorbable antibiotics used for bowel surgery. Too early use of antibiotics (one to two days before) only promotes resistant organisms and therefore may impair the drug's effectiveness in decreasing the postoperative infection rate. The postoperative infection rate has been shown to decrease with the use of prophylactic antibiotics in vaginal hysterectomy and in high-risk cesarean sections, as well as in clean orthopedic surgery for implanting a prosthetic hip. Antibiotics are not indicated in cardiac catheterization, and there are no convincing data on the usefulness of prophylactic antibiotics in clean neurosurgical procedures not involving a shunt. *(Cecil, Chs. 28 and 260; Mandell et al, pp. 1637–1644)*

33.(E) This woman is susceptible to rubella, and if she acquires it during the first trimester there is a 30 to 50% chance that the fetus will suffer significant congenital defects. However, brief exposure to a child with rubella will not always transmit infection. Therefore, she should be re-tested in two to three weeks; if the HI titer has risen significantly, infection has occurred and therapeutic abortion should be advised. Ara-A has no effect on the rubella virus, since it is an RNA virus. Human immunoglobulin may mask infection without protecting the fetus, and should not be given, except in the special case in which it is known at the outset that the mother will certainly refuse an abortion, even if infection occurs. In this circumstance, answer D would be correct, since human gamma globulin probably offers some protection against infection of the fetus. Vaccination during pregnancy is contraindicated, because it is already too late to prevent natural infection from the contact and because the live vaccine virus theoretically could infect the fetus and cause congenital anomalies. *(Cecil, Ch. 337)*

34.(B) Pleocytosis and elevated CSF protein should resolve slowly after successful treatment of neurosyphilis, and VDRL titer in the CSF should fall in most patients. The *serum* VDRL titer is not a reliable indicator of disease activity in the CNS. The FTA-ABS test result is reported only as positive, negative, or equivocal; it is not titered out. FTA-ABS in CSF is of less value than the VDRL titer in assessment of neurosyphilis. CSF glucose is usually normal in neurosyphilis. *(Cecil, Chs. 310 and 482)*

35.(B) Individuals who are far from medical care need maximal protection, but this cannot be attained if the fetus is to be protected from teratogenic drugs and viruses. Live virus vaccines such as yellow fever vaccine should never be given to pregnant women, nor should drugs that have teratogenic potential or have not been thoroughly tested. Pyrimethamine is known to be teratogenic, so pyrimethamine-sulfadoxine (Fansidar) should not be used. In addition, severe hypersensitivity reactions to Fansidar have recently been reported, several of which were fatal. Chloroquine has been extensively used, however, and appears to be safe in pregnant women, although it does not provide complete malaria protection: many strains of falciparum malaria are resistant. Paratyphoid vaccine is not effective and is no longer available. There are only rare cases of cholera in South America, and the immunization is not very effective. This patient should receive immune serum globulin (ISG) for protection against hepatitis A, as well as Salk (inactivated) polio vaccine and tetanus-diphtheria immunization. *(Cecil, Ch. 261)*

36.(D) Multiple parasitized erythrocytes, the presence of appliqué forms, and the high percentage of involved cells strongly suggest that the malaria is falciparum. Falciparum has no hepatic cycle, so primaquine is unnecessary. Quinine is effective therapy for reducing parasitemia, but recrudescent disease occurs if other drugs are not used in conjunction with quinine. It is prudent to give quinine intravenously to ensure adequate blood levels in the case of life-threatening disease. *(Cecil, Ch. 381; Mandell et al, pp. 1519–1521)*

37.(B) Most series show that *Staphylococcus epidermidis* is a common cause of prosthetic valve endocarditis during the two initial postoperative months. In some series it is also a common cause of late prosthetic valve endocarditis. Prognosis for either early or late PVE due to *S. epidermidis* is dismal. It is rarely a cause of endocarditis in native valves. In most situations relating to patients without abnormal valves, epidermidis bacteremia results from contaminated intravenous or intra-arterial lines. Localized *S. epidermidis* disease is very uncommon. In immunosuppressed patients, however, *S. epidermidis* can cause serious localized or systemic disease on occasion. *(Cecil, Chs. 270 and 271; Mandell et al, pp. 1117–1123)*

38.(D) In a peripheral blood smear, *Borrelia,* malaria, or *Babesia* can be seen. The last two organisms are intraerythrocytic and are well visualized with Giemsa or Wright's stain. *Borrelia* are extraerythrocytic and are best seen also by using Wright's or Giemsa stain. Thick smears are very useful in searching for these parasites in large quantities of erythrocytes. *(Cecil, Chs. 312, 381, and 389)*

39.(D) Echocardiograms can identify vegetations that are 3 to 4 mm or larger if the valve is well visualized. Smaller vegetations are often missed by echocardiography but are easily seen at autopsy. The prognostic significance of vegetations visualized by echocardiography is unclear. Very few experienced clinicians would advocate replacing the valve on the basis of echocardiographic data alone. Many patients with previously unrecognized valvular pathology can develop endocarditis, particularly if the organism is invasive and virulent. Therefore, many older patients with *Staphylococcus aureus* bacteremia do in fact develop valvular involvement after a transient bacteremia from a distant site. Blood cultures often remain positive for three to five days after appropriate therapy is instituted. Sensitive viridans streptococci should be very amenable to penicillin treatment; after four to six weeks of treatment, relapses should occur in less than 1% of cases. *(Cecil, Ch. 372; Popp)*

40.(C) The major concern in treating a patient with gram-negative bacillary meningitis is the administration of drugs that are active against the likely pathogens and that penetrate the blood-brain barrier. Non–lactose-fermenting gram-negative bacilli would include *Pseudomonas* species and *Serratia;* these organisms are likely to be susceptible to aminoglycosides but resistant to first- and second-generation cephalosporins. Aminoglycosides do not reliably penetrate the blood-brain barrier, so they should be administered both intravenously and intrathecally. Some authorities prefer insertion of an Ommaya reservoir to intralumbar injection, since drugs administered by the latter route may not circulate over the cerebral convexities or into the ventricles. Carbenicillin and ticarcillin have activity against many gram-negative bacilli. They are usually active against *P. aeruginosa*, but resistance develops when they are used alone; they should be administered in conjunction with an aminoglycoside. Current studies suggest that certain third-generation cephalosporins used as single agents will be effective empiric therapy in this setting. The antimicrobial spectrum of chloramphenicol or piperacillin is too narrow for these drugs to be adequate empiric therapy for non–lactose-fermenting gram-negative rods; chloramphenicol has no anti-*Pseudomonas* activity, and piperacillin cannot be used alone since *Pseudomonas* may develop resistance. Vancomycin has no activity against aerobic gram-negative bacilli. *(Cecil, Ch. 272; Rahal and Simberkoff)*

41.(C) Rapidly spreading soft tissue infections can be caused by mixed aerobic and anaerobic infections, spore-forming anaerobic infections, or non–spore-forming anaerobic infections. In the perirectal region, bowel flora is very likely to be involved. Surgery is essential diagnostically to establish the extent of infection, and therapeutically to remove necrotic tissue and terminate the anaerobic conditions that allow infection to spread. Until the etiologic agent is established, empiric antimicrobial therapy should be directed against coliforms, spore-forming anaerobic organisms, and non–spore-forming anaerobic organisms. Surgical therapy must be performed as quickly as possible if the lethal consequences of these infections are to be avoided. *(Cecil, Ch. 278; Mandell et al, pp. 609–613)*

42.(A) This patient almost certainly has meningococcal meningitis. Other gram-negative cocci almost never cause meningitis, particularly in previously healthy individuals, although caution must be exercised to ensure that the organisms are in fact cocci rather than coccobacilli, which might suggest *Haemophilus*. A substantial proportion of types A and C meningococcal infections can be prevented by immunization. Most co-primary or secondary cases occur within four days of the index case. Secondary cases occur primarily in those who have had very close contact with the patient, e.g., household contacts who share a bedroom with the patient. Rifampin prophylaxis (600 mg orally, twice daily for two days) is preferred until sensitivities of the organisms are known. Sulfa drugs are effective for prophylaxis only if the organisms are susceptible. Minocycline is effective for prophylaxis, but in the United States it is associated with an unacceptably high frequency of dizziness. *(Cecil, Chs. 272 and 273; Peltola)*

43.(E) *Candida* esophagitis occurs almost exclusively in patients with immunologic defects. It is often present in patients who do not have oropharyngeal candidiasis. The mucosal defect that can be seen on barium swallow can be produced by a variety of infectious agents, particularly herpes simplex and cytomegalovirus; a biopsy is needed for a specific diagnosis. Perforation and rupture are recognized complications of *Candida* esophagitis, although they do not occur frequently. Therapy with oral ketoconazole or small doses of intravenous amphotericin B (100 to 300 mg) is usually effective. *(Cecil, Ch. 375; Edwards)*

44.(B) Isoniazid prophylaxis is indicated in any individual who has evidence of subclinical but active disease. Anyone under the age of 35 years who has a positive PPD should receive prophylaxis, as should any older individual whose PPD is converted from negative to positive, or who has a positive PPD and a risk factor such as diabetes mellitus, renal failure, alcoholism, silicosis, or any important immunologic deficiency. Patients with evidence of old, inadequately treated tuberculosis should also receive isoniazid for one year even if no progressive disease is apparent. If the patient has or is suspected to have active clinical (as opposed to subclinical) infection, he or she should receive therapy with two or more drugs, not isoniazid alone, even if the patient has no symptoms. Granulomas alone are not an indication for isoniazid prophylaxis, since there are numerous potential causes. *(Cecil, Ch. 302)*

45.(D) Amphotericin B is effective against all these fungi, but *Sporothrix schenckii* infections often respond to a less toxic drug: saturated solution of potassium iodide (SSKI). Lymphocutaneous sporotrichosis should initially be treated with SSKI. Amphotericin B is effective in many nonresponders. Amphotericin B therapy is clearly preferred to SSKI in disseminated infection; for pulmonary disease, there is no clear difference in response to these two agents. *(Cecil, Ch. 374; Mandell et al, pp. 264–266)*

46.(B) Flucytosine is an oral agent that has fungistatic activity against *Candida, Cryptococcus, Torulopsis,* and chromomycosis. Resistance emerges rapidly when flucytosine is used as a single agent, so it is usually used only in combination with amphotericin B; this combination of flucytosine and amphotericin B has synergy against some cryptococci and some *Candida.* The most convincing study was that of cryptococcal meningitis, which showed that flucytosine (150 mg/kg/day) plus amphotericin B (0.3 mg/kg/day) for six weeks was as effective as ten weeks of amphotericin B alone (0.4 mg/kg/day), and considerably less toxic. There is no convincing evidence that flucytosine contributes to clinical efficacy in regimens designed to treat *Candida* infections. *(Cecil, Chs. 373 and 375; Bennett et al)*

47.(C) *Trichinella spiralis* organisms burrow into the mucosa of the small bowel and disseminate via the lymphatics and bloodstream to virtually all organs. The larvae persist only in skeletal muscle fibers. Organisms can be seen in squash preparations or stained sections of skeletal muscle, but not in the bloodstream at the time of symptomatic muscle disease. A skin test and a bentonite flocculation test show evidence of disease, although they do not distinguish acute from chronic infection. False-positive bentonite flocculation tests do occur. *(Cecil, Ch. 411)*

48.(B) The common cold, a viral syndrome, is characterized as an acute coryza unassociated with fever. A heterogeneous group of viruses can cause the syndrome; no single agent is responsible for more than a small portion of cases. In order of frequency, the following viruses cause colds: picornaviruses (rhinoviruses), paramyxoviruses (parainfluenza and respiratory syncytial virus), myxoviruses (influenza A, B), coronaviruses, reoviruses, and adenoviruses. Rotaviruses do not cause respiratory diseases; they cause gastroenteritis, which usually occurs as acute febrile episodes with nausea, vomiting, cramps, and diarrhea, lasting five to eight days. *(Cecil, Ch. 329)*

49.(D) For individuals exposed by needle stick to a patient who is HBsAG positive, prophylaxis is indicated because of the likelihood of transmission. Two doses of HBIG are generally recommended to be given one month apart, though one dose may be effective. Hepatitis B immunization is not necessary to prevent disease due to the exposure, although some authorities recommend its use in conjunction with HBIG. Prophylactic measures should be instituted as soon as it is known that the patient is HB antigen positive and the injured individual is susceptible (HB antibody negative). *(Cecil, Ch. 121)*

50.(B) Herpetic whitlow, caused by herpes simplex, is an occupational hazard for anyone who puts a finger into the mouth of an individual with herpes simplex. Physicians, nurses, respiratory therapists, and dentists are most often affected, although the disease can be seen in non–health care workers as well. This viral process is often mistaken for a bacterial paronychia. Acyclovir may be effective therapy. *(Cecil, Ch. 340)*

51.(A—True; B—True; C—False; D—False; E—False) Infectious mononucleosis is caused by EBV, which is usually transmitted via oropharyngeal secretions, although transmission can occur by means of blood transfusion. EBV infection occurs more commonly in many developing countries than in developed countries. In developing countries infection is more likely to occur early in life and to be asymptomatic. Asymptomatic infection occurs twice as often as symptomatic infection, at least in middle-class college students. Once an individual is seropositive, he or she is a chronic EBV carrier and may shed the virus intermittently in secretions. *(Cecil, Ch. 342)*

52.(A—True; B—False; C—False; D—False; E—True) Azidothymidine, now known as zidovudine, has activity against certain retroviruses including HIV but not against other common human pathogens such as herpesviruses. In the initial controlled trial done with HIV-infected patients who had experienced one episode of *Pneumocystis* pneumonia, azidothymidine therapy was compared to placebo. Azidothymidine-treated patients had fewer serious opportunistic infections and deaths than did placebo-treated patients. *Pneumocystis* pneumonia continued to occur, however. Subsequent studies suggest that 40% of azidothymidine-treated patients will experience a second episode of *Pneumocystis* pneumonia during their first 12 months of therapy. Anemia has been a major sequela of azidothymidine therapy. *(Cecil, Ch. 346; Fischl et al)*

53.(A—True; B—True; C—True; D—False; E—True) Leprosy is caused by *Mycobacterium leprae.* About 15 million cases exist worldwide, especially in Africa and Asia. In the United States over 85% of cases have occurred in foreign-born individuals in recent years, but there are indigenous cases in Hawaii, Florida, Texas, and Louisiana. It is not clear if man is the only natural reservoir for the organism: certain armadillos and monkeys appear to be infected by *M. leprae.* Prolonged close exposure to a patient with leprosy does increase the likelihood of transmission. Household contacts of lepromatous leprosy patients have an eightfold increased likelihood of developing leprosy; household contacts of tuberculoid leprosy patients have a fourfold increase in susceptibility. *(Cecil, Ch. 304)*

54.(A—True; B—True; C—True; D—False; E—True) Primary tuberculosis refers to tuberculosis in an individual who was not previously infected with a virulent mycobacterium. Previously, primary tuberculosis was common among children; now it is being seen with increasing frequency among adults in the United States. Most primary infections are subclinical and cannot be detected by conventional radiology. The morbidity and mortality of primary infection are age-related: Mortality is much higher in infants than in older children and adults. In adults, primary disease is especially prone to progression and cavitation. *(Cecil, Ch. 302)*

55.(A—True; B—False; C—True; D—True; E—False) Isoniazid is the most important drug for antituberculosis therapy. It is bactericidal for actively multiplying mycobacteria. Primary resistance has remained at low levels in the United States for many years (about 2%) but is much higher in many areas of the developing world, including Asia, Africa, and South America. The drug is well absorbed and well tolerated, but 5% of patients treated with 5 mg/kg/day do develop adverse reactions. Peripheral neuropathy is a common adverse reaction, although it is unlikely to occur in well-nourished younger patients. It is more likely to be seen in slow acetylators and is preventable by pyridoxine administration. Transaminase elevations occur in at least 10% of patients treated with conventional doses of INH, particularly older patients and alcoholics. Transaminase elevations usually resolve during the first few weeks of therapy, but INH hepatitis can be severe or even fatal. *(Cecil, Ch. 302; Pratt and Fekety, pp. 281–288)*

56.(A—True; B—True; C—True; D—False; E—False) Brucellosis can be diagnosed by blood culture in 50–75% of untreated patients, but culturing the organism can be dangerous for laboratory personnel who do not have biosafety level 3 facilities available. When *Brucella* is suspected, the laboratory should be notified. The *Brucella* agglutination test is quite reliable: Within three weeks of illness, about 99% of patients will have serologic evidence of infection. The therapy of choice is a four- to six-week course of tetracycline, with streptomycin added for the initial two weeks to reduce the frequency of relapse. Penicillins and first-generation cephalosporins are generally ineffective. *(Cecil, Ch. 299)*

57.(A—True; B—False; C—True; D—False; E—False) *Nocardia* are aerobic organisms that are gram-positive and weakly acid-fast. Disease results from inhalation of organisms and has been reported in normal patients, patients with chronic obstructive pulmonary disease, and immunosuppressed patients. About 75% of cases present as pneumonia with fever and cough; central nervous system, skin, and subcutaneous involvement are common. The organism grows slowly on many routine media, but it may be overlooked because of overgrowth by normal flora. It is often recognized on fungal or mycobacterial media. The treatment of choice is a sulfonamide for weeks, months, or a year, depending on the clinical situation. Second drugs are often added. *(Cecil, Ch. 298)*

58.(All are False) Actinomycosis is a chronic suppurative and granulomatous disease caused by an anaerobic or facultative gram-positive non–acid-fast bacteria. Several species of *Actinomyces* are normal flora, so their isolation is not an indication of disease. They require mucous membrane disruption to cause diseases. *Actinomyces* abscess produces granules that contain central filaments of the organisms surrounded by an immune complex sheath. There is no serology generally available. Long courses of penicillin are the therapy of choice. *(Cecil, Ch. 297)*

59.(A—True; B—False; C—True; D—False; E—False) Anthrax is caused by a gram-positive bacillus that is acquired by contact with animals, animal products, or airborne particles created by processing animal products. From 1974–1983, the average annual occurrence in the United

States was 1.3 cases. Penicillin is the therapy of choice. About 20% of untreated cases are fatal, and less than 5% of treated cases are fatal. *(Cecil, Ch. 293)*

60.(A—True; B—False; C—True; D—False; E—True) Q fever is a self-limited rickettsial disease that often presents with fever and pulmonary infiltrates. The organism is transmitted by a tick vector to wild and domestic animals. Domestic animals have the organism in their milk and in placental tissue. Aerosolization from these sources can transmit the disease to other animals and humans. Humans appear to become infected from animal contact much more frequently than from ticks. Diagnosis is made by a complement fixation test. Few laboratories have the facilities to safely isolate the organism. Therapy of choice is tetracycline or chloramphenicol. *(Cecil, Ch. 327)*

61.(A—True; B—True; C—False; D—False; E—True) Spinal epidural abscesses have a clinical course that typically progresses through four phases: back pain, radicular pain, muscle weakness, and paralysis. Sensory loss often accompanies the motor loss. The cerebrospinal fluid below the level of the block shows normal glucose typically but almost always shows elevated protein and leukocytes. *Staphylococcus aureus* is the most common cause, but enteric gram-negative rods and streptococci are also recognized. Myelography is abnormal in all cases. *(Cecil, Ch. 481)*

62.(A—True; B—True; C—True; D—True; E—False) Malignant external otitis is a particular concern in diabetics who present with ear pain or purulent discharge. The infection, characteristically caused by *Pseudomonas aeruginosa*, spreads from the outer ear to the temporal bone and its surrounding tissues. Death is often the result of meningitis. Aminoglycoside and a penicillin with anti-*Pseudomonas* activity should be given. Surgery is often necessary to debride the area. *(Cecil, Ch. 481)*

63.(A—True; B—False; C—False; D—False; E—False) *Legionella* are gram-negative bacteria that can be grown on a variety of supplemented media. Over 11 species have been identified which cause disease in man. Two major syndromes occur: a pneumonia and a fever (Pontiac fever) which is unassociated with other organ system involvement. *Legionella* is usually transmitted from environmental sources. Human-to-human transmission has not been documented to occur. Organisms have been cultivated from blood and from a variety of extrapulmonary sources. Although the organism was recognized and named after a 1976 outbreak, the organism had been isolated in the 1940's, and retrospective serologic evidence suggests that infections have always occurred, although only in the past decade have diagnostic tests been available. *(Cecil, Ch. 267)*

64.(A—False; B—False; C—True; D—False; E—True) Aspiration pneumonia is typically caused by mixed aerobic and anaerobic flora from the oropharynx. Foul and purulent sputum can be seen, but it is not an invariable feature. A Gram stain of the sputum is useful for indicating the predominant organism, but a culture will reveal contaminating mouth flora as well as lower respiratory flora: Interpretation is almost impossible. Infiltrates may progress to abscess formation during the initial weeks of infection. Pleural effusions are not typically seen. The role for corticosteroid therapy remains controversial. *(Cecil, Ch. 266; Mandell et al, pp. 1349–1355)*

65.(A—False; B—False; C—True; D—True) Mucormycosis is an opportunistic fungus that causes rhinocerebral, pulmonary, gastrointestinal, cutaneous, and disseminated disease. Infection can be seen in diabetics, burn patients, and malnourished patients, and patients with a variety of intestinal disorders as well as in immunosuppressed patients. Amphotericin B has proven efficacy, but mortality is substantial in any patient population. *(Cecil, Ch. 377)*

66.(A—False; B—True; C—True; D—True; E—True) Paralytic poliomyelitis is caused by three distinct serotypes of poliovirus. About 5–32 cases are reported in the United States per year. Outbreaks occur among immigrants or among religious groups who do not believe in immunization. These infected individuals can transmit the virus to nonimmune individuals by hand-mouth contamination or respiratory spread. Asymptomatic infection commonly occurs. The oral vaccine is quite effective, but fecal excretion of virus poses a risk for secondary cases of polio. This does not occur with the killed vaccine. *(Cecil, Ch. 486)*

67.(A—True; B—False; C—True; D—True; E—False) Zoster and varicella are caused by the identical virus. Exposure to zoster can lead to varicella in the nonimmune host; the reverse rarely if ever occurs. Lesions typically crust over within 5–10 days of appearance. Because host defense depends on cell-mediated immune mechanisms, abnormal cell-mediated immunity is the major risk factor for dissemination. *(Cecil, Ch. 485)*

68.(A—False; B—True; C—True; D—False; E—True) Lyme disease is caused by a tick-borne spirochete and occurs in many areas of the United States, Europe, and Australia. Days to weeks after the tick bite, erythema chronicum migrans usually but not invariably occurs at the site of the bite. Within weeks or months, joint, cardiac, and neurologic sequelae may occur. Tetracycline is effective in eradicating erythema chronicum migrans and in preventing most major symptoms. *(Cecil, Ch. 435; Mandell et al, pp. 1343–1349)*

69.(All are True) Trachoma is a major cause of blindness worldwide, especially in arid areas of Africa and Asia. This chlamydial infection is spread by fingers, fomites, and perhaps flies. In the United States it is occasionally seen in a less severe form among immigrants and on Indian reservations. Tetracycline or erythromycin has a role in therapy as a topical or systemic agent. *(Cecil, Ch. 317)*

70.(A—True; B—True; C—False; D—False; E—False) *Mycoplasma* pneumonia occurs in all ages and is characterized clinically by the insidious onset of a severe paroxysmal cough. The chest roentgenogram is more impressive than the physical examination. Infiltrates are patchy and may be unilateral or bilateral. Pleural effusions are unusual on routine PA and lateral chest roentgenograms. The organism can be grown from respiratory secretions by laboratories that have special media available; the organism does not appear to be present in the blood. *Mycoplasma* pneumonia does not appear to occur with increased frequency or severity in immunosuppressed patients. *(Cecil, Ch. 264)*

71.(A—True; B—False; C—False; D—True; E—False) Dengue virus is an arthropod-borne virus transmitted by the *Aedes* mosquito. It is occurring with increasing frequency in the southern United States. The clinical syndrome characteristically consists of fever, prostration, myalgia, rash, lymphadenopathy, and leukopenia. The disease is usually self-limiting, and only supportive care is available for therapy. Death due to dengue is very unusual in the United States. Hemorrhagic fever can be a fatal form of the disease, however. Hemorrhagic fever is thought to be due to an immunologic reaction in previously infected individuals who were undoubtedly experiencing their first episode of dengue. *(Cecil, Ch. 353)*

72. (A—False; B—True; C—True; D—True; E—True) Tetanus is a clinical syndrome caused by the endotoxin elaborated by *Clostridium tetani.* Principles of therapy include debridement of the wound, eradication of organisms by penicillin or erythromycin therapy, and administration of human tetanus immunoglobulin. The last should be given prior to surgical debridement in case the surgical procedure releases more endotoxin into the circulation. An episode of tetanus does not produce immunity, so active immunization should be completed during the recovery period. *(Cecil, Ch. 281; Centers for Disease Control, 1985b)*

73. (A—True; B—False; C—True; D—True; E—True) In the United States, botulism is most often associated with home-canned foods. In Europe, meat and meat products are common vehicles, while in Japan, preserved fish is usually the responsible product. The incubation period is short. Gastrointestinal symptoms are common. Diplopia, dysphagia, and dry mouth are often the initial symptoms, followed by descending involvement of the motor neurons. *(Cecil, Ch. 280; Merson et al)*

74. (A—False; B—True; C—True; D—False; E—True) *Clostridium difficile* can be found in the stool of asymptomatic individuals, so its presence in the stool does not invariably have clinical implications. *C. difficile* toxin can induce diarrheal illness that can range in severity from mild to life-threatening. The disease can occur spontaneously as a community-acquired process or it can follow almost any antibiotic therapy, clindamycin being the most notorious. The preferred diagnostic test is the toxin assay. Oral vancomycin is the therapy of choice, but oral bacitracin and metronidazole are acceptable alternatives. *(Cecil, Ch. 279; Mandell et al, pp. 664–665)*

75. (A—True; B—True; C—False; D—True; E—True) Cryptosporidia are protozoa that occur in animals including cows. They are spread by fecal-oral contamination. There are occasional cases of diarrhea in travelers and in slaughterhouse workers due to this organism. In immunocompetent individuals the diarrhea is usually self-limiting. In AIDS patients, cryptosporidiosis is unusually common and severe. It is less commonly recognized in other immunosuppressed patients. Only rarely have cryptosporidia been found outside the bowel. There is no effective therapy. *(Cecil, Ch. 391)*

76. (A—True; B—True; C—False; D—True) Osteomyelitis is an infectious process that destroys bone. *Staphylococcus aureus* is responsible for more than 50% of cases, but gram-negative enteric organisms, *Salmonella,* and anaerobic organisms are also responsible for cases. Anaerobic bacteria are likely to cause disease near an anaerobic reservoir such as a sinus, a tooth, or the mastoids. In many developing countries, *Mycobacterium tuberculosis* is still a very common cause of bone infection, especially involving the spine. *(Cecil, Ch. 275)*

77. (A—False; B—True; C—False; D—False; E—False) Acyclovir is generally well tolerated. Thrombophlebitis can occur if the solution extravasates. Acyclovir is not highly soluble and can cause a crystalline nephropathy. Reversible renal dysfunction occurs in 6–25% of patients receiving high-dose therapy (30 mg/kg/day) for herpes zoster infections. Rash and neurologic abormalities are also reported. *(Cecil, Ch. 29; Mandell et al, p. 272)*

78. (A—False; B—False; C—True; D—True; E—False) Rabies can be transmitted to humans in the United States by dogs, bats, foxes, skunks, cats, and raccoons. Most cases are caused by wild animal bites, but rabid dogs along the U.S./Mexican border are a substantial source of concern. The incubation period is usually 20 to 60 days, although a range of 10 days to 19 years has been reported. Human recovery from documented rabies has been reported in very few patients. Infected humans often have rabies virus in their saliva and urine, so caution should be exercised in all patient contacts. For preexposure or postexposure prophylaxis, the human diploid vaccine is much safer than duck embryo vaccine and is therefore preferred. *(Cecil, Ch. 487)*

79. (A—True; B—True; C—False; D—True) Viral meningitis characteristically produces a cerebrospinal fluid that has 10 to 100 cells/mm^3 with a predominance of mononuclear cells. Early in the course of the disease, however, the cells may be predominantly neutrophils. Several thousand cells per mm^3 are occasionally seen in viral meningitides, but such a finding should raise the clinician's suspicions that a bacterial process is present. Coxsackie and echoviruses are spread by a fecal-oral route, and thus often spread from hand to mouth in families. Mumps is the most common recognized cause of viral meningitis. If lumbar punctures are performed on hospitalized patients with parotid swelling, 65% will have CSF abnormalities. *(Cecil, Ch. 484)*

80. (A—False; B—True; C—True; D—True; E—False) Entero-Vioform is toxic to the optic nerve; its efficacy is unproven, and thus it should never be used. Subsalicylate bismuth is effective in preventing traveler's diarrhea when 60 ml is taken four times daily, an impractical quantity to carry on a long trip. Doxycycline and trimethoprim-sulfamethoxazole have been shown to be effective in preventing diarrhea during short trips. Toxigenic *Escherichia coli,* the primary cause of traveler's diarrhea, is often resistant to these antibiotics, however, and each of these drugs has recognized adverse effects. Many physicians advocate care in choice of food and beverages and the judicious use of antimotility drugs rather than prophylactic antibiotics. *(Cecil, Ch. 260; Gorbach and Edelman)*

81. (A—True; B—True; C—False; D—True; E—False) For a witnessed in-hospital aspiration, an appropriate antibiotic regimen should include coverage of anaerobic organisms and gram-negative bacilli. Vancomycin and amikacin provide incomplete anaerobic coverage, although many oral anaerobes are susceptible to vancomycin. Piperacillin provides anaerobic coverage but only limited coverage of gram-negative bacilli. *(Cecil, Ch. 266)*

82. (A—True; B—True; C—True; D—True; E—False) Prosthetic valve endocarditis is often due to *Staphylococcus epidermidis* or diphtheroid species, particularly when the infection is recognized in the early postoperative period. Culture-negative endocarditis can occur in patients with native valves or prosthetic valves, but if the blood is cultured repeatedly with the patient off all antibiotics, the organism can usually be isolated in both patient populations. Prosthetic valve endocarditis characteristically responds to medical therapy alone when the infection occurs more than two months after surgery and is caused by a streptococcus. In other types of prosthetic valve endocarditis, surgery is probably needed. *(Cecil, Ch. 270)*

83. (A—False; B—True; C—True; D—True; E—True) Cat-scratch disease characteristically causes enlargement of single or multiple lymph nodes about two weeks after contact with an animal, usually a young cat. Diagnosis is established by a history of animal exposure, aspiration of sterile pus from the node, a positive test for cat-scratch antigen, and histopathology that reveals a pleomorphic rod with the Warthin-Starry silver stain. Antimicrobial therapy has not proved useful. *(Cecil, Ch. 300)*

84.(A—True; B—True; C—False; D—True; E—False) Encapsulated *Haemophilus influenzae* organisms cause invasive disease; almost all such infections are caused by type B, which does not cause community epidemics but does cause disease among susceptibles exposed to the index case, particularly among family members and children at daycare centers. Nonencapsulated hemophilus can cause localized infection, but rarely does bacteremia occur. Successful treatment of serious *H. influenzae* infections does not invariably lead to eradication of upper respiratory tract organisms. *Haemophilus* species other than influenza can occasionally cause other diseases such as chancroid (*Haemophilus ducreyi*), pneumonia, meningitis, endocarditis, and a wide variety of other processes. *(Cecil, Ch. 274)*

85.(A—True; B—False; C—True; D—True) Tuberculous lymphadenitis can be caused by typical or atypical organisms. Lymph node swelling may occur in the absence of systemic symptoms. It is preferable to remove a node for diagnosis, since aspiration often results in a chronic fistulous tract that may be difficult to heal. In adults, *Mycobacterium tuberculosis* is currently a more common cause of tuberculous cervical lymphadenitis than is *M. bovis,* but atypical mycobacteria (*M. scrofulaceum* and *M. avium-intracellulare*) are much more common, particularly in children. A role for drug therapy has not been clearly established. *(Cecil, Chs. 302 and 303)*

86.(A—True; B—False; C—True; D—False) About 60 to 80% of women who have sexual contact with an infected man will develop gonorrhea, compared with 20 to 30% of men who have sexual contact with an infected woman. About 50% of infected women are asymptomatic, compared with 10% of infected men. Before the use of antibiotics, the infection usually persisted for two to three months before host defenses eradicated the organism. *(Cecil, Ch. 306)*

87.(A—True; B—False; C—False; D—True; E—True) The treatment of choice for psittacosis is tetracycline. The incubation period for this disease is relatively short, 7 to 15 days. Diagnosis can be established by growing the organism in tissue culture, although such cultivation is hazardous to technical personnel. *(Cecil, Ch. 319)*

88.(A—True; B—True; C—False; D—False; E—False) Transmission of HIV among homosexual males correlates directly with the number of sexual partners and with the practice of receptive anal intercourse. Anonymous sexual partners and failure to use condoms probably increase the risk of transmission. No technique of sexual intercourse (active oral-genital, passive oral-genital, active genital-anal) is "safe": Any method can probably be associated with HIV transmission, although receptive anal intercourse probably transmits the virus most efficiently. Although there has been considerable speculation about what role recreational drugs have played in the transmission of HIV or in its subsequent clinical manifestations, no convincing link has been demonstrated. Heterosexual intercourse does not appear to be as efficient for transmitting the HIV as is homosexual rectal intercourse, but male-to-female and female-to-male spread does occur when genital-vaginal intercourse is practiced. The ELISA test for HIV is a very sensitive screening test for blood products, but current technology does not allow 100% sensitivity: some individuals will still, unfortunately, become infected from HIV-infected blood and other biologic products in the United States. *(Cecil, Ch. 346; Friedland and Klein)*

89.(All are False) Congenital syphilis does not cause syphilitic aortitis—this is an unexplained phenomenon. Calcification in the arch of the aorta suggests arteriosclerosis; syphilis causes linear calcifications in the *ascending* aorta. Syphilitic aortitis does not cause dissection and is associated with neurosyphilis in only 10 to 25% of cases. Dilatation of the ascending aorta stretches the aortic valve ring, causing aortic incompetence, not stenosis. *(Cecil, Ch. 310)*

90.(A—True; B—False; C—True; D—False) This patient probably has allergic bronchopulmonary aspergillosis. Such patients usually have eosinophilia, and precipitins to *Aspergillus* are present in serum. CIE has not yet been proved useful for routine detection of *Aspergillus* antigens. Endobronchial colonization with *Aspergillus* does not respond to systemic administration of amphotericin B. *(Cecil, Ch. 376)*

91.(All are True) Amantadine has been shown to be effective in preventing influenza during epidemics in highly susceptible groups such as elderly inpatients. Thiosemicarbazone may be effective as a prophylactic agent after exposure to smallpox. Ara-A can reduce mortality and sequelae in herpes simplex encephalitis if used early, before coma supervenes. Idoxuridine is useful in topical therapy of herpes keratitis (dendritic ulcer). *(Cecil, Ch. 340)*

92.(All are True) In the well-known Oslo Study, 2000 untreated patients with syphilis were followed over a period of 60 years (1891–1951). One or more relapses of secondary syphilis occurred in about 25% of these cases. One third of all patients developed tertiary syphilis. The majority with tertiary disease had gummas involving skin, mucous membrane, or skeleton; about 10% had cardiovascular syphilis; and about 7% developed neurosyphilis. *(Cecil, Ch. 482)*

93.(A—True; B—True; C—False; D—True) Rotaviruses are probably the most common cause of acute gastroenteritis in small children. Rotavirus may affect neonates, is most common between 6 and 24 months of age, and is unusual after 4 years of age. The disease is most common in winter (it is sometimes called "winter vomiting disease") and may occur sporadically or in epidemics. Incubation period during epidemics is one to four days. Fecal leukocytes are usually absent; this helps to differentiate acute viral gastroenteritis from shigellosis. *(Cecil, Ch. 335)*

94.(C); 95.(A); 96.(D); 97.(B); 98.(E) Cutaneous leishmaniasis is caused by a protozoon that involves the skin and mucous membranes. Although work is being done on skin tests and serologies, the diagnosis must be established by biopsy of the lesion. *Diphyllobothrium latum* causes a cestode infection that is confined to the intestinal tract; diagnosis is established by recognizing eggs or proglottids in the stool. Amebic liver abscesses can be diagnosed by aspiration of the abscess, but a positive amebic serology in a patient with a liver abscess is highly suggestive, particularly in a North American patient. *Babesia* species are intraerythrocytic protozoa; diagnosis should be made by thick or thin peripheral blood smears stained with Giemsa technique. Enterobiasis, or pinworm, can be detected on stool exam, but the best technique is to identify ova outside the anus when the patient arises from sleep. *(Cecil, Chs. 384, 389, 393, and 409)*

99.(C); 100.(E); 101.(A); 102.(B); 103.(D) For *Streptococcus viridans* endocarditis involving native (in contrast to prosthetic) heart valves, high-dose penicillin for four weeks or penicillin with streptomycin for two weeks is adequate therapy. For *S. faecalis* endocarditis, ampicillin plus gentamicin for four to six weeks is required, since *S. faecalis* is not nearly as penicillin-sensitive as many *S. viridans.* It should be noted, however, that some viridans streptococci can be relatively resistant to penicillin so that determinations of minimum inhibitory concentrations of penicillin can be useful in guiding therapy. Since many *Staphylococcus aureus* are penicillin-resistant, penicillin may not be adequate therapy. Nafcillin is the drug of choice until the susceptibility pattern of the isolate is determined. For endocarditis of unknown cause, coverage of *S. aureus, S. faecalis,* and *S. viridans* is necessary, utilizing a three-drug regimen. *Candida* endocarditis has a poor prognosis with any therapy. Most authorities recommend prompt valve replacement as well as long courses of amphotericin B. *(Cecil, Ch. 270; Mandell et al, pp. 504–538)*

104.(B); 105.(C); 106.(D); 107.(E); 108.(A) For urinary sepsis, the pathogens of major concern are *Streptococcus faecalis* and gram-negative bacilli. Vancomycin provides activity against *S. faecalis,* while gentamicin provides excellent coverage for gram-negative bacilli. For neutropenic cancer patients, piperacillin and tobramycin provide broad-spectrum gram-positive and gram-negative acitivity with particularly good coverage of *Pseudomonas aeruginosa.* In healthy adults with diffuse pneumonias, major etiologic considerations are *Mycoplasma* and *Legionella,* which are adequately treated by erythromycin. For meningitis of unknown cause in a college student, meningococcus is the major concern, with *Haemophilus influenza* and *Streptococcus pneumoniae* being other considerations. High-dose penicillin or high-dose ampicillin or chloramphenicol, or some combination thereof, is the therapy of choice. Ketoconazole is effective therapy for mucosal *Candida. (Cecil, Chs. 28, 258, 262, 272, 346, and 375)*

109.(F); 110.(B); 111.(A); 112.(D); 113.(C); 114.(E) *Clostridium difficile* is a bowel organism that causes a range of gastrointestinal manifestations varying from asymptomatic carriage to fulminant pseudomembranous colitis. *Pneumocystis* involves only the lungs and causes pneumonia in immunosuppressed patients. *Sporothrix schenckii* causes skin and lymph node disease after inoculation of the organism, often after handling plants. *Leishmania donovani* is a protozoon that involves the bone marrow, liver, and spleen after infection by the bite of a *Phlebotomus. Ochocerca volvulus* transmitted by the simulian fly manifests as nodules containing adult worms in the soft tissues and microfilariae that migrate through skin and corneas. Yellow fever virus causes characteristic histopathologic changes in the liver as well as hemorrhages and petechiae of mucous membranes. *(Cecil, Chs. 279, 361, 374, 384, 386, and 413)*

115.(B); 116.(G); 117.(C); 118.(A); 119.(A); 120.(E) Brucellosis is optimally treated with tetracycline for four to six weeks. The addition of streptomycin will reduce relapse rates. Leptospirosis will probably have a shorter course if tetracycline is administered during the first two to four days of illness. Penicillin may also be effective, although there is less documented experience with this drug. For tularemia, aminoglycosides are recommended, although tetracycline and chloramphenicol are also useful. High-dose penicillin or ampicillin is the mainstay of therapy for listeriosis, although *Listeria* are often sensitive to a wide variety of antibiotics. Conventional therapy to eradicate *Corynebacterium diphtheriae* from the nasopharynx is penicillin or erythromycin, although other agents may be effective. For leprosy, dapsone and rifampin are important therapeutic agents, usually used in combination with clofazimine. *(Cecil, Chs. 277, 292, 295, 299, and 316)*

121.(A); 122.(A); 123.(A); 124.(A); 125.(B) Hard ticks are vectors of several diseases of medical importance, including several arboviral hemorrhagic fevers and encephalitides, tick-borne typhus, tularemia, babesiosis, and Lyme disease. Hard ticks also cause tick paralysis. Soft ticks are of medical concern primarily because they can transmit *Borrelia,* the cause of relapsing fever. Centipedes and lice do not transmit these infectious diseases. *(Cecil, Ch. 414; Mandell et al, pp. 1589–1595)*

126.(C); 127.(A); 128.(A); 129.(A); 130.(B); 131.(D) Diphtheria, polio, and hepatitis A all occur commonly in the developing world. Anyone living or visiting there should be protected. Yellow fever exists only in areas adjacent to the equator in the continents of Africa and South America. There is no reason to receive yellow fever vaccine if the traveler is not going to be in those areas. Tetanus is a problem worldwide. In contrast, smallpox no longer exists in the world, and no one should be subjected to the complications of the vaccine unless he or she is going to have exposure in a research laboratory. *(Cecil, Ch. 261)*

132.(D); 133.(B); 134.(A); 135.(E); 136.(F); 137.(C) Oral leukoplakia presents as whitish, smooth lesions on the lateral aspects of the tongue and is probably caused by Epstein-Barr virus and papillomavirus. *Mycobacterium avium-intracellulare* can be cultivated from at least 40% of patients with AIDS. Blood cultures, using a radiometric or lysis-centrifugation technique, can frequently demonstrate a persistent bacteremia for many months prior to death. Aseptic meningitis, fever, malaise, and lethargy can be recognized within 3–14 days after acquisition of HIV infection in some patients. Clinical manifestations are usually self-limited within days or a few weeks. Toxoplasmosis is almost always confined to the central nervous system in AIDS patients, although retinitis and disseminated disease have been reported. The clinical presentation is usually that of a cerebral inflammatory mass lesion. Cytomegalovirus infection is present in almost all AIDS patients, especially those who are homosexual or bisexual. The role of cytomegalovirus in causing the fever, weight loss, and inanition associated with AIDS is still being delineated, but CMV is by far the most common cause of retinitis among AIDS patients. For reasons that are not currently clear, Kaposi's sarcoma is almost never recognized among AIDS patients who are not homosexual or bisexual. *(Cecil, Ch. 346)*

138.(B); 139.(B); 140.(C); 141.(D); 142.(D); 143.(A) Croup is a viral infection of the upper and lower respiratory tract that occurs only in children. Parainfluenza viruses are the most common causes. The other diseases listed occur in all age groups. Bronchitis is most often viral in etiology, though bacterial infections as primary or secondary agents do occur. Pharyngitis can be caused by viruses, but *Streptococcus pyogenes* is a common cause. All of these infectious processes involving the upper respiratory tract must be distinguished from acute epiglottitis, which is often caused by *Haemophilus influenzae* type b and may require emergency tracheostomy. *(Cecil, Chs. 274 and 330; Mandell et al, pp. 355–375)*

144–148. *(Cecil, Chs. 268 and 269)* **144.(B); 145.(C)** Nephritogenic strains of group A streptococcus cause impetigo and pharyngitis; in contrast, rheumatogenic strains cause only pharyngitis. Thus, glomerulonephritis can follow either pharyngitis or skin infection, but acute rheumatic fever follows pharyngitis only.

146.(A) Treatment of streptococcal pharyngitis with penicillin is effective in preventing rheumatic fever, and this protective effect lasts for several weeks after the acute pharyngitis. Penicillin does not prevent glomerulonephritis.

147.(C) Both acute rheumatic fever and poststreptococcal glomerulonephritis are thought to be immune-mediated diseases, although the responsible streptococcal antigen has not been identified.

148.(A) Patients who have had rheumatic fever are at high risk of developing recurrent disease following significant streptococcal upper respiratory tract disease. Thus, patients with acute rheumatic fever require continuous prophylaxis to prevent recurrences. Because recurrent episodes of glomerulonephritis are extremely rare, prophylaxis is not needed.

149–153. *(Cecil, Chs. 272, 295, and 481)* **149.(D)** The most common causes of fungal meningitis include *Cryptococcus, Coccidioides,* and *Candida. Candida* will be cultured; however, cryptococcal and coccidioidal meningitis are usually diagnosed with serologic testing of the CSF for the antigen of *Cryptococcus* and the antibody for *Coccidioides,* present in more than 90% of cases.

150.(B) Bacterial meningitis is almost always diagnosed by CSF culture (exceptions include *Listeria monocytogenes* meningitis in which blood cultures are positive but CSF is negative, and partially treated bacterial meningitis). The CSF pleocytosis is predominantly PMN's, and the CSF glucose is decreased. Early diagnosis of pneumococcal, meningococcal, and *Haemophilus influenzae* meningitis can be made rapidly with counterimmunoelectrophoresis.

151.(A) Aseptic viral meningitis is usually caused by the enteroviruses, which are rarely cultured from CSF. CSF pleocytosis shows lymphocytes predominantly, although some PMN's can be seen early in the course of a viral meningitis.

152.(E) Brain abscess can cause irritation of the meninges and produces the CSF findings described in E. Spinal tap carries a risk in a patient with a brain abscess, and deaths associated with brain herniation have been described. Unless the abscess ruptures into the CSF, information obtained from the CSF (culture, cell count, and chemical tests) is generally of little help.

153.(C) Tuberculous meningitis may be difficult to diagnose, since acid-fast stains are usually negative and culture of the CSF is positive in only about 50% of cases. Since several weeks are needed for the culture data, the acute illness is often misdiagnosed. The diagnosis should be suspected with CSF data as described in C.

154–159. *(Cecil, Chs. 305–310; Mandell et al, pp. 712–748)* **154.(E)** Lymphogranuloma venereum typically causes marked inguinal adenopathy with suppuration, discharging sinuses, and associated systemic symptoms. Late complications include chronic fibrosis, rectal strictures, and lymphatic obstruction. The LGV chlamydiae may be treated with sulfonamide or tetracycline.

155.(A) This is a classic description of a primary syphilitic chancre. Syphilis, which is now relatively common among promiscuous male homosexuals, should be suspected in all cases of genital or perianal ulceration. Even when the lesions are not typical, dark-field examination and serology are usually advisable to exclude this diagnosis. Inguinal adenopathy is often absent in the presence of a rectal chancre.

156.(B) Multiple shallow, painful ulcers with a strong tendency to recurrence are typical of genital herpes, caused by herpes simplex virus type 2. This distressing disease has increased greatly in frequency in the past 10 years.

157.(D) Chancroid is caused by *Haemophilus ducreyi.* It is characterized by painful, nonindurated ulcers with associated enlarged inguinal nodes, which frequently suppurate. Coexisting syphilis should always be carefully excluded, after which chancroid may be treated with sulfisoxazole.

158.(F) Granuloma inguinale is an indolent granulomatous and ulcerative disease caused by a pleomorphic coccobacillus, *Calymmatobacterium granulomatis,* which is related to *Klebsiella.* These bacilli may be seen within monocytes in scrapings from the genital lesion. After coexisting syphilis has been excluded, this infection may be treated with tetracycline.

159.(C) Scrotal ulcers, often associated with oral ulcerations, venous thromboses, and inflammation of the eye, suggest Behçet's syndrome. This is a vasculitis of unknown etiology that may be associated with a wide spectrum of additional manifestations, including arthritis and gastrointestinal symptoms.

160.(D) Wounds infected with methicillin-resistant *S. aureus* are a risk to other patients, primarily owing to spread via the hands and clothing of hospital personnel. Thus, gloving, gowning, and careful handwashing are sufficient isolation procedures when patient contact is involved. *(Cecil, Ch. 260)*

161.(B) Pulmonary tuberculosis is spread by respiratory droplets, especially when pulmonary cavities or laryngeal involvement is present, which characteristically contain high numbers of organisms. Masks, private room, and strict handwashing are adequate precautions, with masks necessary only to prevent gross contamination by secretions not carefully handled by the patient. *(Cecil, Ch. 260)*

162.(C) Hepatitis A virus is spread primarily by stool. Careful handwashing is adequate for contact with most patients. If patient hygiene is poor, a private room and gowning are recommended. Gloves should be used for contact with infective material. *(Cecil, Ch. 260; Mandell et al, pp. 1608–1609)*

163.(B) Meningococcal infection is spread by close respiratory contact. Thus, the use of masks, a private room, and careful handwashing are appropriate. *(Cecil, Ch. 260)*

164.(A) Susceptible individuals can acquire varicella from patients with herpes zoster. The route of spread is primarily through direct or close contact with the lesion. Respiratory spread is not nearly so likely with localized as with disseminated zoster, probably because less skin and no mucous membrane are usually involved. For immunosuppressed patients, strict isolation is needed for zoster that is either localized or disseminated. *(Mandell et al, p. 959)*

165.(B) Measles is highly contagious. Virus is present in nasopharyngeal secretions early in the course of infection, and epidemiologic evidence is clear that spread is via the respiratory route. Thus, masks, a private room, and handwashing are necessary. *(Cecil, Ch. 260)*

166.(E) Hepatitis B virus is present in blood, less often in stool or other body secretions. The use of gloves when handling or drawing blood and careful handwashing are adequate precautions. A private room is not necessary unless the patient's hygiene is poor. *(Cecil, Ch. 260)*

167. (C); 168. (D); 169. (E); 170. (B) Most patients with syphilis will recognize a chancre 10 to 90 days after exposure if the lesion is on the penis. Rectal or vaginal lesion may produce no symptoms or signs and thus may not be noted by the patient. Secondary syphilis generally appears four to eight weeks after the chancre appears. The incubation period of LGV has been less carefully studied but appears to be several days to several weeks. Gonorrhea usually presents as a symptomatic process relatively soon after exposure, generally two to six days after contact. *(Cecil, Chs. 305–307, 309, and 310)*

BIBLIOGRAPHY

Bennett JE, Dismukes WE, Duma RJ, et al: A collaborative study comparing amphotericin B-5-fluorocytosine versus amphotericin B alone in the treatment of cryptococcal meningitis. N Engl J Med 301:126, 1979.

Bennett JV, Brachman PS: Hospital Infections. 2nd ed. Boston, Little, Brown and Company, 1986.

Braude AI, Davis CE, Fierer J (eds): Infectious Diseases and Medical Microbiology. 2nd ed. Philadelphia, W.B. Saunders Company, 1986.

Bryan JP, Rocha H, Scheld WM: Problems in salmonellosis: Rationale for trials with newer beta lactam agents and quinolones. Rev Infect Dis 89:189–207, 1986.

Cecil Textbook of Medicine. 18th ed. Wyngaarden JB, Smith LH Jr (eds). Philadelphia, W.B. Saunders Company, 1988.

Centers for Disease Control: 1985 STD treatment guidelines. MMWR 34(45):755, 1985a.

Centers for Disease Control: Diphtheria, tetanus, and pertussis: Guidelines for vaccine prophylaxis and other preventive measures. Ann Intern Med 103:896–905, 1985b.

DeVita VT, Broder S, Fauci AS, et al: Developmental therapeutics and the acquired immunodeficiency syndrome. Ann Intern Med 106:568–581, 1987.

Dinarello CA, Wolfe SM: Molecular basis of fever in humans. Am J Med 72:799, 1982.

Edwards JE (moderator): Severe candidal infections. Clinical perspective, immune defense mechanisms, and current concepts of therapy. Ann Intern Med 88:91, 1978.

Fields BN, et al (eds): Virology. New York, Raven Press, 1985.

Fischl M, Richman D, Grieco MH, et al: The efficacy of azidothymidine (AZT) in the treatment of patients with AIDS and AIDS-related complex. N Engl J Med 317:185–191, 1987.

Friedland GH, Klein RS: Transmission of human immunodeficiency virus. N Engl J Med 317:1125–1135, 1987.

Gallin JI, Fauci AS (eds): Advances in Host Defense Mechanisms. Vol. 5, Acquired Immunodeficiency Syndrome (AIDS). New York, Raven Press, 1985.

Gorbach SL, Edelman R: Travelers diarrhea: National Institutes of Health Consensus Development Conference. Rev Infect Dis 1986, Suppl 2.

Karchmer AW, Archer GL, Dismukes WE: *Staphylococcus epidermidis* causing prosthetic valve endocarditis: Microbiologic and clinical observations as guides to therapy. Ann Intern Med 98:447, 1983.

Kovacs JA, Hiemenz JW, Macher AM, et al: *Pneumocystis carinii* pneumonia: A comparison between patients with the acquired immunodeficiency syndrome and patients with other immunodeficiencies. Ann Intern Med 100:663, 1984.

Mandell GL, Douglas RG, Bennett JE: Principles and Practice of Infectious Diseases. 2nd ed. New York, John Wiley & Sons, 1985.

Matthay RA, Moritz ED: Invasive procedures for diagnosing pulmonary infection—a critical review. Clin Chest Med 2:3, 1981.

Merson MH, Hughes JM, Dowell VR, et al: Current trends in botulism in the United States. JAMA 229:1305, 1974.

Morbidity and Mortality Weekly Report: General recommendations on immunizations. 32:1, 1983.

Pearson RD, Guerrant RL: Praziquantel: A major advance in anthelminthic therapy. Ann Intern Med 34(45):755, 1985.

Peltola H: Meningococcal disease: Still with us. Rev Infect Dis 5:71, 1983.

Popp RL: Echocardiography and infectious endocarditis. *In* Remington JS, Swartz MN (eds): Current Clinical Topics in Infectious Diseases, Vol. 4. New York, McGraw-Hill Book Company, 1983, p 98.

Pratt WB, Fekety R: The Antimicrobial Drugs. New York, Oxford University Press, 1986.

Quinn TC, Stamm WE, Goodall SE, et al: The polymicrobial origin of intestinal infections in homosexual men. N Engl J Med 309:576, 1983.

Rahal JJ, Simberkoff MS: Host defense and antimicrobial therapy in gram-negative bacillary meningitis. Ann Intern Med 96:468, 1982.

Richman DD, Fischl MA, Grieco MH: The toxicity of azidothymidine (AZT) in the treatment of patients with AIDS and AIDS-related complex. N Engl J Med 317:192–197, 1987.

Rinaldi MG: Invasive aspergillosis. Rev Infect Dis 5:1061, 1983.

Salter AJ: Trimethoprim-sulfamethoxazole: An assessment of more than 12 years of use. Rev Infect Dis 4:190, 1982.

Seef LB, Koff RS: Passive and active immunoprophylaxis of hepatitis B. Gastroenterology 86:958, 1984.

Spagnuolo PJ, Ellner JJ, Lerner PI, et al: *Haemophilus influenzae* meningitis; the spectrum of disease in adults. Medicine 61:74, 1982.

Wise RI, Kory M (eds): Reassessments of vancomycin—a potentially useful antibiotic. Rev Infect Dis 3:S199, 1981.

Wolinsky E: Non-tuberculous mycobacteria in pulmonary disease. Am Rev Respir Dis 119:107, 1979.

PART 9

CLINICAL IMMUNOLOGY AND RHEUMATOLOGY

JOHN B. IMBODEN, JR.

DIRECTIONS: For questions 1 to 31, choose the ONE BEST answer to each question.

1. A 40-year-old woman has seropositive rheumatoid arthritis. Six months ago, she had several hours of morning stiffness despite optimal salicylate therapy, and gold therapy was begun. Although other joints have improved substantially, she has had persisting synovitis in the dorsum of the right wrist. Four weeks ago, synovial fluid from the right wrist revealed 8000 white blood cells/mm³. Cultures for bacteria, mycobacteria, and fungi showed no growth. Physical examination now shows boggy synovial swelling over the right wrist, unchanged over four weeks. Which of the following is the most appropriate next step?

A. Continue the current regimen
B. Continue current regimen and inject the right wrist with triamcinolone
C. Discontinue gold and begin penicillamine
D. Perform a biopsy of the synovium of the right wrist
E. Discontinue gold and start methotrexate

2. Each of the following is a roentgenographic feature of chondrocalcinosis EXCEPT

A. linear calcification of the symphysis pubis
B. narrowing of the radiocarpal joint
C. juxta-articular demineralization
D. knee involvement restricted to the patellofemoral compartment
E. osteophytosis

3. A 28-year-old man has an eight-month history of pain and swelling of the right knee without antecedent trauma. Arthrocentesis on three separate occasions yielded bloody, nonclotting synovial fluid; white blood cell count was less than 1000/mm³. Cultures of synovial fluid for bacteria, fungi, and mycobacteria showed no growth. The patient is otherwise well and has no history of a bleeding diathesis. Physical examination now shows a moderately swollen right knee which is not tender; the examination is otherwise normal. The knee is stable and has a nearly full range of motion. Which of the following is most likely to be of value in establishing a diagnosis?

A. Arthrogram of the right knee
B. Tuberculin skin test
C. Test for HLA-B27
D. Determination of bleeding time
E. Determination of partial thromboplastin time

4. You are asked to see a 35-year-old man who developed proximal muscle weakness four months ago, associated with marked elevations in muscle enzymes. A muscle biopsy was consistent with polymyositis. Prednisone, 60 mg daily, was prescribed, and over the next six weeks all muscle enzymes became normal. Initially there was a substantial improvement in strength. Over the past two months, however, the proximal muscle weakness has become progressively worse despite continuation of prednisone. Muscle enzymes have stayed normal. On physical examination, the patient has a cushingoid appearance; there is significant proximal muscle weakness, particularly of the lower extremities. Which of the following is the most appropriate next step?

A. Decrease the prednisone dose to 40 mg daily
B. Continue prednisone, 60 mg daily, and begin azathioprine, 2 mg/kg/day
C. Continue prednisone, 60 mg daily, and begin methotrexate, 10 mg orally every week
D. Increase the prednisone dose to 80 mg daily
E. Continue prednisone, 60 mg daily, and begin cyclophosphamide 2 mg/kg/day

5. Which of the following is most likely to be observed in a patient with mixed essential cryoglobulinemia?

A. Glomerulonephritis
B. Palpable purpura
C. Cold intolerance
D. Evidence of prior hepatitis B infection
E. Normal serum complement levels

6. Each of the following is characteristic of Behçet's disease EXCEPT

A. meningoencephalitis
B. erosive arthritis
C. mucosal ulceration of the ileum
D. recurrent thrombophlebitis
E. painless vaginal ulcers

7. A 30-year-old man has had pain and stiffness in his lower back for a year. The pain is particularly bad in the morning but improves as the day progresses. He has no other symptoms. Physical examination shows loss of lumbar lordosis and limited range of motion of the lumbar spine. Which of the following is most likely to be observed on roentgenograms of the pelvis and lumbosacral spine?

A. Bilateral sacroiliitis
B. L2-L3 disk space narrowing

C. Spondylolisthesis of L4 on L5
D. Ossification of the anterior longitudinal ligament at the level of the lumbar spine
E. No detectable abnormality

8. A patient with rheumatoid arthritis was initially given gold sodium thiomalate, 10 mg intramuscularly, without reaction, then received 50 mg weekly. Blood count and urinalysis remained normal. After the third injection of gold, however, she immediately became lightheaded and felt flushed. These symptoms abated within 10 minutes. Which of the following should be done?

A. Continue gold sodium thiomalate, 50 mg weekly
B. Decrease the dose to 25 mg weekly
C. Discontinue gold sodium thiomalate and begin aurothioglucose, 50 mg weekly
D. Discontinue gold sodium thiomalate and begin penicillamine, 250 mg daily
E. Admit patient to the hospital for observation

9. A 47-year-old man is referred to you after a three-month history of sinusitis unresponsive to decongestants and antibiotics. He has had several episodes of serous otitis media as well. During this time he has lost 20 pounds. Physical examination now reveals saddle-nose deformity; the patient is afebrile and appears chronically ill. Blood pressure is 150/100 mm Hg. Roentgenograms of the sinus show opacification of both maxillary sinuses. Roentgenogram of the chest reveals an ill-defined infiltrate in the right lower lobe. Urinalysis shows 3+ proteinuria; microscopic examination of the urine sediment reveals red cells, white cells, granular casts, and occasional red cell casts. Serum creatinine is 1.8 mg/dl. The patient is admitted to the hospital and remains afebrile. Cultures of sputum show only normal flora. Nasal biopsies demonstrate acute and chronic inflammation. A percutaneous renal biopsy reveals a crescentic, proliferative glomerulonephritis without evidence of vasculitis. Which of the following is the most appropriate next step?

A. Begin prednisone, 60 mg daily
B. Begin cyclophosphamide, 2 mg/kg/day
C. Begin prednisone, 60 mg daily, and cyclophosphamide, 2 mg/kg/day
D. Begin cyclophosphamide, 2 mg/kg/day, and perform daily plasmapheresis
E. Perform transbronchial biopsy of the right lower lobe

10. In a patient with psoriatic arthritis and distal interphalangeal joint involvement, which of the following is most likely to be observed?

A. HLA-B27
B. Psoriatic nail changes
C. Asymmetric sacroiliitis
D. Rheumatoid factor in a titer of 1:160
E. Absence of articular involvement elsewhere

11. A 55-year-old man has had recurrent episodes of right shoulder pain over the past two years. For the past two weeks he has had progressively worsening pain in the right shoulder, to the point that he dresses with severe discomfort. There is no history of trauma. Examination of the right shoulder reveals tenderness localized at a point 2 to 3 cm distal to the acromium. Active abduction is limited to 60 degrees by pain, but there is full passive range of motion of the shoulder. The remainder of the musculoskeletal examination shows modest reduction in extension of the cervical spine; it is otherwise normal. Which of the following is the most appropriate next step?

A. Injection of the right glenohumoral joint with triamcinolone, 20 mg
B. Injection of the right subdeltoid bursa with triamcinolone, 20 mg
C. Arthrogram of the right shoulder
D. Roentgenogram of the cervical spine, with anteroposterior and oblique views
E. Order active range of motion exercises

12. Each of the following predisposes to the development of hyperuricemia and/or gout EXCEPT

A. hydrochlorothiazide therapy
B. polycythemia vera
C. chronic high-dose aspirin therapy
D. habitual ingestion of "moonshine" alcohol
E. psoriasis

13. In which one of the following are reducible "swan-neck" deformities (flexion at the distal interphalangeal joints and hyperextension at the proximal interphalangeal joints) characteristically found?

A. Dermatomyositis
B. Reiter's syndrome
C. Psoriatic arthritis
D. Rheumatoid arthritis
E. Systemic lupus erythematosus

14. Each of the following is a roentgenographic feature of neuropathic arthropathy (Charcot joints) EXCEPT

A. subarticular sclerosis
B. heterotopic calcification
C. erosions at the joint margins
D. joint effusion
E. subluxation

15. Each of the following is a side effect of nonsteroidal anti-inflammatory drugs EXCEPT

A. hyperkalemia
B. nephrotic syndrome
C. acute renal failure
D. nephrogenic diabetes insipidus
E. allergic interstitial nephritis

16. Each of the following is associated with an increased incidence of osteonecrosis EXCEPT

A. alcohol abuse
B. deep-sea diving
C. sickle cell disease
D. exposure to vinyl chloride
E. iatrogenic Cushing's syndrome

17. Which one of the following distinguishes lymphokine-activated (LAK) cells from antigen-specific T lymphocytes?

A. Expression of the cell-surface marker T3 (CD3)
B. The ability to lyse target cells
C. The ability to proliferate in vitro
D. The ability to recognize targets across HLA barriers
E. Expression of T11 (sheep red blood cell receptor)

18. In a patient with sarcoidosis of recent onset, who has bilateral hilar adenopathy and erythema nodosum, which of the following is most likely to be observed?

A. Monoarticular arthritis involving the wrist

B. Oligoarticular arthritis of the lower extremities with prominent knee effusions
C. Painful periarthritis and tenosynovitis involving the ankles and knees
D. Asymptomatic cysts of the phalanges and metatarsal heads
E. Bilateral sacroiliitis

19. Which of the following is most characteristic of synovial fluid obtained from a patient with active rheumatoid arthritis?

A. White blood cell count 40,000/mm^3, 80% mononuclear cells; complement normal
B. White blood cell count 20,000/mm^3, 70% polymorphonuclear cells; complement low
C. White blood cell count 15,000/mm^3, 70% mononuclear cells; complement low
D. White blood cell count 10,000/mm^3, 70% polymorphonuclear cells; complement normal
E. White blood cell count 1,000/mm^3, 80% polymorphonuclear leukocytes; complement normal

20. Which of the following is most likely to be associated with anaphylactic reactions to infusion of blood products?

A. Thymic hypoplasia (DiGeorge's syndrome)
B. Hyperimmunoglobulinemia E syndrome
C. Selective IgA deficiency
D. Adenosine deaminase deficiency
E. Purine nucleoside phosphorylase deficiency

21. A patient with progressive systemic sclerosis has blood pressure of 180/120 mm Hg; serum creatinine is 2.5 mg/dl. Which of the following is the most likely associated finding?

A. Urinary protein excretion of 6.2 g/24 hours
B. Microangiopathic appearance on peripheral blood smear
C. Absence of sclerodermatous skin changes
D. Hypocomplementemia
E. Elevated antiribonucleoprotein (RNP) antibody titer

22. Each of the following occurs in relapsing polychondritis EXCEPT

A. aortic regurgitation
B. saddle-nose deformity
C. tracheal stenosis
D. erythema and swelling of the ear lobe
E. arthralgias

23. A 73-year-old woman with a long history of hypertension has a three-week history of steady right-sided headache. She has lost 5 pounds in two weeks. For the past 24 hours, she has noted decreasing visual acuity in the right eye. Blood pressure is 170/90 mm Hg. The temporal arteries are slightly tender. The right eye has a diminished light response; there is pallor and edema of the optic disc. The erythrocyte sedimentation rate (Westergren) is 88 mm/hour. The most appropriate next step is to

A. begin prednisone, 20 mg orally daily
B. begin prednisone, 20 mg orally three times daily
C. perform carotid angiography
D. perform head computed tomography
E. perform a right temporal artery biopsy

24. A 68-year-old woman who is a chronic user of aspirin accidentally overdoses and has a salicylate level of 81 mg/dl (therapeutic level 20 to 30 mg/dl). Which of the following is the most likely presentation of this salicylate overdose?

A. Hepatitis, pneumonia
B. Encephalopathy, coagulopathy
C. Uremia, pericarditis
D. Gastritis, thrombocytopenia
E. Purpura, tinnitus

25. Each of the following is a potential side effect of penicillamine EXCEPT

A. dysgeusia (abnormal sense of taste)
B. polymyositis
C. myasthenia gravis
D. lupus-like syndrome
E. scleroderma

26. A 27-year-old woman has had systemic lupus erythematosus (SLE) for five years, characterized by Raynaud's disease, thrombocytopenia, and skin vasculitis. One year ago she received a three-month course of prednisone, 60 mg daily, for treatment of nephritis. She is now referred to you after having right knee pain for two months. Physical examination shows tenderness along the medial joint space of the right knee; the remaining results of the joint examination are normal. The most likely cause of the knee pain is

A. flare of SLE
B. meniscal tear
C. avascular necrosis
D. gonococcal arthritis
E. chondromalacia patellae

27. A 65-year-old woman abruptly develops hot, painful, bilateral knee effusions 24 hours following hysterectomy for a benign ovarian cyst. In the past she was well except for occasional bilateral knee pain after prolonged ambulation. Temperature is 101°F, respiratory rate 20 per minute, blood pressure 140/80 mm Hg, and pulse 108 per minute. The most likely diagnosis is

A. septic arthritis
B. gout
C. pseudogout
D. acute rheumatoid arthritis
E. ruptured Baker's cyst

28. A 32-year-old woman who jogs 35 miles per week develops right knee pain that worsens while going down stairs and after sitting for a few hours. Physical examination of the right knee shows that movement of the patella over the femur is extremely painful; history and examination are otherwise normal. Which of the following is the most appropriate next step?

A. Arthrogram
B. Roentgenograms of the sacroiliac joints
C. Determination of antinuclear antibody, rheumatoid factor, and sedimentation rate
D. Injection of intra-articular steroids
E. Prescription of aspirin and quadricep exercises

29. In evaluation of the patient whose hands are illustrated, all the following tests might be useful EXCEPT

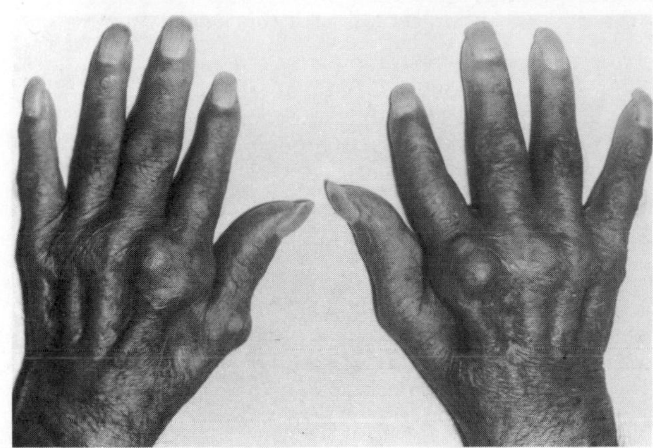

A. serum iron and total iron-binding capacity
B. plain films of the hands
C. serum uric acid level
D. muscle biopsy
E. latex test for rheumatoid factor

30. A patient with systemic lupus erythematosus has fever, maculopapular skin rash, and arthralgias. There is no evidence of other organ involvement. Initial management should include all the following EXCEPT

A. topical sun screens
B. topical corticosteroids
C. systemic corticosteroids
D. acetylsalicylic acid
E. antimalarial drugs

31. A 26-year-old man is stung by a bee, and shortly thereafter a wheal develops at the site of the sting. He soon feels flushed and develops hives, rhinorrhea, and tightness in the chest. He is brought to your office. Immediate therapy should be

A. transfer to a local hospital emergency room
B. cold compress to the site of the sting
C. epinephrine, subcutaneously
D. isoproterenol, sublingually
E. parenteral administration of antihistamines and steroids

DIRECTIONS: For questions 32 to 49, you are to decide whether EACH choice is true or false. Any combination of answers, from all true to all false, may occur. Mark the answer sheet "T" or "F" in the space provided.

32. Which of the following statements concerning T lymphocytes is/are true?

A. Congenital T cell deficiencies are characterized by recurrent pyogenic infections
B. T cells recognize antigen on the surfaces of other cells
C. Resting T cells express HLA-DR antigens
D. Productive rearrangement of the genes encoding the T cell antigen receptor occurs exclusively in T cells
E. The ratio of T4 T cells to T8 T cells in the peripheral blood regulates the T cell response to specific antigens

33. Which of the following statements about HLA-B27 is/are true?

A. It is inherited as an autosomal recessive trait
B. Its incidence is increased in patients with rheumatoid arthritis
C. Its incidence is increased in patients with uveitus in the absence of rheumatic disease
D. Its presence in a patient with roentgenographically demonstrated bilateral sacroiliitis increases the probability that the sacroiliitis is due to ankylosing spondylitis
E. Ninety per cent of Caucasian patients with ankylosing spondylitis are HLA-B27 positive

34. Which of the following statements concerning Reiter's syndrome is/are true?

A. It is associated with acquired immunodeficiency syndrome
B. One of its features is dactylitis ("sausage" digit)
C. Arthritis in the disorder is usually self-limited
D. In articular manifestations unresponsive to nonsteroidal, anti-inflammatory drugs, gold therapy is indicated
E. When urethritis occurs during an acute episode, antibiotic therapy effectively controls other manifestations of the disease

35. Which of the following statements is/are true?

A. The antibody response to protein antigens requires the participation of T lymphocytes
B. The maturation of the antibody response to an antigen is partly due to mutations that occur within the antibody genes of the responding B cell population
C. A minority of B lymphocytes express the cell-surface molecules designated T4 (CD4)
D. B lymphocytes are the primary effector cells in the rejection of allografts
E. IgM is the predominant immunoglobulin expressed on the cell surface of B lymphocytes

36. Which of the following statements regarding interleukin-2 (IL-2) is/are true?

A. It can stimulate T lymphocytes to proliferate
B. Helper T lymphocytes constitutively produce IL-2
C. Resting T lymphocytes express receptors for IL-2
D. Only T lymphocytes produce IL-2

37. Which of the following statements concerning the treatment of rheumatoid arthritis is/are true?

A. Liver function tests are a sensitive indicator of methotrexate-induced hepatotoxicity
B. Methotrexate therapy will produce a clinical response more quickly than parenteral gold therapy
C. Ibuprofen is more efficacious than naproxen
D. Pre-existing proteinuria contraindicates the initiation of gold therapy

38. Which of the following statements regarding gout is/are true?

A. A characteristic radiographic feature of chronic gout is preservation of joint space in the presence of erosions
B. During an acute gout attack, initiation of allopurinol is effective therapy
C. In the treatment of acute gout, intra-articular steroid injections are effective therapy
D. In an acute gout attack that has been untreated for 72 hours, colchicine is more effective therapy than indomethacin

39. Which of the following statements regarding carpal tunnel syndrome is/are true?

A. It is commonly associated with paresthesias and burning pain involving the volar surface of the forearm
B. Nocturnal symptoms are unusual
C. Interosseous muscle wasting is characteristic of severe cases
D. The incidence is increased during pregnancy

40. Which of the following statements concerning polyarteritis nodosa (PAN) is/are true?

A. Amphetamine abuse is a precipitating event for PAN development
B. Elevated antinuclear antibody titer is a characteristic finding
C. Hypertension accompanies renal involvement
D. Pulmonary angiography is likely to reveal characteristic microaneurysms
E. Chronic cutaneous manifestations sometimes occur in the absence of visceral involvement

41. Which of the following statements is/are true concerning human immunodeficiency virus (HIV, HTLV-III, LAV)?

A. In helper T cells, HIV binds to the cell-surface molecule designated T8 (CD8)
B. HIV is a DNA virus
C. In central Africa, transmission of HIV occurs primarily through heterosexual contact
D. The latency period between the time of infection with HIV and the onset of clinical symptoms is generally less than 18 months
E. In vitro 3′-azido-2′,3′-dideoxythymidine (AZT) inhibits viral entry into T cells

42. Which of the following statements is/are true?

A. Lateral stability of the knee is best assessed with the knee in full extension
B. In a normal individual, the skin overlying the

knee is slightly cooler than the skin above or below the knee

C. During a straight-leg raising test in a patient with suspected lumbar disc disease, tightness in the posterior thigh indicates a positive finding
D. Internal rotation is preserved until late in the course of osteoarthritis of the hip
E. Hip disease can cause discomfort that is felt exclusively in the knee

43. A 45-year-old woman who has additive symmetric polyarthritis of one year's duration has tried several nonsteroidal anti-inflammatory drugs, including aspirin, with only modest benefit. Despite her current regimen of naproxen, 250 mg three times daily, she has 5 hours of morning stiffness. Physical examination shows synovitis involving the proximal interphalangeal joints, the metacarpophalangeal joints, the wrists, and the knees. She has several nontender nodules palpable along the exterior surfaces of both forearms. Which of the following statements is/are true?

A. Serum complement levels are probably low
B. A test for rheumatoid factor will be positive
C. A synovial biopsy is likely to reveal pathognomonic changes
D. Roentgenograms are likely to reveal abnormalities of the sacroiliac joints
E. Radiographic erosions should be demonstrated before parenteral gold therapy is begun

44. Which of the following statements about aspirin-drug interactions is/are correct?

A. Oral antacids will elevate the patient's serum salicylate level
B. Reducing the regimen of prednisone will lower the patient's serum salicylate level
C. Aspirin blocks the uricosuric action of both probenecid and sulfinpyrazone
D. Aspirin reduces the hypoglycemic effects of sulfonylurea drugs

45. Which of the following is/are found in patients with Sjögren's syndrome?

A. Renal tubular acidosis
B. Positive rheumatoid factor
C. Positive antinuclear antibody
D. An increased risk of lymphoma
E. An increased frequency of HLA-DR7

46. Which of the following statements about patients with osteoarthritis of the left knee is/are true?

A. They should hold a cane in the right hand
B. The left knee is likely to demonstrate a valgus (knock-kneed) deformity
C. Synovial fluid analysis of the left knee is likely to reveal a glucose level greater than 50% of the serum glucose, and a white blood cell count of 10,000/mm^3
D. Roentgenogram of the left knee is likely to show uniform joint space narrowing
E. Roentgenogram of the left knee may show punctate calcifications in the fibrocartilage

47. Which of the following statements about reflex sympathetic dystrophy is/are true?

A. Precipitating events include trauma and medical illness
B. Swelling of involved extremities is localized to the joints
C. Physical therapy should be avoided until the swelling subsides
D. Roentgenograms of chronically involved areas are usually normal
E. A three-week tapering course of oral prednisone often accelerates resolution of pain and mobilization of the affected area

48. Which of the following statements concerning insect sting allergy is/are true?

A. The radioallergosorbent test (RAST) is the most sensitive diagnostic tool
B. Most patients with this allergy are sensitive to both bee and vespid venom
C. IgG antibodies are protective
D. Whole body extract of the insect is effective in desensitization immunotherapy
E. Desensitization immunotherapy should be administered over a prolonged period to reduce the incidence of side effects

49. Which of the following statements about hereditary angioedema is/are true?

A. Inheritance is sex-linked
B. Serum C3 levels are low
C. Serum C4 levels are low
D. Activity of C1 esterase inhibitor is decreased
E. Danazol is effective preventive therapy

DIRECTIONS: Questions 50 to 83 are matching questions. For each numbered item, choose the most likely associated lettered item from those provided. Each numbered item has ONLY ONE answer. Within each set of questions, each lettered item may be the answer to one, more than one, or none of the numbered items, unless otherwise specified.

QUESTIONS 50–53

For each of the following reactions, select the drug (A–E) with which it is most likely to be associated.

A. Indomethacin
B. Cyclophosphamide
C. Procainamide
D. Prednisone
E. Plaquenil

50. Headache

51. Polyarthritis

52. Hematuria without significant proteinuria

53. Cataracts

QUESTIONS 54–57

For each of the following, select the clinical syndrome (A–E) with which it is most likely to be associated.

A. Oligoarticular arthritis
B. Symmetric polyarthritis
C. Sacroiliitis
D. Anterior erosions of the thoracic spine
E. Erosive arthritis of the sternoclavicular joint

54. Hepatitis B infection

55. Rubella

56. Enteric infection with *Yersinia enterocolitica*

57. *Borrelia burgdorferi* infection

QUESTIONS 58–61

For each of the following, select the disease (A–E) with which it is most likely to be associated.

A. Still's disease
B. Necrotizing venulitis
C. Rheumatoid arthritis
D. Kawasaki disease
E. Dermatomyositis

58. Pyoderma gangrenosum

59. Transient erythematous macular rash that exhibits the Koebner phenomenon

60. Mucosal erythema

61. Urticaria

QUESTIONS 62–65

For each of the following renal histologic findings, select the disease (A–E) with which it is most likely to be associated.

A. Wegener's granulomatosis
B. Systemic lupus erythematosus
C. Rheumatoid arthritis
D. Henoch-Schölein purpura
E. Progressive systemic sclerosis

62. Focal necrotizing glomerulonephritis with diffuse mesangial IgA deposits

63. Proliferative glomerulonephritis without detectable immunoglobulin deposits

64. Proliferative glomerulonephritis with mesangial and subendothelial deposits of IgG, IgM, and IgA

65. Interstitial nephritis

QUESTIONS 66–69

For each of the following, select the autoantibody (A–E) with which it is most likely to be associated.

A. Anti-Sm
B. Lupus anticoagulant
C. Anti-Ro
D. Antiribonucleoprotein (RNP)
E. Rheumatoid factor

66. Recurrent spontaneous abortions

67. Congenital heart block

68. Myositis

69. Subacute cutaneous lupus erythematosus

QUESTIONS 70–73

For each of the following, select the most characteristic roentgenographic finding (A–E).

A. Ankylosis of the carpal bones
B. Metacarpophalangeal arthritis with osteophytosis
C. Narrowing and sclerosis of the first carpometacarpal joint
D. Resorption of the distal phalangeal tufts
E. Ulnar styloid erosions

70. Primary osteoarthritis

71. Rheumatoid arthritis

72. Juvenile rheumatoid arthritis

73. Hemochromatosis

QUESTIONS 74–78

For each of the following complement abnormalities, select the disorder (A–E) with which it is most likely to be associated.

A. Neisserial infections
B. Recurrent pyogenic infections
C. Lupus-like illness
D. Partial lipodystrophy
E. Recurrent abdominal pain

74. C3 nephritis factor

75. Heterozygous C1 esterase inhibitor deficiency

76. Homozygous C2 deficiency

77. Homozygous C7 deficiency

78. Homozygous C3 deficiency

QUESTIONS 79–83

For each of the following ocular lesions, select the diagnosis with which it is most likely to be associated. *(Note: Use each lettered item only once.)*

A. Systemic lupus erythematosus
B. Reiter's syndrome
C. Behçet's syndrome
D. Rheumatoid arthritis
E. Ankylosing spondylitis

79. Conjunctivitis

80. Iritis

81. Posterior uveitis

82. Nodular scleritis

83. Cytoid body

PART 9

CLINICAL IMMUNOLOGY AND RHEUMATOLOGY

ANSWERS

1.(B) Persistent synovitis in the dorsum of the wrist can lead to extensor tendon rupture. Initially, the wrist should be injected with corticosteroid. If this maneuver does not control the synovitis, synovectomy is indicated. Apart from the persistent wrist synovitis, this patient has responded clearly to gold therapy; the current regimen should be continued. *(Cecil Ch. 433; Primer)*

2.(C) Chondrocalcinosis can be associated with a degenerative arthropathy that, unlike primary osteoarthritis, can lead to isolated involvement of the radiocarpal and patellofemoral joints. The roentgenographic features of this chondrocalcinosis-associated arthropathy are otherwise similar to those of primary osteoarthritis and include joint space narrowing, osteophytosis, and discrete subchondral cysts. Eburnation, rather than juxta-articular demineralization (a feature of inflammatory arthritides), is characteristic. Chondrocalcinosis is most commonly observed in the knees, wrists, and symphysis pubis. *(Genant)*

3.(A) Pigmented villonodular synovitis occurs primarily in young adults and generally appears as a monoarthritis, particularly of the knee. A clue to the diagnosis is the aspiration of sanguineous fluid that does not clot. Arthrograms reveal numerous recesses and filling defects characteristic of the disorder. The diagnosis is established by synovial biopsy. In this case, the low white blood cell count makes an infectious etiology or inflammatory arthritis unlikely. Repeated hemarthroses and arthropathy are features of hemophilia, but hemophilia would not appear initially as a hemathrosis at age 28. *(Primer)*

4.(A) The issue is whether the patient's current muscle weakness is due to active polymyositis or to a combination of steroid myopathy and prior muscle damage. The initial clinical response to prednisone favors the latter. Similarly, the combination of normal muscle enzymes and weakness suggests steroid myopathy, although in some cases of active polymyositis muscle enzymes are normal. If superimposed steroid myopathy is contributing to the weakness, a decrease in prednisone dose should lead to improvement. This should be done with careful monitoring of muscle enzymes and muscle strength. *(Cecil, Chs. 30 and 443)*

5.(B) Palpable purpura occurs in the great majority of patients with mixed essential cryoglobulinemia and is an important clue to the diagnosis. Glomerulonephritis occurs in a substantial minority and is a major cause of death. There is an association between hepatitis B infection and mixed essential cryoglobulinemia, but the incidence varies considerably among different series. Cold intolerance is more likely to be a feature of Type I cryoglobulinemia than of mixed essential cryoglobulinemia. Complement levels are usually depressed in mixed essential cryoglobulinemia. *(Cecil, Ch. 81; Gorevic et al)*

6.(B) Frank arthritis, although seen in about 50% of patients with Behçet's disease, is rarely, if ever, deforming. Well-recognized features of the disease include meningoencephalitis, recurrent thromboses, and intestinal lesions that are indistinguishable from those of inflammatory bowel disease. Although the oral ulcers of Behçet's disease are extremely painful, the vaginal ulcers are often asymptomatic. *(Cecil, Ch. 453)*

7.(A) Back pain and stiffness that improve with activity are characteristic of an inflammatory process, not features of low back pain due to mechanical or degenerative causes. The most likely diagnosis is ankylosing spondylitis. In a patient with symptomatic ankylosing spondylitis for one year, roentgenographic evidence of bilateral sacroiliitis should be apparent. Ossification of the anterior longitudinal ligament is a feature of diffuse idiopathic skeletal hyperostosis (DISH). *(Cecil, Ch. 434)*

8.(C) Gold sodium thiomalate can cause vasomotor reactions ("nitritoid" reactions) that occur within minutes of injection and that resolve spontaneously. These symptoms rarely complicate aurothioglucose therapy. Gold therapy can be continued using aurothioglucose. *(Primer)*

9.(C) This patient has chronic sinusitis, pulmonary infiltrates, and a rapidly progressive glomerulonephritis. This set of findings is characteristic of Wegener's granulomatosis. The sinusitis of Wegener's granulomatosis is unresponsive to conventional therapy; it is often associated with destruction of the nasal septum (saddle-nose deformity) and with signs of a systemic illness (weight loss). Biopsies of the nasal mucosa, however, frequently reveal only nonspecific inflammation. The renal histology of Wegener's granulomatosis is that of a focal or diffuse proliferative glomerulonephritis, usually without evidence of granulomatous vasculitis. While the renal histology is not pathognomonic, proliferative glomerulonephritis in association with sinusitis and pulmonary disease is sufficient to establish the diagnosis. Open lung biopsies of involved tissue are an alternative means of establishing a tissue diagnosis. The therapeutic efficacy of cyclophosphamide in this disorder has been convincingly demonstrated. In the presence of a rapidly progressive glomerulonephritis, concomitant therapy with high-dose prednisone is indicated. The therapeutic efficacy of plasmapheresis is uncertain. *(Cecil, Ch. 441; Cupps and Fauci; Fauci et al)*

10.(B) The arthritis that occurs in association with psoriasis can occur in a number of distinct patterns: predominant (but not exclusive) involvement of distal interphalangeal joints; arthritis mutilans; seronegative polyarthritis indistinguishable from rheumatoid arthritis; oligoarthritis; and ankylosing spondylitis (in association with HLA-B27). Nail changes often accompany articular changes, particularly when distal interphalangeal joints are involved. *(Cecil, Ch. 434; Primer)*

11.(B) The age of onset, the location of the tenderness, and the pain upon abduction all point to degenerative supraspinatus tendinitis as the etiology of the shoulder pain. Appropriate therapy consists of either nonsteroidal anti-inflammatory agents, local injection of the subdeltoid bursa with a corticosteroid, or a combination of the two. Passive range of motion exercises are essential. Failure of active abduction to return following pain relief raises the possibility of a rotator cuff tear, which can be confirmed by arthrography. Surgical treatment of a rotator cuff tear associated with chronic tendinitis, however, is rarely successful. *(Cecil, Ch. 447)*

12.(C) In low doses, aspirin blocks the urinary secretion of urate and may increase serum uric acid. In high doses, however, aspirin also inhibits the tubular reabsorption of urate and has a net uricosuric effect, lowering serum uric acid levels. Hydrochlorothiazide, polycythemia vera, and psoriasis are frequently associated with hyperuricemia. Habitual consumption of "moonshine" alcohol can lead to chronic lead intoxication and saturnine gout. *(Cecil, Ch. 195)*

13.(E) Rheumatoid arthritis, psoriatic arthritis, and systemic lupus erythematosus (SLE) all can cause "swan-neck" deformities. In SLE the deformity reflects tendon laxity rather than joint destruction and thus is reducible. Reducible swan-neck deformities also occur in Jaccoud's syndrome (chronic post–rheumatic fever arthropathy). *(Cecil, Ch. 436)*

14.(C) The roentgenographic features of neuropathic arthropathy include subarticular sclerosis, marginal osteophytosis, effusion, subluxation, fracture, and fragmentation. Heterotopic calcification and ossification can be striking. Erosions, which are the hallmark of certain inflammatory arthritides, do not occur. *(Genant)*

15.(D) Renal side effects account for much of the toxicity of nonsteroidal anti-inflammatory drugs (NSAID's). These drugs can cause marked hyperkalemia, particularly in elderly patients with mild antecedent renal failure. NSAID-induced hemodynamic alterations can lead to acute renal failure. Predisposing conditions include pre-existing renal insufficiency, diuretic therapy, congestive heart failure, and liver disease. An unusual syndrome of renal failure with nephrotic-range proteinuria is also associated with NSAID's, particularly after chronic use. Renal biopsies reveal allergic interstitial nephritis and epithelial foot process fusion. NSAID's potentiate the effects of antidiuretic hormone (prostaglandins can antagonize the effects of antidiuretic hormone) and have been used to limit free water excretion in patients with nephrogenic diabetes insipidus. Edema is the most common clinically evident renal side effect of NSAID's. *(Clive and Stoff)*

16.(D) A number of conditions predispose to the development of osteonecrosis, including sickle cell disease, corticosteroid therapy, and alcoholism. Failure to follow decompression procedures can lead to dysbarism-related osteonecrosis (caisson disease), presumably due to the formation of nitrogen bubbles in terminal vessels. Vinyl chloride exposure can cause distal tuft resorption and Raynaud's phenomenon but is not associated with osteonecrosis. *(Cecil, Chs. 252 and 437)*

17.(D) Both LAK cells and T cells express T3 (a component of the T cell antigen receptor) and rosette sheep red blood cells and can proliferate in vitro in response to interleukin-2. Cytotoxic T cells lyse target cells but, unlike LAK cells, can only recognize specific antigen in association with a particular HLA gene product. *(Rosenberg et al)*

18.(C) Sarcoidosis can cause all these rheumatic syndromes. The arthritis that occurs as an initial manifestation of the disease, however, is distinctive. This form of sarcoid arthritis is a self-limited polyarthritis of acute onset that involves the ankles, knees, and hands. Painful periarthritis and tenosynovitis with minimal joint effusion are characteristic. Acute sarcoid arthritis is commonly associated with bilateral hilar adenopathy and erythema nodosum (Lofgren's syndrome). Sacroiliitis is not a feature of sarcoidosis. *(Cecil, Ch. 449; Primer)*

19.(B) The synovial fluid in rheumatoid arthritis is inflammatory with mean white blood cell count/mm^3 of 20,000 (range 1,000 to 100,000), with a predominance of polymorphonuclear cells. Although serum complement levels are usually normal in rheumatoid arthritis, complement levels in the synovial fluid are low. *(Cecil, Ch. 432)*

20.(C) Selective IgA deficiency is the most common primary immunodeficiency syndrome. This disorder is associated with increased infections of the respiratory and gastrointestinal tracts and an increased incidence of atopy. Severe anaphylactic reactions to infusion of blood products have been reported. DiGeorge's syndrome and purine nucleoside phosphorylase deficiency have deficient cell-mediated immunity. Adenosine deaminase deficiency is associated with combined cellular and humoral immunodeficiency. Hyperimmunogobulinemia E syndrome is characterized by recurrent staphylococcal abscesses with an increase in serum IgE. *(Cecil, Ch. 419)*

21.(B) Microangiopathic changes in the peripheral blood frequently are associated with scleroderma renal crisis; this is an ominous finding. Renal disease in scleroderma resembles the nephropathy of malignant hypertension. Proliferative glomerulonephritis is not seen, and the nephrotic syndrome and hypocomplementemia are not features of progressive systemic sclerosis. The presence of early, extensive skin involvement of the trunk identifies a subgroup of patients at greater risk for severe visceral involvement. An elevated anti-RNP antibody titer is associated with the mixed connective tissue syndrome. *(Cecil, Ch. 437).*

22.(D) Relapsing polychondritis is characterized by inflammation and destruction of cartilage. Ear inflammation is characteristic of this disorder, but involves the cartilaginous pinna and spares the lobe. Erythema and swelling of the lobe is more likely to be due to cellulitis. Aortic regurgitation and lower airway involvement are serious complications of this disease. *(Cecil, Ch. 445)*

23.(B) Giant cell arteritis is a treatable disease that must be considered in an elderly patient with headache and/or visual symptoms. Eye involvement is a medical emergency, and treatment should be started prior to an extensive diagnostic evaluation. In contrast to visual loss due to atherosclerosis of the carotid artery, visual loss in giant cell arteritis is usually irreversible; it is due to ischemia of the optic nerve rather than involvement of the retinal artery. *(Cecil, Ch. 442)*

24.(B) There are two clinical patterns of salicylate overdose. One involves generally young patients who ingest salicylate and other medications during a suicide attempt. The diagnosis in this group is usually made promptly. The second pattern involves older patients with a history of various medical illnesses and chronic salicylate use, who overdose accidentally. The diagnosis in this group is frequently missed or delayed and is associated with high morbidity and mortality. The most frequent admission diagnoses in this second group are cardiopulmonary disease or encephalopathy of unknown origin. Elevation of PT and PTT also is often found. Thus, unexplained encephalopathy with coagulopathy should raise the question of salicylate overdose. *(Anderson et al)*

25.(E) Rashes, proteinuria, and cytopenia are side effects common to both penicillamine and gold. Potential side effects unique to penicillamine include dysgeusia and a variety of autoimmune disorders. Penicillamine has been used to treat scleroderma; it does not cause the disease. *(Cecil, Ch. 84)*

26.(C) Avascular necrosis is a common complication of SLE, affecting more than 30% of all patients in some series. Raynaud's disease, myositis, vasculitis, and steroid use appear to be risk factors. Hips, knees, shoulders, and elbows can be affected. Bilateral involvement is common. Avascular necrosis of the knee is usually localized to the medial aspect of the femoral head, thereby producing pain in the medial joint space. Joint flares of SLE are polyarticular. The chronicity of joint pain and the absence of effusion argue against gonococcal arthritis. Meniscal tears in a young person are usually secondary to identifiable trauma. Chondromalacia patellae is a common cause of pain beneath the patella. *(Cecil, Ch. 447)*

27.(C) Pseudogout is due to calcium pyrophosphate dihydrate crystals. It tends to strike the knees or wrists, and episodes frequently occur following surgery, trauma, or major medical illness. Attacks of pseudogout are usually monoarticular, but two or more joints may be involved simultaneously. The diagnosis is established by the finding in synovial fluid of rod or rhomboidal crystals that are weakly positive for birefringence. Gout is more likely to strike the foot, especially the base of the great toe. Septic arthritis is usually monoarticular and would be a very unusual complication of "clean" surgery. Rupture of a Baker's cyst can produce a pseudothrombophlebitis syndrome. Abrupt knee swelling would be a very unusual initial presentation for rheumatoid arthritis. *(Cecil, Ch. 444)*

28.(E) These symptoms and findings are typical of chondromalacia patellae—a syndrome of pain and crepitus over the anterior aspect of the knee that is found in young adults, especially athletic women. The involved knee usually shows a normal range of motion and no effusion. The diagnosis is suspected on the basis of the typical symptoms and the presence of a positive patella inhibition test. (The test is performed while the patient is supine, with the knee extended and relaxed. Use the thumb and second finger to push the patella in the direction of the foot. While keeping the patella in this position, ask the patient to raise the entire leg. Such raising of the leg will cause acute pain at the patella if chondromalacia patellae is present.) Aspirin and quadricep exercises are the standard therapy. *(Cecil, Ch. 446)*

29.(D) The differential diagnosis of a symmetric polyarthritis with involvement of the wrist and metacarpophalangeal and proximal interphalangeal joints includes rheumatoid arthritis, gout, and hemochromatosis. Arthritis of this extent and distribution would not be associated with polymyositis. *(Cecil, Ch. 433)*

30.(C) Not all patients with SLE require therapy with systemic corticosteroids. Skin disease will often respond to sun avoidance and to topical corticosteroids. Nondeforming arthritis may be helped by salicylates or alternate antiinflammatory drugs. Antimalarial drugs are useful in the treatment of both skin and joint manifestations. *(Cecil, Ch. 436)*

31.(C) Systemic hypersensitivity reactions can result from stings of insects of the order Hymenoptera. Immediate therapy for systemic reactions is epinephrine given subcutaneously if there is no evidence of shock, or intravenously if vascular collapse has occurred. Antihistamines and steroids may be beneficial in the treatment of some urticarial reactions, but the possibility of a severe anaphylactic reaction demands prompt administration of epinephrine. *(Cecil, Ch. 423)*

32.(A–False; B—True; C–False; D—True; E—False) T cell deficiencies lead to recurrent infections with such low-grade pathogens as fungi, viruses, and *Pneumocystis carinii*. Antibody deficiencies cause recurrent infections with extracellular encapsulated pathogens. Mature T cells express either T4 or T8. T4 T cells recognize antigen in association with class II HLA gene products (e.g., HLA-DR), while T8 T cells recognize antigen in association with class I HLA gene products (e.g., HLA-A,B,C). Both subsets of T cells are functionally heterogeneous, although T4 cells tend to be helper cells and T8 cells generally have cytotoxic or suppressor functions. Although the ratio of $T4^+$ to $T8^+$ peripheral T cells is abnormal in a number of diseases, this ratio does not regulate the responses of antigen-specific T cells. Unlike B cells, which recognize soluble antigen, T cells recognize antigen in association with HLA gene products on the surfaces of other cells. When T cells are activated, as occurs following specific antigen recognition, the cell-surface phenotype of the T cell changes. Among the new molecules expressed by activated T cells are products of the HLA-D region. Productive rearrangement of the T cell antigen receptor genes occurs exclusively in T cells and has been used to identify the T cell nature of certain lymphoid malignancies. *(Cecil, Chs. 417 and 419; Acuto and Reinherz)*

33.(A—False; B—False; C—True; D—False; E—True) HLA-B27, which is inherited as an autosomal codominant, is associated with ankylosing spondylitis, Reiter's disease, and the spondyloarthropathies of inflammatory bowel disease, psoriasis, and juvenile chronic arthritis. The association between ankylosing spondylitis and HLA-B27 varies among racial groups and is particularly striking in Caucasians. Although uveitis is a feature of the rheumatic diseases with which HLA-B27 is associated, HLA-B27 is found in approximately 50% of patients who have uveitis in the absence of rheumatic disease. The presence of HLA-B27 would not be helpful in establishing the diagnosis of ankylosing spondylitis if roentgenograms demonstrated bilateral sacroiliitis. The differential diagnosis of bilateral sacroiliitis consists entirely of diseases that are associated with HLA-B27. *(Cecil, Chs. 425 and 434)*

34.(A—True; B—True; C—False; D—False; E—False) A particularly severe form of Reiter's syndrome appears to occur in association with acquired immunodeficiency syndrome. Dactylitis reflects the presence of tenosynovitis in Reiter's syndrome. Although earlier reports indicated that Reiter's syndrome was a self-limited disorder, it is now quite clear that the arthritis is often chronic. Gold therapy is ineffective; patients whose symptoms are unresponsive to nonsteroidal anti-inflammatory agents have responded to methotrexate. There is no evidence that antibiotic treatment of the urethritis of Reiter's syndrome has a beneficial effect on the disease. *(Cecil, Ch. 434; Winchester et al)*

35.(A—True; B—True; C—False; D—False; E—True) The antibody response to protein antigens requires the participation of "helper" T cells; antibody responses to certain polysaccharides are relatively T cell–independent. Somatic mutation in the antibody genes contributes to the increased avidity of the mature antibody response to an antigen. T4, the HIV "receptor," is expressed by T cells and in brain tissue but not by B cells. T cells, not B cells, are the major effector cells in the rejection of allografts. The presence of cell-surface IgM is a distinguishing feature of B cells. *(Cecil, Ch. 417)*

36.(A—True; B—False; C—False; D—True) IL-2 is produced by helper T cells when these cells are activated by antigen or mitogens. Originally known as T cell growth factor, IL-2 causes T cells to proliferate. The receptor that binds IL-2 is expressed by activated, but not resting, T cells. Thus, the effect of IL-2 is to selectively expand the T cells that are actively participating in a specific immune response. *(Greene et al)*

37.(A—False; B—True; C—False; D—True) During methotrexate therapy, hepatotoxicity can occur despite normal liver function tests, and abnormal liver function tests do not necessarily indicate significant hepatotoxicity. Liver biopsy may be required to monitor chronic methotrexate therapy. One advantage of methotrexate in the treatment of rheumatoid arthritis is that a clinical response, if it occurs, occurs sooner than with gold, penicillamine, or Plaquenil. Although an individual patient may respond better to certain nonsteroidal anti-inflammatory drugs (NSAID's) than to others, the various NSAID's appear to have equal efficacy in the treatment of rheumatoid arthritis. Because pre-existent proteinuria would make detection of gold nephropathy impossible, proteinuria is a contradiction to instituting gold therapy. *(Cecil, Ch. 433; Primer)*

38.(A—True; B—False; C—True; D—False) Fluctuations in the serum uric acid level can precipitate gouty attacks or exacerbate ongoing gouty arthritis; therefore, allopurinol therapy should not be instituted during an acute attack. Intra-articular steroids are effective in acute gout and are particularly useful when neither indomethacin nor colchicine can be used. The distinctive roentgenographic features of chronic gout include the absence of osteopenia, the relative maintenance of joint space, and the presence of sharply marginated erosions. Colchicine is most effective if used within the first 12 hours of a gouty attack. *(Cecil, Ch. 195)*

39.(A—True; B—False; C—False; D—True) Carpal tunnel syndrome is due to compression of the median nerve at the wrist. Initial symptoms include pain and paresthesias of the middle fingers, especially at night. Discomfort is commonly felt along the volar surface of the forearm as well as in the hand. Motor involvement, which leads to wasting of the thenar eminence (not the interossei), is an indication for surgical intervention. Pregnancy is the most common predisposing condition. Carpal tunnel syndrome is also associated with amyloidosis, myxedema, acromegaly, and wrist arthritis of any etiology. *(Cecil, Chs. 451 and 511; Primer)*

40.(A—True; B—False; C—True; D—False; E—True) A variety of precipitating events have been implicated in the development of PAN, including amphetamine abuse, hepatitis B infection, serous otitis media, hairy cell leukemia, and allergic hyposensitization therapy. PAN is not associated with antinuclear antibodies. Renal disease due either to vasculitis or to glomerulonephritis is almost always associated with hypertension. PAN characteristically spares the pulmonary circulation; microaneurysms are most commonly observed in the distribution of the renal and superior mesenteric arteries. Chronic cutaneous PAN is a well-recognized entity. *(Cecil, Ch. 440; Cupps and Fauci)*

41.(A—False; B—False; C—True; D—False; E—False) HIV, a retrovirus (RNA virus), preferentially infects helper T cells because it binds to the cell-surface molecule designated T4; expression of T4 and T8 on mature T cells is mutually exclusive. The heterosexual transmission of HIV in central Africa is well-established. The latency period between the time of HIV infection and onset of clinical symptoms is usually of several years' duration. AZT does not affect viral entry into cells: the antiviral effects of AZT are due to its ability to inhibit viral reverse transcriptase (HIV infection requires the action of reverse transcriptase, which transcribes viral RNA into DNA). *(Cecil, Ch. 346; Broder and Gallo; Yarchoan and Broder)*

42.(A—False; B—True; C—False; D—False; E—True) When the knee is fully extended, the anterior and posterior cruciate ligaments can confer lateral stability. The knee should be in slight flexion for examination of medial and lateral ligamentous laxity. The skin overlying the knee is typically cooler than the skin above or below the joint; this point should be kept in mind while determining whether a knee is inflamed. A positive straight-leg raising test reproduces sciatic pain and/or low back pain; a tight sensation in the hamstrings is common and has no diagnostic value. Pain with internal rotation and diminished internal rotation are often the earliest signs of hip disease of any cause. Pain due to hip disease can be felt exclusively in the knee. A patient with knee pain and a normal knee examination should be evaluated carefully for hip disease. *(Polley and Hunder)*

43.(A—False; B—True; C—False; D—False; E—False) The additive nature of the polyarthritis, the joints involved, and the presence of nodules on extensor surfaces are characteristic of rheumatoid arthritis. Rheumatoid factor is present in the great majority of patients with nodular rheumatoid arthritis. Complement levels are normal in the serum but depressed in synovial fluid. Rheumatoid arthritis does not cause sacroiliitis. Significant synovitis, unresponsive to nonsteroidal anti-inflammatory drugs, is the major indication for the addition of a so-called remittive agent such as gold. Synovial biopsies reveal a hyperplastic inflammatory synovitis that is characteristic of rheumatoid arthritis but that can be observed in other inflammatory arthropathies. *(Cecil, Ch. 433)*

44.(A—False; B—False; C—True; D—False) Antacids—even "nonabsorbable" antacids—raise the urine pH, thereby increasing renal excretion of salicylate and lowering the serum salicylate level. Corticosteroids can lower the salicylate level. Consequently, for a patient with a therapeutic salicylate level, a reduction in the prednisone dose can increase the salicylate level to a toxic level. Aspirin blocks the effect of uricosuric agents and spironolactone; it potentiates the hypoglycemic effects of sulfonylurea drugs. *(Plotz)*

45.(A—True; B—True; C—True; D—True; E—False) Sjögren's syndrome is not simply a disease of lacrimal and salivary glands; vasculitis, pulmonary disease, central and peripheral neurologic disease, myositis, and various forms of renal disease (including renal tubular acidosis) have been reported. The risk of developing non-Hodgkin's lymphoma in Sjögren's syndrome is 44 times greater than normal. Most patients with Sjögren's have both a positive rheumatoid factor and antinuclear antibody test. Primary Sjögren's is associated with an increased frequency of HLA-DR3; when associated with rheumatoid arthritis, Sjögren's is associated with an increased frequency of HLA-DR4. *(Cecil, Ch. 438)*

46.(A—True; B—False; C—False; D—False; E—True) A cane should be held on the side opposite the arthritic knee. The most common deformity at the knees from osteoarthritis is a varus deformity (bow-legged; 90%). Valgus deformity (knock-knees) due to osteoarthritis is uncommon (10%). In rheumatoid arthritis the frequency of these deformities is reversed. Osteoarthritis produces noninflammatory synovial fluid with a glucose level greater than 50% of serum and a white blood cell count of less than 3000. A radiographic hallmark of osteoarthritis is irregular joint space loss; uniform joint space narrowing is a feature of rheumatoid arthritis. Punctate cartilage calcifications, associated with calcium pyrophosphate crystal deposition, may be seen in osteoarthritis. *(Cecil, Ch. 446)*

47.(A—True; B—False; C—False; D—False; E—True) Reflex sympathetic dystrophy is a syndrome characterized by (1) pain and tenderness in an extremity, (2) diffuse swelling of soft tissues, (3) diminished motor function, (4) trophic skin changes, (5) vasomotor instability, and (6) patchy osteoporosis. It is commonly precipitated by trauma or a medical illness (e.g., myocardial infarction). Aggressive physical therapy will reverse the condition in most patients. A brief course of prednisone can accelerate the improvement, but it is not usually required. *(Cecil, Ch. 466)*

48.(A—False; B—False; C—True; D—False; E—False) Because of the severe and sometimes fatal results of allergic reactions to insect stings, physicians must be aware of the proper approach to diagnosis, treatment, and prevention. There are multiple antigens borne by insects of the order Hymenoptera, and use of improved antigen preparations and immunologic testing have allowed investigation of patterns of susceptibility to these materials. The skin test is the most sensitive and specific technique for documenting allergy. This and the RAST show that only about 10% of patients with such allergies are sensitive to both bee and vespid venom. After the nature of the antigen to which a sensitive patient is allergic has been documented, immunotherapy can be undertaken. This treatment presumably leads to the production of IgG antibodies; these are protective, unlike IgE antibodies, which lead to anaphylactic reactions. Venom therapy should be employed, as whole body extract has been shown to be ineffective. Desensitization therapy should be performed rapidly over a six- to eight-week period, since this schedule is associated with both improved responsiveness and a lower incidence of adverse reactions. *(Cecil, Ch. 423)*

49.(A—False; B—False; C—True; D—True; E—True) Hereditary angioneurotic edema results from absence of the inhibitor of activated C1. Acute attacks may be marked by angioedema or acute abdominal pain that sometimes mimics a surgical abdominal condition. Low levels of C4 result from spontaneous activation of the complement cascade. Specific therapy for termination of acute attacks is not well established, but anabolic steroids such as danazol are effective in preventing them. The inheritance of this condition is autosomal dominant; however, the absence of a family history should not exclude the diagnosis. *(Cecil, Chs. 418 and 420)*

50.(A); 51.(C); 52.(B); 53.(D) A common side effect of indomethacin is headache; patients may also complain of drowsiness, loss of concentration, and feeling of confusion. Polyarthritis is a manifestation of procainamide-induced lupus and resolves when the drug is withdrawn. A potentially devastating side effect of cyclophosphamide is hemorrhagic cystitis; the risk can be minimized by frequent bladder-emptying and maintenance of a large urine output. Posterior subcapsular cataracts occur with prolonged use of corticosteroids. *(Cecil, Ch. 436; Cupps and Fauci; Simon and Mills)*

54.(B); 55.(B); 56.(A); 57.(A) Both hepatitis B and rubella infections can cause a transient, symmetric polyarthritis. Rubella arthritis occurs primarily in adult women; rubella vaccine can cause a similar syndrome in women and children. Enteric infection with *Yersinia enterocolitica* can lead to a "reactive" oligoarthritis. *Borrelia burgdorferi* is the etiologic agent of Lyme disease. This spirochete can cause recurrent monoarticular or oligoarticular arthritis, usually of large joints. *(Cecil, Chs. 435 and 436; Steere et al)*

58.(C); 59.(A); 60.(D); 61.(B) An association between pyoderma gangrenosum and rheumatoid arthritis is well established. The characteristic rash of Still's disease is an evanescent (often coinciding with fever), nonpruritic, erythematous, macular eruption that is most commonly seen on the trunk and can be precipitated by scratching the skin (Koebner phenomenon). Kawasaki disease (mucocutaneous lymph node disease) is a febrile illness of children characterized by a desquamating rash of the distal extremities, erythematous oral mucosa, exanthem of the trunk, congested conjunctivae, and cervical adenopathy. Coronary arteritis with aneurysm formation can occur. Urticaria can be due to necrotizing venulitis. Clues to the underlying vasculitis include foci of purpura, associated arthralgias, and an elevated erythrocyte sedimentation rate. *(Cecil, Chs. 420, 433, and 439; Cupps and Fauci)*

62.(D); 63.(A); 64.(B); 65.(B) Although systemic lupus erythematosus, Wegener's granulomatosis, and Henoch-Schönlein purpura all cause glomerulonephritis, the presence of extensive IgA deposits is most characteristic of Henoch-Schönlein purpura. The renal manifestations of lupus include proliferative glomerulonephritis and interstitial nephritis; mesangial and subendothelial deposits of all immunoglobulin classes occur in proliferative lupus glomerulonephritis. In contrast to lupus and Henoch-Schönlein purpura (in which immunoglobulin deposits are always present), the proliferative glomerulonephritis of Wegener's granulomatosis often occurs in the absence of demonstrable immune complex deposits. Rheumatoid arthritis is not associated with either interstitial nephritis or glomerulonephritis; the renal changes in scleroderma result from progressive arterial lesions rather than a proliferative glomerulonephritis. *(Cecil, Chs. 81, 436, 437 and 441)*

66.(B); 67.(C); 68.(D); 69.(C) Antibodies to Ro, a nuclear antigen, are found in the majority of patients with primary Sjögren's syndrome; they are also seen in secondary Sjögren's syndrome, systemic lupus, subacute cutaneous lupus, and primary biliary cirrhosis. There is a strong association between neonatal lupus and maternal antibodies to Ro; the two major manifestations of neonatal lupus are congenital heart block and transient cutaneous lupus. Patients with mixed connective tissue disease have high titers of antibodies to RNP, an extractable nuclear antigen, and a clinical syndrome with features of systemic lupus, scleroderma, and polymyositis. The lupus anticoagulant is an autoantibody that prolongs phospholipid-dependent coagulation tumor. Lupus anticoagulant is associated with recurrent spontaneous abortions and an increased incidence of thrombotic events. Sm is another extractable nuclear antigen; antibodies to Sm are specific for systemic lupus. *(Cecil, Chs. 436 and 437; Reichlin; Branch et al)*

70.(C); 71.(E); 72.(A); 73.(B) The roentgenographic features of osteoarthritis include irregular joint space narrowing, subchondral sclerosis, and osteophyte formation. Primary osteoarthritis of the hand involves the proximal and distal interphalangeal joints and the first carpometacarpal joints. Degenerative changes involving the metacarpophalangeal joints are characteristic of hemochromatosis, not primary osteoarthritis. Rheumatoid arthritis causes juxta-articular demineralization, uniform cartilage loss, and erosion; it commonly involves the metacarpophalangeal joints but does not cause osteophyte formation. The ulnar styloid is a common site for early erosive changes in rheumatoid arthritis. Juvenile rheumatoid arthritis can lead to bony ankylosis of joints, particularly the carpus and tarsus. *(Genant)*

74.(D); 75.(E); 76.(C); 77.(A); 78.(B) C3 nephritic factor, an acquired complement abnormality, is an IgG antibody that stabilizes the alternative pathway C3 convertase. It is associated with idiopathic membranoproliferative (mesangiocapillary) glomerulonephritis as well as with partial lipodystrophy. Lupus-like syndromes have been associated with complete absence of several different complement components; the most common is C2 deficiency. Recurrent neisserial infections are associated with several homozygous deficiencies of components of the membrane attack unit; C6, C7, and C8; the reasons for the selective susceptibility are uncertain. In contrast, complete absence of C3 removes the opsonizing capacity of the complement system and prevents the generation of chemotactic and lytic activities. Serious pyogenic infections result. Heterozygous deficiency of C1 esterase inhibitor is the abnormality in hereditary angioedema and is characterized by recurrent submucosal edema of the respiratory and gastrointestinal tracts. *(Cecil, Ch. 418)*

79.(B); 80.(E); 81.(C); 82.(D); 83.(A) Reiter's syndrome is more frequently associated with conjunctivitis than with iritis. Iritis is the most frequent ocular lesion in ankylosing spondylitis. Behçet's syndrome is the only choice associated with posterior uveitis. Nodular scleritis is a complication of rheumatoid arthritis. Cytoid bodies are "cotton-wool spots" that represent retinal microinfarcts; they are seen with SLE. *(Cecil, Chs. 433, 434 and 436)*

BIBLIOGRAPHY

Acuto O, Reinherz EL: The human T-cell receptor: Structure and function. N Engl J Med 312:1100, 1985.

Anderson RJ, Potts DE, Gabow PA, et al: Unrecognized adult salicylate intoxication. Ann Intern Med 85:745, 1976.

Branch DW, Scott JR, Kochenour NK, et al: Obstetric complications associated with the lupus anticoagulant. N Engl J Med 313:1322, 1985.

Broder S, Gallo RC: A pathogenic retrovirus (HTLV-III) linked to AIDS. N Engl J Med 311:1292, 1984.

Cecil Textbook of Medicine. 18th ed. Wyngaarden JB, Smith LH Jr (eds). Philadelphia, W.B. Saunders Company, 1988.

Clive DM, Stoff JS: Renal syndromes associated with nonsteroidal antiinflammatory drugs. N Engl J Med 310:563, 1984.

Cupps TR, Fauci AS: The Vasculitides. Philadelphia, W.B. Saunders Company, 1981.

Fauci AS, Haynes BF, Katz P, et al: Wegener's granulomatosis: Prospective clinical and therapeutic experience with 85 patients for 21 years. Ann Intern Med 98:76, 1983.

Genant HK: Radiology of rheumatic diseases. *In* McCarty DJ (ed): Arthritis and Allied Conditions: A Textbook of Rheumatology. 10th ed. Philadelphia, Lea & Febiger, 1985, pp. 76–147.

Gorevic PD, Kassab HJ, Levo Y, et al: Mixed cryoglobulinemia: Clinical aspects and long-term followup of 40 patients. Am J Med 69:287, 1980.

Greene WC, Leonard WJ, Depper JM, et al: The human interleukin-2 receptor: Normal and abnormal expression in T cells and in leukemias induced by the human T-lymphotropic retroviruses. Ann Intern Med 105:560, 1986.

Plotz PH: Aspirin and salicylate. *In* Kelley WN, Harris ED Jr, Ruddy S, et al (eds): Textbook of Rheumatology. 2nd ed. Philadelphia, W.B. Saunders Company, 1985, pp. 725–752.

Polley HF, Hunder GG: Rheumatologic Interviewing and Physical Examination of the Joints. 2nd ed. Philadelphia, W.B. Saunders Company, 1978.

Primer on the Rheumatic Diseases. 8th ed. Atlanta, Arthritis Foundation, 1983.

Reichlin M: Significance of the Ro antigen system. J Clin Immunol 6:339, 1986.

Rosenberg SA, Lotze MT, Muul LM, et al: Observations on the systemic administration of autologous lymphokine-activated killer cells and recombinant interleukin-2 to patients with metastatic cancer. N Engl J Med 313:1485, 1985.

Simon LS, Mills JA: Nonsteroidal antiinflammatory drugs (first of two parts). N Engl J Med 302:1179, 1980.

Steere AC, Grodzicki RL, Kornblatt AN, et al: The spirochetal etiology of Lyme disease. N Engl J Med 308:733, 1983.

Winchester R, Bernstein DH, Fischer HD, et al: The co-occurrence of Reiter's syndrome and acquired immunodeficiency. Ann Intern Med 106:19, 1987.

Yarchoan R, Broder S: Development of antiretroviral therapy for the acquired immunodeficiency syndrome and related disorders: A progress report. N Engl J Med 316:557, 1987.

PART 10

NEUROLOGIC DISEASE

BARRIE J. HURWITZ and MICHAEL H. BOWMAN

DIRECTIONS: For questions 1 to 54 choose the ONE BEST answer to each question.

1. Each of the following has been implicated in producing parkinsonism EXCEPT

A. MPTP
B. reserpine
C. haloperidol
D. chlorpromazine
E. trihexyphenidyl

2. A 72-year-old man has progressive difficulty with balance together with abrupt falling, slurred speech, dysphagia, emotional lability, and vague changes in personality. When examined he cannot voluntarily gaze upward or downward; however, fixation of the eyes on a target, followed by tipping the head up and down, shows that the eyes move. Optokinetic and caloric-induced tests fail to demonstrate the fast component of the resulting nystagmus. The neck is stiff and extended and the limbs show some cogwheel rigidity. The face is expressionless and the gait is festinating. When pushed, the patient topples over easily. Finger-to-nose dysmetria is absent. Which of the following is the most likely diagnosis?

A. Parkinson's disease
B. Striatonigral degeneration
C. Dystonia musculorum deformans
D. Progressive supranuclear palsy
E. Olivopontocerebellar degeneration

3. A 63-year-old woman is referred to you with progressive headache of two weeks' duration. Her husband states that she is unable to sleep, cries frequently, and is very depressed. Past medical history is unremarkable. Her local physician has prescribed diazepam and aspirin. Two weeks ago, the hemoglobin was 13.1 g/dl and white blood cell count was 6,700/mm.^{3} The patient is awake, alert, and weepy and has mild pallor. Physical examination shows that the temporalis, trapezius, masseter, and posterior cervical muscles are all tender to palpation. The neck is supple and Kernig's and Brudzinski's signs are absent. Funduscopic examination is benign. The remainder of the examination is unremarkable. Which one of the following would most likely be of assistance in establishing a diagnosis?

A. Lumbar puncture
B. Dexamethasone suppression test
C. Computed tomography (CT scan) of the brain
D. Repeat complete blood count and sedimentation rate
E. Thyroid function tests, rheumatoid factor, and cervical spine roentgenogram

4. A 52-year-old woman has a four-year history of a progressive "pulling sensation" in the right neck muscles which has spread to the right upper extremity this past year. Three years ago she began to have periodic turning of her chin toward the right side, the frequency and severity of which have increased. She has found that placing her hand on her chin partially relieves this painful "muscle spasm." She has also noticed episodic but progressive slowing of her voice. Which of the following has NOT been found to be helpful in the treatment of this disorder?

A. Carbamazepine
B. Trihexyphenidyl
C. Dorsal column stimulation
D. Dorsal root entry zone (DREZ) surgery
E. Surgical section of the accessory nerve

5. Computed tomography (CT scan) of the brain of a 64-year-old man is shown below. Which of the following is the most likely clinical history?

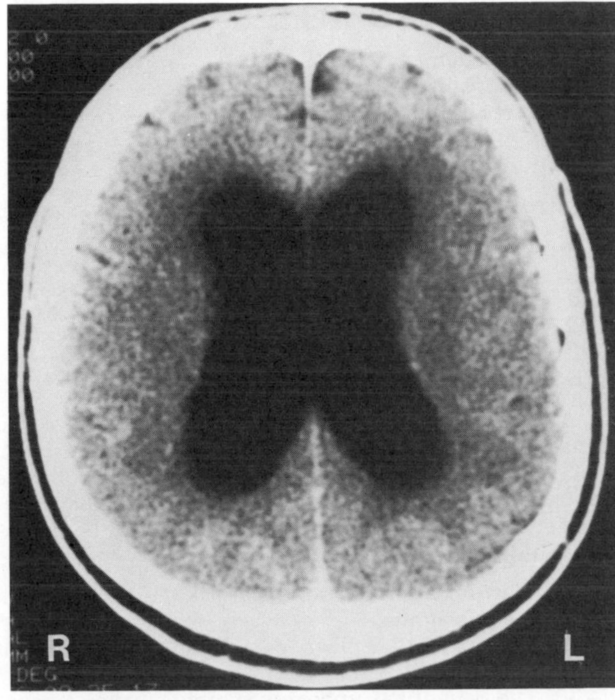

A. Papilledema, dementia, and aphasia
B. Papilledema, seizures, and urinary incontinence

C. Gait ataxia, dementia, and urinary incontinence
D. Aphasia, right hemiparesis, and urinary incontinence
E. History and examination are normal

6. A 42-year-old man is brought to the hospital by his wife because of diplopia. He awakened 30 minutes ago and, while putting on his shoes, noted that he could not see his left foot. On physical examination, the patient appears slightly lethargic and has a supple neck. Pulse rate is 82 per minute; blood pressure is 140/90 mm Hg. Ocular examination shows minimal right ptosis. The right pupil is 1 mm larger than the left and both are reactive. The fundi are benign. There is a left homonymous hemianopsia. While you are examining the patient's reflexes, he becomes progressively drowsy and obtunded. There is a left hemiparesis. Rechecking his eyes you find the right eye deviated laterally. The left eye shows brisk doll's eye movements, but the right eye shows no doll's eye movements, up, down, or medially. The patient becomes rigid with diffuse muscular shivering. Which one of the following would be most appropriate to do next?

A. Check the oculovestibular reflexes with ice water
B. Order computed tomography (CT scan) of the brain immediately
C. Perform a lumbar puncture
D. Intubate, hyperventilate, and administer mannitol intravenously
E. Administer 40% nasal oxygen; then complete the neurologic examination

7. Each of the following may produce hearing loss EXCEPT

A. furosemide
B. gentamicin
C. salicylates
D. erythromycin
E. *cis*-platinum

8. Subacute bacterial endocarditis often presents with each of the following EXCEPT

A. papilledema
B. personality changes
C. cerebral infarction
D. intracerebral hemorrhage
E. transient ischemic attacks

9. When obtaining a neurologic history, the examiner should heed each of the following EXCEPT

A. Avoid interrupting the patient
B. Always obtain a complete history
C. Attempt to formulate a diagnosis
D. Summarize the history to the patient
E. Demonstrate reassurance and support

10. A 39-year-old woman has abrupt onset of vertigo and a sense that she is falling or being pulled to the right. Associated with this are nausea and vomiting. All of these symptoms subside when she remains lying quietly on her left side. Which of the following would NOT be an expected finding in this patient?

A. Visual fixation during the attack tends to dampen the nystagmus
B. The patient displays past-pointing to the right during an attack
C. The patient has upbeat nystagmus during a spontaneous attack of vertigo
D. The Barany maneuver with head down to the right causes a left-beating horizontal and rotatory nystagmus
E. Cold caloric testing of the right ear shows decreased velocity and decreased duration of the slow component of the nystagmus

11. Which of the following statements about multi-infarct dementia is INCORRECT?

A. Depression is rarely a prominent feature
B. It represents approximately 20% of all patients with dementia
C. Prominent disturbances of gait, station, and limb motor function are seen
D. It appears most often in concert with diabetes mellitus and/or hypertension
E. Steplike progression with partial recovery between periodic losses of function is typical

12. A 72-year-old man is brought to the emergency room by his wife because of confusion. He abruptly became confused eight hours ago while working with her in the garden. He has had no alteration in consciousness and has remained alert and seemingly frustrated with this problem. Physical examination shows vital signs to be normal. The patient knows his name and his wife's name, but does not know where he is, the date, or the time. He is alert, articulate, and attentive and has a normal neurologic examination. The most likely diagnosis is

A. hysteria
B. hepatic encephalopathy
C. transient global amnesia
D. partial complex status epilepticus
E. absence (petit mal) status epilepticus

13. Which of the following statements regarding Alzheimer's disease is FALSE?

A. Focal or generalized seizures occur in 10 to 15% of cases
B. Memory disturbance for recent events is usually an early finding
C. Senile plaques and neurofibrillary tangles are found in the cerebral cortex
D. The disease is rapidly progressive, usually advancing to a fatal termination within a year
E. Most examples occur sporadically, but a family history of dementia and Down's syndrome is seen in up to 25% of cases

14. A 36-year-old woman was referred to you with a three-week history of blurred vision and unsteady gait. She has experienced progressive fatigue for the past six months; one year ago, she abruptly lost vision in the right eye which returned to normal after 10 days. She has lost 5 lbs in the past week and has developed insomnia. On examination, vital signs are normal and the patient is awake, alert, and oriented with no evidence of dementia or aphasia but with an inappropriate euphoric affect. She has bilateral horizontal nystagmus with mild clumsiness of rapid alternating movements in the right upper extremity. Generalized hyper-reflexia is present. Vibration sense is slightly decreased in both feet. The brain MRI scan is shown on page 235. Which of the following is the most likely diagnosis?

A. Multiple sclerosis
B. Multiple cerebral infarcts
C. Metastatic choriocarcinoma

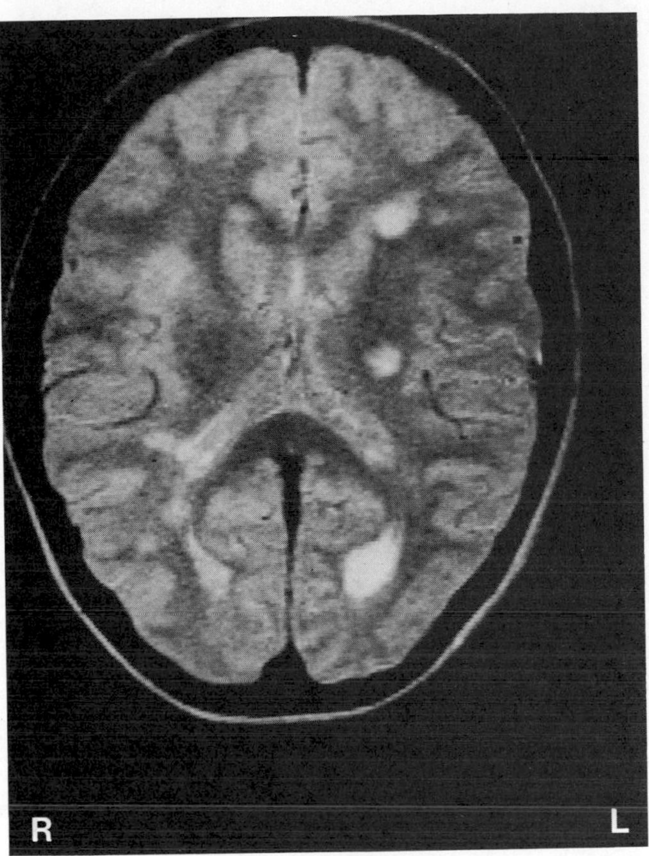

D. Amyotrophic lateral sclerosis
E. Acquired immunodeficiency syndrome

15. A 49-year-old man is referred to you because of difficulty staying asleep at night. He states that he awakens repetitively at night and feels sleepy in the daytime. He was recently involved in an automobile accident and thinks he may have fallen asleep at the wheel. His wife moved to another bedroom two years ago because of his continued snoring. She has noted a personality change in him during this period of time, characterized by poor temper control, anger, and depression. The patient has become impotent and frequently removes the bed linen during the night. On physical examination, the blood pressure is 160/98 mm Hg; the pulse rate is 70 beats per minute; respiratory rate is 28 per minute. Height is 5′10″ and weight is 269 lbs. The patient has a mild recent memory loss; the neurologic examination is otherwise normal. Which of the following would be most appropriate for this patient?

A. No studies are needed; amitriptyline should be administered to help him sleep at night while he undergoes a weight-reduction program
B. A sleep-deprived EEG should be performed; a trial of phenobarbital or ethosuximide should be administered
C. A multiple sleep latency test should be performed; a long-acting benzodiazepine should be administered to help him sleep
D. An overnight sleep EEG study should be performed; continuous positive airway pressure should be administered at night while he undergoes weight reduction
E. Computed tomography (CT scan) of the brain should be performed with views of the posterior fossa; if normal, he should be treated with methylphenidate

16. Which of the following bony abnormalities has the highest incidence of associated neurologic abnormalities?

A. Facet tropism
B. Spondylolisthesis
C. Basilar impression
D. Spina bifida occulta
E. Klippel-Feil syndrome

17. Which of the following findings is NOT seen as a result of chronic excessive alcohol intake?

A. The commonly noted triad of confusion, ataxia, and ophthalmoplegia
B. An abrupt onset of muscle pain, cramps, tenderness, weakness, and swelling of the legs
C. Progressive ophthalmoplegia, nuchal dystonia, a dystonic smile with deep nasolabial folds, and a shuffling gait with masked facial expression
D. Slowly developing unsteadiness of gait with rapid turning of the body that occurs early, although progressive worsening of station and gait lead to severe truncal ataxia
E. Progressive dementia over several years accompanied by agitation or apathy, hallucinations, and emotional lability that is replaced by seizures, stupor, and eventually coma

18. A 38-year-old woman is brought to the emergency room after suffering a seizure. There is a two-day history of headache and lethargy, but no previous seizures. On examination, she has a poor attention span and decreased memory. The plantar response on the left is extensor. CT scan of the brain is normal. Which of the following is the most likely diagnosis?

A. Herpes simplex encephalitis
B. Glioblastoma multiforme
C. Intracerebral hemorrhage
D. Embolic occlusion at the trifurcation of the right middle cerebral artery
E. Todd's paralysis

19. The computed tomography (CT scan) of the brain shown above is that of a 32-year-old female nurse who has had two recent grand mal seizures. There is a history of intermittent dull frontal headaches for the past 10 years. She had a mild learning disorder as a child and was diagnosed in her teens as having a personality disorder. Which of the following is the most likely diagnosis?

A. Glioblastoma multiforme
B. Cystic astrocytoma
C. Pituitary adenoma
D. Pinealoma
E. Dermoid

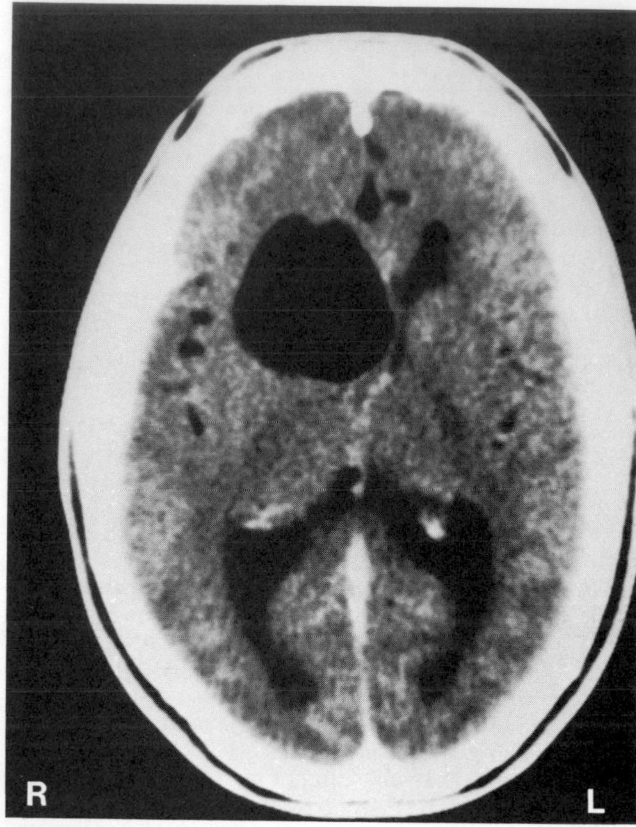

20. Which of the following statements concerning schizophrenia is NOT correct?

A. The occurrence of visual hallucinations is common
B. Prolonged abnormal posturing and grimacing may occur
C. The patient often feels under the control of some outside force
D. The patient often expresses thoughts awkwardly and unclearly
E. The emotional attitude of the patient is often blunted or inappropriate.

21. Which of the following about the difference between Alzheimer's and Pick's disease is NOT correct?

A. Memory is lost early in Alzheimer's and late in Pick's
B. Acalculia occurs early in Alzheimer's and late in Pick's
C. Personality changes occur early in Pick's and late in Alzheimer's
D. Klüver-Bucy syndrome develops early in Pick's and late in Alzheimer's
E. Visuospatial disturbances occur early in Pick's and late in Alzheimer's

22. Permanent loss of smell is most likely associated with which of the following?

A. Basal skull fracture
B. Vitamin B_{12} deficiency
C. Chronic purulent sinusitis
D. Astrocytoma of the amygdala
E. Meningioma of the posterior wall of the frontal sinus

23. Each of the following statements regarding the management of parkinsonism is true EXCEPT

A. Psychotherapy is important
B. Physical therapy is important
C. Early treatment will halt progression
D. The introduction of levodopa has significantly lowered the mortality rate
E. The "on-off" phenomenon is a disabling complication of chronic levodopa therapy

24. Which of the following is NOT characteristic of depression?

A. Frequent suicidal ideations
B. Diminished appetite and weight loss
C. Recurrent insomnia and increased appetite
D. Social disorganization and ineffectiveness in work
E. Heightened sexual interest and overconcern with personal appearance

25. A 58-year-old man has a six-month history of difficulty in walking and of numbness on the left side of his body. Four years ago, a squamous cell carcinoma of his epiglottis was excised and he received radiation therapy to this area. Physical examination shows diffuse fasciculations throughout the right upper extremity with generalized atrophy, decreased tone, hyporeflexia, and weakness of this limb. There is loss of proprioception in the right upper and lower extremities, together with loss of pain and temperature in the left upper and lower extremities. There is weakness, increased tone, hyper-reflexia, and a Babinski sign in the right lower extremity. He has a right-sided hemiparetic gait. Each of the following is true EXCEPT

A. The Brown-Séquard syndrome is a common presentation in radiation myelopathy
B. The upper motor neuron weakness is the result of damage to the right corticospinal tract, which is located in the lateral funiculus
C. The right upper extremity fasciculations, atrophy, and weakness are the result of anterior horn cell damage in the cervical region from C5 to T1
D. Proprioception on the right side is interrupted because of involvement of the fasciculus gracilis and fasciculus cuneatus, which are located in the dorsal funiculus
E. Pain and temperature sensation from the left half of the body is interrupted because it is carried in the right spinothalamic tract, which is located in the ventral funiculus

26. Which of the following statements concerning the management of chronic pain is correct?

A. Drug combinations are to be avoided
B. Tolerance develops to all narcotic analgesics
C. Minor analgesics are of little benefit and should be avoided
D. Antidepressants should be reserved for patients with concomitant depression
E. Analgesic doses should be spaced as far apart as possible to prevent drug abuse

27. A 36-year-old woman is amused by a friend, laughs heartily, and then suddenly falls to the ground without losing consciousness. Such attacks have occurred repeatedly over the past three years. Which of the following will most likely prevent these from recurring?

A. Diazepam
B. Imipramine

C. Methylphenidate
D. Phenytoin
E. Psychiatric counseling

28. Which of the following signs is NOT indicative of Parkinson's disease?

A. Rigidity
B. Bradykinesia
C. Micrographia
D. Action tremor
E. Loss of postural reflexes

29. Which of the following statements concerning subarachnoid hemorrhage is INCORRECT?

A. Inappropriate antidiuretic hormone secretion frequently occurs
B. Electrocardiographic abnormalities simulating myocardial infarction frequently occur
C. Vasospasm is the usual cause of initial lateralizing signs
D. CT scan of the brain frequently identifies blood in the subarachnoid space
E. The prognosis for a ruptured aneurysm is worse than for a bleeding arteriovenous malformation (AVM)

30. In a patient with disordered thinking and behavior, which of the following suggests an organic delirium rather than a psychiatric disease?

A. Auditory hallucinations
B. Asterixis and myoclonus
C. A normal awake electroencephalogram
D. Confusion as to personal identity, place, and time
E. Normal cognitive function (e.g., abstractions, calculations)

31. A 30-year-old man has a one-week history of low back pain that intermittently radiates into the left leg and is associated with numbness of the left foot. Which one of the following signs would most reliably indicate a herniated low lumbar intervertebral disc in this patient?

A. Low back pain exacerbated by forward flexion of the trunk and relieved by lying down
B. Point tenderness on percussion over the lumbar spine
C. Pain radiating from the back into the left leg when the nonpainful extended right leg is raised
D. Pain radiating from the back into the extended left leg when it is raised
E. Pain in the lumbar area produced by neck flexion

32. The parasomnias include each of the following EXCEPT

A. narcolepsy
B. nightmares
C. night terrors
D. somnambulism
E. sleep-talking

33. In a patient with the acquired immunodeficiency syndrome (AIDS), the most common CNS infection is due to

A. *Candida albicans*
B. *Toxoplasma gondii*
C. *Cryptococcus neoformans*
D. *Listeria monocytogenes*
E. *Coccidioides immitis*

34. Which of the following statements about patients with cerebral transient ischemic attacks (TIAs) is INCORRECT?

A. Angiography is indicated if the clinical picture suggests carotid artery disease
B. Transient unilateral visual loss is highly suggestive of carotid artery disease
C. The chance of recurring stroke after a TIA is approximately 5% per year
D. Aspirin appears effective in preventing stroke in many TIA patients
E. Stroke is the most likely cause of death

35. Each of the following statements regarding muscle cramps is correct EXCEPT

A. They are caused by motor units firing at a very fast rate (300+/sec)
B. The pain is often relieved by contracting the affected muscle
C. The pain may be effectively treated with quinine
D. They may be effectively treated with phenytoin
E. They may be effectively treated with diazepam

36. Which of the following statements concerning multiple sclerosis is INCORRECT?

A. Many patients worsen with an intercurrent febrile illness
B. Many patients worsen during pregnancy
C. Migration from high-incidence areas to low-incidence areas during childhood diminishes the risk of developing the disease
D. Prevalence is higher in the northern United States and in Canada than in the southern United States and in Mexico
E. The average interval from clinical onset to death is 30 to 40 years

37. Manifestations of neurosyphilis include each of the following EXCEPT

A. meningitis
B. dementia
C. optic atrophy
D. pupils that react to light but do not accommodate
E. cerebral infarction

38. The basal ganglia comprise each of the following nuclei EXCEPT

A. caudate
B. putamen
C. amygdala
D. substantia nigra
E. subthalamic nuclei

39. Typical characteristics of nontraumatic brachial plexus neuropathy (brachial plexitis) include each of the following EXCEPT

A. pain in the affected extremity
B. complete recovery to be expected
C. prominent wasting of the involved muscles
D. distal muscles more involved than proximal muscles
E. motor impairment much greater than sensory impairment

40. A 69-year-old man has a six-month history of progressive difficulty with ambulation. Examination of his gait reveals that the feet appear glued to the floor and that he has great difficulty initiating movement. Once he starts walking, his gait is a halting, frequently broad-based movement that is done more easily with guidance and support. Retropulsion does occur and he has difficulty turning. The most likely cause of this gait disorder is

A. vestibular disease
B. cerebellar disease
C. sensory deprivation
D. frontal lobe disease
E. corticospinal tract disease

41. Which of the following is NOT characteristic of acute poliomyelitis?

A. Sensory dysfunction is rare
B. Autonomic dysfunction is rare
C. Fever to 39°C often marks the onset
D. Muscle pain often antedates paralysis
E. Cranial nerve palsies may occur early

42. A 19-year-old man has a six-year history of progressive loss of hearing and visual acuity. His ability to walk has slowly worsened. On examination he is noted to be short in stature and to display ataxia of gait. Incomplete external ophthalmoplegia is seen, together with pigmentary degeneration of the retina. Bilateral sensorineural hearing loss is also present. The toes are extensor to plantar stimulation. An EKG shows first-degree heart block and the CSF protein is 140 mg/dl. Which of the following is the most likely diagnosis?

A. Krabbe's disease
B. Kearns-Sayre syndrome
C. Pelizaeus-Merzbacher disease
D. Metachromatic leukodystrophy
E. Wohlfart-Kugelberg-Welander disease

43. You are called to the emergency room one morning to see a 65-year-old man who had several episodes of blindness in the left eye lasting up to five minutes the evening before. He now has persisting headache; he has just recovered from difficulty with expression and partial weakness of the right face and right hand lasting five minutes. The most appropriate diagnostic test is

A. digital subtraction angiography
B. 24-hour cardiac Holter monitor
C. electroencephalogram with sleep
D. ultrasound examination of the left carotid artery
E. computed tomography (CT scan) of the brain

44. A 59-year-old woman has a six-week history of progressive right hemiparesis which has lead to quadriparesis. She displays cortical blindness, dysarthria, dementia, and dysphasia. She was treated for chronic lymphocytic leukemia two years ago. Computed tomography (CT scan) of the brain shows many low-density, nonenhancing white matter lesions. The CSF is normal. The JC virus has been isolated from the brain biopsy sample. Which of the following is the appropriate diagnosis?

A. Multiple sclerosis
B. Alzheimer's disease
C. Creutzfeldt-Jakob disease
D. Subacute sclerosing panencephalitis
E. Progressive multifocal leukoencephalopathy

45. Complications of chronic benzodiazepine administration include each of the following EXCEPT

A. addiction
B. rebound insomnia
C. active metabolite accumulation
D. suppression of rapid eye movement (REM) sleep
E. suppression of stages III and IV of non-REM sleep

46. A 62-year-old woman is brought to the emergency room by a relative who describes her as confused. The relative leaves soon thereafter and no other history is available. The patient is confused, agitated, and knows neither where she is nor the month or year but can tell you her name. Immediate recall is good and remote memory is fair, but she cannot remember any newly learned items after three minutes. A lack of judgment and insight is noted. She tends to insert fabricated stories within answers as if to fill in the gaps in her memory. Examination shows a thin, frail patient with dry skin having poor turgor. Blood pressure is 130/70 mm Hg (supine); it falls to 90/50 mm Hg upon standing. Eye movements are hindered by a total inability to abduct the left eye and partial inability to abduct the right eye. Nystagmus is seen with upgaze. The pupils are 6 mm reacting to 4 mm bilaterally. The liver is hard, non-tender, and palpable 3 cm below the costal margin. The reflexes are brisk except for absent ankle jerks. Pain and temperature sensation are decreased in the hands and feet; the gait is ataxic. Serum sodium is 119 mEq/L. Which of the following is the most appropriate treatment for this patient?

A. Administer naloxone, 0.4 mg intravenously
B. Administer thiamine, 100 mg intramuscularly
C. Administer phenytoin, 1 g intravenously, not to exceed 50 mg/minute
D. Administer 10% sodium chloride solution intravenously, at 500 cc/hour
E. Administer 50% dextrose solution intravenously, followed by a maintenance infusion of 5% dextrose water solution

47. Which of the following statements concerning syringomyelia is INCORRECT?

A. It is frequently associated with a spinal neoplasm
B. It may be associated with vocal cord paralysis and lingual atrophy
C. It is frequently associated with congenital craniocervical malformations
D. It is characterized by loss of pain and position sense, with preservation of temperature and touch
E. Although surgical decompression of the syrinx may slow disease progression, it is *not* curative

48. A 78-year-old woman has a four-year history of slowly worsening gait disorder. She reports no pain but has noted slowly developing weakness in the arms and hands for the past two years. Examination shows atrophy, weakness, and fasciculations of the intrinsic hand muscles with mild weakness of the triceps and brachioradialis muscles bilaterally. There is diminished proprioception and vibration sense in both feet. The gait is spastic with mild weakness of the hip flexors, foot dorsiflexors, and hamstrings, but no atrophy or fasciculations are seen in the lower extremities. EMG reveals spontaneous activity in the intrinsic muscles of both hands and chronic reinnervative changes in the biceps and triceps muscles bilaterally. EMG of the lower limbs is normal. Which of the following is the most likely diagnosis?

A. Cervical spondylosis
B. Peripheral neuropathy
C. Scapuloperoneal dystrophy
D. Bilateral C8 radiculopathies
E. Amyotrophic lateral sclerosis

49. You see a 7-year-old boy because of problems with decreased school performance; poor attention span with periods of inattentiveness; and unpredictable, sudden, shocklike muscular contractions of the upper arms. The parents are distraught because a maternal first cousin has subacute sclerosing panencephalitis. On neurologic examination the child appears to be normal. Which of the following is the most likely diagnosis?

A. Early autism with self-stimulating behavior
B. Familial subacute sclerosing panencephalitis
C. Juvenile epileptic myoclonus
D. Absence (petit mal) seizures with complex motor manifestations
E. Childhood adjustment reaction manifested as school phobia

50. Which of the following is correct concerning uremic neuropathy?

A. Chronic hemodialysis frequently reverses the neuropathy
B. Renal transplantation frequently reverses the neuropathy
C. Distal motor weakness is the most consistent feature
D. Segmental demyelination is characteristic pathologically
E. The molecular weight of the responsible agent(s) is less than that of urea or creatinine

51. The febrile convulsion syndrome is generally considered to be benign, but a complete neurologic work-up, including CT scan of the brain, should be instituted in each of the following circumstances EXCEPT

A. when the child is younger than 2 years
B. when the child is older than 5 years
C. when focal posturing occurs during seizure
D. when the seizures last longer than 10 minutes
E. when the neurologic examination is abnormal after the seizure

52. In a patient who has been comatose for 48 hours following an episode of cerebral hypoxemia, each of the following neurologic signs is compatible with a poor prognosis EXCEPT

A. dysconjugate eye movements
B. mid-position (3 mm) fixed pupils
C. absent corneal responses
D. absent deep tendon reflexes
E. absent oculovestibular responses

53. A 54-year-old woman has a six-week history of progressive difficulty getting out of a chair, climbing stairs, and arising from a sitting position. The muscles and joints ache and she has developed difficulty swallowing. Examination shows tenderness and mild weakness of the pectoral and pelvic girdle musculature. The deep tendon reflexes are preserved and sensation is normal. Erythrocyte sedimentation rate is 25 mm/hour; creatinine phosphokinase is 550 units. EMG reveals florid spontaneous activity with highly complex, small motor unit potentials which are easily recruited. Which of the following statements is correct?

A. Muscle biopsy will reveal neuropathic changes
B. Pyridostigmine is the treatment of choice
C. An erythematous rash is an important diagnostic finding
D. The disorder is inherited as an autosomal recessive trait
E. The majority of patients with this disorder succumb within one year

54. A 55-year-old man suddenly collapses at home with a groan, falls unconscious, and is rushed to the emergency room. He did not report headache or any other symptoms before the attack. Although he had been taking two types of "medicine for hypertension," his wife believes he may have stopped taking these during the past month. On examination the patient is comatose with a respiratory rate of 12 per minute characterized by sustained periods of inspiration followed by sustained periods of expiration. Pulse rate is 50 per minute and blood pressure is 220/126 mm Hg. The eyes are tonically deviated to the right and the pupils measure 2 mm; they are equal but nonreactive to light. Corneal reflexes are absent on the left and diminished on the right. Ice-water calorics of the right ear show no response. There is no motor response to painful stimulation on the right half of the body; bilateral Babinski signs are present. The most likely diagnosis is

A. left pontine hemorrhage
B. right basal ganglia hemorrhage
C. Hemorrhage into the left parietal lobe
D. right middle cerebral artery ischemic infarction
E. ischemic infarction of the right lateral medullary region

DIRECTIONS: For questions 55 to 100, you are to decide whether EACH choice is true or false. Any combination of answers, from all true to all false, may occur. Mark the answer sheet "T" or "F" in the space provided.

55. Which of the following is/are true concerning aphasia?

A. Fluent expression with full comprehension but inability to repeat spoken phrases is localized to the parietal operculum
B. Nonfluent expression with inability to comprehend or to repeat spoken phrases is called expressive (Broca's) aphasia
C. Fluent expression with ability both to comprehend and to repeat spoken phrases but inability to name objects is localized to the angular gyrus
D. Nonfluent expression with ability both to comprehend and to repeat spoken phrases is called transcortical motor aphasia
E. Fluent expression with inability to comprehend or to repeat spoken phrases is localized to the posterior superior temporal area

56. Which of the following is/are effective in the treatment of myasthenia gravis?

A. Azathioprine
B. Thymectomy
C. Pyridostigmine
D. Prednisolone
E. Plasmapheresis

57. Essential tremor

A. is improved with intentional movements
B. often is suppressed by propranolol
C. often is suppressed by alcohol
D. often involves the voice
E. persists in REM sleep

58. Which of the following statements concerning use of cannabis is/are true?

A. It has an antinauseant effect
B. It has a peripheral vasoconstrictor effect
C. Depression and acute panic reactions are common adverse effects
D. Driving performance is usually significantly impaired
E. Excessive use is likely to produce stupor and coma

59. Which of the following is/are among the neurologic complications of vitamin B_{12} deficiency?

A. Absent ankle reflexes
B. Bilateral Babinski signs
C. Generalized seizures
D. Urinary retention
E. Loss of smell

60. Which of the following conditions is/are associated with myoglobulinuria?

A. Vigorous exercise
B. Malignant hyperthermia
C. Acute intermittent porphyria
D. Acid maltase deficiency (Pompe's disease)
E. Carnitine palmityl transferase deficiency (DiMauro's disease)

61. Electrophysiologic studies in a patient with amyotrophic lateral sclerosis are likely to show which of the following?

A. Normal F-responses
B. Normal H-reflexes
C. Fasciculations on EMG
D. Fibrillation potentials on EMG
E. Normal nerve conduction velocity

62. Which of the following is/are true of asterixis?

A. It is rhythmic
B. It is likely to affect the feet
C. It is likely to affect the tongue
D. It cannot be controlled by the patient
E. Its presence usually implies metabolic brain disease

63. Which of the following statements regarding lumbar puncture is/are true?

A. A platelet count below 30,000/mm^3 is an absolute contraindication
B. It is the procedure of choice to evaluate subarachnoid bleeding
C. The opening pressure should be measured with the patient relaxed and with knees extended
D. Lateral decubitus position with knees flexed is the ideal patient position
E. The 20-gauge stylet needle is rapidly introduced between the L4–L5 interspace

64. Insomnia is frequently associated with which of the following?

A. Sleep apnea
B. Depression
C. Chronic alcohol use
D. Kleine-Levin syndrome
E. Schizophrenia

65. Which of the following statements concerning AIDS is/are true?

A. HIV is associated with acute "aseptic" meningitis
B. HIV is associated with chronic "aseptic" meningitis
C. HIV is associated with a subacute encephalitis
D. HIV is associated with a chronic myelopathy
E. Early central nervous system involvement suggests opportunistic infection

66. Which of the following statements concerning the cerebral circulation is/are true?

A. Both the posterior and middle cerebral arteries supply the posterior limb of the internal capsule
B. The middle cerebral artery supplies the primary motor and sensory cortical areas for face and hand, together with the optic radiations
C. The anterior cerebral artery supplies the medial and superior surfaces of the cerebral hemisphere, together with Broca's area
D. The vertebral arteries arise from the subclavian arteries, traverse the bony canals in the transverse processes from the sixth to the second cervical vertebrae, and enter the skull through the jugular foramina
E. The basilar artery arises at the lower border of the pons and extends along the ventral aspect of the midbrain, supplying the corticospinal tracts, medial lemnisci, and medial longitudinal fasciculi in the pons and midbrain

67. Which of the following statements regarding the Eaton-Lambert syndrome is/are true?

A. Impaired release of acetylcholine occurs at nerve terminals
B. Impaired binding of acetylcholine occurs at muscle receptors
C. Circulating antibodies to acetylcholine receptors are present
D. Repetitive nerve stimulation produces an increase in action potential amplitude
E. An underlying malignancy is often present

68. Which of the following pharmaceutical agents is likely to cause peripheral neuropathy?

A. *Cis*-platinum
B. Vincristine
C. Isoniazid
D. Pyridoxine
E. Cyclophosphamide

69. Which of the following statements concerning basilar skull fracture is/are true?

A. Epidural hematomas occur more frequently than with other nondisplacing linear fractures
B. Prophylactic antibiotics are indicated when CSF rhinorrhea is present
C. Hemotympanum may precede Battle's sign
D. Cranial nerve palsies, primarily involving the optic, oculomotor, trochlear, and facial nerves, are common
E. The presence of intracranial air on skull roentgenograms requires surgical intervention

70. Electrophysiologic studies in a patient with acute Guillain-Barré syndrome of seven days' duration would be expected to show which of the following?

A. Delayed F-responses
B. Delayed H-reflexes
C. Normal sensory nerve conduction velocities
D. No spontaneous activity on EMG
E. A predominance of small motor units on EMG during voluntary muscle contraction

71. An MRI scan of a 56-year-old woman is shown above; the only abnormality is indicated by the arrow. Which of the following statements concerning this patient's disorder is/are true?

A. It is prevented by the rapid correction of profound hyponatremia
B. It commonly occurs in alcoholics and severely ill patients
C. An inflammatory cell infiltrate and nerve cell destruction occur in the central pons
D. Altered consciousness and sensory loss commonly occur
E. Quadriparesis with dysphagia and dysarthria commonly occurs

72. Pharmacologic properties of phenytoin include which of the following?

A. Erratic absorption from the gastrointestinal tract
B. Saturation kinetics, once steady state is attained
C. Hypotension after intramuscular administration
D. Shortness of refractory period and reduced automaticity in His-Purkinje tissue
E. Pyorrhea associated with long-term administration

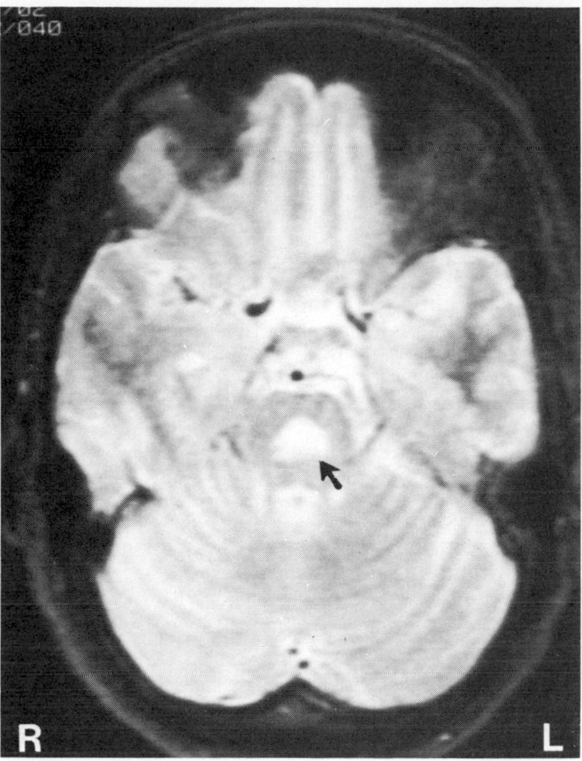

73. Which of the following statements regarding peripheral nervous system complications of AIDS is/are true?

A. Acute inflammatory demyelinating polyneuropathy (Guillain-Barré syndrome) occurs
B. Chronic inflammatory demyelinating polyneuropathy occurs
C. Painful distal sensory neuropathy occurs
D. Multiple mononeuropathies occur
E. Peripheral nervous system involvement occurs in otherwise asymptomatic patients

74. Which of the following is/are characteristic of the Shy-Drager syndrome (idiopathic autonomic insufficiency)?

A. Progressive bradykinesia, coarse tremor, and rigidity
B. Sexual impotence and anhidrosis
C. Urinary hesitancy, urgency, or incontinence
D. Blood pressure change from 140/180 mm Hg supine to 125/70 mm Hg standing
E. Fecal incontinence, chronic diarrhea, or constipation and dysphagia

75. A 40-year-old man is brought to see you by his wife. She states that he has recently become restless and overactive; he has incessant disjointed speech, has grandiose ideas, and is easy to anger. His sexual desires have increased, he has become reckless with money, and he has not been sleeping for the past week. He has a past history of intermittent depression dating back four years. Five years ago he had a similar episode of the present symptoms. His late father apparently had similar symptomatology. Detailed neurologic examination is otherwise normal. The most appropriate management of this patient would include which of the following?

A. Immediate hospitalization
B. Urgent CT scan of the brain

C. Administration of imipramine
D. Administration of lithium carbonate
E. Electroconvulsive treatment

76. Which of the following is/are true of post–lumbar puncture headache?

A. A frontal and occipital throbbing headache occurs in the upright position
B. The headache rapidly subsides in the recumbent position
C. The headache usually occurs within one day of the lumbar puncture
D. Prompt bed rest after the procedure will significantly reduce the incidence of these headaches
E. An epidural blood patch helps resolve persistent cases

77. Which of the following is/are among the predisposing causes of carpal tunnel syndrome?

A. Myxedema
B. Acromegaly
C. Amyloidosis
D. Pregnancy
E. Excessive use of the hands

78. Which of the following statements concerning trigeminal neuralgia is/are true?

A. It is characterized by sudden, lightning-like paroxysms of pain in the distribution of one or more divisions of the trigeminal nerve
B. Pain may be precipitated by touching the lip, talking, chewing, or brushing the teeth
C. There is variable sensory loss in the trigeminal distribution, but the neurologic examination is otherwise normal
D. Phenytoin is the drug of choice
E. Surgical intervention for the relief of intractable pain is of dubious value

79. Which of the following is/are included among signs of a lower motor neuron lesion?

A. Clonus
B. Atrophy
C. Hypotonia
D. Hyper-reflexia
E. Fasciculations

80. Which of the following statements concerning peripheral neuropathy is/are true?

A. Diphtheria is a rare cause of a pure demyelinating neuropathy
B. Glucocorticoids are often efficacious in treating chronic inflammatory neuropathy
C. Progressive, painful, asymmetric weakness of the anterior thigh muscles with loss of the knee jerk is often due to diabetes
D. Childhood onset of a slowly progressive weakness with atrophy of the anterolateral muscles of the legs, along with a pes cavus deformity of the feet and extremely slow motor conduction velocities, strongly suggests Type I hereditary motor and sensory neuropathy
E. Patients with known myeloma who develop bilateral carpal tunnel syndrome should be evaluated for systemic amyloidosis

81. Which of the following statements regarding cortical vein thrombosis is/are true?

A. Focal seizures are a common presentation
B. It commonly occurs during the puerperium
C. It may be mistaken for subarachnoid hemorrhage
D. The presence of major neurologic deficits indicates a poor prognosis
E. Early cases may mimic transient ischemic attacks

82. Which of the following is/are true of intracranial hypertension?

A. It is sometimes produced by sagittal sinus thrombosis
B. It is sometimes produced by the Guillain-Barré syndrome
C. Papilledema is usually present
D. Retinal venous pulsations are sometimes present
E. Headaches of varying severity usually occur in the early morning
F. Severe headache is usually present

83. A 38-year-old male alcoholic comes to the emergency room and reports that he had a stroke. After spending the night in an all-night theater, he noted weakness of the right hand this morning. Physical examination shows a total inability to extend the fingers and wrist on the right side with normal elbow extension and triceps reflex. When the arm is held outward there is marked difficulty abducting and adducting the fingers of the right hand. Hypesthesia is noted on the dorsal surface of the right hand extending onto the thumb, index, and middle fingers. No sign of injury is found and the remainder of the examination is normal. Which of the following is/are true?

A. The prognosis for complete recovery is good
B. The probably site of the lesion is the posterior cord of the brachial plexus
C. The lesion most likely involves demyelination
D. The loss of finger abduction/adduction suggests ulnar nerve impairment
E. The normal elbow extension and triceps reflex rule out a radial nerve palsy

84. A 30-year-old woman has gradual worsening of vision in the right eye. Ophthalmologic examination shows bright, colored, highly refractile opacities beneath the posterior lens capsule, and the patient is referred to a neurologist. She reports a long history of "stiffness" in her hands and of trouble relaxing her grip. She is noted to have slight male pattern baldness and a long, thin face with mild bilateral ptosis. The voice is markedly nasal in quality. Atrophy of the intrinsic hand and forearm muscles is noted. When the thenar muscles are struck with a percussion hammer, there is abduction and flexion of the thumb with very slow relaxation. Which of the following is/are true of this patient's disorder?

A. Intelligence is often found to be low normal
B. An EKG is likely to show first-degree heart block
C. It is transmitted as a sex-linked recessive trait
D. Hypothyroidism is often found to be present
E. Laboratory measurements of creatine phosphokinase and aldolase are likely to be 20 times the normal value

85. Which of the following statements concerning rabies is/are true?

A. Active vaccination of domestic animals helps eradicate the disease
B. It is enzootic in skunks, foxes, raccoons, wolves, and bats
C. Prompt debridement and cleansing of a bite is the most effective way of preventing rabies
D. Vaccination after a rabid bite is *not* effective in preventing rabies
E. The incubation period usually ranges from 20 to 60 days

86. Which of the following statements concerning the malignant hyperthermia syndrome is/are true?

A. It is often associated with the use of halothane
B. It is often associated with the use of succinylcholine
C. Muscle stiffness should be relieved by dantrolene
D. An autosomal dominant inheritance occurs in some families
E. Elevated creatine phosphokinase is found in some patients at risk

87. Elevated cerebrospinal fluid gamma globulin concentration is sometimes seen in

A. neurosyphilis
B. Reye's syndrome
C. multiple sclerosis
D. Guillain-Barré syndrome
E. subacute sclerosing panencephalitis

88. Which of the following is/are true of post-poliomyelitis motor neuron disease?

A. It is an early complication of paralytic poliomyelitis
B. It is characterized by increasing weakness in previously affected muscles
C. Spasticity commonly develops in the affected limbs
D. Progressive muscular atrophy is commonly present
E. Fasciculations are commonly present

89. Which of the following is/are useful in differentiating papilledema from acute papillitis (optic neuritis)?

A. Bedside measurement of visual acuity
B. Bedside measurement of visual fields
C. Bedside evaluation of ocular motility
D. Bedside evaluation of the pupillary light reflex
E. Ophthalmoscopic examination of the retina

90. Which of the following statements regarding the neurologic complications of AIDS is/are true?

A. The incidence of bacterial meningitis is increased
B. Lymphoma of the brain and meninges is the most common CNS neoplasm
C. Vascular events with associated hemorrhage occur frequently
D. Unexplained focal neurologic deficits with no clear etiology have been reported
E. Peripheral neuropathy occurs frequently

91. A 56-year-old man and three of his four children (two sons and one daughter) have repeated episodes of weakness that developed during adolescence. These attacks always begin with weakness of the legs followed by gradually progressive weakness of the arms. They have found that avoidance of exercise is helpful, since an attack always occurs when they are recovering from vigorous exercise. The attacks occur frequently at night; when they do, the patient may wake up unable to move for one or more days. Which of the following is/are true of this disorder?

A. During an attack, the ECG shows peaked T-waves
B. During an attack, serum potassium is usually in the range of 2.5–3.5 mEq per liter
C. Persistent proximal muscle weakness is not found between attacks
D. Acetazolamide is the drug of choice to prevent the attacks
E. Intravenous administration of glucose, 100 g, and regular insulin, 20 units, will reproduce the symptoms in an affected patient

92. Which of the following statements concerning the treatment of postherpetic neuralgia is/are true?

A. Direct cutaneous stimulation over the involved area provides relief
B. Amitriptyline appears to be beneficial
C. The early administration of corticosteroids may reduce the severity
D. Epidural and paraspinal nerve blocks provide relief
E. Surgical division of the involved intercostal nerve is curative

93. Which of the following is compatible with a mitochondrial myopathy?

A. Proximal limb weakness
B. A low serum carnitine concentration
C. A low muscle carnitine concentration
D. Ragged red muscle fibers
E. Ophthalmoplegia, pigmentary degeneration of the retina, and heart block

94. Which of the following statements regarding reflex sympathetic dystrophy is/are true?

A. Muscle atrophy and osteoporosis are early features
B. Continuous burning pain is characteristic
C. A sympathetic block relieves the pain
D. A surgical sympathectomy relieves the pain
E. An antecedent major traumatic injury usually occurs

95. Which of the following clinical features is/are compatible with a lacunar infarction?

A. Pure motor hemiplegia
B. Hemisensory loss on face, arm, and leg
C. Unilateral ataxia and hemiparesis
D. Receptive aphasia and right arm paresis
E. Left homonymous hemianopsia and right arm paresis

96. Which of the following drugs is/are useful in the prophylaxis of migraine?

A. Oxycodone
B. Ergotamine
C. Propranolol
D. Methysergide
E. Amitriptyline

97. Which of the following is/are included among features of Friedreich's ataxia?

A. Nystagmus
B. Pes cavus
C. Impaired position sense

D. Absent deep tendon reflexes
E. Extensor plantar response (Babinski sign)

98. Which of the following has/have been shown to be of benefit in the treatment of multiple sclerosis?

A. Adrenocorticotropic hormone (ACTH)
B. Glucocorticoids
C. Cyclosporine
D. Plasmapheresis
E. Hyperbaric oxygenation

99. A 37-year-old woman reports diminished hearing in the right ear; she gradually lost vision in the left eye 20 years ago. Physical examination shows that the tongue deviates to the right, speech is slurred, and the palate elevates poorly on the right side, with the gag reflex absent on the right. Seven flat, nontender pigmented skin lesions, each 2–3 cm in size, are seen on the torso. In this patient, which of the following is/are likely now or in the future?

A. Meningioma
B. Primary glioma
C. Oligodendroglioma
D. Metastatic tumor to brain
E. Primary CNS lymphoma

100. Which of the following statements concerning acute transverse myelitis is/are true?

A. Most cases are due to multiple sclerosis
B. Most cases are due to vascular occlusion
C. Urinary incontinence is frequent but retention is rare
D. If used early, glucocorticoids produce significant resolution
E. Rapid onset of paraplegia is accompanied by sparing of vibration and position sense distally

DIRECTIONS: Questions 101 to 155 are matching questions. For each numbered item, choose the most likely associated lettered item from those provided. Each numbered item has ONLY ONE answer. Within each set of questions, each lettered item may be the answer to one, more than one, or none of the numbered items.

QUESTIONS 101–105

For each patient described below, select the most appropriate anticonvulsant drug. (*NOTE: Unless otherwise noted, use each lettered item only once.*)

A. Phenytoin
B. Sodium valproate
C. Carbamazepine
D. Ethosuximide
E. None of the above

101. A 2-year-old boy with generalized seizures and a temperature of 39.5°C

102. A 5-year-old girl who has been mistakenly considered "inattentive" and "a daydreamer"

103. A 20-year-old woman who jerks involuntarily in response to sensory stimulation or movement

104. A 24-year-old man who persistently smacks the lips with an arrest of other activities

105. A 37-year-old man with focal motor seizures that spread up the extremities toward the trunk

QUESTIONS 106–110

For each of the following clinical descriptions select the most appropriate diagnosis.

A. Duchenne dystrophy
B. Limb-girdle dystrophy
C. Myotonia congenita
D. Myotonic dystrophy
E. Facioscapulohumeral dystrophy

106. An autosomal dominant inheritance; there is difficulty in relaxing muscles but no weakness

107. An autosomal dominant inheritance; it is associated with cataracts, testicular atrophy, and baldness in males

108. An autosomal recessive inheritance; it begins in adolescence with normal or slightly increased muscle enzymes

109. An autosomal dominant inheritance; it begins in adolescence and occasionally involves the truncal muscles

110. An X-linked recessive inheritance; it begins in childhood and muscle enlargement is common

QUESTIONS 111–115

For each of the following headache syndromes, select the most appropriate treatment. (*NOTE: Use each lettered item only once.*)

A. Carbamazepine
B. Ergotamine
C. Lithium
D. Indomethacin
E. Biofeedback

111. Migraine

112. Cluster

113. Tension

114. Trigeminal neuralgia

115. Paroxysmal hemicrania

QUESTIONS 116–120

For each of the following stroke syndromes, select the artery that is most likely to be involved.

A. Right vertebral
B. Left anterior cerebral
C. Left middle cerebral
D. Left posterior cerebral
E. Right paramedian branch of the basilar

116. Loss of abduction of the right eye with a left hemiplegia and diminished tactile and proprioceptive sense in the left half of the body

117. Diplopia with gaze to the right, ptosis and pupillary mydriasis on the left, and a right hemiplegia

118. Loss of pain and temperature in the right half of the face and left half of the body; ataxia with falling to the right, right ptosis and miosis, dysphagia, hoarseness, and diminished gag reflex on the right

119. Aphasia with paralysis and diminished sensation of the right face and right upper extremity

120. Paresis and diminished sensation of the right leg along with urinary retention, mild confusion, agitation, and dysphasic speech

QUESTIONS 121–125

For each of the following descriptions of drug overdose, select the most appropriate treatment.

A. Intubation and ventilation
B. Hydration and hemodialysis
C. Administration of naloxone
D. Administration of chlorpromazine
E. Administration of physostigmine

121. A hyperactive, agitated patient with dilated pupils, hyperthermia, and tachycardia

122. A drowsy patient with small pupils, shallow respirations, hypothermia, and hypotension

123. A restless, drowsy patient with tachyarrhythmias, hyperpyrexia, and convulsions

124. A confused patient with progressive drowsiness and slightly constricted but reactive pupils

125. A lethargic patient who is mute and has multifocal seizures

QUESTIONS 126–130

For each of the following pupillary abnormalities, select the most likely diagnosis.

A. Syphilis
B. Pancoast tumor

C. Multiple sclerosis
D. Holmes-Adie syndrome
E. Posterior communicating artery aneurysm

126. The pupil is 3–6 mm and constricts little or not at all to light and slowly to accommodation, but constricts well with instillation of dilute (0.02%) pilocarpine

127. The pupil is 2 mm, reactive to light, and associated with ipsilateral slight ptosis and anhidrosis

128. The pupil is 1–2 mm and nonreactive to light, but constricts with accommodation

129. The pupil is equal to or slightly larger than the contralateral pupil and constricts to consensual light but not to direct light stimulation

130. The pupil is 5–6 mm, unreactive to light, and associated with ipsilateral ptosis and mild exotropia

QUESTIONS 131–135

For each of the following clinical syndromes, select the most appropriate site of the lesion.

A. Musculocutaneous nerve
B. Peroneal nerve
C. Median nerve
D. Femoral nerve
E. C6 nerve root

131. Decreased sensation on volar aspect of thumb and index and middle fingers; weakness of wrist flexors, long finger flexors (thumb, index and middle fingers), pronators of forearm, and the abductor pollicus brevis; loss of finger reflexes

132. Decreased sensation over the lateral forearm excluding the thumb; weakness of biceps and brachialis; absent biceps reflex

133. Decreased sensation over the dorsum of foot; weakness of foot and toe dorsiflexion; no reflex changes

134. Decreased sensation on lateral forearm including the thumb; weakness of biceps, brachialis, and brachioradialis; absent supinator reflex

135. Decreased sensation on anterior thigh and medial leg; weakness of extension at the knee; absent knee reflex

QUESTIONS 136–140

From the description of each of the following choreiform disorders, find the most likely diagnosis.

A. Huntington's disease
B. Wilson's disease
C. Ataxia-telangiectasia
D. Lesch-Nyhan syndrome
E. Chorea-acanthocytosis

136. A 7-year-old boy with chorea, athetosis, spasticity, aggression, and compulsive self-multilation of the lips; hyperuricemia is present

137. A 14-year-old girl with recurrent pulmonary infections and a 10-year history of progressive ataxia and choreoathetoid movements, dysarthria, and myoclonic jerks; she is areflexic with a peripheral neuropathy and spider-like vascular abnormalities on the ears, nose, and forearms

138. A 36-year-old man with a seven-year history of tremor of the arms and head progressing to choreiform movements, with dysarthria, dysphagia, drooling, muscle rigidity, and mental dulling; ophthalmologic and hepatic dysfunctions are present

139. A 42-year-old woman with a four-year history of progressive chorea, orofacial tics, self-mutilation of the lips and tongue, areflexia, elevated serum creatine phosphokinase, "burr cells" on peripheral blood smear, and atrophy of the caudate nuclei on CT scan

140. A 49-year-old woman with a seven-year history of progressive clumsiness leading to chorea of arms, legs, and bulbar musculature. The gait is characterized by hesitation, stuttering steps, and frequent falls. Emotional problems in earlier years have progressed to delusions, paranoia, impulsiveness, and agitation, with recent impairment of memory and judgment

QUESTIONS 141–145

For each of the following syndromes, select the most appropriate treatment.

A. Reserpine
B. Guanidine
C. Haloperidol
D. Thiamine
E. Insulin
F. Glucose
G. Symptomatic

141. Eaton-Lambert syndrome

142. Tourette's syndrome

143. Reye's syndrome

144. Tardive dyskinesia syndrome

145. Korsakoff's syndrome

QUESTIONS 146–150

For each of the following clinical descriptions of peripheral neuropathy, select the most likely causative toxin.

A. Lead
B. Acrylamide
C. Thallium
D. Arsenic
E. Organophosphates

146. Sensory loss, hyperkeratosis, brown skin, Mees' lines, and pitting edema of the feet and ankles

147. Painful paresthesias of the feet and hands, alopecia, Mees' lines, ataxia, chorea, and cranial neuropathies

148. Wrist drop, abdominal colic, constipation, fatigue, anorexia, and weight loss

149. Truncal ataxia and skin peeling, and excessive sweating of feet and hands

150. Cholinergic symptoms may occur first with slightly delayed onset of neuropathy that maximizes within two weeks

QUESTIONS 151–155

For each of the following descriptions, select the most likely diagnosis.

A. Lateral sinus thrombosis
B. Cavernous sinus thrombosis
C. Sagittal sinus thrombosis

D. Temporal lobe abscess
E. Subdural empyema

151. A 14-year-old girl with right facial pain, high fever, left hemiparesis, nuchal rigidity, and progressive obtundation

152. A 30-year-old man with prostration, fever, headache, papilledema, and edema of the right forehead and anterior scalp, with left focal motor seizures

153. A 47-year-old man with a one-week history of left forehead and temporal headache along with nausea and vomiting. Brief episodes of altered awareness with normal consciousness and an inability to follow commands began two days ago. He now speaks fluently, but the speech is remarkably devoid of meaning with much paraphasia

154. A 51-year-old man with high fever and a generalized headache with malaise, who has chemosis, edema, and cyanosis of the upper face with a right oculomotor palsy and hypesthesia of the right forehead

155. A 69-year-old man with fever, right-sided headache felt maximally behind the right ear, tenderness over the right mastoid process, right abducens palsy, and right facial numbness

PART 10

NEUROLOGIC DISEASE

ANSWERS

1.(E) Trihexyphenidyl is a commonly employed anticholinergic agent that is useful in Parkinson's disease as adjunctive therapy to levodopa, especially to suppress tremor. It may also be used in mildly affected patients before levodopa is administered and is the agent of choice in drug-induced parkinsonism. In contrast, reserpine depletes the storage of dopamine in dopaminergic nerve terminals in the striatum; chlorpromazine (a phenothiazine) and haloperidol (a butyrophenone) block postsynaptic dopamine receptors in the striatum. These latter two agents are well-recognized potential causes of drug-induced parkinsonism. The synthetic opiate by-product, MPTP, produces selective destruction of cells within the substantia nigra, leading to parkinsonism that is identical to idiopathic Parkinson's disease. *(Cecil, Ch. 468; Burns et al)*

2.(D) Progressive supranuclear palsy (PSP) resembles Parkinson's disease, but tremor is rare. Progressive ophthalmoplegia occurs and vertical eye movements are lost first. Impairment of downward gaze clearly differentiates this from Parkinson's disease, in which upgaze alone may be limited in some cases. Eventually, horizontal eye movements become totally restricted, yet a full range of reflex eye movements exists because the ophthalmoplegia is supranuclear. Hyperextension of the neck in PSP is unlike the more typically flexed position of the parkinsonian patient. Striatonigral degeneration may present clinically as Parkinson's disease, but, with time, signs of cerebellar ataxia and laryngeal stridor usually appear. Failure to respond to levodopa therapy also suggests striatonigral degeneration. Dystonia musculorum deformans comprises a group of twisting movement disorders (torsion spasm). One characteristic is the propensity of these spasms to be maintained at the end of the movement for a second or two (dystonic movements) or for minutes to hours (dystonic postures). The olivopontocerebellar degenerations represent a group of adult-onset disorders characterized by progressive cerebellar dysfunction, nystagmus, and loss of fast saccadic eye movements. Later in the course, patients develop spasticity, optic nerve atrophy, distal sensory impairment, and intellectual dysfunction. *(Cecil, Chs. 467, 468, and 471)*

3.(D) This patient has giant cell arteritis. Recent onset of progressive headache in the elderly may indicate giant cell arteritis. Many patients have pain in the facial muscles with few or no other symptoms. A mild anemia may coexist. The Westergren sedimentation rate is invariably elevated, and temporal artery biopsy confirms the diagnosis. The normal neurologic examination with the history of progressive headache is not suggestive of an expanding intracranial lesion. The absence of pyrexia and signs of meningeal irritation with normal mentation argue against meningitis or subarachnoid hemorrhage. Coexistence of depression may be common, but is not the cause of this headache. Depressive headache is usually a generalized headache of variable intensity and may indeed be prominent with depression in older individuals. This, however, is a diagnosis of exclusion. Rheumatoid arthritis and thyroid disorders rarely cause isolated severe headaches. *(Cecil, Chs. 442 and 466)*

4.(D) Spasmodic torticollis is the most common form of focal torsion dystonia. It usually begins in adulthood and remains limited to this region of the body. Occasionally there is spread to involve the vocal cords (spasmodic dysphonia) and one or both arms (segmental dystonia). Various treatments have been tried: surgical section of cranial nerve XI produces inconsistent relief; dorsal column stimulation is sometimes helpful, as is sensory biofeedback therapy. Anticholinergics in high doses are often effective, and the drug of choice is trihexyphenidyl. Some benefit may be found with carbamazepine, diazepam, and, rarely, levodopa. Although dorsal root entry zone surgery has been reported to be effective in chronic pain following root avulsion injuries, it has not been effectively employed in the treatment of spasmodic torticollis. *(Cecil, Ch. 471)*

5.(C) Brain CT scan reveals hydrocephalus with ventricular enlargement, no significant cortical atrophy, and no evidence of focal intracerebral structural disease. This most likely represents chronic hydrocephalus of a normal pressure variety. Gait ataxia, dementia, and urinary incontinence are the triad of common presenting features. With acute hydrocephalus, raised intracranial pressure and papilledema may occur; however, focal brain symptoms such as seizures, aphasia, and hemiparesis are not seen unless a focal cause of the obstruction is present. Detailed history and neurologic examination should not be normal with hydrocephalus of this degree. *(Cecil, Ch. 495)*

6.(D) The initial clinical picture of visuospatial neglect is that of a right parieto-occipital expanding mass lesion. Displacement of the hemisphere causes the uncus of the right temporal lobe to squeeze into the tentorial notch and against the midbrain. As this occurs the ipsilateral third nerve becomes compressed, resulting in partial ptosis, pupillary dilatation, and eventual loss of extraocular movements. Compression of the ipsilateral peduncle produces contralateral signs (left hemiplegia) and, as the rostrocaudal pressure continues, diffuse decerebrate posturing and shivering begin. The initial management is to rapidly reduce the raised intracranial pressure. Hyperventilation producing hypocapnia will reduce cerebral blood flow and thus help reduce intracranial pressure, as will intravenous osmotic agents such as mannitol. This is the treatment of choice for acute herniation, and it should not be delayed pending further examination or special investigations. *(Cecil, Ch. 457; Plum and Posner, pp. 97–101)*

7.(D) The aminoglycosides (gentamicin, tobramycin, kanamycin, streptomycin, neomycin, and amikacin) are all toxic to the cochlea, but this does not include erythromycin. These agents destroy the cochlear hair cells in direct relation to their serum concentrations, and cumulative drug exposure may produce permanent hearing loss. Salicylates, furosemide, and ethacrynic acid produce transient deafness when taken in high doses. *Cis*-platinum may produce severe ototoxicity. *(Cecil, Ch. 464)*

8.(A) Neurologic symptoms and signs occur in 25–30% of patients with subacute bacterial endocarditis. The most common neurologic manifestation is cerebrovascular disease, which occurs in about half the patients. Embolic lesions, such as cerebral infarction, intracerebral hemorrhage, and transient ischemic attacks, occur and behave like similar lesions from other kinds of emboli. A subacute toxic encephalopathy with confusion, delirium, hallucinations, confabulation, disorientation, and paranoid ideation may occur. Milder manifestations include drowsiness, insomnia, apathy, irritability, and personality changes. As is the case with other types of embolic cerebrovascular disease, papilledema is not a typical presenting sign. *(Cecil, Ch. 481)*

9.(A) The purpose of the neurologic history is to obtain diagnostic information that will direct the physical and laboratory examinations and lead to an appropriate diagnosis. To establish a satisfactory doctor-patient relationship and thus manage the patient's illness satisfactorily, reassurance, support, and confidence should be instilled in the patient from the beginning. The history often suggests the anatomic site of the lesion, and the rate and character of progression may frequently suggest the pathophysiology. Completeness in history-taking is essential to avoid missing symptoms that the patient may deem unimportant. The history should always be summarized to the patient to correct any misinformation or misunderstanding on the physician's part. It is important to elicit the history in the patient's own words and to allow the patient whenever possible to tell the story without excessive interruptions. However, it is essential that the patient's history have relevance and precision. Therefore, interruptions to direct the patient back to the main complaint, and to identify qualities such as frequency and intensity of symptoms together with aggravating and relieving factors, may be essential. *(Cecil, Ch. 456)*

10.(C) The patient most likely has right-sided peripheral end-organ vestibular dysfunction. Vertigo accompanied by vertical nystagmus is highly suggestive of central nervous system pathology and would not be expected in this case. With peripheral vertigo one expects the Barany maneuver to show rotatory and horizontal nystagmus with a fast component away from the affected ear when it is placed downward. Absent or decreased response to cold water caloric testing of the affected labyrinth (vestibular paresis) is typical of peripheral pathology. Visual fixation during vertigo dampens the nystagmus produced by labyrinthine dysfunction but has no effect upon central nystagmus. In peripheral labyrinthine dysfunction, past-pointing will be toward the side of the affected end organ. *(Cecil, Ch. 464; Asbury et al, Ch. 42; Baloh, pp. 73–95)*

11.(A) Multi-infarct dementia describes dementia resulting from cerebrovascular disease. The decline in intellectual function results from multifocal occlusion of cerebral arteries and arterioles, either from remotely arising emboli or from intrinsic cerebral arteriolar occlusive disease. As is typical of subcortical dementias, insight is often retained and accompanied by depression of mood. Disturbances of gait, station, and motor function accompanied by abnormalities in language, mood, and attention may also be seen, depending upon the location of the cerebral infarcts. The condition appears most often in association with diabetic or hypertensive vascular disease that produces both large and small infarcts. This dementia characteristically progresses in steps with partial recovery occurring between the periodic losses of neurologic function. The disorder accounts for approximately 20% of all dementias and thus represents about one-half the number of patients with Alzheimer's disease (40% of all dementias). *(Cecil, Ch. 461; Asbury et al, Ch. 71; Cummings, pp. 125–143)*

12.(C) Transient global amnesia is marked by fully alert periods lasting from several minutes to as long as one day of acute confusion, during which the affected person can identify himself but is severely disoriented with regard to time and place. Status epilepticus with complex partial or nonconvulsive, generalized (absence or petit mal) seizures can produce a somewhat similar amnestic state, but convulsions are distinguished by dull, slow-witted, and inattentive behavior. With organic memory loss, disorientation is greatest for time, less for place and person, and rarely for self. In contrast, psychogenic amnesia tends to be greatest for emotionally important events, and the patient may claim loss of well-defined blocks of past events while leaving intact the recall of preceding or following material; it tends to affect remote memory equally with recent memory, resists improvement with cues, and sometimes even includes disorientation to self. With hepatic encephalopathy, the patient becomes drowsy and finally stuporous or comatose; the alteration in memory and other cognitive function parallels this decrease in level of consciousness. *(Cecil, Chs. 457 and 460)*

13.(D) Alzheimer's disease usually presents with a recent memory disturbance that is gradually progressive.The illness slowly advances over many years, in contrast to Creutzfeldt-Jakob disease, and rapidly advancing dementia that results in death usually within a year. Seizures do occur in up to 15% of patients with Alzheimer's disease. The pathologic hallmarks are senile plaques and neurofibrillary tangles in the cerebral cortex. The cause of Alzheimer's disease is unknown, but up to 25% of patients do have a family history of dementia and/or Down's syndrome. *(Cecil, Ch. 461; Heyman et al)*

14.(A) The clinical picture (history and physical) indicates multifocal neurologic dysfunction involving the right eye (optic nerve), corticospinal tracts (hyper-reflexia), cerebellum (right upper extremity dysmetria and bilateral nystagmus), and the posterior columns of the spinal cord (diminished vibration sense). The MRI scan reveals multiple white matter lesions compatible with a diagnosis of multiple sclerosis. An inappropriate euphoric effect is common in this condition. Amyotrophic lateral sclerosis results from loss of anterior horn cells and cortical motor neurons but does not show multiple focal abnormalities on MRI scan. Cerebral infarction rarely involves the white matter alone. The characteristic appearance is that of distal wedge-shaped lesions involving the gray as well as the white matter. Metastatic carcinoma is usually associated with significant surrounding edema and distortion of adjacent brain which is not present in this scan. AIDS may be associated with various opportunistic infections, but neither the clinical history nor the scan appearance is strongly suggestive of any of these. *(Cecil, Chs. 456, 492, and 494)*

15.(D) This man has almost all the symptoms and signs of obstructive sleep apnea. An overnight sleep EEG study with the use of nasal and oral thermistors as well as monitoring of chest and abdominal wall movement is the test of choice. Continuous nasal positive airway pressure is often helpful in relieving the obstruction during sleep.

The apnea often improves markedly or disappears after the patient loses weight. In recalcitrant cases tracheostomy may be necessary. It is unwise to suppress central respiratory centers, as many of these patients also have concomitant central nervous system dysfunction. Thus, amitriptyline and benzodiazepines are contraindicated. The multiple sleep latency test is useful in the diagnosis of narcolepsy. Sleep-deprived EEG is useful in the diagnosis of epilepsy. Although methylphenidate (Ritalin) may help with daytime somnolence, it does not treat the underlying cause of this condition. *(Cecil, Ch. 458; Parkes, pp. 383–386)*

16. (C) Congenital anomalies of the spine are common and are often encountered on radiographs of patients suffering from neck or back pain. Some congenital abnormalities, such as spina bifida occulta, are so common as to be considered normal variants. Other congenital anomalies, such as the Klippel-Feil syndrome (congenital fusion of two or more cervical vertebrae), are usually not responsible for neck pain or any neurologic symptom. Although facet tropism (misalignment of the facets on the two sides of the corresponding vertebral body) may lead to neck pain, it is not thought to be associated with neuropathology. Spondylolisthesis (forward slipping of one vertebral body over another, caused by a defect between the articular facets) may result in back pain, but only rarely is it associated with true neurologic abnormalities. Basilar impression, however, is frequently associated with the Arnold-Chiari malformation (downward displacement of the cerebellum in the foramen magnum) as well as with cerebellar dysfunction, lower cranial nerve abnormalities, pyramidal tract signs, and posterior column deficits. *(Cecil, Ch. 503)*

17. (C) Unlike the ophthalmoplegia in Wernicke's encephalopathy, that seen in progressive supranuclear palsy is supranuclear, such that a full range of reflex eye movements can be demonstrated by the doll's eye maneuver or by cold caloric testing. Cerebellar degeneration occurs in chronic alcoholics. Initially, unsteadiness with turning rapidly and abnormal tandem walking are seen and progress to a wide-based hesitant gait with truncal ataxia. This may develop abruptly, rapidly over several weeks, or sometimes more slowly with exacerbations following binge drinking or during intercurrent illnesses. Wernicke's encephalopathy, characterized by ophthalmoplegia, ataxia, and global confusion, commonly occurs. Marchiafava-Bignami disease is a rare disorder of symmetric demyelination of the corpus callosum and adjacent white matter affecting severely alcoholic middle-aged men with progressive dementia; it is accompanied by root, suck, and grasp reflexes along with paratonic rigidity, incontinence, and a slow hesitant gait suggesting frontal lobe dysfunction. Acute alcoholic myopathy is a dramatic and life-threatening condition developing in chronic alcoholics during prolonged drinking bouts. Creatine phosphokinase is elevated and acute rhabdomyolysis occurs. Myoglobulinuria may lead to acute renal failure, hyperkalemia, and death. Recovery usually follows days to weeks of abstinence but may leave residual proximal muscle weakness. *(Cecil, Chs. 467 and 468)*

18. (A) Herpes simplex encephalitis is a sporadic disease with a highly variable clinical course. Neurologic dysfunction can range from a mild encephalitis with confusion to widespread neurologic devastation. The onset is often abrupt and is frequently associated with seizures and focal neurologic findings on examination. The CT scan is often normal in the first four to five days of the disease, and cerebral biopsy is often indicated for confirmation. The EEG may be more reliable in indicating focal temporal lobe slowing and sometimes epileptiform discharges. Intracerebral blood and large invasive tumors rarely escape detection by CT scan. The preseizure symptoms argue against a Todd's paralysis. Occlusion of the middle cerebral artery would be expected to result in major sensory and motor impairment of the contralateral half of the body. *(Cecil, Ch. 485)*

19. (E) The history is of a longstanding problem and the scan demonstrates multiple cystic lesions without attendant edema or infiltration. Glioblastomas are rapidly malignant tumors that are occasionally cystic but are usually solitary and invasive. Astrocytomas usually diffusely infiltrate the brain, often with significant edema and distortion of the surrounding brain. Pituitary adenomas arise from the sella and may present as a suprasellar mass. Pinealomas do not arise from the frontal lobes and are usually not cystic tumors, but may produce hydrocephalus. Thus, by a process of elimination, multiple dermoid cysts is correct. *(Cecil, Ch. 494)*

20. (A) Schizophrenia is a disturbance of mind and personality marked by hallucinations, delusions, and altered behavior. Auditory hallucinations are common in schizophrenia, but visual hallucinations are more commonly seen in acute toxic delirium, as caused by alcohol or drugs. Delusions about bodily control frequently occur in schizophrenia, and the patient's language is frequently abnormal, lacking clarity and showing a tendency to wander. Emotional expression may vary from inappropriate to markedly blunted. Catatonic posturing is not infrequent, and dyskinetic grimacing due to antipsychotic drugs may be seen. *(Cecil, Ch. 462)*

21. (E) A cardinal feature of Alzheimer's disease is early loss of visuospatial orientation, which may lead to the patient's becoming lost in unfamiliar environments and can be demonstrated by an inability to copy three-dimensional drawings. Along with this, acalculia and memory disturbances occur early in Alzheimer's disease. Klüver-Bucy syndrome and personality changes occur early in Pick's disease but late in Alzheimer's disease. Unlike Alzheimer's disease, acalculia, memory loss, and visuospatial disturbances occur late in Pick's disease. *(Cecil, Ch. 461; Cummings, pp. 35–72)*

22. (A) Head trauma associated with basal skull fracture often produces significant sheering forces with tearing of the olfactory nerve fibrils as they traverse the cribriform plate to reach the olfactory bulb located on the ventral surface of the frontal lobe. This commonly produces permanent loss of smell. Chronic sinus infection, as well as vitamin B_{12} deficiency, herpes zoster, and multiple sclerosis, less commonly produce loss of smell. Tumors of the amygdala may result in hallucinations of smell but usually not loss of smell. Tumors arising from the cribriform plate may produce loss of smell, but tumors from the posterior wall of the frontal sinus commonly do not. *(Cecil, Ch. 464)*

23. (C) Psychotherapy and physical therapy are valuable adjunctive treatments. Levodopa has halved the mortality rate in parkinsonism, but the disease invariably progresses in spite of any form of treatment. Levodopa increases functional capacity and delays disabling symptoms, but because of the relentless progress of the disease it is advised that this drug be used only when the patient is significantly disabled. The "on-off" phenomenon occurs with levodopa usage in approximately 40% of patients, possibly owing to desensitization of dopamine receptors. *(Cecil, Ch. 468)*

24. (E) Depression denotes a mood of sadness and gloom. The patient appears miserable, the face expressive of sadness and perhaps tension. Sexual interest is greatly reduced. Appetite is usually lessened but may be increased, and weight may be increased or decreased. The patient may seem socially disorganized and prove inefficient in work, failing in duties, and neglectful of appearance. Sleep is typically restless and diminished. Acknowledged inadequacies in these respects may add to a sense of misery and may prompt thoughts of resigning from work, leaving the family, or even committing suicide. *(Cecil, Ch. 462)*

25. (E) Pain and temperature sensation from the left half of the body has been interrupted in the spinothalamic tract located in the right *lateral* funiculus. Proprioception is carried in the ipsilateral dorsal columns. The Brown-Séquard syndrome is sometimes seen with tumors either compressing or invading the spinal cord and is a common presenting syndrome in radiation myelopathy. The upper motor neuron weakness seen in this patient is due chiefly to damage of the descending corticospinal tract of the lateral funiculus. This tract is located on the side of the weakness, since the descending corticospinal fibers decussate at the craniovertebral junction. Anterior horn cell damage results in lower motor neuron findings, which include weakness, hypotonicity, hyporeflexia, atrophy, and fasciculations. Cord levels C5–T1 are responsible for supplying innervation to the musculature of the upper extremity. *(Cecil, Ch. 466; Carpenter, pp. 265–314)*

26. (B) Clinical and experimental evidence suggests that early prompt treatment is the most effective means of controlling chronic pain. Combination treatment is often better than a single agent alone, and the effects of minor analgesics and/or tricyclic antidepressants are often additive to the pain relief obtained from narcotics, to which tolerance will always develop. *(Cecil, Ch. 466)*

27. (B) This patient has cataplexy, which is part of the narcolepsy syndrome. This condition is difficult to control, and patients frequently develop depression and anxiety. Psychiatric counseling will not help the condition, and neither will benzodiazepines or anticonvulsants. Amphetamines, including methylphenidate, frequently help control the sleep attacks of narcolepsy, but the best pharmacologic agents for the treatment of cataplexy are such tricyclic antidepressants as imipramine. *(Cecil, Ch. 458)*

28. (D) Cardinal features of parkinsonism include tremor at rest, rigidity, bradykinesia, and loss of postural reflexes. Micrographia is a frequent occurrence. Most other types of tremor occur during action and these may signify cerebellar disease, benign familial tremor, drug effect, or metabolic illness. *(Cecil, Ch. 468)*

29. (C) Initial lateralizing signs, including hemiplegia, are usually due to an intracerebral hematoma, a large subdural hematoma, or a large subarachnoid hematoma. Vasospasm is usually a delayed phenomenon, producing ischemia and subsequent infarction during the first few days after a bleed. Excessive outpouring of catecholamines may cause multifocal micronecrosis of the myocardium, producing EKG abnormalities simulating myocardial infarction. SIADH may also occur. CT scan of the brain identifies blood in the subarachnoid space and/or ventricles in the majority of cases. The prognosis in subarachnoid hemorrhage from a ruptured aneurysm is grave, but that from a bleeding AVM is better. *(Cecil, Ch. 480; Heros et al)*

30. (B) Psychiatric disease can be distinguished in the awake patient by examination of the mental status and motor function. Psychotic patients are oriented and have normal cognitive functions. Delirious patients are disoriented and confused but never forget their personal identities. Hallucinations in psychiatric illness are usually auditory, but in metabolic illness they are usually visual. Asterixis and myoclonus indicate metabolic encephalopathy. *(Cecil, Ch. 457; Adams and Victor, pp. 306–308; Morse and Litin)*

31. (C) Pain referred to the contralateral back or leg when the nonpainful leg is raised (crossed straight leg raising) implies root compression within the spinal canal, and is the most accurate mechanical sign of a herniated intervertebral disc. The straight leg raising sign (i.e., pain radiating into an extended lower extremity when it is raised) occurs in most patients with severe low back pain, but does not indicate the underlying cause. Point tenderness over a spinous process raises the suspicion of vertebral tumor or infection. Point tenderness over muscles may indicate severe muscle spasm, which again is not diagnostic of the underlying etiology. Low back pain exacerbated by forward flexion and relieved by lying down occurs with any cause of spasm of the paravertebral back muscles. Pain in the lumbar area produced by neck flexion suggests cervical spinal cord disease or compression. *(Cecil, Ch. 499)*

32. (A) Narcolepsy is a pathologic syndrome characterized by a disordered sleep pattern; it is primarily attributed to increased excitability of the REM-regulating mechanism. The parasomnias, however, are sleep-associated processes that occur intermittently but do not represent a disorganization of normal sleep patterns and thus do not indicate a chronic pathologic state. Night terrors, somnambulism, bruxism, and sleep-talking are frequently associated with stages III and IV of sleep. Threatening nightmares frequently occur during REM sleep but occasionally may be seen in non-REM sleep. Narcolepsy represents a disorganization of the normal non-REM and REM sleep regulatory mechanism. *(Cecil, Ch. 458)*

33. (B) The usual CNS infection in a patient with AIDS is opportunistic, and this may be the mode of initial presentation for 10% of all AIDS patients. CNS toxoplasmosis is the most common cause, accounting for about one third of all CNS infections in AIDS. Cryptococcosis, candidiasis, coccidioidomycosis, and other opportunistic infections may also be expected, but at lower frequencies. *(Cecil, Ch. 491)*

34. (E) Most deaths in patients with TIAs appear to result from myocardial infarction. TIA therefore is a major risk factor for both stroke and myocardial infarction. Angiography with a view to endarterectomy may be indicated if the symptoms suggest carotid artery disease. Unilateral blindness is frequently an indicator of proximal carotid artery disease, as the ophthalmic artery is the first branch of the internal carotid artery and thus may be the site for termination of a carotid embolus. There is a 5 to 6% chance per year of stroke occurring after a TIA. Several clinical trials have indicated that aspirin is effective in preventing stroke and death in a significant number of men with TIAs. *(Cecil, Ch. 479; Heyman et al)*

35. (B) Muscle cramp is caused by a painful abrupt shortening of the muscle. EMG reveals that motor units fire at a very rapid rate, much higher than the most vigorous voluntary contractions, and usually at about 300 times/sec.

It is presumably this high rate of discharge that causes the palpable muscle tautness and pain. The pain can be relieved by stretching the affected muscle or by massage. Cramps occur not uncommonly in motor neuron disease, pregnancy, and electrolyte disturbances, particularly hyponatremia. They also occur in normal individuals. Cramps may be prevented at night by the use of quinine and during the day by the use of phenytoin or diazepam. *(Cecil, Ch. 517)*

36.(B) Any intercurrent febrile illness may lead to a temporary worsening of multiple sclerosis (MS), since a decrease in axonal conduction is often induced by heating. There is no evidence that pregnancy causes exacerbation of the disease. The average lifespan is approximately 35 years after the clinical onset. Epidemiologically, it appears that the risk of developing MS is related to the age of immigration: that is, those moving after puberty have the same chance of developing the illness as they would have in their country of origin. This is felt to be the case since a presumptive exposure to an environmental agent occurs at about the age of 8 to 15 years. *(Cecil, Ch. 492)*

37.(D) Central nervous system involvement by syphilis may be that of acute syphilitic meningitis, general paresis (dementia), or tabes dorsalis with optic atrophy. Argyll Robertson pupils, which accommodate but fail to react to light, are characteristic of this illness. Cerebral infarction, now uncommon, was once a frequent finding in untreated cases. *(Cecil, Ch. 482; Adams and Victor, pp. 529–535)*

38.(C) Basal ganglia comprise five paired nuclei: caudate, putamen, globus pallidus, subthalamic nucleus, and substantia nigra. They lie deep within the white matter of the cerebral hemispheres, with the exception of the subthalamic nuclei, which are in the diencephalon, and the substantia nigra, which is located in the midbrain. The amygdala are located in the anteromedial temporal lobes and are part of the limbic system. *(Cecil, Ch. 467)*

39.(D) This disorder typically begins with pain in the involved extremity, which is most often proximal. There is progression to weakness of proximal muscles with minimal sensory loss. Wasting follows, but complete recovery usually occurs over many months. *(Cecil, Ch. 510; Adams and Victor, pp. 994–999; Tsairis et al)*

40.(D) Disease of the frontal lobes frequently produces a gait apraxia, in which the feet appeared glued to the floor. Attempts at walking consist of short shuffles or even hops. Retropulsion is common, and minimal guidance or support frequently leads to marked improvement. Midline cerebellar dysfunction produces a wide-based reeling gait with arms and legs widely thrust apart. With sensory deprivation (proprioceptive ataxia) the patient develops a broad-based gait with severe lurching that is accentuated by eye closure. The patient with vestibular ataxia frequently complains of dizziness. Spasticity, as seen in corticospinal tract disease, produces a broad-based, tottering, and pounding gait with the knees held high and the legs moving stiffly. *(Cecil, Ch. 465)*

41.(B) Autonomic dysfunction complicates acute poliomyelitis in many cases, and over 50% of adults suffer at least transient urinary retention. Blood pressure may be markedly elevated. Tachycardia and fatal pulmonary edema together with cardiac arrhythmias may occur. Poliomyelitis produces an acute febrile illness, the temperature usually ranging from 38.5° to 40° C. Sensory involvement is extremely rare and usually minimal. Progressive motor weakness may occur rapidly and is often preceded by intense muscle aches. *(Cecil, Ch. 486)*

42.(B) The Kearns-Sayre syndrome comprises neuromyopathy and ataxia, retinitis pigmentosa, ophthalmoplegia, and cardiac arrhythmias, usually beginning in adolescence or adulthood. This is a mitochondrial myopathy; ragged red muscle fibers are seen on trichrome stain. Wohlfart-Kugelberg-Welander disease is an autosomal recessive disorder beginning typically in late childhood, adolescence, or early adulthood and includes slowly progressive proximal muscular atrophy, weakness, and fasciculations. Pelizaeus-Merzbacher disease is a rare leukodystrophy inherited as a sex-linked recessive trait beginning early in infancy. It progresses slowly, producing extensive, diffuse, symmetric disturbances of myelin associated with gliosis in the cerebrum and cerebellum. The peripheral nervous system is not affected. Metachromatic leukodystrophy is the most common of the leukodystrophies, producing diffuse dysmyelination; it usually starts in the first 10 years of life. Progressive personality changes lead to dementia along with convulsions, cranial nerve abnormalities, and finally, severe spasticity and rigidity. Krabbe's disease (globoid cell leukodystrophy) affects infants in the first two to three months of life, initially producing irritability and unexplained episodes of crying. Also seen is sensitivity to light and noise and failure to achieve developmental milestones. In the second year of life these children become opisthotonic and develop myoclonic jerks, atypical seizures, and optic atrophy. *(Cecil, Chs. 492 and 516)*

43.(A) Partial obstruction of the internal carotid artery at its origin is suggested by intermittent blindness in the eye on the ipsilateral side, combined with a contralateral hemiparesis and sensory loss. This clinical picture often begins with a series of transient ischemic attacks or amaurosis fugax (transient monocular blindness), and only later do permanent weakness and sensory loss develop. The presence of either a partial obstruction at the carotid bifurcation or an ulcerated plaque in the same location can best be demonstrated by angiography. Carotid artery ultrasound is not as reliable as angiography in defining such lesions. Brain CT scans frequently are normal for 24 to 48 hours after cerebral infarction. Neither the electroencephalogram nor the cardiac holter monitor can assess the patency of the carotid artery. *(Cecil, Ch. 479)*

44.(E) Progressive multifocal leukoencephalopathy is a rare demyelinating disease usually developing either in patients with such pre-existing reticuloendothelial diseases as leukemia, lymphoma, sarcoidosis, and AIDS, or in those who are immunosuppressed. The onset is sudden, with a subacute progression comprising abnormalities of motor function, sensation, vision, speech, and mentation. The CT scan of the brain typically shows multiple areas of demyelination. The JC virus, a newly recognized human papovavirus to which most persons develop antibodies during childhood, is the causative agent. In contrast, subacute sclerosing panencephalitis is an uncommon condition affecting children or young adults. Behavioral disorders or deterioration in schoolwork is often followed by weeks or months of mental deterioration and neurologic signs, the most characteristic of which is myoclonus. The illness terminates after a third stage of stupor, blindness, dementia, and decorticate rigidity which may last months to years. Creutzfeldt-Jakob disease is an uncommon form of rapidly progressive dementia accompanied by myoclonus, pyramidal tract findings, cerebellar ataxia, visual disturbances, and muscle wasting with fasciculations. Alzheimer's disease is a cortical dementia that slowly progresses over many years, and only in the late stages are subcortical features of spasticity, rigidity, dysarthria, and dysphagia seen. Multiple sclerosis is an episodic disorder in which different sites of the nervous system are damaged by demyelination. It would be unusual for this disease to progress over so brief a period of time as seen in this patient. *(Cecil, Chs. 461, 488, and 492)*

45.(D) The benzodiazepines do not suppress REM sleep, but they do reduce total sleep time in stages III and IV of non-REM sleep. Because of the accumulation of active metabolites, the benzodiazepines with longer half-lives tend to accumulate with chronic administration. Short-acting agents tend to lessen the interference with daytime alertness. Addiction has been associated with chronic administration of the benzodiazepines, especially with long-term use of diazepam. Rebound insomnia is more common with intermediate-term use of benzodiazepines. *(Cecil, Ch. 458)*

46.(B) The patient shows evidence of the Wernicke-Korsakoff syndrome with ophthalmoplegia, gait ataxia, and global confusion. Hepatomegaly, dry skin with poor turgor, and other associated physical abnormalities that may be seen in chronic ethanol abuse are present. Thiamine is the necessary cofactor in the metabolism of glucose, so it is necessary to avoid administering excessive glucose prior to giving thiamine, as this may precipitate or worsen the encephalopathy in these patients. Anticonvulsants are not indicated, as the patient has not had seizures. There is no evidence of opiate overdose and thus naloxone is not indicated. Although the patient has severe hyponatremia, this should be corrected slowly with lesser concentrations of salt solution, since central pontine myelinolysis is a catastrophic disorder that can occur when profound hyponatremia in alcoholic patients is returned to normal by rapid osmolal correction. *(Cecil, Chs. 77, 457, and 467)*

47.(D) A syrinx develops within the spinal cord, usually in the central region at the cervical level, and often extends to the medulla, where pharyngeal and vocal cord paralysis together with lingual atrophy are typically seen. Syringomyelia is frequently associated with congenital malformations at the craniocervical junction, such as the Arnold-Chiari malformation. It may also be seen with intramedullary neoplasms, of which approximately 25% are associated with a syrinx. The symptoms typically include a selective impairment of pain and temperature sensations with a preservation of touch. The posterior columns in the upper extremities are spared and position sense impairment does not occur. Late involvement of vibratory and position sense in the lower extremities may occur as the syrinx extends into the posterior columns of the lower spinal cord. This rarely occurs in the upper cervical cord. *(Cecil, Ch. 476)*

48.(A) Cervical spondylosis typically appears with little or no pain but with slowly developing weakness, atrophy, and fasciculations in the upper extremities, together with a spastic paraparesis and decreased proprioception in the legs. Sensory changes differentiate this from amyotrophic lateral sclerosis, in which fasciculations are seen in the upper and lower extremities as well as in bulbar muscles. Bilateral C8 radiculopathy may produce intrinsic hand weakness and atrophy, but it is accompanied by sensory impairment on the ulnar side of the hand and ulnar two fingers; the lower extremities are characteristically normal. Peripheral neuropathy implies sensory and/or motor changes distally in both legs as well as in the arms. Upper motor neuron findings are not present in peripheral neuropathy. In scapuloperoneal dystrophy there is leg weakness resembling neurogenic peroneal muscular atrophy, but sensory loss is lacking and there is proximal weakness of the shoulder girdle musculature. *(Cecil, Chs. 500, 513, and 514)*

49.(D) Petit mal is a genetically transmitted disorder beginning exclusively in childhood and characterized by brief absence attacks that may occur as often as 100 or more times daily. These absence spells are often easily induced by hyperventilation. Autism almost invariably occurs before the age of 3 and is associated with repetitive self-stimulating behavior. Juvenile epileptic myoclonus usually begins in late adolescence. Subacute sclerosing panencephalopathy has not been shown to have any hereditary pattern; by the time the patient comes for clinical evaluation, the neurologic examination is abnormal. *(Cecil, Ch. 493)*

50.(B) Uremic neuropathy is characteristically an axonal degeneration in which sensory symptoms of burning, restlessness, and paresthesia predominate. Chronic hemodialysis is usually ineffective in reversing the neuropathy, but successful renal transplantation often does. The cause is unknown but appears to be related to retention of dialyzable toxins or metabolites that are normally excreted by the kidneys and that have molecular weights exceeding those of urea and creatinine. *(Cecil, Ch. 508)*

51.(A) One or more febrile convulsions occur in up to 4% of otherwise healthy children between the ages of 6 months and 5 years. These episodes consist of brief tonic-clonic generalized seizures. A genetic basis may be present. Affected children outgrow their vulnerability between 3 and 5 years of age. Weighing against the diagnosis of benign febrile convulsions are seizures lasting longer than 10 minutes, focal abnormalities during or after the seizure, or an abnormal neurologic examination. In such instances investigation and treatment are required. *(Cecil, Ch. 493)*

52.(D) Persistent signs of severe brain stem dysfunction in patients who remain unconscious for up to 48 hours generally imply a poor chance for short-term survival or for a good ultimate outcome. Such signs would include bilateral pupillary abnormalities, absent corneal responses, dysconjugate or dysjunctive eye movements, and impaired or absent oculovestibular or oculocephalic responses. The deep tendon reflexes are not a good indicator of brain stem dysfunction, and their absence or hyperactivity does not significantly affect the prognosis. *(Cecil, Ch. 457; Plum and Posner, Ch. 7)*

53.(C) The clinical picture is that of an inflammatory myopathy (polymyositis), which may occur with or without cutaneous lesions. When lesions are present, the disorder is termed dermatomyositis. Patients typically have no family history and present in a subacute state with weeks or months of progressive disability. Dysphagia and neck weakness are common, and arthralgias or Raynaud's phenomenon may be seen. Muscle biopsy typically shows an inflammatory reaction. Spontaneous electrical activity with small myopathic motor unit potentials is seen on EMG. The treatment of choice is immunosuppression (prednisone, azathioprine, or methotrexate). Since neuromuscular transmission is normal, pyridostigmine is not effective. This acquired myopathy occurs most often in patients over

35 years; long-term prognosis with immunosuppression is good. *(Cecil, Chs. 443 and 517)*

54.(A) A pontine hemorrhage often occurs abruptly with uncontrolled hypertension and results in apneustic breathing, miotic and unreactive pupils, and, with expanding pressure and herniation, a Cushing reflex during which the pulse slows as the blood pressure rises. Destruction of the parapontine reticular formation causes the eyes to tonically deviate away from the lesion, and ice-water caloric testing on the side opposite the lesion shows no response. With destruction of the fifth cranial nerve nucleus and associated tracts, the corneal reflex is absent ipsilaterally and diminished contralaterally. Hemiplegia exists contralateral to the site of hemorrhage, and milder corticospinal tract dysfunction may be seen on the side opposite the lesion. The lateral medullary syndrome does not typically lead to the coma, pyramidal tract signs, or eye movement abnormalities described in this case. Alteration in the level of consciousness may occur with a large hemorrhage into the parietal lobe or with middle cerebral artery infarction, but brain stem signs are generally absent, with the exception of corticobulbar abnormalities involving the contralateral seventh and twelfth cranial nerves. A large basal ganglia hemorrhage may interfere with the level of consciousness, but it typically produces contralateral disturbances in sensory and motor function with minimal disturbances of lower brain stem function, unless it progresses to uncal herniation. *(Cecil, Chs. 457, 478, 479, and 480)*

55.(A—True; B—False; C—True; D—True; E—True) The lesion producing conductive aphasia is usually in the parietal operculum. Global aphasia has nonfluent expression with inability to comprehend or to repeat spoken phrases and is typically due to massive peri-Sylvian lesions. In contrast, Broca's aphasia is usually localized to the lower posterior frontal area. Wernicke's (receptive) aphasia is due to a lesion in the posterior superior temporal area. The angular gyrus is believed to be the site of the lesion in anomic aphasia. The supplementary speech area anterior to Broca's area is believed to be the site of involvement in transcortical motor aphasia. *(Cecil, Ch. 460)*

56.(All are True) The medical treatment of myasthenia falls into two categories: those that affect symptoms without influencing the course of the disease (plasmapheresis and anticholinesterase drugs), and those designed to induce remission of the disease itself (thymectomy, steroids, immunosuppressive drugs). Plasmapheresis often produces prompt but unsustained improvement. The severity of the patient's disease often dictates the initial approaches to the therapy. Frequently, generalized myasthenia is treated with thymectomy, whereas ocular myasthenia is treated with more conservative measures. *(Cecil, Ch. 518)*

57.(A—False; B—True; C—True; D—True; E—False) Essential tremor may involve the hands, head, and least frequently the voice. It is aggravated by writing and diminished by alcohol. It is exacerbated by volitional movement and is quiet at rest. It disappears during all stages of sleep and is often suppressed with the use of propranolol as well as benzodiazepines. The age of onset is variable, but it usually begins in early adulthood. It usually persists throughout life with an increase in intensity. There is a strong familial incidence. *(Cecil, Ch. 469)*

58.(A—True; B—False; C—True; D—True; E—False) Cannabis has been shown to be effective in reducing the nausea in patients undergoing cancer chemotherapy. It also reduces intraocular pressure in glaucoma. It causes peripheral vascular dilatation, increases airway conduction, produces dryness of the mouth and throat, and causes fine tremor of the fingers. Orthostatic hypotension occurs infrequently. Driving performance and fine motor performance are significantly impaired, as is reaction time. There are no documented reports of human fatalities caused by overdose. Stupor and coma are not produced by the drug, which by itself may produce agitation, apathy, and acute panic attacks. *(Cecil, Ch. 16)*

59.(A—True; B—True; C—False; D—False; E—True) Neurologic manifestations of vitamin B_{12} deficiency include a sensory peripheral neuropathy, absent distal reflexes, and distal sensory impairment. The loss of smell may occur as well. As the illness progresses, subacute combined degeneration of the cord develops and the patient may develop bilateral Babinski signs. Urinary retention is uncommon, and generalized seizures do not occur. *(Cecil, Ch. 467; Rundles)*

60.(A—True; B—True; C—False; D—False; E—True) The most common cause of inherited myoglobulinuria is probably DiMauro's disease, or deficiency of the enzyme carnitine palmityl transferase, which plays a vital role in the oxygenation of long chain fatty acids. Pompe's disease is an infantile form of glycogen storage disease presenting with weakness and wasting resembling infantile motor neuron disease, but myoglobulinuria does not occur. Malignant hyperthermia generally occurs in reaction to general anesthesia, with succinylcholine and/or halothane being the precipitating agent(s). Severe metabolic acidosis because of lactic acidemia occurs along with myoglobulinuria. The most common cause of myoglobulinuria is probably unusually vigorous exercise by an otherwise normal person. Acute intermittent porphyria produces a red-brown urine because of accumulation of porphyrins, but the urine does not contain myoglobulin. Porphyria would not give a positive test with benzidine, but would give a positive Watson-Schwartz test. *(Cecil, Ch. 516)*

61.(All are True) In amyotrophic lateral sclerosis, there is death of motor neuron cells with a resultant pure motor axonopathy. All the features described are characteristic of an axonopathy. *(Cecil, Ch. 475)*

62.(A—False; B—True; C—True; D—True; E—True) Asterixis is an abnormal, involuntary jerking movement seen most prominently in the hands when the patient is asked to dorsiflex the wrist and extend the fingers. In its mildest form it involves irregular random lateral jerking movements of the fingers at the metacarpophalangeal joints. When fully developed there may be sudden plantar flexion at the wrist. The movements are asynchronous and nonrhythmic, and they may be seen in the tongue and feet. They cannot be controlled by the patient and their presence usually implies metabolic brain disease. *(Cecil, Ch. 516)*

63.(A—True; B—True; C—True; D—True; E—False) Lumbar puncture is a simple procedure when the patient is correctly positioned in the lateral decubitus position, with knees flexed, to allow for full extension of the space between the spinous processes. The 20-gauge stylet needle should be *slowly* introduced between the interspaces until it pierces the dura. If the needle is advanced too far, trauma to the ventrally located epidural venous plexus will yield a bloody tap. A platelet count below 30,000/mm^3 is an absolute contraindication. Lumbar puncture is the most sensitive procedure to evaluate a patient for possible subarachnoid bleeding, although greater degrees of subarachnoid hemorrhage may indeed be seen on cranial computed tomography. The opening pressure should always be measured while the patient is relaxed, the knees extended, and the neck in a neutral position. *(Cecil, Ch. 456; Petito and Plum)*

64. (A—True; B—True; C—True; D—False; E—True) Insomnia may be produced by fever, pain, and numerous psychiatric disturbances, including anxiety, stress, depression, and schizophrenia. Chronic alcohol abuse may also result in insomnia. Kleine-Levin syndrome is a rare disorder occurring in adolescent males; it is characterized by episodic periods of excessive sleep and overeating. The cause of this syndrome is unknown, but the condition usually remits in adulthood. The sleep apnea syndromes do result in too little sleep (insomnia) but are usually characterized by excessive daytime sleepiness. *(Cecil, Ch. 458)*

65. (All are True) HIV is believed to be neurotropic, and early direct central nervous system involvement may occur. This may take the form of encephalitis (subacute), aseptic meningitis (acute and chronic), and myelopathy (noninflammatory). In all of these syndromes, however, opportunistic infections and neoplasia need to be excluded. These neurologic complications are not uncommon. Subacute encephalitis has been seen in 90% of patients dying with AIDS. *(Cecil, Ch. 491; Hollander et al; Johnson et al)*

66. (A—True; B—True; C—False; D—False; E—True) Broca's area, on the lateral aspect of the posterior frontal lobe, is supplied by the middle cerebral artery. The vertebral arteries arise from subclavian arteries, pass through the bony canals in the transverse processes from the sixth to the second cervical vertebrae, and then enter the skull through the foramen magnum. The jugular vein leaves the skull through the jugular foramen. *(Cecil, Chs. 478 and 479)*

67. (A—True; B—False; C—False; D—True; E—False) The Eaton-Lambert syndrome is a facilitating disorder of neuromuscular transmission in which the amplitude of the first evoked muscle action potential is reduced; with repetitive stimulation the amplitude of the action potential increases to more than three times the original height. Underlying malignancy is usually present but not invariably so. The defect is due to impaired release of acetylcholine at the nerve terminals. Antibodies to components of nerve terminals may be responsible, but antibodies to acetylcholine receptors have not been found. There is no evidence of any impaired binding of acetylcholine at the muscle membrane receptors. *(Cecil, Ch. 518)*

68. (A—True; B—True; C—True; D—True; E—False) Numerous pharmaceutical agents may cause peripheral neuropathy. Careful experimental studies have confirmed causation with isoniazid, pyridoxine, and vincristine. *Cis*-platinum has been reported to cause severe permanent peripheral neuropathy in a number of cases, but cyclophosphamide has not been shown to do so. *(Cecil, Ch. 509)*

69. (A—False; B—False; C—True; D—True; E—False) Fractures across the base of the skull often lacerate the thin and firmly adherent dura in that area. The leakage of blood from such a dural tear across the floor of the anterior fossa results in bilateral periorbital ecchymosis. Linear, nondisplaced skull fractures extending across the groove of the middle meningeal artery more commonly cause an extradural hematoma than do linear basilar skull fractures. With fractures of the middle fossa, hemotympanum is the earliest sign, frequently followed by accumulation of subcutaneous blood over the mastoid bone (Battle's sign). Evidence does not indicate that prophylactic antibiotics reduce the incidence of meningitis when CSF rhinorrhea is present. Multiple cranial nerve palsies are frequent, but the abducens nerve is usually spared, perhaps because of its long intracranial course. The involvement of cranial nerves 7 and 8 in addition to 2, 3, and 4 is much more common. The presence of intracranial air merely means that the fracture traverses an air sinus of the middle or external ear canal. Although patients are at higher risk for infection, surgical intervention is not indicated unless a persistent CSF leak exists for longer than 7 to 10 days. *(Cecil, Ch. 496)*

70. (A—True; B—True; C—True; D—True; E—False) Acute Guillain-Barré syndrome is a demyelinating neuropathy. The characteristics of such a condition include slow nerve conduction velocities. However, in early cases of up to 7 to 10 days' duration, nerve conduction velocities may be normal. The earliest changes seen are delayed F-responses and H-reflexes, as would be expected with the proximal (nerve and root) demyelination. EMG is typically normal without spontaneous activity (a sign of denervation) or with small myopathic motor potentials. *(Cecil, Chs. 456 and 506)*

71. (A—False; B—True; C—False; D—True; E—True) Central pontine myelinolysis is a rare disorder affecting primarily alcoholics and patients with severe electrolyte disorders, liver disease, malnutrition, anorexia, burns, cancer, Addison's disease, sepsis, and Wilson's disease. The signs and symptoms relate to symmetric focal myelin destruction involving the basal central pons, with similar lesions occasionally affecting extrapontine areas. There is no associated inflammation or nerve cell destruction, and the lesions appear to be reversible with time and proper nutrition and fluid balance. This disorder commonly follows a period of profound hyponatremia followed by rapid osmolar correction of greater than 20 mEq/L. Mental symptoms are often prominent, with clouded consciousness or an increase in a post-alcoholic delirious state. Flaccid or spastic quadriparesis with bulbar involvement may occur, but sensory abnormalities are usually absent. *(Cecil, Ch. 467)*

72. (A—True; B—True; C—False; D—True; E—False) Phenytoin undergoes erratic absorption from the gastrointestinal tract and is extensively bound to serum albumin. The drug is unusual in that the hepatic enzymes that metabolize phenytoin conform to first-order kinetics up to the point at which they are saturated; thereafter, only a fixed amount of drug is eliminated per unit time, suggesting that when this occurs a small increase in dose can cause a large increase in the serum blood level and result in drug toxicity. Hypotension occurs following intravenous, not intramuscular, administration. In addition to hypotension, the vehicle has a markedly alkaline pH, which readily causes phlebitis. The drug is useful in digitalis-toxic arrhythmias in humans because it shortens the refractory period in both atrial and His-Purkinje tissue. Although gingival hyperplasia occurs with long-term administration, pyorrhea is a result of poor dental hygiene and is not a side effect of the medication. *(Cecil, Ch. 493)*

73. (All are True) HIV has been isolated from affected peripheral nerves in some persons. CSF pleocytosis, an unusual feature of acute and chronic inflammatory demyelinating polyneuropathies, is more commonly seen when these syndromes are associated with HIV infection. Painful distal sensory neuropathy, distal sensorimotor neuropathy, and mononeuritis multiplex have all been associated with HIV infection. All these neuropathies have occurred in both symptomatic and asymptomatic HIV-infected persons. *(Cecil, Ch. 488.2; Snider et al; Cornblath et al)*

74.(All are True) The Shy-Drager syndrome (idiopathic autonomic insufficiency) is a rare degenerative disorder of unknown etiology which strikes during middle age, causing progressive autonomic dysfunction. Severe debility or death may occur within 5–15 years of onset. Associated extrapyramidal abnormalities and lesions of pigmented brain nuclei play a prominent role in the genesis of symptoms. Pathologic examination at autopsy has disclosed degeneration of peripheral autonomic ganglia as well as central nervous system autonomic symptoms in the hypothalamus, nigrostriatal system, pontine nuclei, and globus pallidus. Postmortem biochemical studies have revealed marked depression of dopamine-beta-hydroxylase, which converts dopamine or norepinephrine. Orthostatic hypotension, bladder and bowel symptoms, impotence, and loss of sweating are among the features of parkinsonism. *(Cecil, Ch. 463)*

75.(A—True; B—False; C—False; D—True; E—False) The clinical picture strongly suggests mania. The past history of intermittent depression and a similar episode of mania strongly points to a diagnosis of manic-depressive psychosis. In this condition a positive family history is frequently present. Hospitalization is usually necessary to avoid catastrophic injury to the patients or their families. Tricyclic antidepressants, such as imipramine, and electroconvulsive therapy are useful treatments in severe depression, but are not indicated in mania. Lithium carbonate is an effective agent in controlling mania. *(Cecil, Ch. 462)*

76.(A—True; B—True; C—False; D—False; E—True) The clinical syndrome of low spinal fluid pressure is characterized by a severe throbbing frontal and occipital headache that is brought on when the patient is upright and subsides on lying down. Dizziness, nausea, stiff neck and photophobia may also occur. The disorder often arises 3–21 days after lumbar puncture and rarely may be accompanied by an abducens nerve palsy. The symptoms and signs probably result from chronic CSF leakage, loss of the normal CSF cushion, and cortical displacement of the brain within the cranial vault. Traction on pain-sensitive intracranial structures probably accounts for the headache and diplopia. When symptoms are persistent an epidural "blood patch" may be indicated. This involves the injection of 10 ml of the patient's own blood into the epidural space to seal a presumed dural leak. Contrary to popular belief, bed rest after the procedure has no effect on the incidence or duration of post–lumbar puncture headache. *(Cecil, Ch. 495)*

77.(All are True) In carpal tunnel syndrome the median nerve becomes compressed at the wrist as it passes deep to the flexor retinaculum. It is commonly associated with excessive use of the hands and may be seen in cases of arthritis and in relation to an old carpal bone fracture. Other predisposing causes are pregnancy, myxedema, acromegaly, infiltration of the transverse carpal ligament in primary amyloidosis, and chronic hemodialysis treatments. When the condition is severe or intractable, surgical decompression is advisable. *(Cecil, Ch. 511)*

78.(A—True; B—True; C—False; D—False; E—False) The neurologic examination must be exquisitely normal for the diagnosis to be entertained. Any sensory impairment implies an underlying structural lesion that must be searched for. Carbamazepine is the drug of choice in the relief of pain. Phenytoin is also useful, but usually less effective. If medical treatment fails, surgical intervention is frequently beneficial in relieving pain for a time. Radiofrequency lesions of the gasserian ganglion and posterior fossa craniotomy to relieve pressure on the trigeminal nerve from small blood vessels appear beneficial. *(Cecil, Ch. 466)*

79.(A—False; B—True; C—True; D—False; E—True) Signs of lower motor neuron disease include weakness, atrophy, fasciculations, hypotonicity, and hyporeflexia. In contrast, upper motor neuron lesions typically result in weakness, little or no atrophy, no fasciculations, hypertonicity with associated clonus, and hyper-reflexia. (*Cecil, Chs. 475 and 504*)

80.(All are True) Myelinopathy refers to conditions in which the lesion affects primarily the myelin sheath of the peripheral nerve. The Guillain-Barré syndrome is the most commonly encountered disease that affects primarily the peripheral nerve myelin. A few genetic leukodystrophies also result in myelinopathy, as does infection with diphtheria. Chronic inflammatory polyneuropathy generally has a protracted onset and an indolent steady progression, but glucocorticoids are often efficacious in producing a remission. Hereditary motor and sensory neuropathy, Type I (Charcot-Marie-Tooth disease) is an autosomal dominant disorder. Pes cavus deformity of the feet and extreme distal lower limb atrophy are found along with very slow motor conduction velocities. The peripheral neuropathy of amyloidosis affects the distal lower extremities more than the upper extremities and includes small fibers more than large fibers. The diagnosis of primary amyloidosis should be strongly suspected when this type of neuropathy is associated with cardiac enlargement, nephropathology, or microglossia. Patients with multiple myeloma who develop carpal tunnel syndrome may have systemic amyloidosis. (*Cecil, Chs. 504 to 511; Schaumburg, pp. 25–39, 41–55, 99–118, 167–172*)

81.(A—True; B—True; C—True; D—False; E—True) Premonitory headaches and transient ischemic events usually herald more florid signs and symptoms in intracranial venous thrombosis. Focal and generalized seizures occur in at least half the cases. Mild and occasionally marked evidence of subarachnoid hemorrhage may be present. Despite the presence of major focal neurologic deficits, the prognosis is good, usually with complete resolution. Conditions in which phlebothrombosis of cortical veins develops are identical to the conditions that predispose to deep vein thrombosis in the lower extremities. This would include the postpartum or pregnancy state; as a complication of estrogen contraceptive therapy; in cachectic and wasting conditions, but also in some patients with cancer and ulcerative colitis; in patients with congestive heart failure; in hypopyrexia; and with abnormalities of the coagulation system. (*Cecil, Ch. 479*)

82.(A—True; B—True; C—False; D—False; E—True; F—False) When present, papilledema is the most reliable sign of intracranial hypertension; however, many patients with raised intracranial pressure fail to develop papilledema. Retinal venous pulsations, when present, imply that CSF pressure is normal or not significantly elevated. Most of the signs and symptoms associated with intracranial hypertension are related to traction on cerebral blood vessels and distortion of the pain-sensitive structures within the head. Headache is therefore variable in nature and occurrence but frequently is found in the early morning. Sagittal sinus thrombosis may be associated with increased intracranial pressure and papilledema. Increased intracranial pressure and papilledema may rarely occur in the Guillain-Barré syndrome. (*Cecil, Chs. 495 and 506*)

83.(A—True; B—False; C—True; D—False, E—False) This radial nerve palsy (Saturday night palsy) is a neuropraxic injury that involves focal demyelination. There should be a gradual but complete recovery over several weeks. The location of the lesion is the spiral groove of the humerus through which the radial nerve passes from the medial to the lateral aspect of the arm. Innervation of the triceps occurs above this lesion, at a point just distal to the division of the posterior cord into the radial and axillary nerves. Because of this, there is no abnormality of the triceps muscle and the triceps reflex is preserved. The extensor muscles of the wrist and forearm, however, receive innervation distal to the site of injury and are therefore impaired. The terminal cutaneous branch of the radial nerve also is damaged, and this explains the moderate sensory loss in the distribution of this nerve. It is necessary that the fingers be locked in an extended position so that the interosseous muscles of the hand can abduct and adduct the fingers at the metacarpophalangeal joints. Therefore, patients with radial nerve palsies may give the false impression of intrinsic hand muscle weakness, suggesting ulnar nerve injury. (*Cecil, Ch. 511; Schaumberg, pp. 19–23, 187–208*)

84.(A—True; B—True; C—False; D—False; E—False) Myotonic muscular dystrophy diverges from other human muscular dystrophies in several respects. The distribution of weakness differs in that cranial muscles are often affected and limb weakness is initially more marked in distal muscles. Ptosis, dysarthria, and facial weakness with a characteristic long, lean facial appearance are signs not seen in other forms of dystrophy. Myotonia, or difficulty in muscle relaxation, may be evident on examination of the grip and can also be elicited by percussing the thenar eminence, whereupon a sustained contraction of the abductor pollicis muscle persists for several seconds, then gradually relaxes. This disorder is transmitted as an autosomal dominant trait, and thus each offspring has a 50% chance of being affected. Conduction defects are common in the EKG and typically are noted first by evidence of first-degree heart block. These defects may eventually lead to clinically significant dysrhythmias or congestive heart failure. Many other body systems are involved in this pleomorphic disorder, and patients are often found to have low normal intelligence, with testicular atrophy and baldness in men (with some male pattern baldness seen in women) and cataracts. The basal metabolic rate is often low, but other tests of thyroid function are normal. The incidence of diabetes mellitus may be increased, and insulin resistance may be due to decreased affinity of insulin receptors. This slowly progressing dystrophy characteristically has slight or no increase in the serum muscle enzymes. (*Cecil, Ch. 513*)

85.(A—True; B—True; C—True; D—False; E—True) Rabies is enzootic in warm-blooded animals, including skunks, foxes, bats, raccoons, mongooses, wolves, and vampire bats (in which it is maintained by bite transmission). In areas where domestic animal rabies has been inadequately controlled, dog and cat rabies account for more than 90% of reported cases. The most important aspect of control is the prevention of spread between domestic animals by active vaccination and elimination of stray animals. This disease has been eradicated in England and Japan by these means. Rabies virus can be inactivated by soap, quaternary ammonium compounds, alcohol, and other viricidal chemicals. Prompt local debridement and cleansing of wounds with soap and water is probably the most effective measure for preventing rabies. Two patients have recovered following postexposure prophylaxis, which should include passive immunization with hyperimmune rabies globulin or antirabies serum and rabies vaccination. The incubation period normally ranges from 20 to 60 days. (*Cecil, Ch. 487*)

86.(All are True) Malignant hyperthermia is a rare illness characterized by catastrophic reaction to general anesthesia with succinylcholine and halothane. Muscles become very stiff and the body temperature rapidly rises. Aborting the anesthesia, cooling the patient rapidly, neutralizing acidosis, and giving dantrolene resolves most cases. Autosomal dominant inheritance appears to occur in some families. Some patients at risk may have high serum creatine phosphokinase activity between attacks. (*Cecil, Ch. 516*)

87.(A—True; B—False; C—True; D—False; E—True) A selective increase in the CSF gamma globulin concentration may be found in cases of neurosyphilis, subacute sclerosing panencephalitis, and multiple sclerosis, reflecting ongoing immunologic dysfunction. In Guillain-Barré syndrome the CNS protein content is elevated, but this is largely albumin and not gamma globulin. In Reye's syndrome the cerebrospinal fluid is under increased pressure but is acellular with normal protein and normal gamma globulin concentration. (*Cecil, Chs. 482, 488, 490, 492, and 506*)

88.(A—False; B—True; C—False, D—True; E—True) Many years after paralytic poliomyelitis, a few patients, usually in their fifth or sixth decades, develop increased weakness that may be associated with muscle loss and fasciculations. This weakness is often in the area of original paralysis. The weakness has a more benign course than the original case of poliomyelitis; upper motor neuron findings are lacking and this helps to differentiate the late post-poliomyelitis motor neuron disease from such primary motor neuron diseases as amyotrophic lateral sclerosis. It has been postulated that this may result from persistence of the polio virus, but it may more likely represent an aging process superimposed upon a depleted anterior horn cell population. (*Cecil, Ch. 486*)

89.(A—True; B—True; C—False; D—True; E—False) Demyelinating disease (optic neuritis or papillitis) produces papilledema along with loss of central vision in the affected eye. Bedside measurement of visual acuity, visual fields, and the pupillary light reflex will help to differentiate this disorder, since each of these should be abnormal in a case of acute papillitis. Ocular motility is not dependent on raised intracranial pressure or optic nerve dysfunction and should be normal. Ophthalmoscopic examination of the retina may reveal papilledema in both cases. (*Cecil, Chs. 464 and 492*)

90.(A—False; B—True; C—True; D—True; E—True) Patients with AIDS have an increased incidence of central nervous system infections, but these are not primarily bacterial in nature. They consist of infection with *Toxoplasma gondii*, cytomegalovirus, and *Cryptococcus.* In addition, patients also have developed progressive multifocal leukoencephalopathy and a subacute encephalitis of unknown cause. Primary lymphoma of the brain and meninges is the neoplasm seen most frequently. Vascular complications often occur and are frequently associated with hemorrhage. Peripheral neuropathy is one of the major neurologic complications. (*Cecil, Ch. 488.2; Snider et al*)

91.(A—False; B—True; C—False; D—True; E—True) Familial periodic paralysis is characterized by recurrent attacks of flaccid weakness, usually associated with abnormally high or low serum potassium. This family has the hypokalemic form—in general, the hypokalemic variety tends to begin in later life (late childhood or adolescence versus early childhood in the hyperkalemic form), occurs frequently at night, is more severe, and tends to last longer (one or more days versus minutes to hours for the hyperkalemic form). In the hypokalemic form, low T-waves are seen on the EKG, versus peaked T-waves in the hyperkalemic form. Provocative testing in suspected individuals is done by the intravenous administration of 100 g of glucose mixed with 20 units of regular insulin. Hypokalemia is induced as the blood sugar falls, usually within 1 hour after the infusion is completed. If an attack is induced, it can be terminated with the administration of 7–10 g of potassium chloride or 90–130 mEq of mixed potassium salts. In the hypokalemic form, serum potassium falls to 2.5–3.5 mEq per liter, while in the hyperkalemic form the potassium rises to 5.0–7.0 mEq per liter. Between attacks, serum potassium levels are usually normal. Persistent proximal muscle weakness exists in both forms. Acetazolamide is equally effective in preventing both hypokalemic and hyperkalemic periodic paralysis. (*Cecil, Ch. 516*)

92.(A—True; B—True; C—True; D—True; E—False) Although treatment of postherpetic neuralgia is difficult, cutaneous stimulation of the involved area, administration of tricyclic antidepressants and mild analgesics, administration of corticosteroids early in the course of herpes zoster, and epidural and paraspinal nerve blocks are all reported to reduce the incidence and severity of the illness. The results of surgical therapy are poor. (*Cecil, Chs. 466 and 506*)

93.(All are True) In the diverse group of conditions known as mitochondrial myopathies, the mitochrondria are too numerous or too large or contain abnormal crystalline inclusions. Histologic abnormalities described as ragged red fibers are seen on trichrome staining. These findings are associated with a variety of clinical syndromes. Proximal limb weakness is a prominent feature. Some patients may present with an isolated muscle carnitine deficiency, and others may have systemic carnitine deficiency. Kearns-Sayre syndrome describes the association of ophthalmoplegia, pigmentary degeneration of the retina, heart block, high CSF protein, and other neural disorders with this myopathy. (*Cecil, Ch. 516*)

94.(A—False; B—True; C—True; D—True; E—False) Reflex sympathetic dystrophy refers to pain, hyperalgesia, hyperesthesia, and autonomic changes, usually after injury to an extremity. The injury may be major or mild. Muscular atrophy and osteoporosis are late features. Both sympathetic block with lidocaine and surgical sympathectomy may produce benefit. The pain is characteristically burning and continuous. (*Cecil, Ch. 466*)

95.(A—True; B—True; C—True; D—False; E—False) A lacunar infarct is associated with small vessel disease and produces a small area of infarction and subsequent cavitation. These lesions are less than 3 mm in diameter but may be multiple and occasionally coalesce to form larger areas visible by CT scanning. The most important of the clinical syndromes produced by lacunar infarction are (a) pure motor hemiplegia; (b) pure sensory stroke involving the face, arm, and leg; and (c) the ataxic hemiparesis syndrome with unilateral ataxia and hemiparesis. Receptive aphasia and right arm paresis would be produced by a large lesion involving the dominant hemisphere that measures much greater than 3 mm or multiple lesions involving both parietal and frontal lobes. Similarly, a left homonymous hemianopsia implies a lesion of the right parieto-occipital lobe, whereas a right arm paresis implies a left frontal lobe or capsular lesion. (*Cecil, Ch. 479*)

96.(A—False; B—False; C—True; D—True, E—True) Beta-adrenergic blockers (propranolol), amitriptyline, and methysergide have all been shown to be effective in the prophylaxis of migraine. Ergotamine is useful in the abortive treatment of migraine but is not recommended for regular prophylactic use because of the risk of ergotism. Oxycodone is a potent analgesic that may lead to habituation and addiction if used regularly. (*Cecil, Ch. 466*)

97.(All are True) Friedreich's ataxia, the most common form of spinocerebellar degeneration, begins in childhood and is inherited mainly as an autosomal recessive, but also as an autosomal dominant, disorder. Nystagmus occurs early, as does gait ataxia. Optic atrophy may develop and there is distal sensory impairment, including vibration and position sense. The deep tendon reflexes are usually absent, but Babinski signs do occur. The pathology includes demyelination with gliosis in the spinocerebellar tracts, lateral corticospinal tracts, posterior columns, and peripheral nerves. (*Cecil, Ch. 473*)

98.(A—True; B—True; C—False; D—False; E—False) There is evidence that administration of ACTH or glucocorticoids (prednisone) may shorten an exacerbation of multiple sclerosis. There is no evidence to date that plasmapheresis or hyperbaric oxygenation plays a role in the treatment of this disorder. Therapeutic trials to evaluate various immunosuppressants, including cyclosporine, are currently under way. However, this drug has potent nephrotoxic side effects and cannot be recommended for the treatment of multiple sclerosis at this time. (*Cecil, Ch. 492*)

99.(A—True; B—True; C—False; D—False; E—False) The clinical picture is that of neurofibromatosis. The patient has multiple café au lait spots that are at least 1.5 cm in diameter; these are characteristic of the disorder. The multiple neurologic abnormalities refer to different locations and are compatible with multiple neurofibromas. Visual loss in the left eye is due to an optic nerve glioma, which not uncommonly occurs in this condition. The cranial neuropathies on the right are due to a jugular foramen meningioma. There is an increased association with pheochromocytomas, cystic lung disease, and renal vascular lesions causing hypertension, fibrous dysplasia of bone, gastrointestinal neurofibromas, gliomas of the brain, and intracranial meningiomas. There is no increased association with oligodendroglioma, primary CNS lymphoma, or metastatic brain tumor. (*Cecil, Ch. 477*)

100.(All are False) Acute transverse myelitis is a clinical syndrome often affecting the mid- to upper thoracic level of the cord. It is characterized by rapid onset of severe paraparesis or paraplegia, usually affecting all motor and sensory pathways distal to the lesion. The cause is unknown in most cases and only a minority of patients develop multiple sclerosis. A vascular cause is suggested in some cases, but the clinical picture is not typically that of anterior spinal artery thrombosis. Both urinary incontinence and retention commonly occur. Treatment is supportive and there is no evidence that glucocorticoids or ACTH is effective. (*Cecil, Ch. 492*)

101.(E); 102.(D); 103.(B); 104.(C); 105.(A) Febrile convulsions in a 2-year-old child do not of themselves necessitate long-term anticonvulsant treatment. They may be either watched without any treatment or treated for a short time with phenobarbital. Ethosuximide is the treatment of choice for absence (petit mal) epilepsy, which may be mistaken for daydreaming or inattention in children. Sodium valproate may also be used in this disorder. Myoclonic jerk or myoclonic seizures may respond well to sodium valproate. Carbamazepine is the drug of choice for complex partial seizures in which cessation of activity, lip-smacking, chewing, or other aimless behavior may occur. Focal motor seizures or jacksonian seizures usually imply an underlying structural lesion. The treatment of choice here is phenytoin, but carbamazepine or phenobarbital may be used. (*Cecil, Ch. 493; Solomon and Plum; Penry and Newmark*)

106.(C); 107.(D); 108.(B); 109.(E); 110.(A) Muscular dystrophies are inherited myopathies characterized by progressive severe weakness. There is no specific treatment for any form of muscular dystrophy. The gene for Duchenne dystrophy is on the short arm of the X-chromosome. The gene for myotonic dystrophy is on chromosome 19. Myotonia congenita is a rare disorder present from early childhood and commonly inherited in an autosomal dominant fashion. It is differentiated from myotonic dystrophy in that the only symptoms and signs are those related to myotonia. Muscular weakness, cataracts, baldness, and testicular atrophy do not occur. Many patients with Duchenne dystrophy have pseudohypertrophy of muscles. Patients with facioscapulohumeral dystrophy always have facial involvement. (*Cecil, Ch. 513*)

111.(B); 112.(C); 113.(E); 114.(A); 115.(D) Ergotamine is most effective in aborting common migraine and may also be effective in cluster headache. Lithium carbonate is quite effective in the treatment of cluster headache; indomethacin is very effective in the treatment of paroxysmal hemicrania, which appears to be a variant of cluster headache. Trigeminal neuralgia is frequently aborted by the use of carbamazepine or phenytoin. Biofeedback treatments may effectively relieve muscle contraction and thus help treat chronic tension headaches. (*Cecil, Ch. 466*)

116.(E); 117.(D); 118.(A); 119.(C); 120(B) An occlusion of the paramedian branch of the basilar artery in the caudal part of the pons interrupts the ipsilateral abducens nerve along with the descending corticospinal tract prior to its decussation at the craniocervical junction. The former leads to ipsilateral loss of eye abduction, whereas the latter leads to contralateral hemiplegia. Tactile and proprioceptive impulses carried from the contralateral half of the body are affected as they pass cephalad in the medial lemniscus. This constellation of findings is sometimes termed the Millard-Gubler syndrome. Branches of the posterior cerebral artery supply the cerebral peduncle and midbrain tegmentum. Occlusion here leads to Weber's syndrome, in which an ipsilateral third nerve palsy is combined with contralateral hemiplegia. The lateral medullary syndrome may occur from occlusion of the homolateral vertebral artery, with resulting damage to the descending tract and nucleus of cranial nerve V, causing sensory loss of the ipsilateral side of the face. The spinothalamic tract is affected, resulting in loss of sensation of pain and temperature on the contralateral side of the body. Ataxia results from involvement of the inferior cerebellar peduncle (restiform body). The descending sympathetic fibers are interrupted, leading to an ipsilateral Horner's syndrome. The patient may have dysphagia, hoarseness, and paralysis of the ipsilateral vocal cord along with a diminished gag reflex because of involvement of cranial nerves IX and X. Middle cerebral artery strokes result in contralateral hemiplegia and hemisensory deficits that are most marked in the upper limb and face, with relative sparing of the leg. Dominant hemisphere involvement produces aphasia. Anterior cerebral artery occlusion typically results in partial contralateral leg weakness and sensory loss with minimal arm involvement and total sparing of the face. Voluntary control of urination is commonly disturbed, and mental confusion and behavioral disorders may be encountered. Since the branches of this artery contribute to the supply of the cortical white matter beneath the motor speech area of the dominant hemisphere, dysphasic symptoms also may result from occlusion of this artery. (*Cecil, Chs. 478 to 480*)

121.(D); 122.(C); 123.(E); 124.(A); 125.(B) Chlorpromazine will counteract severe agitation and hyperactivity in amphetamine overdose, which is marked by hyperthermia, tachycardia, and dilated pupils. Hypothermia can occur in severe cases. Naloxone frequently reverses the effect of an overdose with opiates, including heroin, morphine, and methadone. This condition is marked by drowsiness, miotic pupils, shallow respirations, hypotension, hypothermia, and coma. Physostigmine is the drug of choice for a tricyclic antidepressant overdose, in which tachyarrhythmias, hyperpyrexia, restlessness, and drowsiness are usually seen. The reaction may progress to convulsions. CNS depressants, such as alcohol, barbiturates, and benzodiazepines, produce progressive drowsiness and confusion, but the pupils remain reactive although slightly constricted. There is no specific antidote and the patient should be intubated and ventilated. An excellent recovery should occur if hypoxia is avoided. An overdose of lithium may result in muteness, lethargy, and multifocal seizures. This compound can be hemodialyzed. Adequate hydration may suffice in mild cases. (*Cecil, Ch. 457*)

126.(D); 127.(B); 128.(A); 129.(C); 130.(E) The pupil in the Holmes-Adie syndrome is the result of an affection of the postganglionic parasympathetic fibers, which normally constrict the pupil and cause accommodation. The patient may report blurring of vision or may have suddenly noticed that one pupil is larger than the other. Reaction to light and sometimes to accommodation is absent if tested in the customary manner, although the size of the pupil will change slowly on prolonged maximal stimulation as well as after instillation of dilute pilocarpine. Pancoast's syndrome results when a neoplasm in the apex of the lung invades contiguous structures. Pain in the shoulder area is the most common initial complaint and findings will typically include an ipsilateral Horner's syndrome. The Argyll Robertson pupil is a small, often unequal and irregular pupil that is fixed to light but constricts to accommodation. The principal cause for this is tertiary neurosyphilis, although partial Argyll Robertson changes occur with diabetes and certain autonomic neuropathies. The Marcus-Gunn pupil is seen frequently in multiple sclerosis and results from a defect in the anterior optic pathway. Thus, stimulation of the unaffected eye with light reflexly constricts the affected pupil, but when the light stimulus is placed in front of the affected eye, there is neither direct nor consensual constriction. A third cranial nerve palsy that includes the parasympathetic fibers is often due to local compression of the proximal portion of the oculomotor nerve. The most common cause of this disorder is an aneurysm of the posterior communicating artery of the circle of Willis. (*Cecil, Chs. 310, 464, 480, and 492; Alexandridis, pp. 49–75*)

131.(C); 132.(A); 133.(B); 134.(E); 135.(D) The median nerve innervates the thenar muscles of the hand, the lumbrical muscles of the index and long fingers, the superficial and deep forearm flexor muscles with the exception of the flexor carpi ulnaris and the flexor digitorum profundus muscle that pass to the ring and little fingers, the deep flexor of the thumb, and the pronators of the forearm. Sensation mediated by this nerve is distributed over the radial half of the palm out onto the thumb and the index and middle fingers. The musculocutaneous nerve innervates the coracobrachialis, brachialis, and biceps brachii muscles and provides sensation to the lateral half of the forearm but not the thumb. The peroneal nerve innervates the musculature of the anterior and lateral compartments of the leg and the extensor digitorum brevus muscle of the foot. Sensation from the dorsum of the foot and toes is carried by this nerve. The dermatomal distribution of the C6 root is along the lateral forearm and includes the thumb. A lesion of the motor fibers in this root leads to weakness of the flexor muscles at the elbow as well as the supinator muscle. The femoral nerve innervates the flexor muscles of the hip along with the extensor muscles of the knee and carries sensation from the anterior thigh and the medial aspect of the leg. Because it supplies the quadriceps muscle, a lesion of this nerve causes loss of the knee jerk. (*Cecil, Ch. 498; Schaumburg, pp. 187–208*)

136.(D); 137.(C); 138.(B); 139.(E); 140.(A) The Lesch-Nyhan syndrome is an X-linked disorder caused by a deficiency of hypoxanthine-guanine phosphoribosyltransferase (HPRT) activity. It is manifested by hyperuricemia, excessive production of uric acid, and neurologic features including self-mutilation, choreoathetosis, spasticity, and mental retardation. Children with the syndrome are normal at birth, but delay in motor development begins at 3–4 months, followed by extrapyramidal and pyramidal tract signs within one year. Compulsive self-destructive behavior appears any time between early childhood and adolescence. Wilson's disease is a rare autosomal recessive disorder characterized by degenerative changes in the brain, particularly the basal ganglia, and cirrhosis of the liver. A defect in biliary excretion of copper leads to accumulations in the liver, brain, and other tissues. Kayser-Fleischer rings, prolonged prothrombin time, intention tremor, difficulty with speech and swallowing, incoordination, personality changes, and dementia may be seen. Chorea-acanthocytosis is an uncommon sporadic or autosomal recessive disorder that may mimic Huntington's disease. It begins in the third to fourth decade with progressive chorea, orofacial dyskinetic movements often accompanied by self-mutilation of the lips and tongue, a loss of tendon reflexes, vocal tics, acanthocytes in the peripheral blood, elevated CPK, and caudate nucleus atrophy. Huntington's disease, an autosomal dominant disorder with complete penetrance, is the most common of the hereditary choreas. It is manifested by the triad of choreic movements, intellectual decline leading to dementia, and emotional disturbances. Caudate nucleus atrophy is present, but unlike chorea-acanthocytosis there is usually a family history, normal muscle enzymes, preserved DTRs, and absence of acanthocytes. Ataxia-telangiectasia is an autosomal recessive neurocutaneous disorder that begins in the first decade of life with prominent telangiectatic lesions involving the bulbar conjunctiva, malar eminences, earlobes, and occasionally the upper neck regions; it is associated with cerebellar ataxia, nystagmus, and thymic hypoplasia. Recurrent pulmonary infections, deficiency of IgA and IgE as well as lymphocytopenia, a reduced response to skin test antigens, and a lack of sensitization to dinitrochlorobenzene (DNCB) all occur. (*Cecil, Chs. 196, 205, 470, and 477*)

141.(B); 142.(C); 143.(G); 144.(A); 145.(D) The Eaton-Lambert syndrome (myasthenic syndrome) is a facilitating disorder of neuromuscular transmission characterized by weakness and defective release of acetylcholine at the nerve terminals. Guanidine promotes the release of acetylcholine and is effective in daily doses of 35 mg/kg body weight. Tourette's syndrome is characterized by multiple tics and involuntary vocalizations that are often obscene. Haloperidol is the most effective drug in this disorder. Reye's syndrome is an acute and sometimes fatal encephalopathy associated with acute hepatic dysfunction. Hypoglycemia may occur, but the treatment is supportive with control of hypoglycemia and any electrolyte disturbance. Tardive dyskinesia is associated with chronic administration of antipsychotic drugs, particularly phenothiazines and butyrophenones. Withdrawal of the offending agent is the treatment of choice, but if the problem persists, dopamine-depleting drugs (reserpine and alpha-methyl-paratyrosine) that act presynaptically are the preferred agents to relieve both the dyskinesia and akathisia. Korsakoff's amnestic syndrome is associated with chronic thiamine deprivation and is commonly seen in alcoholics. Although Wernicke's encephalopathy often improves after thiamine treatment, Korsakoff's amnestic syndrome may resolve in only about 20% of patients similarly treated. All patients with Korsakoff's syndrome, however, should be given thiamine to treat possible coexistent Wernicke's encephalopathy and to prevent progression of amnesia. (*Cecil, Chs. 467, 470, 471, 490, and 518*)

146.(D); 147.(C); 148.(A); 149.(B); 150.(E) Many toxic chemicals have been implicated as causes of peripheral neuropathy. The neuropathy is usually a distal axonopathy. A careful occupational and environmental history is most important when dealing with any type of neuropathy. The notation of specific features may help to identify certain specific chemical causes. (*Cecil, Ch. 509; Schaumburg, pp. 131–155*)

151.(E); 152.(C); 153.(D); 154.(B); 155.(A) Superior sagittal sinus thrombosis may occur because of infection that extends from the nasal cavity, by secondary spread from the lateral or cavernous sinuses, by extension from osteomyelitis, or from an epidural or subdural infection. Subdural empyema refers to an intracranial collection of pus in the subdural space. This often occurs in children and adolescents and is often the result of rupture of a paranasal sinus with spillage of infected material into the subdural space. Thrombosis or thrombophlebitis of superficial cortical veins produces hemorrhagic infarction of the area drained by the diseased vessels and leads to focal neurologic disease that may accompany generalized progressive obtundation. Lateral sinus thrombosis is almost always a complication of acute or chronic otitis media, mastoiditis, or cholesteatoma formation. Fever, headache, nausea, and vomiting, accompanied by progressive drowsiness and eventual coma, are typically seen. Spread of the infection to the inferior petrosal sinus may lead to abducens nerve paralysis and trigeminal nerve involvement (Gradenigo's syndrome). The symptoms of brain abscess are generally those of a space-occupying intracranial lesion. Increased intracranial pressure usually develops rapidly, and headache, nausea, and vomiting are common early symptoms. Temporal lobe abscesses often lead to complex partial seizures and such language difficulties as Wernicke's aphasia. Cavernous sinus thrombosis is usually due to a suppurative process in the orbit, nasal sinuses, or upper half of the face. This disorder usually produces an illness of desperate severity with high fever, headache, malaise, prostration, nausea, vomiting, convulsions, and tachycardia. Chemosis, edema, and cyanosis of the upper face are due to obstruction of the ophthalmic vein as it enters the cavernous sinus. The ophthalmic division of cranial nerve V may be involved and lead to pain and hypesthesia of the forehead. The pupil may be dilated from parasympathetic paralysis or may be small and immobile if both parasympathetic and sympathetic fibers are involved. Ophthalmoplegia, often affecting the sixth cranial nerve, is common, but the fourth and third cranial nerves also pass through the cavernous sinus and may be affected as well. (*Cecil, Ch. 481*)

BIBLIOGRAPHY

Adams RD, Victor M: Principles of Neurology. 3rd ed. New York, McGraw-Hill Book Company, 1984.

Alexandridis E: The Pupil. New York, Springer-Verlag, 1985.

Asbury AK, McKhann GM, McDonald WI: Diseases of the Nervous System. Philadelphia, Ardmore Medical Books (W.B. Saunders Company), 1986.

Baloh RW: Dizziness, Hearing Loss, and Tinnitus: The Essentials of Neurotology. Philadelphia, F.A. Davis Company, 1984.

Burns RS, Lewitt PA, Ebert MH, et al: The clinical syndrome of striatal dopamine deficiency parkinsonism induced by 1-methyl-4-phenyl-1,2,3,-tetrahydropyridine (MPTP). N Engl J Med 312:1418–1421, 1985.

Carpenter MB, Sutin J: Human Neuroanatomy. 8th ed. Baltimore, Williams and Wilkins, 1983.

Cecil Textbook of Medicine. 18th ed. Wyngaarden JB, Smith LH Jr (eds). Philadelphia, W.B. Saunders Company, 1988.

Cornblath DR, McArthur JC, Kennedy PGE, et al: Inflammatory demyelinating peripheral neuropathies associated with human T-cell lymphotropic virus type III infection. Ann Neurol 21:32–40, 1987.

Cummings JL, Benson DF: Dementia: A Clinical Approach. Boston, Butterworths, 1983.

Heros RC, Zervas NT, Varsos V: Cerebral vasospasm after subarachnoid hemorrhage: An update. Ann Neurol 14:599–608, 1983.

Heyman A, Wilkinson WE, Hurwitz BJ, et al: Risk of ischemic heart disease in patients with TIA. Neurology 34:626–630, 1984.

Heyman A, Wilkinson WE, Hurwitz BJ, et al: Alzheimer's disease: Genetic aspects and associated clinical disorders. Ann Neurol 14:507–515, 1983.

Hollander H, Stringari S: Human immunodeficiency virus–associated meningitis. Am J Med 83:813–816, 1987.

Johnson RT, McArthur JC: Myelopathies and retroviral infections. Ann Neurol 21:113–116, 1987.

Morse RM, Litin EM: Postoperative delirium: A study of etiologic factors. Am J Psychiatry 126:388, 1969.

Parkes JD: Sleep and Its Disorders. Philadelphia, W.B. Saunders Company, 1985.

Penry JK, Newmark ME: The use of antiepileptic drugs. Ann Intern Med 90:207, 1979.

Petito F, Plum F: The lumbar puncture. N Engl J Med 290:225–226, 1974.

Plum F, Posner JB: The Diagnosis of Stupor and Coma. 3rd ed. Philadelphia, F.A. Davis Company, 1980.

Rundles RW: Prognosis in the neurologic manifestations of pernicious anemia. Blood 1:209–219, 1946.

Schaumburg HH, Spencer PS, Thomas PK: Disorders of Peripheral Nerves. Philadelphia, F.A. Davis Company, 1983.

Snider WD, Simpson DM, Nielsen S, et al: Neurological complications of acquired immune deficiency syndrome: Analysis of 50 patients. Ann Neurol 14:403–418, 1983.

Solomon GE, Plum F: Clinical Management of Seizures. Philadelphia, W.B. Saunders Company, 1976.

Tsairis P, Dyck PJ, Mulder DW: Natural history of brachial plexus neuropathy. Arch Neurol 27:109, 1972.

PART 11

DERMATOLOGY

EDWARD E. BONDI

DIRECTIONS: For questions 1 to 21, choose the ONE BEST answer to each question.

1. A 36-year-old man comes to you for evaluation of a pigmented lesion which he says has changed in size and color over the past year. Examination reveals a 1.5-cm irregularly pigmented red-brown-black plaque with irregular, notched borders. Which of the following is the best diagnostic procedure?

A. Wide surgical excision (3-5 cm border)
B. Incisional biopsy
C. Exfoliative cytology
D. Excisional biopsy
E. Serologic testing

2. A 57-year-old man notes diffuse hyperpigmentation of the skin. Each of the following is a possible explanation EXCEPT

A. drug reaction
B. pemphigus vulgaris
C. biliary cirrhosis
D. underlying malignancy
E. metastatic melanoma

3. A 22-year-old woman receiving thiazide diuretic and Bactrim therapy has an acute erythematous eruption in a **V**-shaped pattern over the chest and diffusely over the face with sparing of the eyelids and the area under the chin. Each of the following is a possible diagnosis EXCEPT

A. a thiazide reaction
B. a Bactrim reaction
C. lupus erythematosus
D. a photosensitivity reaction
E. psoriasis

4. Telogen effluvium, the temporary shedding of increased numbers of resting hair, can be caused by each of the following EXCEPT

A. normal delivery
B. severe malnutrition
C. a myocardial infarction
D. an anesthesia stress
E. seborrheic dermatitis

5. The Tzanck smear can aid in the diagnosis of each of the following diseases EXCEPT

A. vitiligo
B. herpes zoster
C. pemphigus vulgaris
D. herpes simplex
E. varicella

6. The cutaneous manifestations of acquired immunodeficiency syndrome (AIDS) include an increased incidence of all of the following EXCEPT

A. herpes simplex infections
B. oral candidiasis
C. diffuse Kaposi's sarcoma
D. oral hairy leukoplakia
E. melanoma

7. A 4-year-old boy is admitted to the hospital with severe prostration, high fever, conjunctivitis, enlarged cervical lymph nodes, ulcerative gingivitis, and prominent erythema of the palms and soles with desquamation of the fingers. Which of the following is the most likely diagnosis?

A. Mastocytosis
B. Lupus erythematosus
C. Mucocutaneous lymph node syndrome
D. Malignant acanthosis nigricans
E. Allergic contact dermatitis

8. Each of the following is characteristic of atopic dermatitis EXCEPT

A. blanching response to injections of acetylcholine
B. increased susceptibility to cutaneous viral infections
C. association with increased risk for cataracts
D. increased risk of melanoma
E. deficiency of T-cell function

9. You are asked to see a 23-year-old woman, in the third trimester of her first pregnancy, who has an extremely pruritic bullous eruption. She is otherwise healthy. Which of the following is the most likely diagnosis?

A. Herpes gestationis
B. Psoriasis
C. Lichen planus
D. Mucocutaneous lymph node syndrome
E. Rosacea

10. Which of the following is characteristic of *both* the major form of erythema multiforme (Stevens-Johnson syndrome) and the minor form?

A. Prominent oral mucosal lesions
B. Iris or target lesions
C. High fever and prostration
D. Conjunctival involvement
E. Erosions of the esophagus and colon

11. A 10-year-old girl has hepatosplenomegaly and a chronic eruption of diffuse, red-brown pigmented macules that become hivelike when rubbed. Each of the following is associated with the disease described EXCEPT

A. peptic ulcer
B. skin biopsy revealing large numbers of mast cells
C. flushing episodes and headaches following aspirin ingestion
D. significant incidence of gluten sensitivity
E. significantly increased risk of leukemia

12. From which one of the following sites would squamous cell carcinoma be LEAST likely to metastasize to the local lymph node?

A. The lower lip
B. An area of previous x-ray damage
C. An old burn scar
D. The tip of the nose
E. The oral mucosa

13. The order of classic progression of mycosis fungoides is

A. lymphadenopathy, erythematous scaling patch, indurated plaques, tumor formation
B. tumor formation, lymphadenopathy, visceral involvement, indurated plaques
C. erythematous scaling patch, indurated plaques, tumor formation, lymphadenopathy
D. erythematous scaling patch, tumor formation, indurated plaques, lymphadenopathy
E. indurated plaques, erythematous scaling patch, tumor formation, lymphadenopathy

14. Each of the following is characteristic of congenital nevi EXCEPT

A. They are generally larger than normal acquired nevi
B. They often display increased hair growth
C. They are the site for almost half the melanomas occurring in childhood
D. They represent less than 0.1% of the nevi present in an average young adult
E. There is no correlation between the size of a congenital nevus and its risk for malignant transformation

15. An 87-year-old woman, a collector of violins, has a tense bullous eruption over the abdomen, inner thighs, and flexoral surface of the forearms. Which of the following is the most likely diagnosis?

A. Pemphigus
B. Dermatitis herpetiformis
C. Allergic contact dermatitis
D. Lichen planus
E. Bullous pemphigoid

16. Vitiligo has been associated with each of the following EXCEPT

A. peptic ulcer
B. pernicious anemia
C. thyroid dysfunction
D. Addison's disease
E. alopecia areata

17. Pemphigus vulgaris is characterized by all of the following EXCEPT

A. frequent oral ulcerations
B. subepidermal bullae
C. flaccid bullae
D. high mortality if left untreated
E. higher incidence among Jews

18. All of the following are true regarding the classic (non-AIDS) form of Kaposi's sarcoma EXCEPT

A. It may present as a purple cutaneous nodule
B. It occurs more frequently in males than in females
C. It usually follows an aggressive course, with death resulting within two years of diagnosis
D. It is more prevalent in Jews and those of Mediterranean descent
E. Initial cutaneous lesions are frequently located on the lower extremities

19. Which of the following is the facial eruption most frequently associated with AIDS?

A. Lupus
B. Acne
C. Seborrheic dermatitis
D. Melasma
E. Rosacea

20. Each of the following is associated with an exfoliative erythroderma EXCEPT

A. drug allergy
B. psoriasis
C. contact dermatitis
D. lymphoma
E. Sweet's syndrome

21. The risk of sudden death in the mucocutaneous lymph node syndrome is usually secondary to

A. renal complications
B. underlying malignancy
C. anaphylaxis
D. myocardial complications
E. secondary infections

DIRECTIONS: For questions 22 to 28, decide whether EACH choice is true or false. Any combination of answers, from all true to all false, may occur. Mark the answer sheet "T" or "F" in the space provided.

22. Which of the following is/are true concerning sweat gland functioning?

A. A normal individual can produce as much as 2 liters of sweat per hour
B. The detection of increased body temperature by the hypothalamus stimulates eccrine glands via sympathetic fibers
C. Blockage or rupture of the eccrine sweat duct can produce miliaria (prickly heat)
D. Body odor results mainly from the decomposition of apocrine sweat by bacteria
E. Eccrine sweat is *not* formed in the axilla

23. Which of the following is/are true regarding basal cell carcinoma?

A. It is the most common form of skin cancer
B. It is the cause of more deaths each year than melanoma
C. It can be treated with x-rays
D. It commonly presents as a painful nodule in a sun-exposed area
E. If not treated early, it commonly will metastasize

24. Which of the following is/are true regarding the staphylococcal scaled skin syndrome (SSSS)?

A. It usually affects young children
B. Clinical eruption is characterized by diffuse erythema and loss of skin in large sheets
C. Level of the cleavage is subepidermal
D. Cleavage is caused by a staphylococcal toxin
E. The treatment of choice is high-dose systemic steroids

25. Which of the following is/are characteristic of benign mucosal pemphigoid?

A. Subepidermal bullae formation
B. Prominent involvement of mucous membranes
C. Possible complication of blindness
D. Associated malabsorptive enteropathy
E. Rapid response to systemic steroid therapy

26. Which of the following is/are associated with neurofibromatosis?

A. Increased incidence of psoriasis
B. Café au lait spots
C. Axillary freckles
D. Darier's sign
E. Diabetes

27. Which of the following is/are true regarding *Candida albicans*?

A. It frequently causes infections in patients with acrodermatitis enteropathica
B. It is sensitive to treatment with nystatin
C. It causes a skin eruption characterized by satellite pustules
D. It is likely to be associated with endocrinopathies
E. It will fluoresce under Wood's light

28. Which of the following is/are true regarding psoriasis?

A. It is associated with a seronegative arthritis
B. It is associated with remission in response to the Goeckerman regimen
C. It has an accelerated epidermal turnover rate
D. It may be cured by psoralin and ultraviolet A light (PUVA) therapy
E. It is associated with an increased incidence of internal malignancy

DIRECTIONS: Questions 29 to 50 are matching questions. For each numbered item, choose the most likely associated lettered item from those provided. Each numbered item has ONLY ONE answer. Within each set of questions, each lettered item may be the answer to one, more than one, or none of the numbered items.

QUESTIONS 29–33

For each of the following numbered descriptions, select the appropriate skin lesion.

A. Superficial spreading melanoma
B. Nodular melanoma
C. Lentigo maligna melanoma
D. Acral lentiginous melanoma
E. Dysplastic nevus (B-K mole)

29. Cutaneous marker of the familial melanoma syndrome
30. Malignancy with no radial growth phase
31. Benign mole
32. Melanoma most commonly located on the face
33. Presents as enlarging black nodule

QUESTIONS 34–37

For each of the following numbered descriptions, select the appropriate lettered item.

A. Erythema nodosum
B. Erythema induratum
C. Both
D. Neither

34. Commonly appears on the posterior aspect of the legs
35. A form of panniculitis
36. A common presenting sign of sarcoidosis
37. Tendency for malignant transformation

QUESTIONS 38–41

For each of the following diseases select the appropriate lettered item.

A. Positive direct immunofluorescence
B. Positive indirect immunofluorescence
C. Both
D. Neither

38. Pemphigus vulgaris
39. Bullous pemphigoid
40. Dermatitis herpetiformis
41. Erythema multiforme

QUESTIONS 42–46

For each of the following diseases select the most appropriate therapy.

A. Zinc
B. Electron beam therapy
C. Gold therapy
D. Goeckerman therapy
E. Dapsone

42. Psoriasis
43. Acrodermatitis enteropathica
44. Mycosis fungoides
45. Pemphigus vulgaris
46. Dermatitis herpetiformis

QUESTIONS 47–50

For each of the following descriptions choose the most appropriate cell type.

A. Langerhans' cell
B. Melanocyte
C. Basal cell
D. Sézary cell
E. Horny cell

47. No nucleus
48. Pigment-forming dendritic cell
49. Dendritic immunocompetent cell
50. Epidermal germinative cell

PART 11

DERMATOLOGY

ANSWERS

1.(D) The description is typical of a melanoma, and the clinical diagnosis should always be confirmed by an excisional biopsy. It is preferable to an incisional biopsy because it permits the analysis of the entire lesion, the determination of the deepest level of inclusion, and the planning of definitive therapy. Wide surgical excision is usually the appropriate treatment but it should be preceded by a diagnostic biopsy. Exfoliative cytology is not a dependable method of diagnosing melanoma. Serologic tests are usually not abnormal unless metastatic disease is present. (*Cecil, Ch. 534*)

2.(B) Drugs such as chlorpromazine, metabolic disturbances such as hemochromatosis and biliary cirrhosis, and endocrinopathies such as Addison's disease and Cushing's syndrome can cause diffuse hyperpigmentation. On rare occasions, diffuse metastatic melanoma and lung tumors producing MSH-like peptides can cause hyperpigmentation. Pemphigus vulgaris is an intraepidermal blistering disease that is not associated with diffuse hyperpigmentation. (*Cecil, Ch. 534*)

3.(E) The distribution indicates a photosensitivity eruption (phototoxic or photoallergic). Thiazides and sulfa drugs are both common causes of photosensitivity. Lupus erythematosus could also cause acute onset of an eruption in a photo distribution. Although psoriasis can occasionally involve the face, it would not display this photo distribution. On the contrary, sun-exposed areas are often spared in psoriasis. (*Cecil, Ch. 534*)

4.(E) Any severe physical or psychologic stress may trigger large numbers of hairs to enter a resting phase followed two to three months later by their loss, or telogen effluvium. Cutaneous eruptions of the scalp such as seborrheic dermatitis do not cause hair loss. (*Cecil, Ch. 534*)

5.(A) The Tzanck smear is a technique of rapid cytologic examination that is useful in analyzing vesicles and bullae. The detection of multinucleated giant cells of viral disease and acantholytic cells of pemphigus are important diagnostic points. It is of no use in diagnosing vitiligo. (*Cecil, Ch. 532*)

6.(E) The cutaneous manifestations of AIDS include an increased incidence of cutaneous neoplasms (Kaposi's sarcoma, lymphoma, squamous cell carcinoma, and basal cell carcinoma), infections (verruca, condyloma molluscum, oral hairy leukoplakia, oral candidiasis, herpes simplex, and onychomycosis), and miscellaneous inflammatory diseases (seborrheic dermatitis, psoriasis, and an erythematous papular eruption). Melanoma is not seen more frequently. (*Cecil, Chs. 346 and 534*)

7.(C) Mucocutaneous lymph node syndrome, or Kawasaki's disease, is characterized by high fever, prostration, and oral mucosal lesions. The cutaneous eruption prominently involves palms and soles with desquamation of fingers and toes. (*Cecil, Ch. 534*)

8.(D) Atopic dermatitis is a poorly understood condition, characterized by a defect in T-cell function, manifested by an increased susceptibility to cutaneous viral infections. An abnormal blanching response is also noted in response to intradermal injections of acetylcholine. An increased incidence of cataracts has been noted in patients with atopic dermatitis, and this is further increased by the frequent use of systemic steroids. There is no known increased incidence of melanoma. (*Cecil, Ch. 534*)

9.(A) Herpes gestationis is a bullous eruption that occurs specifically during pregnancy and may persist briefly in the puerperium. Psoriasis, mucocutaneous lymph node syndrome, and rosacea do not produce bullae. Lichen planus can occasionally take a bullous form, but its occurrence during pregnancy would be coincidental. (*Cecil, Ch. 534*)

10.(B) Target or iris lesions are seen in both the major and minor forms of erythema multiforme. Mucosal lesions (oral, genital, and conjunctival), high fever, and prostration are all characteristics of the Stevens-Johnson syndrome (erythema multiforme major). (*Cecil, Ch. 534*)

11.(D) This patient suffers from mastocytosis. The urticarial reaction to rubbing of the cutaneous lesion is an example of Darier's sign. Each of the findings is associated with mastocytosis except gluten sensitivity, which is a characteristic of dermatitis herpetiformis. (*Cecil, Ch. 534*)

12.(D) Squamous cell carcinomas occurring on sun-exposed skin, except for the ears and mucosal surfaces, have a very low incidence of metastasis. (*Cecil, Ch. 534*)

13.(C) Although the presentation and progression of mycosis fungoides can vary greatly, the classic progression is from an erythematous patch premycotic stage, to an indurated plaque stage, to a tumor stage, and finally to lymphadenopathy and visceral involvement. (*Cecil, Ch. 534*)

14.(E) There clearly is some correlation between the size of a congenital nevus and its risk of malignant transformation. The larger giant congenital nevi are at the highest risk, and controversy remains regarding the potential risk of smaller congenital nevi. (*Cecil, Ch. 534*)

15.(E) Although all these diseases can cause bullae, the age of the patient and the tense quality of the bullae are characteristic of bullous pemphigoid. This diagnosis could be confirmed by a skin biopsy and direct immunofluorescent study. (*Cecil, Ch. 534*)

16.(A) Peptic ulcer is not associated with vitiligo. In keeping with its suspected autoimmune pathogenesis, vitiligo has been associated with pernicious anemia, thyroid dysfunction, Addison's disease, alopecia areata, and diabetes. (*Cecil, Ch. 534*)

17.(B) Pemphigus is characterized by a flaccid bullous eruption and oral lesions. Histology of the bullae reveals that they are intraepidermal acantholytic bullae; they are not subepidermal. Without treatment, there is a greater than 95% mortality from pemphigus. Pemphigus has a higher incidence among Jews. (*Cecil, Ch. 534*)

18.(C) The classic (non-AIDS) form of Kaposi's sarcoma seen in the United States usually presents as a purple nodule developing on the lower extremity of an elderly male. It is more common in Jews and those of Mediterranean descent. Unlike Kaposi's sarcoma in AIDS patients, the classic form of Kaposi's sarcoma usually follows a slowly progressive course with death not occurring for 10 years. (*Cecil, Chs. 346 and 534*)

19.(C) Patients with AIDS frequently manifest the facial eruption of seborrheic dermatitis. Some reports have displayed positive potassium hydroxide preparations from these patients, suggesting a primary or secondary fungal colonization, but this has not been seen in all cases. (*Cecil, Chs. 346 and 534*)

20.(E) Drug allergy, psoriasis, contact dermatitis, eczema, and lymphomas may all appear as an exfoliative erythroderma. Even after a careful evaluation, a significant percentage of cases go unexplained. Sweet's syndrome, or acute febrile neutrophilic dermatosis, is a nodular or plaque eruption of the face, neck, and extremities. It is not an erythroderma. (*Cecil, Ch. 534*)

21.(D) Sudden death occurs in 1 to 2% of patients with the mucocutaneous lymph node syndrome; it is generally attributed to myocardial involvement and coronary occlusion. (*Cecil, Ch. 534*)

22.(A—True; B—True; C—True; D—True; E—False) Well-trained athletes can produce in excess of 3 liters of sweat per hour. The hypothalamus, after sensing increased body temperature, stimulates the eccrine glands via the sympathetic nervous system. Blockage of the eccrine ducts can cause miliaria. The eccrine glands are present over the entire body surface except for specialized mucocutaneous junctions and under nails. The apocrine sweat glands are located in the axilla and groin; body odor is produced by the decomposition of apocrine sweat by bacteria. (*Cecil, Ch. 531*)

23.(A—True; B—False; C—True; D—False; E—False) Basal cell carcinomas are the most common form of skin cancer. They present as asymptomatic translucent nodules with telangiectasias; even without treatment they almost never metastasize and rarely are lethal. Treatment modalities including surgery, cryosurgery, and x-rays may be used. (*Cecil, Ch. 534*)

24.(A—True; B—True; C—False; D—True; E—False) Staphylococcal scalded skin syndrome occurs predominantly in neonates and is characterized by diffuse erythema with sloughing of sheets of skin. A toxin produced by phage type 71 staphylococcal bacteria produces a cleavage high in the epidermis at about the granular cell layer. Treatment with antibiotics is indicated; systemic steroids are not indicated. (*Cecil, Ch. 534*)

25.(A—True; B—True; C—True; D—False; E—False) Benign mucosal pemphigoid is a form of subepidermal bullous disease that produces prominent involvement of mucous membranes, resulting in scarring and sometimes blindness. It is notoriously refractory to therapy and there is no associated malabsorptive enteropathy. (*Cecil, Ch. 534*)

26.(A—False; B—True; C—True; D—False; E—False) Neurofibromatosis is characterized by the development of cutaneous neurofibromas, café au lait spots, and axillary freckles. There is no increased incidence of psoriasis or diabetes. Darier's sign is observed in mastocytosis, not in neurofibromatosis. (*Cecil, Ch. 534*)

27.(A—True; B—True; C—True; D—True; E—False) *Candida albicans* will frequently cause an erythematous scaling eruption in intertriginous areas with "satellite" pustules surrounding the edge. This infection occurs more frequently in patients with endocrinopathies. It can occur as chronic mucocutaneous candidiasis and it may act as a secondary infection in such conditions as angular cheilitis (perlèche) or acrodermatitis enteropathica. *Candida albicans* does not fluoresce under Wood's light. (*Cecil, Ch. 534*)

28.(A—True; B—True; C—True; D—False; E—False) Psoriasis is a common papulosquamous eruption characterized by an accelerated epidermal turnover rate. It is a chronic disease, but remissions can frequently be produced by treatment with tar and light (Goeckerman regimen or psoralin and ultraviolet A light [PUVA] therapy). There is no known cure. Psoriasis may be complicated by a seronegative arthritis that classically involves the DIP joints but can be clinically indistinguishable from rheumatoid arthritis. There is no increased risk of internal malignancy. (*Cecil, Ch. 534*)

29.(E); 30.(B); 31.(E); 32.(C); 33.(B) The dysplastic nevus (B-K mole) is a benign but atypical mole that is seen in large numbers in the hereditary melanoma syndrome. Of the four forms of melanoma, only nodular melanoma lacks a radial growth phase. It usually presents as a solitary black nodule on the skin which slowly enlarges. Lentigo maligna melanoma almost always evolves in an area of severe sun damage, most frequently on the face. It evolves from a premalignant lentigo maligna to a lentigo maligna melanoma. (*Cecil, Ch. 534*)

34.(B); 35.(C); 36.(A); 37.(D) Both erythema nodosum and erythema induratum are forms of panniculitis. Erythema nodosum usually presents on the anterior shin and often is a presenting sign of sarcoidosis. Erythema induratum develops on the posterior calf and may be associated with tuberculosis. Neither form of panniculitis displays a tendency for malignant transformation. (*Cecil, Ch. 534*)

38.(C); 39.(C); 40.(A); 41.(D) Pemphigus vulgaris usually has antibodies directed at the epidermal intercellular spaces present both in the blood and in the skin. Bullous pemphigoid displays antibodies both in the blood and in the skin directed at the basement membrane zone. Dermatitis herpetiformis displays IGA in the skin on direct immunofluorescence only. Erythema multiforme usually has negative immunofluorescence. (*Cecil, Ch. 531*)

42.(D); 43.(A); 44.(B); 45.(C); 46.(E) Psoriasis is usually responsive to ultraviolet light (UVL) therapy, and the Goeckerman regimen combines tar and UVL. Acrodermatitis enteropathica is a hereditary disorder of zinc absorption. It is usually treated with zinc supplements. Mycosis fungoides is usually treated with topical nitrogen mustard or electron beam therapy. Pemphigus vulgaris is usually treated with systemic steroids and/or immunosuppressive therapy or systemic gold therapy. Dermatitis herpetiformis is usually treated with a gluten-free diet and dapsone. (*Cecil, Ch. 534*)

47.(E); 48.(B); 49.(A); 50.(C) The Langerhans cell is an immunocompetent cell that is important in allergic contact dermatitis. The melanocyte produces melanin in melanosomes; the melanin moves out of the dendrites to be picked up by the squamous cells. The basal cell layer of the epidermis is the germinative layer. The Sèzary cell is an atypical mononuclear cell that appears in large numbers in the blood of patients with Sèzary cell syndrome, the leukemic phase of mycosis fungoides. The horny cell is the anucleated stratum corneum cell. (*Cecil, Ch. 531*)

BIBLIOGRAPHY

Cecil Textbook of Medicine. 18th ed. Wyngaarden JB, Smith LH Jr (eds). Philadelphia, W.B. Saunders Company, 1988.

ANSWERS

PART 1. CARDIOVASCULAR DISEASES

1. D
2. C
3. B
4. E
5. B
6. B
7. D
8. E
9. D
10. E
11. A
12. D
13. C
14. B
15. D
16. B
17. D
18. D
19. D
20. E
21. A
22. B
23. C
24. C
25. A
26. E
27. D
28. E
29. D
30. D
31. C
32. D
33. C
34. C
35. A
36. E
37. A
38. D
39. C
40. E
41. E
42. E
43. D
44. C
45. D
46. E
47. C
48. C
49. D
50. B
51. B
52. C
53. D
54. E
55. D
56. B
57. C
58. D
59. B
60. A
61. A
62. D
63. D
64. D
65. B
66. E
67. D
68. D
69. B

70. A–T; B–T; C–F; D–T; E–T
71. A–F; B–T; C–F; D–F; E–F
72. A–T; B–T; C–T; D–T; E–F
73. A–F; B–F; C–T; D–F; E–F
74. A–T; B–T; C–T; D–F; E–T
75. A–F; B–F; C–F; D–T; E–F
76. A–F; B–T; C–F; D–F; E–F
77. A–F; B–F; C–F; D–T; E–T
78. All are False
79. A–T; B–T; C–F; D–F; E–F
80. A–T; B–T; C–F; D–F; E–F
81. A–T; B–F; C–T; D–F; E–F
82. A–F; B–T; C–F; D–F; E–F
83. A–F; B–T; C–F; D–T; E–F
84. A–F; B–F; C–F; D–T; E–T
85. A–T; B–F; C–F; D–T; E–T
86. A–F; B–F; C–F; D–T; E–T
87. A–T; B–F; C–F; D–F; E–T
88. A–T; B–F; C–F; D–T; E–T
89. All are True
90. A–F; B–T; C–T; D–F; E–T
91. A–T; B–T; C–T; D–F; E–T
92. A–T; B–T; C–F; D–F; E–T
93. A–T; B–T; C–F; D–T; E–F
94. A–T; B–T; C–T; D–F; E–T
95. A–T; B–F; C–T; D–T; E–F
96. A–T; B–T; C–F; D–T; E–F
97. A–T; B–T; C–T; D–T; E–F
98. A–T; B–F; C–F; D–F; E–T
99. A–T; B–T; C–T; D–F; E–T
100. A–F; B–T; C–T; D–T; E–F
101. A–F; B–T; C–F; D–F; E–T
102. A–F; B–T; C–T; D–T; E–F
103. All are True
104. A–T; B–F; C–T; D–T; E–F
105. A–F; B–T; C–F; D–T; E–F
106. A–T; B–F; C–T; D–T; E–F
107. A–F; B–T; C–F; D–T; E–F
108. All are True
109. A–T; B–T; C–T; D–T; E–F
110. All are True
111. All are True
112. A–T; B–F; C–T; D–F; E–T
113. A–T; B–F; C–F; D–F; E–F
114. A–T; B–T; C–T; D–F; E–F
115. A–T; B–F; C–T; D–T; E–F
116. A–F; B–T; C–F; D–T; E–T
117. A–F; B–F; C–F; D–F; E–T
118. A–T; B–F; C–F; D–F; E–F
119. A–T; B–F; C–T; D–T; E–F
120. A–T; B–F; C–T; D–T; E–F

121. C
122. B
123. A
124. E
125. D
126. C
127. A
128. B
129. E
130. D
131. B
132. A
133. C
134. E
135. D
136. D
137. A
138. C
139. D
140. B
141. B
142. B
143. A
144. E
145. B
146. D
147. C
148. B
149. E
150. A
151. B
152. C
153. C
154. C
155. B
156. A
157. C
158. A
159. C
160. B
161. D
162. A
163. B
164. C
165. D
166. F
167. B
168. C
169. E
170. B
171. D
172. A
173. E
174. C
175. A
176. E
177. D
178. B
179. D
180. C
181. D
182. F
183. B
184. E
185. A
186. B
187. E
188. D
189. A
190. C
191. C
192. E
193. D
194. A
195. B

PART 2. RESPIRATORY DISEASE

1. C
2. B
3. D
4. A
5. E
6. B
7. B
8. D
9. E
10. E
11. C
12. C
13. C
14. D
15. D
16. A
17. D
18. C
19. E
20. A
21. C
22. E
23. C
24. B
25. C
26. A
27. C
28. D
29. C
30. B
31. A
32. D
33. B
34. E
35. C
36. E
37. A
38. B
39. E
40. B
41. C
42. A

43. A–T; B–F; C–F; D–T; E–F
44. A–F; B–T; C–F; D–F; E–F
45. A–T; B–F; C–T; D–T; E–T
46. A–F; B–F; C–F; D–T; E–T
47. A–F; B–T; C–F; D–T; E–T
48. A–T; B–F; C–T; D–F; E–T
49. A–T; B–F; C–T; D–T; E–T
50. A–T; B–F; C–F; D–F; E–F
51. A–F; B–F; C–T; D–F; E–T
52. A–F; B–F; C–F; D–T; E–T
53. A–T; B–T; C–F; D–F; E–F
54. A–F; B–T; C–F; D–T; E–T
55. A–T; B–F; C–F; D–T; E–T
56. A–T; B–F; C–T; D–T; E–F
57. All are True
58. A–F; B–T; C–F; D–F; E–T
59. A–T; B–F; C–F; D–F; E–T
60. A–F; B–T; C–F; D–F; E–T
61. A–T; B–F; C–T; D–F; E–T
62. All are True
63. A–T; B–F; C–T; D–F; E–T
64. All are False
65. A–F; B–T; C–F; D–T; E–T
66. A–F; B–F; C–T; D–T; E–T
67. A–F; B–T; C–T; D–F; E–T
68. A–F; B–T; C–F; D–T; E–F
69. A–T; B–F; C–T; D–F; E–F
70. A–F; B–T; C–T; D–T; E–F
71. A–T; B–F; C–F; D–T; E–T
72. A–T; B–F; C–F; D–F; E–T
73. A–T; B–T; C–F; D–F; E–T
74. A–T; B–F; C–T; D–T; E–T
75. A–F; B–T; C–F; D–F; E–F
76. A–T; B–T; C–F; D–T; E–T
77. A–F; B–T; C–F; D–F; E–F
78. A–F; B–T; C–F; D–T; E–T
79. A–F; B–T; C–T; D–T; E–F
80. A–F; B–F; C–T; D–T; E–T
81. A–F; B–T; C–F; D–T; E–F
82. A–T; B–F; C–F; D–T; E–F
83. A–F; B–F; C–F; D–F; E–T
84. A–F; B–T; C–T; D–T; E–T
85. A–T; B–F; C–F; D–F; E–F
86. A–F; B–T; C–F; D–T; E–T

87. C
88. D
89. A
90. B
91. E
92. D
93. B
94. E
95. A
96. C
97. E
98. D
99. B
100. A
101. C
102. D
103. C
104. E
105. B
106. A
107. C
108. E
109. A
110. D
111. B
112. C
113. D
114. A
115. B
116. E
117. A
118. B
119. D
120. E
121. C
122. C
123. A
124. D
125. B
126. E
127. A
128. C
129. D
130. B
131. B
132. D
133. C
134. E
135. A
136. C
137. D
138. B
139. A

PART 3. RENAL DISEASE

1. C
2. B
3. A
4. C
5. B
6. B
7. C
8. B
9. A
10. D
11. A
12. B
13. E
14. B
15. D
16. D
17. A
18. E
19. E
20. E
21. A
22. E
23. D
24. B
25. D
26. E
27. C
28. A
29. D
30. B
31. A
32. D
33. D
34. B
35. D
36. E

37. All are False
38. A–F; B–T; C–F; D–F; E–T
39. A–F; B–T; C–T; D–F; E–T
40. A–F; B–T; C–T; D–T; E–F
41. A–F; B–F; C–T; D–T; E–F
42. A–T; B–F; C–F; D–F; E–F
43. A–F; B–F; C–F; D–F; E–T
44. A–F; B–F; C–T; D–T; E–T
45. A–T; B–T; C–F; D–F; E–T
46. A–T; B–T; C–T; D–F; E–F
47. A–F; B–F; C–T; D–T; E–T
48. A–F; B–F; C–F; D–T; E–F
49. A–T; B–T; C–F; D–F; E–F
50. A–F; B–T; C–F; D–T; E–F
51. A–T; B–F; C–F; D–F; E–F
52. A–T; B–T; C–F; D–T; E–F
53. A–T; B–F; C–T; D–T; E–F
54. A–F; B–F; C–F; D–T; E–F
55. A–T; B–T; C–F; D–F; E–F
56. A–F; B–F; C–F; D–T; E–T
57. A–T; B–F; C–T; D–F; E–F
58. A–F; B–T; C–T; D–F; E–T
59. A–F; B–F; C–F; D–F; E–T
60. A–F; B–F; C–T; D–T; E–T
61. A–F; B–F; C–F; D–F; E–T
62. A–F; B–T; C–F; D–T; E–F
63. A–F; B–F; C–T; D–T; E–T
64. A–T; B–F; C–F; D–T; E–T
65. A–F; B–F; C–F; D–T; E–T
66. A–T; B–F; C–F; D–F; E–T
67. A–T; B–F; C–T; D–F; E–T
68. A–T; B–F; C–T; D–F; E–T
69. A–F; B–T; C–F; D–T; E–F
70. A–T; B–F; C–T; D–T; E–T
71. A–T; B–F; C–F; D–F; E–F
72. A–T; B–F; C–T; D–F; E–F
73. A–T; B–F; C–T; D–T; E–F

74. C
75. A
76. B
77. D
78. E
79. C
80. E
81. E
82. D
83. B
84. C
85. A

PART 4. GASTROINTESTINAL DISEASE

1. D
2. D
3. C
4. D
5. A
6. D
7. C
8. C
9. C
10. C
11. A
12. D
13. B
14. C
15. B
16. C
17. C
18. D
19. A
20. D
21. D
22. E
23. E
24. D
25. C
26. C
27. E
28. D
29. E
30. A
31. D
32. C
33. B
34. D
35. D
36. C
37. E
38. B
39. D
40. B
41. D
42. D
43. B
44. C
45. E
46. C
47. B
48. A
49. C
50. E

51. A–T; B–T; C–F; D–F; E–F
52. A–T; B–F; C–F; D–T; E–T
53. A–T; B–F; C–F; D–F; E–T
54. A–F; B–F; C–T; D–F; E–T
55. A–T; B–T; C–F; D–T; E–T
56. A–F; B–T; C–F; D–T; E–F
57. A–F; B–F; C–F; D–T; E–T
58. A–T; B–F; C–T; D–T; E–F; F–T
59. All are False
60. A–F; B–T; C–F; D–F; E–T
61. A–F; B–F; C–F; D–T; E–F
62. A–T; B–F; C–T; D–F; E–T
63. A–F; B–F; C–T; D–F; E–F
64. A–F; B–T; C–F; D–F; E–F
65. A–T; B–T; C–F; D–F; E–T
66. A–T; B–F; C–F; D–T; E–T
67. A–T; B–F; C–F; D–F; E–T
68. A–F; B–T; C–F; D–F; E–T
69. A–F; B–T; C–T; D–F; E–T
70. A–F; B–F; C–F; D–F; E–T
71. A–T; B–T; C–F; D–F; E–T
72. A–F; B–T; C–F; D–T; E–T
73. A–T; B–F; C–F; D–T; E–F
74. A–F; B–F; C–T; D–T; E–F
75. A–T; B–T; C–F; D–T; E–F
76. A–T; B–T; C–T; D–T; E–F
77. A–F; B–T; C–F; D–T; E–T
78. All are True
79. A–F; B–T; C–T; D–F; E–T; F–T
80. A–F; B–T; C–F; D–T; E–F
81. A–T; B–F; C–F; D–T; E–F
82. A–T; B–T; C–F; D–T; E–F
83. A–T; B–T; C–F; D–F
84. A–F; B–T; C–T; D–F; E–T
85. A–T; B–T; C–F; D–F; E–T
86. A–T; B–T; C–F; D–T; E–F
87. A–T; B–F; C–F; D–T; E–F
88. A–T; B–T; C–F; D–T; E–T
89. A–F; B–T; C–F; D–T; E–T
90. A–F; B–T; C–T; D–F; E–T
91. A–T; B–F; C–F; D–T; E–F
92. A–F; B–F; C–T; D–F; E–T; F–F
93. A–T; B–F; C–F; D–F; E–F
94. A–T; B–F; C–F; D–T
95. A–T; B–T; C–T; D–F; E–F
96. All are False

97. B
98. G
99. D
100. H
101. A
102. F
103. C
104. E
105. B
106. D
107. C
108. A
109. A
110. B
111. D
112. A
113. E
114. C
115. C
116. E
117. A
118. B
119. C
120. A
121. B
122. E
123. B
124. C
125. A
126. B
127. E
128. D
129. A
130. A
131. F
132. D
133. E
134. B
135. C
136. E
137. B
138. C
139. G
140. A
141. C
142. E
143. H
144. F
145. D
146. C
147. A
148. B
149. E
150. D
151. C
152. A
153. B
154. A
155. B
156. D
157. E
158. C
159. A
160. C
161. D
162. B
163. E
164. E
165. B
166. C
167. E
168. D
169. F
170. C
171. B
172. A
173. B
174. E
175. C
176. A
177. D
178. B
179. A
180. C
181. D
182. D

PART 5. HEMATOLOGY AND ONCOLOGY

1. B
2. C
3. C
4. C
5. B
6. A
7. C
8. B
9. B
10. C
11. C
12. C
13. A
14. D
15. C
16. D
17. D
18. C
19. A
20. C
21. D
22. C
23. C
24. A
25. B
26. D
27. C
28. B
29. C

30. A–F; B–T; C–T; D–F; E–F
31. A–T; B–F; C–F; D–T
32. All are True
33. A–T; B–T; C–T; D–F
34. A–T; B–T; C–F; D–T
35. A–T; B–F; C–T; D–T; E–F
36. A–T; B–F; C–F; D–F
37. A–T; B–F; C–F; D–T
38. A–T; B–F; C–T; D–F; E–F
39. A–T; B–T; C–F; D–T
40. A–F; B–F; C–T; D–T
41. A–T; B–F; C–T; D–F; E–F

42. A–F; B–T; C–F; D–F
43. A–T; B–F; C–F; D–T
44. A–F; B–F; C–F; D–T
45. A–T; B–F; C–F; D–F
46. A–F; B–T; C–T; D–F
47. A–T; B–T; C–F; D–T
48. A–T; B–F; C–T; D–T
49. A–T; B–T; C–T; D–F
50. A–F; B–T; C–F; D–T
51. A–T; B–F; C–F; D–F
52. A–F; B–F; C–T; D–F
53. A–T; B–T; C–F; D–T
54. A–T; B–F; C–T; D–F
55. A–F; B–T; C–T; D–T
56. A–F; B–F; C–F; D–F; E–T
57. A–F; B–T; C–T; D–T; E–T
58. A–F; B–T; C–F; D–T; E–F
59. A–T; B–F; C–T; D–F; E–F
60. A–T; B–F; C–T; D–F
61. A–T; B–T; C–T; D–F
62. A–F; B–F; C–F; D–T
63. A–T; B–T; C–F; D–T
64. A–F; B–T; C–F; D–T
65. A–T; B–F; C–F; D–T
66. A–T; B–T; C–F; D–F
67. A–T; B–F; C–T; D–F
68. A–T; B–F; C–F; D–T
69. All are True
70. A–F; B–F; C–F; D–T
71. A–T; B–T; C–F; D–T
72. A–T; B–T; C–T; D–F
73. A–T; B–F; C–F; D–T
74. A–T; B–F; C–T; D–T

75. G
76. F
77. C
78. E
79. B
80. H
81. D
82. F
83. A
84. C
85. B
86. C
87. A
88. D
89. B
90. D
91. A
92. A
93. D
94. C
95. B
96. C
97. A
98. B
99. C
100. E
101. D
102. B
103. G
104. F
105. C
106. C
107. B
108. A
109. E
110. B
111. C
112. A
113. B
114. A
115. B
116. B
117. A
118. B
119. C
120. D
121. A
122. C
123. C
124. A
125. A
126. B
127. D
128. A
129. C
130. D
131. B
132. E
133. C
134. B
135. A

PART 6. GENETIC AND METABOLIC DISEASE

1. A
2. D
3. C
4. C
5. A
6. A
7. E
8. D
9. A
10. C
11. C
12. A
13. B
14. D
15. E
16. C
17. D
18. C
19. B
20. D
21. D
22. D
23. C
24. A
25. D
26. A
27. C
28. C
29. D
30. C
31. C
32. C

33. A–T; B–T; C–F; D–F
34. A–F; B–F; C–T; D–T
35. A–F; B–T; C–F; D–F
36. A–F; B–F; C–F; D–T
37. A–F; B–T; C–T; D–T
38. All are True
39. A–F; B–T; C–F; D–F
40. A–F; B–T; C–F; D–F
41. A–F; B–T; C–T; D–T
42. All are True
43. All are True
44. A–T; B–T; C–T; D–F
45. A–T; B–T; C–F; D–T; E–F
46. All are True
47. A–T; B–T; C–T; D–F; E–F
48. A–F; B–T; C–T; D–F; E–T
49. A–T; B–F; C–T; D–T
50. A–T; B–F; C–F; D–T
51. A–F; B–T; C–F; D–T
52. A–F; B–F; C–T; D–T; E–F
53. A–T; B–T; C–F; D–F
54. A–F; B–T; C–T; D–T
55. A–T; B–F; C–F; D–T; E–F
56. A–T; B–F; C–T; D–F
57. A–F; B–F; C–F; D–T; E–F
58. A–F; B–T; C–T; D–F
59. A–F; B–F; C–T; D–F
60. A–F; B–T; C–T; D–T

61. C
62. C
63. B
64. B
65. B
66. A
67. C
68. A
69. C
70. A
71. D
72. C
73. B
74. A
75. D
76. C
77. E
78. A
79. C
80. D
81. B
82. A
83. C
84. B
85. A
86. C
87. B
88. A
89. A
90. C
91. B
92. C
93. A
94. B

PART 7. ENDOCRINOLOGY AND DIABETES MELLITUS

1. C
2. E
3. D
4. C
5. C
6. E
7. D
8. C
9. D
10. A
11. E
12. E
13. D
14. E
15. C
16. C
17. D
18. E
19. A
20. B
21. D
22. D
23. A
24. E
25. D
26. E
27. D
28. C
29. D
30. B
31. A
32. D
33. E
34. D
35. C
36. D
37. D
38. B
39. E
40. D

41. D
42. E
43. B
44. A
45. C
46. E
47. D
48. E
49. D
50. D
51. D
52. D
53. D
54. B
55. C
56. E
57. B
58. A
59. E
60. E
61. D
62. E
63. A–T; B–F; C–T; D–T; E–F
64. A–T; B–T; C–T; D–F; E–F
65. A–T; B–T; C–F; D–T; E–F
66. A–F; B–T; C–F; D–T; E–T

67. A–T; B–F; C–F; D–F; E–T
68. A–T; B–F; C–F; D–T; E–F
69. A–T; B–T; C–F; D–F; E–T
70. A–T; B–F; C–T; D–T; E–T
71. A–F; B–F; C–T; D–F; E–F
72. A–T; B–T; C–F; D–F; E–F
73. A–T; B–F; C–F; D–T; E–T
74. A–F; B–T; C–T; D–F; E–F
75. A–T; B–T; C–T; D–F; E–F
76. A–F; B–T; C–F; D–T; E–T
77. A–F; B–T; C–T; D–F; E–F
78. A–T; B–T; C–F; D–F; E–T
79. A–F; B–T; C–T; D–F; E–F
80. A–F; B–T; C–F; D–T; E–F
81. A–F; B–F; C–F; D–T; E–T
82. A–T; B–F; C–T; D–F; E–T
83. A–T; B–T; C–T; D–F; E–T
84. A–F; B–T; C–T; D–T; E–T
85. A–F; B–T; C–T; D–T; E–T
86. A–F; B–T; C–F; D–T; E–F
87. A–F; B–F; C–T; D–F; E–F
88. All are True
89. A–F; B–T; C–T; D–T; E–T
90. A–T; B–F; C–T; D–T; E–T
91. A–T; B–F; C–F; D–T; E–T
92. A–F; B–F; C–T; D–T; E–F
93. A–T; B–F; C–T; D–T; E–F
94. All are True
95. A–T; B–T; C–T; D–F; E–T
96. A–F; B–T; C–F; D–T; E–F
97. A–T; B–F; C–F; D–T; E–T
98. A–F; B–T; C–T; D–T; E–T
99. A–F; B–F; C–F; D–F; E–T
100. A–T; B–F; C–F; D–T; E–T
101. A–F; B–T; C–T; D–T; E–T
102. A–T; B–T; C–F; D–T; E–T
103. A–F; B–T; C–T; D–T; E–T

104. B
105. C
106. B
107. A
108. C
109. A
110. B
111. D
112. E
113. E
114. B
115. C
116. A
117. D
118. E
119. A
120. C
121. D
122. B
123. B
124. D
125. A
126. C
127. E
128. C
129. A
130. D
131. B
132. C
133. B
134. F
135. D
136. A
137. E

PART 8. INFECTIOUS DISEASE

1. E
2. A
3. B
4. B
5. C
6. A
7. C
8. D
9. C
10. C
11. A
12. D
13. E
14. D
15. C
16. A
17. D
18. E
19. D
20. B
21. A
22. E
23. E
24. E
25. D
26. E
27. A
28. D
29. E
30. D
31. C
32. C
33. E
34. B
35. B
36. D
37. B
38. D
39. D
40. C
41. C
42. A
43. E
44. B
45. D
46. B
47. C
48. B
49. D
50. B

51. A–T; B–T; C–F; D–F; E–F
52. A–T; B–F; C–F; D–F; E–T
53. A–T; B–T; C–T; D–F; E–T
54. A–T; B–T; C–T; D–F; E–T
55. A–T; B–F; C–T; D–T; E–F
56. A–T; B–T; C–T; D–F; E–F
57. A–T; B–F; C–T; D–F; E–F
58. All are False
59. A–T; B–F; C–T; D–F; E–F
60. A–T; B–F; C–T; D–F; E–T
61. A–T; B–T; C–F; D–F; E–T
62. A–T; B–T; C–T; D–T; E–F
63. A–T; B–F; C–F; D–F; E–F
64. A–F; B–F; C–T; D–F; E–T
65. A–F; B–F; C–T; D–T
66. A–F; B–T; C–T; D–T; E–T
67. A–T; B–F; C–T; D–T; E–F
68. A–F; B–T; C–T; D–F; E–T
69. All are True
70. A–T; B–T; C–F; D–F; E–F
71. A–T; B–F; C–F; D–T; E–F
72. A–F; B–T; C–T; D–T; E–F
73. A–T; B–F; C–T; D–T; E–T
74. A–F; B–T; C–T; D–F; E–T
75. A–T; B–T; C–F; D–T; E–T
76. A–T; B–T; C–F; D–T
77. A–F; B–T; C–F; D–F; E–F
78. A–F; B–F; C–T; D–T; E–F
79. A–T; B–T; C–F; D–T
80. A–F; B–T; C–T; D–T; E–F
81. A–T; B–T; C–F; D–T; E–F
82. A–T; B–T; C–T; D–T; E–F
83. A–F; B–T; C–T; D–T; E–T
84. A–T; B–T; C–F; D–T; E–F
85. A–T; B–F; C–T; D–T
86. A–T; B–T; C–T; D–F
87. A–T; B–F; C–F; D–T; E–T
88. A–T; B–T; C–F; D–F; E–F
89. All are False
90. A–T; B–F; C–T; D–F
91. All are True
92. All are True
93. A–T; B–T; C–F; D–T
94. C
95. A
96. D
97. B
98. E
99. C
100. E
101. A
102. B
103. D

104. B
105. C
106. D
107. E
108. A
109. F
110. B
111. A
112. D
113. C
114. E
115. B
116. G
117. C
118. A
119. A
120. E
121. A
122. A
123. A
124. A
125. B
126. C
127. A
128. A
129. A
130. B
131. D
132. D
133. B
134. A
135. E
136. F
137. C
138. B
139. B
140. C
141. D
142. D
143. A
144. B
145. C
146. A
147. C
148. A
149. D
150. B
151. A
152. E
153. C
154. E
155. A
156. B
157. D
158. F
159. C
160. D
161. B
162. C
163. B
164. A
165. B
166. E
167. C
168. D
169. E
170. B

PART 9. CLINICAL IMMUNOLOGY AND RHEUMATOLOGY

1. B
2. C
3. A
4. A
5. B
6. B
7. A
8. C
9. C
10. B
11. B
12. C
13. E
14. C
15. D
16. D
17. D
18. C
19. B
20. C
21. B
22. D
23. B
24. B
25. E
26. C
27. C
28. E
29. D
30. C
31. C

32. A–F; B–T; C–F; D–T; E–F
33. A–F; B–F; C–T; D–F; E–T
34. A–T; B–T; C–F; D–F; E–F
35. A–T; B–T; C–F; D–F; E–T
36. A–T; B–F; C–F; D–T
37. A–F; B–T; C–F; D–T
38. A–T; B–F; C–T; D–F
39. A–T; B–F; C–F; D–T
40. A–T; B–F; C–T; D–F; E–T
41. A–F; B–F; C–T; D–F; E–F
42. A–F; B–T; C–F; D–F; E–T
43. A–F; B–T; C–F; D–F; E–F
44. A–F; B–F; C–T; D–F
45. A–T; B–T; C–T; D–T; E–F
46. A–T; B–F; C–F; D–F; E–T
47. A–T; B–F; C–F; D–F; E–T
48. A–F; B–F; C–T; D–F; E–F
49. A–F; B–F; C–T; D–T; E–T

50. A
51. C
52. B
53. D
54. B
55. B
56. A
57. A
58. C
59. A
60. D
61. B
62. D
63. A
64. B
65. B
66. B
67. C
68. D
69. C
70. C
71. E
72. A
73. B
74. D
75. E
76. C
77. A
78. B
79. B
80. E
81. C
82. D
83. A

PART 10. NEUROLOGIC DISEASE

1. E
2. D
3. D
4. D
5. C
6. D
7. D
8. A
9. A
10. C
11. A
12. C
13. D
14. A
15. D
16. C
17. C
18. A
19. E
20. A
21. E
22. A
23. C
24. E
25. E
26. B
27. B
28. D
29. C
30. B
31. C
32. A
33. B
34. E
35. B
36. B
37. D
38. C
39. D
40. D
41. B
42. B
43. A
44. E
45. D
46. B
47. D
48. A
49. D
50. B
51. A
52. D
53. C
54. A

55. A–T; B–F; C–T; D–T; E–T
56. All are True
57. A–F; B–T; C–T; D–T; E–F
58. A–T; B–F; C–T; D–T; E–F
59. A–T; B–T; C–F; D–F; E–T
60. A–T; B–T; C–F; D–F; E–T
61. All are True
62. A–F; B–T; C–T; D–T; E–T
63. A–T; B–T; C–T; D–T; E–F
64. A–T; B–T; C–T; D–F; E–T
65. All are True
66. A–T; B–T; C–F; D–F; E–T
67. A–T; B–F; C–F; D–T; E–F
68. A–T; B–T; C–T; D–T; E–F
69. A–F; B–F; C–T; D–T; E–F
70. A–T; B–T; C–T; D–T; E–F
71. A–F; B–T; C–F; D–T; E–T
72. A–T; B–T; C–F; D–T; E–F
73. All are True
74. All are True
75. A–T; B–F; C–F; D–T; E–F
76. A–T; B–T; C–F; D–F; E–T
77. All are True
78. A–T; B–T; C–F; D–F; E–F
79. A–F; B–T; C–T; D–F; E–T
80. All are True
81. A–T; B–T; C–T; D–F; E–T
82. A–T; B–T; C–F; D–F; E–T; F–F
83. A–T; B–F; C–T; D–F; E–F
84. A–T; B–T; C–F; D–F; E–F
85. A–T; B–T; C–T; D–F; E–T
86. All are True
87. A–T; B–F; C–T; D–F; E–T
88. A–F; B–T; C–F; D–T; E–T
89. A–T; B–T; C–F; D–T; E–F
90. A–F; B–T; C–T; D–T; E–T
91. A–F; B–T; C–F; D–T; E–T
92. A–T; B–T; C–T; D–T; E–F
93. All are True
94. A–F; B–T; C–T; D–T; E–F
95. A–T; B–T; C–T; D–F; E–F
96. A–F; B–F; C–T; D–T; E–T
97. All are True
98. A–T; B–T; C–F; D–F; E–F
99. A–T; B–T; C–F; D–F; E–F
100. All are False
101. E
102. D
103. B
104. C
105. A
106. C
107. D
108. B

109. E
110. A
111. B
112. C
113. E
114. A
115. D
116. E
117. D
118. A
119. C
120. B
121. D
122. C
123. E
124. A
125. B
126. D
127. B
128. A
129. C
130. E
131. C
132. A
133. B
134. E
135. D
136. D
137. C
138. B
139. E
140. A
141. B
142. C
143. G
144. A
145. D
146. D
147. C
148. A
149. B
150. E
151. E
152. C
153. D
154. B
155. A

PART 11. DERMATOLOGY

1. D
2. B
3. E
4. E
5. A
6. E
7. C
8. D
9. A
10. B
11. D
12. D
13. C
14. E
15. E
16. A
17. B
18. C
19. C
20. E
21. D
22. A–T; B–T; C–T; D–T; E–F
23. A–T; B–F; C–T; D–F; E–F
24. A–T; B–T; C–F; D–T; E–F
25. A–T; B–T; C–T; D–F; E–F
26. A–F; B–T; C–T; D–F; E–F
27. A–T; B–T; C–T; D–T; E–F
28. A–T; B–T; C–T; D–F; E–F
29. E
30. B
31. E
32. C
33. B
34. B
35. C
36. A
37. D
38. C
39. C
40. A
41. D
42. D
43. A
44. B
45. C
46. E
47. E
48. B
49. A
50. C

PART 1. CARDIOVASCULAR DISEASES

1. A B C D E F G H
2. A B C D E F G H
3. A B C D E F G H
4. A B C D E F G H
5. A B C D E F G H
6. A B C D E F G H
7. A B C D E F G H
8. A B C D E F G H
9. A B C D E F G H
10. A B C D E F G H
11. A B C D E F G H
12. A B C D E F G H
13. A B C D E F G H
14. A B C D E F G H
15. A B C D E F G H
16. A B C D E F G H
17. A B C D E F G H
18. A B C D E F G H
19. A B C D E F G H
20. A B C D E F G H
21. A B C D E F G H
22. A B C D E F G H
23. A B C D E F G H
24. A B C D E F G H
25. A B C D E F G H
26. A B C D E F G H
27. A B C D E F G H
28. A B C D E F G H
29. A B C D E F G H
30. A B C D E F G H
31. A B C D E F G H
32. A B C D E F G H
33. A B C D E F G H
34. A B C D E F G H
35. A B C D E F G H
36. A B C D E F G H
37. A B C D E F G H
38. A B C D E F G H
39. A B C D E F G H
40. A B C D E F G H
41. A B C D E F G H
42. A B C D E F G H
43. A B C D E F G H
44. A B C D E F G H
45. A B C D E F G H
46. A B C D E F G H
47. A B C D E F G H
48. A B C D E F G H
49. A B C D E F G H
50. A B C D E F G H
51. A B C D E F G H
52. A B C D E F G H
53. A B C D E F G H
54. A B C D E F G H
55. A B C D E F G H
56. A B C D E F G H
57. A B C D E F G H
58. A B C D E F G H
59. A B C D E F G H
60. A B C D E F G H
61. A B C D E F G H
62. A B C D E F G H
63. A B C D E F G H
64. A B C D E F G H
65. A B C D E F G H
66. A B C D E F G H
67. A B C D E F G H
68. A B C D E F G H
69. A B C D E F G H
70. A B C D E F G H
71. A B C D E F G H
72. A B C D E F G H
73. A B C D E F G H
74. A B C D E F G H
75. A B C D E F G H
76. A B C D E F G H
77. A B C D E F G H
78. A B C D E F G H
79. A B C D E F G H
80. A B C D E F G H
81. A B C D E F G H
82. A B C D E F G H
83. A B C D E F G H
84. A B C D E F G H
85. A B C D E F G H
86. A B C D E F G H
87. A B C D E F G H
88. A B C D E F G H
89. A B C D E F G H
90. A B C D E F G H
91. A B C D E F G H
92. A B C D E F G H
93. A B C D E F G H
94. A B C D E F G H
95. A B C D E F G H
96. A B C D E F G H
97. A B C D E F G H
98. A B C D E F G H
99. A B C D E F G H
100. A B C D E F G H
101. A B C D E F G H
102. A B C D E F G H

PART 1. CARDIOVASCULAR DISEASES

103. A B C D E F G H
104. A B C D E F G H
105. A B C D E F G H
106. A B C D E F G H
107. A B C D E F G H
108. A B C D E F G H
109. A B C D E F G H
110. A B C D E F G H
111. A B C D E F G H
112. A B C D E F G H
113. A B C D E F G H
114. A B C D E F G H
115. A B C D E F G H
116. A B C D E F G H
117. A B C D E F G H
118. A B C D E F G H
119. A B C D E F G H
120. A B C D E F G H
121. A B C D E F G H
122. A B C D E F G H
123. A B C D E F G H
124. A B C D E F G H
125. A B C D E F G H
126. A B C D E F G H
127. A B C D E F G H
128. A B C D E F G H
129. A B C D E F G H
130. A B C D E F G H
131. A B C D E F G H
132. A B C D E F G H
133. A B C D E F G H
134. A B C D E F G H
135. A B C D E F G H
136. A B C D E F G H
137. A B C D E F G H
138. A B C D E F G H
139. A B C D E F G H
140. A B C D E F G H
141. A B C D E F G H
142. A B C D E F G H
143. A B C D E F G H
144. A B C D E F G H
145. A B C D E F G H
146. A B C D E F G H
147. A B C D E F G H
148. A B C D E F G H
149. A B C D E F G H
150. A B C D E F G H
151. A B C D E F G H
152. A B C D E F G H
153. A B C D E F G H
154. A B C D E F G H
155. A B C D E F G H
156. A B C D E F G H
157. A B C D E F G H
158. A B C D E F G H
159. A B C D E F G H
160. A B C D E F G H
161. A B C D E F G H
162. A B C D E F G H
163. A B C D E F G H
164. A B C D E F G H
165. A B C D E F G H
166. A B C D E F G H
167. A B C D E F G H
168. A B C D E F G H
169. A B C D E F G H
170. A B C D E F G H
171. A B C D E F G H
172. A B C D E F G H
173. A B C D E F G H
174. A B C D E F G H
175. A B C D E F G H
176. A B C D E F G H
177. A B C D E F G H
178. A B C D E F G H
179. A B C D E F G H
180. A B C D E F G H
181. A B C D E F G H
182. A B C D E F G H
183. A B C D E F G H
184. A B C D E F G H
185. A B C D E F G H
186. A B C D E F G H
187. A B C D E F G H
188. A B C D E F G H
189. A B C D E F G H
190. A B C D E F G H
191. A B C D E F G H
192. A B C D E F G H
193. A B C D E F G H
194. A B C D E F G H
195. A B C D E F G H

PART 2. RESPIRATORY DISEASE

1. A B C D E F G H
2. A B C D E F G H
3. A B C D E F G H
4. A B C D E F G H
5. A B C D E F G H
6. A B C D E F G H
7. A B C D E F G H
8. A B C D E F G H
9. A B C D E F G H
10. A B C D E F G H
11. A B C D E F G H
12. A B C D E F G H
13. A B C D E F G H
14. A B C D E F G H
15. A B C D E F G H
16. A B C D E F G H
17. A B C D E F G H
18. A B C D E F G H
19. A B C D E F G H
20. A B C D E F G H
21. A B C D E F G H
22. A B C D E F G H
23. A B C D E F G H
24. A B C D E F G H
25. A B C D E F G H
26. A B C D E F G H
27. A B C D E F G H
28. A B C D E F G H
29. A B C D E F G H
30. A B C D E F G H
31. A B C D E F G H
32. A B C D E F G H
33. A B C D E F G H
34. A B C D E F G H
35. A B C D E F G H
36. A B C D E F G H
37. A B C D E F G H
38. A B C D E F G H
39. A B C D E F G H
40. A B C D E F G H
41. A B C D E F G H
42. A B C D E F G H
43. A B C D E F G H
44. A B C D E F G H
45. A B C D E F G H
46. A B C D E F G H
47. A B C D E F G H
48. A B C D E F G H
49. A B C D E F G H
50. A B C D E F G H
51. A B C D E F G H
52. A B C D E F G H
53. A B C D E F G H
54. A B C D E F G H
55. A B C D E F G H
56. A B C D E F G H
57. A B C D E F G H
58. A B C D E F G H
59. A B C D E F G H
60. A B C D E F G H
61. A B C D E F G H
62. A B C D E F G H
63. A B C D E F G H
64. A B C D E F G H
65. A B C D E F G H
66. A B C D E F G H
67. A B C D E F G H
68. A B C D E F G H
69. A B C D E F G H
70. A B C D E F G H
71. A B C D E F G H
72. A B C D E F G H
73. A B C D E F G H
74. A B C D E F G H
75. A B C D E F G H
76. A B C D E F G H
77. A B C D E F G H
78. A B C D E F G H
79. A B C D E F G H
80. A B C D E F G H
81. A B C D E F G H
82. A B C D E F G H
83. A B C D E F G H
84. A B C D E F G H
85. A B C D E F G H
86. A B C D E F G H
87. A B C D E F G H
88. A B C D E F G H
89. A B C D E F G H
90. A B C D E F G H
91. A B C D E F G H
92. A B C D E F G H
93. A B C D E F G H
94. A B C D E F G H
95. A B C D E F G H
96. A B C D E F G H
97. A B C D E F G H
98. A B C D E F G H
99. A B C D E F G H
100. A B C D E F G H
101. A B C D E F G H
102. A B C D E F G H

PART 2. RESPIRATORY DISEASE

103. A B C D E F G H
104. A B C D E F G H
105. A B C D E F G H
106. A B C D E F G H
107. A B C D E F G H
108. A B C D E F G H
109. A B C D E F G H
110. A B C D E F G H
111. A B C D E F G H
112. A B C D E F G H
113. A B C D E F G H
114. A B C D E F G H
115. A B C D E F G H
116. A B C D E F G H
117. A B C D E F G H
118. A B C D E F G H
119. A B C D E F G H
120. A B C D E F G H
121. A B C D E F G H
122. A B C D E F G H
123. A B C D E F G H
124. A B C D E F G H
125. A B C D E F G H
126. A B C D E F G H
127. A B C D E F G H
128. A B C D E F G H
129. A B C D E F G H
130. A B C D E F G H
131. A B C D E F G H
132. A B C D E F G H
133. A B C D E F G H
134. A B C D E F G H
135. A B C D E F G H
136. A B C D E F G H
137. A B C D E F G H
138. A B C D E F G H
139. A B C D E F G H

PART 3. RENAL DISEASE

1. A B C D E F G H
2. A B C D E F G H
3. A B C D E F G H
4. A B C D E F G H
5. A B C D E F G H
6. A B C D E F G H
7. A B C D E F G H
8. A B C D E F G H
9. A B C D E F G H
10. A B C D E F G H
11. A B C D E F G H
12. A B C D E F G H
13. A B C D E F G H
14. A B C D E F G H
15. A B C D E F G H
16. A B C D E F G H
17. A B C D E F G H
18. A B C D E F G H
19. A B C D E F G H
20. A B C D E F G H
21. A B C D E F G H
22. A B C D E F G H
23. A B C D E F G H
24. A B C D E F G H
25. A B C D E F G H
26. A B C D E F G H
27. A B C D E F G H
28. A B C D E F G H
29. A B C D E F G H
30. A B C D E F G H
31. A B C D E F G H
32. A B C D E F G H
33. A B C D E F G H
34. A B C D E F G H
35. A B C D E F G H
36. A B C D E F G H
37. A B C D E F G H
38. A B C D E F G H
39. A B C D E F G H
40. A B C D E F G H
41. A B C D E F G H
42. A B C D E F G H
43. A B C D E F G H
44. A B C D E F G H
45. A B C D E F G H
46. A B C D E F G H
47. A B C D E F G H
48. A B C D E F G H
49. A B C D E F G H
50. A B C D E F G H
51. A B C D E F G H
52. A B C D E F G H
53. A B C D E F G H
54. A B C D E F G H
55. A B C D E F G H
56. A B C D E F G H
57. A B C D E F G H
58. A B C D E F G H
59. A B C D E F G H
60. A B C D E F G H
61. A B C D E F G H
62. A B C D E F G H
63. A B C D E F G H
64. A B C D E F G H
65. A B C D E F G H
66. A B C D E F G H
67. A B C D E F G H
68. A B C D E F G H
69. A B C D E F G H
70. A B C D E F G H
71. A B C D E F G H
72. A B C D E F G H
73. A B C D E F G H
74. A B C D E F G H
75. A B C D E F G H
76. A B C D E F G H
77. A B C D E F G H
78. A B C D E F G H
79. A B C D E F G H
80. A B C D E F G H
81. A B C D E F G H
82. A B C D E F G H
83. A B C D E F G H
84. A B C D E F G H
85. A B C D E F G H

PART 4. GASTROINTESTINAL DISEASE

1. A B C D E F G H
2. A B C D E F G H
3. A B C D E F G H
4. A B C D E F G H
5. A B C D E F G H
6. A B C D E F G H
7. A B C D E F G H
8. A B C D E F G H
9. A B C D E F G H
10. A B C D E F G H
11. A B C D E F G H
12. A B C D E F G H
13. A B C D E F G H
14. A B C D E F G H
15. A B C D E F G H
16. A B C D E F G H
17. A B C D E F G H
18. A B C D E F G H
19. A B C D E F G H
20. A B C D E F G H
21. A B C D E F G H
22. A B C D E F G H
23. A B C D E F G H
24. A B C D E F G H
25. A B C D E F G H
26. A B C D E F G H
27. A B C D E F G H
28. A B C D E F G H
29. A B C D E F G H
30. A B C D E F G H
31. A B C D E F G H
32. A B C D E F G H
33. A B C D E F G H
34. A B C D E F G H
35. A B C D E F G H
36. A B C D E F G H
37. A B C D E F G H
38. A B C D E F G H
39. A B C D E F G H
40. A B C D E F G H
41. A B C D E F G H
42. A B C D E F G H
43. A B C D E F G H
44. A B C D E F G H
45. A B C D E F G H
46. A B C D E F G H
47. A B C D E F G H
48. A B C D E F G H
49. A B C D E F G H
50. A B C D E F G H
51. A B C D E F G H
52. A B C D E F G H
53. A B C D E F G H
54. A B C D E F G H
55. A B C D E F G H
56. A B C D E F G H
57. A B C D E F G H
58. A B C D E F G H
59. A B C D E F G H
60. A B C D E F G H
61. A B C D E F G H
62. A B C D E F G H
63. A B C D E F G H
64. A B C D E F G H
65. A B C D E F G H
66. A B C D E F G H
67. A B C D E F G H
68. A B C D E F G H
69. A B C D E F G H
70. A B C D E F G H
71. A B C D E F G H
72. A B C D E F G H
73. A B C D E F G H
74. A B C D E F G H
75. A B C D E F G H
76. A B C D E F G H
77. A B C D E F G H
78. A B C D E F G H
79. A B C D E F G H
80. A B C D E F G H
81. A B C D E F G H
82. A B C D E F G H
83. A B C D E F G H
84. A B C D E F G H
85. A B C D E F G H
86. A B C D E F G H
87. A B C D E F G H
88. A B C D E F G H
89. A B C D E F G H
90. A B C D E F G H
91. A B C D E F G H
92. A B C D E F G H
93. A B C D E F G H
94. A B C D E F G H
95. A B C D E F G H
96. A B C D E F G H
97. A B C D E F G H
98. A B C D E F G H
99. A B C D E F G H

PART 4. GASTROINTESTINAL DISEASE

100. A B C D E F G H
101. A B C D E F G H
102. A B C D E F G H
103. A B C D E F G H
104. A B C D E F G H
105. A B C D E F G H
106. A B C D E F G H
107. A B C D E F G H
108. A B C D E F G H
109. A B C D E F G H
110. A B C D E F G H
111. A B C D E F G H
112. A B C D E F G H
113. A B C D E F G H
114. A B C D E F G H
115. A B C D E F G H
116. A B C D E F G H
117. A B C D E F G H
118. A B C D E F G H
119. A B C D E F G H
120. A B C D E F G H
121. A B C D E F G H
122. A B C D E F G H
123. A B C D E F G H
124. A B C D E F G H
125. A B C D E F G H
126. A B C D E F G H
127. A B C D E F G H
128. A B C D E F G H
129. A B C D E F G H
130. A B C D E F G H
131. A B C D E F G H
132. A B C D E F G H
133. A B C D E F G H
134. A B C D E F G H
135. A B C D E F G H
136. A B C D E F G H
137. A B C D E F G H
138. A B C D E F G H
139. A B C D E F G H
140. A B C D E F G H
141. A B C D E F G H
142. A B C D E F G H
143. A B C D E F G H
144. A B C D E F G H
145. A B C D E F G H
146. A B C D E F G H
147. A B C D E F G H
148. A B C D E F G H
149. A B C D E F G H
150. A B C D E F G H
151. A B C D E F G H
152. A B C D E F G H
153. A B C D E F G H
154. A B C D E F G H
155. A B C D E F G H
156. A B C D E F G H
157. A B C D E F G H
158. A B C D E F G H
159. A B C D E F G H
160. A B C D E F G H
161. A B C D E F G H
162. A B C D E F G H
163. A B C D E F G H
164. A B C D E F G H
165. A B C D E F G H
166. A B C D E F G H
167. A B C D E F G H
168. A B C D E F G H
169. A B C D E F G H
170. A B C D E F G H
171. A B C D E F G H
172. A B C D E F G H
173. A B C D E F G H
174. A B C D E F G H
175. A B C D E F G H
176. A B C D E F G H
177. A B C D E F G H
178. A B C D E F G H
179. A B C D E F G H
180. A B C D E F G H
181. A B C D E F G H
182. A B C D E F G H

PART 5. HEMATOLOGY AND ONCOLOGY

1. A B C D E F G H
2. A B C D E F G H
3. A B C D E F G H
4. A B C D E F G H
5. A B C D E F G H
6. A B C D E F G H
7. A B C D E F G H
8. A B C D E F G H
9. A B C D E F G H
10. A B C D E F G H
11. A B C D E F G H
12. A B C D E F G H
13. A B C D E F G H
14. A B C D E F G H
15. A B C D E F G H
16. A B C D E F G H
17. A B C D E F G H
18. A B C D E F G H
19. A B C D E F G H
20. A B C D E F G H
21. A B C D E F G H
22. A B C D E F G H
23. A B C D E F G H
24. A B C D E F G H
25. A B C D E F G H
26. A B C D E F G H
27. A B C D E F G H
28. A B C D E F G H
29. A B C D E F G H
30. A B C D E F G H
31. A B C D E F G H
32. A B C D E F G H
33. A B C D E F G H
34. A B C D E F G H
35. A B C D E F G H
36. A B C D E F G H
37. A B C D E F G H
38. A B C D E F G H
39. A B C D E F G H
40. A B C D E F G H
41. A B C D E F G H
42. A B C D E F G H
43. A B C D E F G H
44. A B C D E F G H
45. A B C D E F G H
46. A B C D E F G H
47. A B C D E F G H
48. A B C D E F G H
49. A B C D E F G H
50. A B C D E F G H
51. A B C D E F G H
52. A B C D E F G H
53. A B C D E F G H
54. A B C D E F G H
55. A B C D E F G H
56. A B C D E F G H
57. A B C D E F G H
58. A B C D E F G H
59. A B C D E F G H
60. A B C D E F G H
61. A B C D E F G H
62. A B C D E F G H
63. A B C D E F G H
64. A B C D E F G H
65. A B C D E F G H
66. A B C D E F G H
67. A B C D E F G H
68. A B C D E F G H
69. A B C D E F G H
70. A B C D E F G H
71. A B C D E F G H
72. A B C D E F G H
73. A B C D E F G H
74. A B C D E F G H
75. A B C D E F G H
76. A B C D E F G H
77. A B C D E F G H
78. A B C D E F G H
79. A B C D E F G H
80. A B C D E F G H
81. A B C D E F G H
82. A B C D E F G H
83. A B C D E F G H
84. A B C D E F G H
85. A B C D E F G H
86. A B C D E F G H
87. A B C D E F G H
88. A B C D E F G H
89. A B C D E F G H
90. A B C D E F G H
91. A B C D E F G H
92. A B C D E F G H
93. A B C D E F G H
94. A B C D E F G H
95. A B C D E F G H
96. A B C D E F G H
97. A B C D E F G H
98. A B C D E F G H
99. A B C D E F G H

PART 5. HEMATOLOGY AND ONCOLOGY

100. A B C D E F G H
101. A B C D E F G H
102. A B C D E F G H
103. A B C D E F G H
104. A B C D E F G H
105. A B C D E F G H
106. A B C D E F G H
107. A B C D E F G H
108. A B C D E F G H
109. A B C D E F G H
110. A B C D E F G H
111. A B C D E F G H
112. A B C D E F G H
113. A B C D E F G H
114. A B C D E F G H
115. A B C D E F G H
116. A B C D E F G H
117. A B C D E F G H
118. A B C D E F G H
119. A B C D E F G H
120. A B C D E F G H
121. A B C D E F G H
122. A B C D E F G H
123. A B C D E F G H
124. A B C D E F G H
125. A B C D E F G H
126. A B C D E F G H
127. A B C D E F G H
128. A B C D E F G H
129. A B C D E F G H
130. A B C D E F G H
131. A B C D E F G H
132. A B C D E F G H
133. A B C D E F G H
134. A B C D E F G H
135. A B C D E F G H

PART 6. GENETIC AND METABOLIC DISEASE

1. A B C D E F G H
2. A B C D E F G H
3. A B C D E F G H
4. A B C D E F G H
5. A B C D E F G H
6. A B C D E F G H
7. A B C D E F G H
8. A B C D E F G H
9. A B C D E F G H
10. A B C D E F G H
11. A B C D E F G H
12. A B C D E F G H
13. A B C D E F G H
14. A B C D E F G H
15. A B C D E F G H
16. A B C D E F G H
17. A B C D E F G H
18. A B C D E F G H
19. A B C D E F G H
20. A B C D E F G H
21. A B C D E F G H
22. A B C D E F G H
23. A B C D E F G H
24. A B C D E F G H
25. A B C D E F G H
26. A B C D E F G H
27. A B C D E F G H
28. A B C D E F G H
29. A B C D E F G H
30. A B C D E F G H
31. A B C D E F G H
32. A B C D E F G H
33. A B C D E F G H
34. A B C D E F G H
35. A B C D E F G H
36. A B C D E F G H
37. A B C D E F G H
38. A B C D E F G H
39. A B C D E F G H
40. A B C D E F G H
41. A B C D E F G H
42. A B C D E F G H
43. A B C D E F G H
44. A B C D E F G H
45. A B C D E F G H
46. A B C D E F G H
47. A B C D E F G H
48. A B C D E F G H
49. A B C D E F G H
50. A B C D E F G H
51. A B C D E F G H
52. A B C D E F G H
53. A B C D E F G H
54. A B C D E F G H
55. A B C D E F G H
56. A B C D E F G H
57. A B C D E F G H
58. A B C D E F G H
59. A B C D E F G H
60. A B C D E F G H
61. A B C D E F G H
62. A B C D E F G H
63. A B C D E F G H
64. A B C D E F G H
65. A B C D E F G H
66. A B C D E F G H
67. A B C D E F G H
68. A B C D E F G H
69. A B C D E F G H
70. A B C D E F G H
71. A B C D E F G H
72. A B C D E F G H
73. A B C D E F G H
74. A B C D E F G H
75. A B C D E F G H
76. A B C D E F G H
77. A B C D E F G H
78. A B C D E F G H
79. A B C D E F G H
80. A B C D E F G H
81. A B C D E F G H
82. A B C D E F G H
83. A B C D E F G H
84. A B C D E F G H
85. A B C D E F G H
86. A B C D E F G H
87. A B C D E F G H
88. A B C D E F G H
89. A B C D E F G H
90. A B C D E F G H
91. A B C D E F G H
92. A B C D E F G H
93. A B C D E F G H
94. A B C D E F G H

PART 7. ENDOCRINOLOGY AND DIABETES MELLITUS

1. A B C D E F G H
2. A B C D E F G H
3. A B C D E F G H
4. A B C D E F G H
5. A B C D E F G H
6. A B C D E F G H
7. A B C D E F G H
8. A B C D E F G H
9. A B C D E F G H
10. A B C D E F G H
11. A B C D E F G H
12. A B C D E F G H
13. A B C D E F G H
14. A B C D E F G H
15. A B C D E F G H
16. A B C D E F G H
17. A B C D E F G H
18. A B C D E F G H
19. A B C D E F G H
20. A B C D E F G H
21. A B C D E F G H
22. A B C D E F G H
23. A B C D E F G H
24. A B C D E F G H
25. A B C D E F G H
26. A B C D E F G H
27. A B C D E F G H
28. A B C D E F G H
29. A B C D E F G H
30. A B C D E F G H
31. A B C D E F G H
32. A B C D E F G H
33. A B C D E F G H
34. A B C D E F G H
35. A B C D E F G H
36. A B C D E F G H
37. A B C D E F G H
38. A B C D E F G H
39. A B C D E F G H
40. A B C D E F G H
41. A B C D E F G H
42. A B C D E F G H
43. A B C D E F G H
44. A B C D E F G H
45. A B C D E F G H
46. A B C D E F G H
47. A B C D E F G H
48. A B C D E F G H
49. A B C D E F G H
50. A B C D E F G H
51. A B C D E F G H
52. A B C D E F G H
53. A B C D E F G H
54. A B C D E F G H
55. A B C D E F G H
56. A B C D E F G H
57. A B C D E F G H
58. A B C D E F G H
59. A B C D E F G H
60. A B C D E F G H
61. A B C D E F G H
62. A B C D E F G H
63. A B C D E F G H
64. A B C D E F G H
65. A B C D E F G H
66. A B C D E F G H
67. A B C D E F G H
68. A B C D E F G H
69. A B C D E F G H
70. A B C D E F G H
71. A B C D E F G H
72. A B C D E F G H
73. A B C D E F G H
74. A B C D E F G H
75. A B C D E F G H
76. A B C D E F G H
77. A B C D E F G H
78. A B C D E F G H
79. A B C D E F G H
80. A B C D E F G H
81. A B C D E F G H
82. A B C D E F G H
83. A B C D E F G H
84. A B C D E F G H
85. A B C D E F G H
86. A B C D E F G H
87. A B C D E F G H
88. A B C D E F G H
89. A B C D E F G H
90. A B C D E F G H
91. A B C D E F G H
92. A B C D E F G H
93. A B C D E F G H
94. A B C D E F G H
95. A B C D E F G H
96. A B C D E F G H
97. A B C D E F G H
98. A B C D E F G H
99. A B C D E F G H

PART 7. ENDOCRINOLOGY AND DIABETES MELLITUS

No.								
100.	A	B	C	D	E	F	G	H
101.	A	B	C	D	E	F	G	H
102.	A	B	C	D	E	F	G	H
103.	A	B	C	D	E	F	G	H
104.	A	B	C	D	E	F	G	H
105.	A	B	C	D	E	F	G	H
106.	A	B	C	D	E	F	G	H
107.	A	B	C	D	E	F	G	H
108.	A	B	C	D	E	F	G	H
109.	A	B	C	D	E	F	G	H
110.	A	B	C	D	E	F	G	H
111.	A	B	C	D	E	F	G	H
112.	A	B	C	D	E	F	G	H
113.	A	B	C	D	E	F	G	H
114.	A	B	C	D	E	F	G	H
115.	A	B	C	D	E	F	G	H
116.	A	B	C	D	E	F	G	H
117.	A	B	C	D	E	F	G	H
118.	A	B	C	D	E	F	G	H
119.	A	B	C	D	E	F	G	H
120.	A	B	C	D	E	F	G	H
121.	A	B	C	D	E	F	G	H
122.	A	B	C	D	E	F	G	H
123.	A	B	C	D	E	F	G	H
124.	A	B	C	D	E	F	G	H
125.	A	B	C	D	E	F	G	H
126.	A	B	C	D	E	F	G	H
127.	A	B	C	D	E	F	G	H
128.	A	B	C	D	E	F	G	H
129.	A	B	C	D	E	F	G	H
130.	A	B	C	D	E	F	G	H
131.	A	B	C	D	E	F	G	H
132.	A	B	C	D	E	F	G	H
133.	A	B	C	D	E	F	G	H
134.	A	B	C	D	E	F	G	H
135.	A	B	C	D	E	F	G	H
136.	A	B	C	D	E	F	G	H
137.	A	B	C	D	E	F	G	H

PART 8. INFECTIOUS DISEASE

1. A B C D E F G H
2. A B C D E F G H
3. A B C D E F G H
4. A B C D E F G H
5. A B C D E F G H
6. A B C D E F G H
7. A B C D E F G H
8. A B C D E F G H
9. A B C D E F G H
10. A B C D E F G H
11. A B C D E F G H
12. A B C D E F G H
13. A B C D E F G H
14. A B C D E F G H
15. A B C D E F G H
16. A B C D E F G H
17. A B C D E F G H
18. A B C D E F G H
19. A B C D E F G H
20. A B C D E F G H
21. A B C D E F G H
22. A B C D E F G H
23. A B C D E F G H
24. A B C D E F G H
25. A B C D E F G H
26. A B C D E F G H
27. A B C D E F G H
28. A B C D E F G H
29. A B C D E F G H
30. A B C D E F G H
31. A B C D E F G H
32. A B C D E F G H
33. A B C D E F G H
34. A B C D E F G H
35. A B C D E F G H
36. A B C D E F G H
37. A B C D E F G H
38. A B C D E F G H
39. A B C D E F G H
40. A B C D E F G H
41. A B C D E F G H
42. A B C D E F G H
43. A B C D E F G H
44. A B C D E F G H
45. A B C D E F G H
46. A B C D E F G H
47. A B C D E F G H
48. A B C D E F G H
49. A B C D E F G H
50. A B C D E F G H
51. A B C D E F G H
52. A B C D E F G H
53. A B C D E F G H
54. A B C D E F G H
55. A B C D E F G H
56. A B C D E F G H
57. A B C D E F G H
58. A B C D E F G H
59. A B C D E F G H
60. A B C D E F G H
61. A B C D E F G H
62. A B C D E F G H
63. A B C D E F G H
64. A B C D E F G H
65. A B C D E F G H
66. A B C D E F G H
67. A B C D E F G H
68. A B C D E F G H
69. A B C D E F G H
70. A B C D E F G H
71. A B C D E F G H
72. A B C D E F G H
73. A B C D E F G H
74. A B C D E F G H
75. A B C D E F G H
76. A B C D E F G H
77. A B C D E F G H
78. A B C D E F G H
79. A B C D E F G H
80. A B C D E F G H
81. A B C D E F G H
82. A B C D E F G H
83. A B C D E F G H
84. A B C D E F G H
85. A B C D E F G H
86. A B C D E F G H
87. A B C D E F G H
88. A B C D E F G H
89. A B C D E F G H
90. A B C D E F G H
91. A B C D E F G H
92. A B C D E F G H
93. A B C D E F G H
94. A B C D E F G H
95. A B C D E F G H
96. A B C D E F G H
97. A B C D E F G H
98. A B C D E F G H
99. A B C D E F G H

PART 8. INFECTIOUS DISEASE

100. A B C D E F G H
101. A B C D E F G H
102. A B C D E F G H
103. A B C D E F G H
104. A B C D E F G H
105. A B C D E F G H
106. A B C D E F G H
107. A B C D E F G H
108. A B C D E F G H
109. A B C D E F G H
110. A B C D E F G H
111. A B C D E F G H
112. A B C D E F G H
113. A B C D E F G H
114. A B C D E F G H
115. A B C D E F G H
116. A B C D E F G H
117. A B C D E F G H
118. A B C D E F G H
119. A B C D E F G H
120. A B C D E F G H
121. A B C D E F G H
122. A B C D E F G H
123. A B C D E F G H
124. A B C D E F G H
125. A B C D E F G H
126. A B C D E F G H
127. A B C D E F G H
128. A B C D E F G H
129. A B C D E F G H
130. A B C D E F G H
131. A B C D E F G H
132. A B C D E F G H
133. A B C D E F G H
134. A B C D E F G H
135. A B C D E F G H
136. A B C D E F G H
137. A B C D E F G H
138. A B C D E F G H
139. A B C D E F G H
140. A B C D E F G H
141. A B C D E F G H
142. A B C D E F G H
143. A B C D E F G H
144. A B C D E F G H
145. A B C D E F G H
146. A B C D E F G H
147. A B C D E F G H
148. A B C D E F G H
149. A B C D E F G H
150. A B C D E F G H
151. A B C D E F G H
152. A B C D E F G H
153. A B C D E F G H
154. A B C D E F G H
155. A B C D E F G H
156. A B C D E F G H
157. A B C D E F G H
158. A B C D E F G H
159. A B C D E F G H
160. A B C D E F G H
161. A B C D E F G H
162. A B C D E F G H
163. A B C D E F G H
164. A B C D E F G H
165. A B C D E F G H
166. A B C D E F G H
167. A B C D E F G H
168. A B C D E F G H
169. A B C D E F G H
170. A B C D E F G H

PART 9. CLINICAL IMMUNOLOGY AND RHEUMATOLOGY

1. A B C D E F G H
2. A B C D E F G H
3. A B C D E F G H
4. A B C D E F G H
5. A B C D E F G H
6. A B C D E F G H
7. A B C D E F G H
8. A B C D E F G H
9. A B C D E F G H
10. A B C D E F G H
11. A B C D E F G H
12. A B C D E F G H
13. A B C D E F G H
14. A B C D E F G H
15. A B C D E F G H
16. A B C D E F G H
17. A B C D E F G H
18. A B C D E F G H
19. A B C D E F G H
20. A B C D E F G H
21. A B C D E F G H
22. A B C D E F G H
23. A B C D E F G H
24. A B C D E F G H
25. A B C D E F G H
26. A B C D E F G H
27. A B C D E F G H
28. A B C D E F G H
29. A B C D E F G H
30. A B C D E F G H
31. A B C D E F G H
32. A B C D E F G H
33. A B C D E F G H
34. A B C D E F G H
35. A B C D E F G H
36. A B C D E F G H
37. A B C D E F G H
38. A B C D E F G H
39. A B C D E F G H
40. A B C D E F G H
41. A B C D E F G H
42. A B C D E F G H
43. A B C D E F G H
44. A B C D E F G H
45. A B C D E F G H
46. A B C D E F G H
47. A B C D E F G H
48. A B C D E F G H
49. A B C D E F G H
50. A B C D E F G H
51. A B C D E F G H
52. A B C D E F G H
53. A B C D E F G H
54. A B C D E F G H
55. A B C D E F G H
56. A B C D E F G H
57. A B C D E F G H
58. A B C D E F G H
59. A B C D E F G H
60. A B C D E F G H
61. A B C D E F G H
62. A B C D E F G H
63. A B C D E F G H
64. A B C D E F G H
65. A B C D E F G H
66. A B C D E F G H
67. A B C D E F G H
68. A B C D E F G H
69. A B C D E F G H
70. A B C D E F G H
71. A B C D E F G H
72. A B C D E F G H
73. A B C D E F G H
74. A B C D E F G H
75. A B C D E F G H
76. A B C D E F G H
77. A B C D E F G H
78. A B C D E F G H
79. A B C D E F G H
80. A B C D E F G H
81. A B C D E F G H
82. A B C D E F G H
83. A B C D E F G H

PART 10. NEUROLOGIC DISEASE

1. A B C D E F G H
2. A B C D E F G H
3. A B C D E F G H
4. A B C D E F G H
5. A B C D E F G H
6. A B C D E F G H
7. A B C D E F G H
8. A B C D E F G H
9. A B C D E F G H
10. A B C D E F G H
11. A B C D E F G H
12. A B C D E F G H
13. A B C D E F G H
14. A B C D E F G H
15. A B C D E F G H
16. A B C D E F G H
17. A B C D E F G H
18. A B C D E F G H
19. A B C D E F G H
20. A B C D E F G H
21. A B C D E F G H
22. A B C D E F G H
23. A B C D E F G H
24. A B C D E F G H
25. A B C D E F G H
26. A B C D E F G H
27. A B C D E F G H
28. A B C D E F G H
29. A B C D E F G H
30. A B C D E F G H
31. A B C D E F G H
32. A B C D E F G H
33. A B C D E F G H
34. A B C D E F G H
35. A B C D E F G H
36. A B C D E F G H
37. A B C D E F G H
38. A B C D E F G H
39. A B C D E F G H
40. A B C D E F G H
41. A B C D E F G H
42. A B C D E F G H
43. A B C D E F G H
44. A B C D E F G H
45. A B C D E F G H
46. A B C D E F G H
47. A B C D E F G H
48. A B C D E F G H
49. A B C D E F G H
50. A B C D E F G H
51. A B C D E F G H
52. A B C D E F G H
53. A B C D E F G H
54. A B C D E F G H
55. A B C D E F G H
56. A B C D E F G H
57. A B C D E F G H
58. A B C D E F G H
59. A B C D E F G H
60. A B C D E F G H
61. A B C D E F G H
62. A B C D E F G H
63. A B C D E F G H
64. A B C D E F G H
65. A B C D E F G H
66. A B C D E F G H
67. A B C D E F G H
68. A B C D E F G H
69. A B C D E F G H
70. A B C D E F G H
71. A B C D E F G H
72. A B C D E F G H
73. A B C D E F G H
74. A B C D E F G H
75. A B C D E F G H
76. A B C D E F G H
77. A B C D E F G H
78. A B C D E F G H
79. A B C D E F G H
80. A B C D E F G H
81. A B C D E F G H
82. A B C D E F G H
83. A B C D E F G H
84. A B C D E F G H
85. A B C D E F G H
86. A B C D E F G H
87. A B C D E F G H
88. A B C D E F G H
89. A B C D E F G H
90. A B C D E F G H
91. A B C D E F G H
92. A B C D E F G H
93. A B C D E F G H
94. A B C D E F G H
95. A B C D E F G H
96. A B C D E F G H
97. A B C D E F G H
98. A B C D E F G H
99. A B C D E F G H

PART 10. NEUROLOGIC DISEASE

100. A B C D E F G H
101. A B C D E F G H
102. A B C D E F G H
103. A B C D E F G H
104. A B C D E F G H
105. A B C D E F G H
106. A B C D E F G H
107. A B C D E F G H
108. A B C D E F G H
109. A B C D E F G H
110. A B C D E F G H
111. A B C D E F G H
112. A B C D E F G H
113. A B C D E F G H
114. A B C D E F G H
115. A B C D E F G H
116. A B C D E F G H
117. A B C D E F G H
118. A B C D E F G H
119. A B C D E F G H
120. A B C D E F G H
121. A B C D E F G H
122. A B C D E F G H
123. A B C D E F G H
124. A B C D E F G H
125. A B C D E F G H
126. A B C D E F G H
127. A B C D E F G H
128. A B C D E F G H
129. A B C D E F G H
130. A B C D E F G H
131. A B C D E F G H
132. A B C D E F G H
133. A B C D E F G H
134. A B C D E F G H
135. A B C D E F G H
136. A B C D E F G H
137. A B C D E F G H
138. A B C D E F G H
139. A B C D E F G H
140. A B C D E F G H
141. A B C D E F G H
142. A B C D E F G H
143. A B C D E F G H
144. A B C D E F G H
145. A B C D E F G H
146. A B C D E F G H
147. A B C D E F G H
148. A B C D E F G H
149. A B C D E F G H
150. A B C D E F G H
151. A B C D E F G H
152. A B C D E F G H
153. A B C D E F G H
154. A B C D E F G H
155. A B C D E F G H

PART 11. DERMATOLOGY

No.	A	B	C	D	E	F	G	H
1.	A	B	C	D	E	F	G	H
2.	A	B	C	D	E	F	G	H
3.	A	B	C	D	E	F	G	H
4.	A	B	C	D	E	F	G	H
5.	A	B	C	D	E	F	G	H
6.	A	B	C	D	E	F	G	H
7.	A	B	C	D	E	F	G	H
8.	A	B	C	D	E	F	G	H
9.	A	B	C	D	E	F	G	H
10.	A	B	C	D	E	F	G	H
11.	A	B	C	D	E	F	G	H
12.	A	B	C	D	E	F	G	H
13.	A	B	C	D	E	F	G	H
14.	A	B	C	D	E	F	G	H
15.	A	B	C	D	E	F	G	H
16.	A	B	C	D	E	F	G	H
17.	A	B	C	D	E	F	G	H
18.	A	B	C	D	E	F	G	H
19.	A	B	C	D	E	F	G	H
20.	A	B	C	D	E	F	G	H
21.	A	B	C	D	E	F	G	H
22.	A	B	C	D	E	F	G	H
23.	A	B	C	D	E	F	G	H
24.	A	B	C	D	E	F	G	H
25.	A	B	C	D	E	F	G	H
26.	A	B	C	D	E	F	G	H
27.	A	B	C	D	E	F	G	H
28.	A	B	C	D	E	F	G	H
29.	A	B	C	D	E	F	G	H
30.	A	B	C	D	E	F	G	H
31.	A	B	C	D	E	F	G	H
32.	A	B	C	D	E	F	G	H
33.	A	B	C	D	E	F	G	H
34.	A	B	C	D	E	F	G	H
35.	A	B	C	D	E	F	G	H
36.	A	B	C	D	E	F	G	H
37.	A	B	C	D	E	F	G	H
38.	A	B	C	D	E	F	G	H
39.	A	B	C	D	E	F	G	H
40.	A	B	C	D	E	F	G	H
41.	A	B	C	D	E	F	G	H
42.	A	B	C	D	E	F	G	H
43.	A	B	C	D	E	F	G	H
44.	A	B	C	D	E	F	G	H
45.	A	B	C	D	E	F	G	H
46.	A	B	C	D	E	F	G	H
47.	A	B	C	D	E	F	G	H
48.	A	B	C	D	E	F	G	H
49.	A	B	C	D	E	F	G	H
50.	A	B	C	D	E	F	G	H